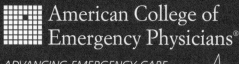

American College of
Emergency Physicians®

ADVANCING EMERGENCY CARE

MW00845299

Tactical Medicine
ESSENTIALS

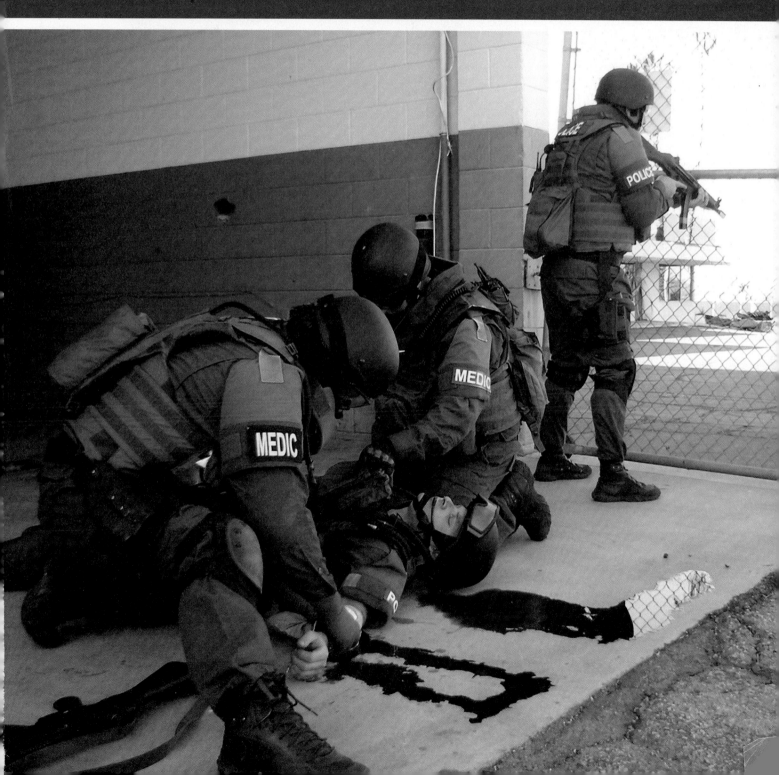

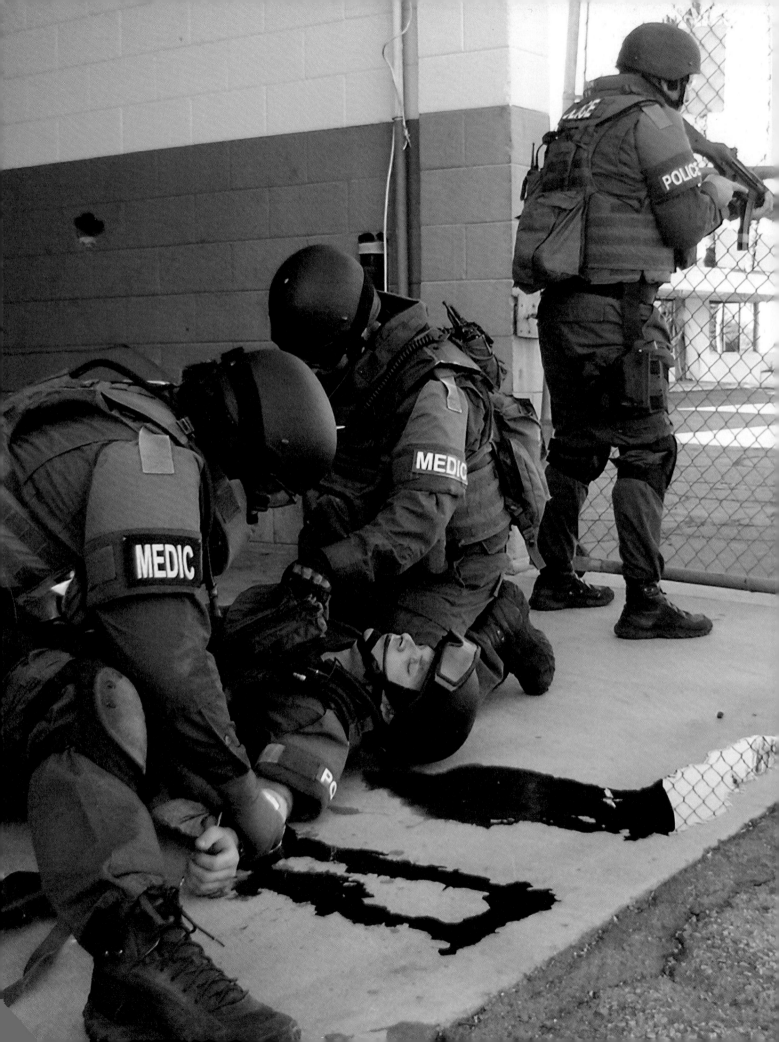

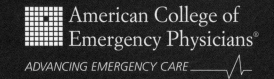
American College of
Emergency Physicians®

ADVANCING EMERGENCY CARE

Tactical Medicine
ESSENTIALS

John E. Campbell, MD, FACEP
Lawrence E. Heiskell, MD, FACEP, FAAFP
Jim Smith, ASEMT, BS, MSS, NREMTP
E. John Wipfler III, MD, FACEP

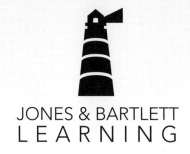

JONES & BARTLETT
L E A R N I N G

World Headquarters

Jones & Bartlett Learning
40 Tall Pine Drive
Sudbury, MA 01776
978-443-5000
info@jblearning.com
www.jblearning.com

Jones & Bartlett Learning Canada
6339 Ormindale Way
Mississauga, Ontario L5V 1J2
Canada

Jones & Bartlett Learning International
Barb House, Barb Mews
London W6 7PA
United Kingdom

Jones & Bartlett Learning books and products are available through most bookstores and online booksellers. To contact Jones & Bartlett Learning directly, call 800-832-0034, fax 978-443-8000, or visit our website, www.jblearning.com.

Substantial discounts on bulk quantities of Jones & Bartlett Learning publications are available to corporations, professional associations, and other qualified organizations. For details and specific discount information, contact the special sales department at Jones & Bartlett Learning via the above contact information or send an email to specialsales@jblearning.com.

Some images in this book feature models. These models do not necessarily endorse, represent, or participate in the activities represented in the images.

The procedures and protocols in this book are based on the most current recommendations of responsible medical sources. The American College of Emergency Physicians and the publisher, however, make no guarantee as to, and assume no responsibility for, the correctness, sufficiency, or completeness of such information or recommendations. Other or additional safety measures may be required under particular circumstances.

This textbook is intended solely as a guide to the appropriate procedures to be employed when rendering emergency care to the sick and injured. It is not intended as a statement of the standards of care required in any particular situation, because circumstances and the patient's physical condition can vary widely from one emergency to another. Nor is it intended that this textbook shall in any way advise emergency personnel concerning legal authority to perform the activities or procedures discussed. Such local determination should be made only with the aid of legal counsel.

Production Credits

Chief Executive Officer: Ty Field
President: James Homer
SVP, Chief Operating Officer: Don Jones, Jr.
SVP, Chief Technology Officer: Dean Fossella
SVP, Chief Marketing Officer: Alison M. Pendergast
SVP, Chief Financial Officer: Ruth Siporin
Executive Publisher: Kimberly Brophy
Executive Acqusitions Editor, EMS: Christine Emerton
Senior Editor: Jennifer Deforge-Kling
Associate Editor: Laura Burns
Senior Production Editor: Susan Schultz
Associate Production Editor: Tina Chen
Director of Marketing: Alisha Weisman
Marketing Manager: Brian Rooney

Associate Marketing Manager: Meagan Norlund
VP, Sales—Public Safety Group: Matthew Maniscalco
VP, Manufacturing and Inventory Control:
    Therese Connell
Composition: Shepherd, Inc.
Text Design: Composure Graphics
Cover Design: Kristin E. Parker
Photo Research and Permissions Manager:
    Kimberly Potvin
Associate Photo Researcher: Jessica Elias
Cover Image: Courtesy of Lawrence Heiskell
Printing and Binding: Courier Companies
Cover Printing: Courier Companies

Library of Congress Cataloging-in-Publication Data

Wipfler, E. John.
    Tactical medicine essentials / American College of Emergency Physicians, E. John Wipfler III.
        p. ; cm.
    Includes index.
    ISBN 978-0-7637-7821-7 (pbk.)
    1. Emergency medicine. 2. Police—Special weapons and tactics units—Medical care. I. American College of Emergency Physicians II. Title.
    [DNLM: 1. Emergency Medical Technicians. 2. Emergency Medicine—methods. 3. Emergency Treatment—methods. 4. Law Enforcement. WB 105]
    RC86.7.W57 2012
    616.02'5—dc22

2010039525

6048

Printed in the United States of America
14 13 10 9 8 7 6 5 4 3 2

BRIEF CONTENTS

CONTENTS

Chapter 3   SWAT Unit Essentials 30

Chapter 4   Equipment of the Tactical Medical Provider 40

Chapter 8   Self-Defense and Close Quarters Battle 94

Chapter 9   Operational Tactics...104

Section 2   Assessment and Management of Injuries

INSTRUCTOR RESOURCES

Instructor's ToolKit CD-ROM

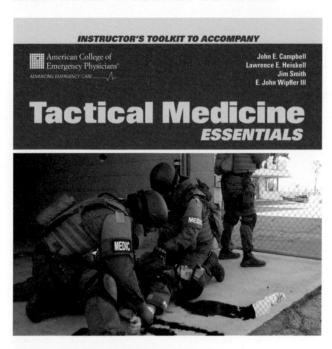

ISBN: 978-0-7637-9444-6

The Instructor's ToolKit CD-ROM includes practical, hands-on, time-saving tools, including:

- PowerPoint Presentations
- Lecture Outlines
- Skill Sheets
- Exams

AUTHOR BIOGRAPHIES

John E. Campbell, MD, FACEP Dr. Campbell has been a practicing emergency physician for over 30 years. He currently serves as the State Medical Director of Emergency Medical Services and Trauma for Alabama. Dr. Campbell is the founder, president, and editor of *International Trauma Life Support* (formerly *BTLS—Basic Trauma Life Support*), an organization of teachers of prehospital trauma care whose course is taught worldwide. He is recognized internationally as a teacher of prehospital trauma care. He is the author of the original *Basic Trauma Life Support* textbook and he and Chief Jim Smith co-authored, *Homeland Security and EMS Response*.

The son of a United States Deputy Marshal, he worked part-time as a guard for the Marshals Service while he was in college. He was once a member of the Opelika, Alabama, police pistol team and is currently the medical director for a tactical EMS squad.

He is an active member of the Alabama Terrorism and Tactical Operations Medical Support Course Advisory Committee and the Alabama State Trauma Advisory Committee. He currently serves on the Board of Directors of the Alabama Chapter of the American College of Emergency Physicians and in the past served as Councilor and President.

He served with the United States Army National Guard for over 20 years, attaining the rank of Captain. He has received numerous awards, including the EMS Award (first recipient) from the American College of Emergency Physicians, and a Certificate of Appreciation from the Surgeon General of the United States for services to the Medical Department Regiment. He is currently writing a history of the 2nd Marine Division in World War II.

Lawrence E. Heiskell, MD, FACEP, FAAFP Dr. Lawrence Heiskell is the founder of and medical director for the International School of Tactical Medicine, the first and only state and federally approved tactical medicine school by the California Commission on Peace Officers Standards and Training (POST) and the United States Department of Homeland Security. Dr. Heiskell is residency trained and board certified in emergency medicine and family practice and has been a full-time practicing emergency physician for more than 23 years in California.

Prior to attending medical school, Dr. Heiskell spent 5 years with the United States Antarctic Research Program and served on three expeditions to Antarctica and the South Pole. He was awarded the Congressional Antarctic Service Medal in 1979. He has 19 years of experience as a reserve police officer and SWAT team physician beginning with the Kern County Sheriff's Department in Bakersfield, California. Dr. Heiskell is currently a reserve police officer and a tactical physician with the Palm Springs Police Department in Palm Springs, California.

Dr. Heiskell served on an 18-agency member tactical medicine coalition under the auspices of the California Commission on Police Officer Standards and Training and California EMS Authority (EMSA) to create the State of California Tactical Medicine Operational Programs and Standardized Training Recommendations.

He is a graduate of California Commission on Peace Officers Standards and Training and Department of Justice (POST/DOJ) school, National Tactical Officers Association (NTOA) school, Heckler & Koch school, and Federal Bureau of Investigation (FBI) SWAT school.

Dr. Heiskell has lectured extensively in the United States and abroad on tactical emergency medicine and has published over 60 articles and other publications on tactical medicine topics.

He is a Heckler & Koch-certified MP5 Master Instructor and a four-time GUNSITE graduate. Dr. Heiskell has provided special operations emergency medical support for the FBI, Drug Enforcement Administration (DEA), and the Bureau of Alcohol, Tobacco, and Firearms (ATF).

Jim Smith, ASEMT, BS, MSS, NREMTP Chief Jim Smith's background includes more than 30 years of public safety experience, which includes working in a variety of settings, including law enforcement with professional involvement as a fire fighter and paramedic, to operating a nuclear power facility where he was a former health physics technician. He has served as 9-1-1 district communications director for a center dispatching more than 30 agencies, as commander of an FBI-certified bomb squad and clandestine drug laboratory entry and assessment team, on a law enforcement rescue dive team, and on a police planning and research section. He continues to serve as police chief, EMT-Paramedic, and fire fighter in a rural town. Chief Smith also teaches criminal justice courses as an adjunct faculty member for Troy University Dothan and University of Phoenix.

Chief Smith's academic background includes a master of science in safety from the University of Southern California, a bachelor of science in chemistry and biology, and an associate's degree in emergency medical technology. Chief Smith is also a certified emergency manager, certified advanced law enforcement planner, and a certified police chief. He is a graduate of the United States Army Chemical School Domestic Countermeasures program. He is also a hazardous materials technician, weapons of mass destruction (WMD) technician, and clandestine drug laboratory safety certified.

Chief Smith has published three textbooks including a text on responding to bomb and WMD threats, a text on addressing law enforcement management and supervision, and a text on homeland security emergency response. Chief Smith's publications include more than 50 articles in peer-reviewed journals, including articles on practical research in blast mitigation, pipe-bomb fragment propagation, and blast suppression. This research led to the issuance of a United States patent and the production of specialized blast mitigation equipment.

Chief Smith is a member of the International Society of Explosive Engineers, International Association of Bomb Technicians and Investigators, a professional member of the American Society of Safety Engineers, and is Certified Homeland Security Level III by the American Board for Homeland Security Certification.

E. John Wipfler III, MD, FACEP   Dr. John Wipfler is a residency-trained, board-certified attending emergency physician and a clinical associate professor of surgery at the University of Illinois College of Medicine. He has taught tactical medicine for over 17 years and teaches several week-long courses annually as an instructor with the International School of Tactical Medicine, the only tactical medicine training school certified by the United States Department of Homeland Security. He served in the military reserves for 14 years, attaining the rank of Major in the United States Army Medical Corps, serving in Panama and volunteering for Desert Storm. He has been involved with law enforcement since 1994, supporting tactical operations as a SWAT team physician and medical director for a TEMS element for three tactical teams in central Illinois. Since completing his internship in surgery and residency in emergency medicine, he teaches and practices medicine with

the Department of Emergency Medicine at OSF Saint Francis Medical Center, a Level I Trauma Center in Peoria, Illinois.

Dr. Wipfler cofounded the first tactical EMS unit in the state of Illinois, the Special Tactical Assistance Trauma Team (STATT). He is a sworn Sheriff's Physician and Auxiliary Deputy Sheriff who has been involved in tactical operations during more than 110 SWAT callouts. The STATT Tactical EMS unit (three physicians, one nurse, two paramedics) supports three law enforcement tactical teams: Central Illinois Emergency Response Team (CIERT), Illinois Law Enforcement Alarm Services team (ILEAS region 6), and the Peoria City Police Department Special Response Team (SRT). He also supports callouts and/or training with the United States Secret Service for presidential motorcade escorts, United States Marshals Service, and the Drug Enforcement Agency (DEA). He has flown helicopter missions with the United States Marshals Service Special Operations Group during high-risk prisoner transport.

As a certified firearms instructor who is also a qualified expert in pistol, small-bore, and high-power rifle marksmanship, Dr. Wipfler routinely teaches firearms safety classes integrated with tactical medicine principles. He has completed multiple military and civilian tactical/medical courses, including the Chapman Academy (Basic and Advanced Pistol, Tactical Rifle), Combat Casualty Care Course, Counter Narcotics & Terrorism Operational Medical Support (CONTOMS), Radiation Emergency Assistance Center /Training Site (REAC/TS) radioactive injury management course, Heckler & Koch Basic and Advanced Tactical EMS courses, United States Army Medical Research Institute for Infectious Disease (USAMRIID) Chemical and Biological Warfare School, InSights Training, and Strike Tactical Solutions close quarters combat courses.

Dr. Wipfler was one of the original founders and medical director of the Region 2 RMERT disaster response team in central Illinois, and has deployed on multiple real-world disasters including several large tornado strikes with mass casualties. Dr. Wipfler served with 12 others on the founding executive council for the sole state-wide disaster response agency in Illinois, the Illinois Medical Emergency Response Team (IMERT). He served for 5 years as medical director of Life Flight.

He has coauthored textbooks on emergency medicine and firearms safety, written chapters for textbooks—including the tactical medicine chapter in the *International Trauma Life Support* (ITLS) text—as well as multiple tactical medicine and research papers. Dr. Wipfler lectures nationally and teaches tactical medicine, disaster preparedness, bioterrorism/WMD response, and advanced emergency ultrasound at the University of Illinois College of Medicine. In 1999, Dr. Wipfler developed one of the first emergency medicine residency program tactical medicine elective rotations in the United States.

As the co-chair of the Illinois Tactical Officers Association (ITOA) tactical EMS committee, he has been involved in instructing Tactical EMS with the ITOA and other law agencies, and has co-chaired the annual ITOA Tactical Medicine Conference for 6 years.

He was asked to serve with an 18-agency member tactical medicine coalition in California, representing the Illinois Department of Public Health Tactical Medicine Committee. This committee worked with the California Commission on Police Officer Standards and Training and California EMS Authority (EMSA) to create the State of California Tactical Medicine Operational Program and Standardized Training Recommendations, approved in March 2010. He currently is working with a task force to further integrate tactical medicine into the EMS system with the Illinois Department of Public Health and other states.

ACKNOWLEDGMENTS

ACEP Review Board

Glenn A. Bollard, MD, FACEP
Past-Chair and Current Section Development Coordinator,
Tactical Emergency Medicine Section
American College of Emergency Physicians
Special Certification, Forensic Medicine and Ballistics
Meadville, Pennsylvania

Stewart R. Coffman, MD, MBA, FACEP
Chief Medical Officer
Questcare Partners
Dallas, Texas

Melissa Wysong Costello, MD, FACEP
Associate Medical Director, Baptist LifeFlight
Adjunct Associate Professor of Emergency Medicine
University of South Alabama
Mobile, Alabama

Richard Kamin, MD, FACEP
EMS Program Director
Assistant Professor of Emergency Medicine
University of Connecticut Health Center
Farmington, Connecticut

Rick Murray, EMT-P, LP
Director, EMS and Disaster Preparedness Department
American College of Emergency Physicians
Former Police Officer
Dallas, Texas

Jeffery C. Metzger, MD, FACEP
Assistant Professor, Division of Emergency Medicine
University of Texas, Southwestern Medical Center
Medical Director/Reserve Police Officer
Dallas Police Department
Dallas, Texas

Wendy Ruggeri, MD
Clinical Assistant Professor
University of Texas Southwestern
Division of Emergency Medicine
Dallas, Texas

Reviewers

The authors would like to extend a special thanks to Doctor
Glenn Bollard, Doctor Martin Greenberg, and Michael R. Meoli
for their exceptional contributions to the text.

Paul Abdey, Dip IMC RCS (Ed), Paramedic
Tactical Medicine Unit Manager
Kent Police
Maidstone, Kent, United Kingdom

Jeff W. Adams
Lieutenant (ret), Special Response Team Commander
Peoria Police Department
Peoria, Illinois

James Bender, BS, EMT-P, HEM
Tactical Paramedic
Healthcare Emergency Manager
Medical Horizons Consulting
Washington, Illinois

Sean Benson
Firearms Tactical Advisor, Bronze Commander, and Trainer
Firearms Training and Development Unit
Rotherham Police Station
Rotherham, South Yorkshire, United Kingdom

Neil P. Blackington, EMT-Tactical
Deputy Superintendent, Commander, Support Services
   Division
Boston EMS
Boston, Massachusetts

William P. Bozeman, MD, FACEP, FAAEM
Associate Professor, Director of Prehospital Research
Wake Forest University, Department of Emergency Medicine
Winston-Salem, North Carolina

Walter J. Bradley, MD, MBA, FACEP
Physician Advisor, Trinity Medical CenterMedical
Director, Illinois State Police Tactical Response Team
Medical Director, Tactical Medicine Team, Moline Police
   Department
Moline, Illinois

Dale Carrison, DO
Professor of Emergency Medicine
Chair, Department of Emergency Medicine
University of Nevada School of Medicine
Las Vegas, Nevada

Matthew Clark
State Registered Paramedic
Police Specialist Firearms Officer
United Kingdom

Keith F. Collins, NREMT-P, CIC
Tactical Medic
Rotterdam Police Department
Rotterdam, New York

Jeff Chudwin, JD
Chief of Police
Olympia Fields Police Department
Olympia Fields, Illinois

Michael Colvard, DDS, MS, M O Med RCSEd
Associate Professor of Oral Medicine and
   Diagnostic Sciences
Director, Disaster/Emergency Medicine Readiness
   Training Center
University of Illinois at Chicago
Chicago, Illinois

John H. Cottey II, MD
Emergency Physician
University Medical Center Brackenridge
Austin, Texas

John Croushorn, MD, FACEP
Chair, Department of Emergency Medicine,
   Trinity Medical Center
Tactical Physician, Federal Bureau of Investigation
Major, United States Army Medical Corp (vet)
Birmingham, Alabama

W. Scott Crowley, BA, EMT-P
EMT Program Director
Phoenix College
Phoenix, Arizona

Fabrice Czarnecki, MD, MA, MPH
Director of Medical-Legal Research, The Gables Group, Inc.
Attending Physician, Emergency Department,
    St. Joseph Medical Center
Towson, Maryland

Tony Damiano
Tactical Medic
Polk County Sheriff Department
Bartow, Florida

Andrew Dennis, DO, FACOS, DME
Trauma Surgery/Burn Surgery/Critical Care
The Cook County Trauma Unit, Cook County Hospital
Cook County Sheriff's Police Hostage and Barricade Team
Chairman, Department of Surgery, Chicago College of
Osteopathic Medicine of Midwestern University
Medical Director/Team Surgeon/Police Officer
Cook County Sheriff's Police Department,
    Emergency Services Bureau
Northern Illinois Police Alarm System Emergency Services
    Team, Des Plaines, Illinois Police Department
Chicago, Illinois

**Raffaele DiGiorgio, NREMT-P, UK HPC Registered
Paramedic**
Owner
Global Options & Solutions
Knoxville, Tennessee

Chris Dinsdale
Senior Lecturer, Prehospital Medicine
Tactical Medicine Specialist
Sheffield Hallam University
Sheffield, South Yorkshire, United Kingdom

Franco Dillena
Training Officer
Miramar Police Department
Miramar, Florida

Steve Erwin, BS, NREMT-I, Tactical EMT-I, EMSI
Program Manager, Emergency Medical Service
Louisiana Department of Health and Hospitals
Baton Rouge, Louisiana

Alexander L. Eastman, MD, MPH
Deputy Medical Director, Police Officer, Tactical Physician
Dallas Police Department
Assistant Professor of Surgery, Division of Burns, Trauma,
    and Critical Care
University of Texas Southwestern Medical Center
Dallas, Texas

Michael Eby, MD, FACOG
Chief, Surgical Critical Care, Jerry L. Pettis Memorial
    Veterans Affairs Medical Center
Loma Linda, California
Tactical Physician/Reserve Officer, San Bernardino
    Police Department
San Bernardino, California

Richard C. Frederick, MD, FACEP
Vice Chair, Department of Emergency Medicine, OSF Saint
    Francis Medical Center
Clinical Associate Professor of Surgery, University of Illinois
    College of Medicine

Tactical Physician, Special Tactical Assistance Trauma
    Team (STATT)
Auxiliary Deputy Sheriff, Peoria County Sheriff's Office
Peoria, Illinois

Martin Greenberg, MD, FACS
Chief, Section of Hand Surgery, Illinois Masonic
    Medical Center
Clinical Assistant Professor of Orthopedic Surgery,
    University of Illinois
Chair, EMS Advisory Council TEMS Committee
Tactical Physician, South Suburban Emergency Response
    Team (SSERT)
Reserve Police Officer, Village of Tinley Park, Illinois
Chicago, Illinois

Mark Griffeth, EMT-P
Manager, Facilities Division, Medical Programs
Illinois Law Enforcement Alarm System (ILEAS)
Urbana, Illinois

Russell J. Graham, BA, AAS, EMT-P
Staff Sergeant
United States of America

Stephen Grasso, BA, EMT-P
Battalion Chief/SWAT Medical Team Leader
Lauderhill Fire-Rescue
Lauderhill, Florida

David Halliwell, MSc Paramedic, FIFL, MIFPA
Head of Education
South Western Ambulance NHS Trust
Bournemouth, Dorset, United Kingdom

Brendan E. Hartford, EMT-Tactical
SWAT Team Training Coordinator, Chicago SWAT
Chicago Police Department
Chicago, Illinois

George Z. Hevesy, MD
Chair, Department of Emergency Medicine
Director of Emergency Medical Services, OSF Saint Francis
    Medical Center
Clinical Associate Professor of Surgery, University of Illinois
    College of Medicine
Tactical Physician, Special Tactical Assistance Trauma
    Team (STATT)
Auxiliary Deputy Sheriff, Peoria County Sheriff's Office
Peoria, Illinois

John Holschen, EMT-P, Tactical Paramedic
United States Army Special Forces Medical Sergeant (ret)
Heiho Consulting Group, LLC
Bothell, Washington

Matthew N. Jackson, MD, FACEP, FAAEM
Attending Emergency Physician, Department of
    Emergency Medicine
OSF Saint Francis Medical Center
Clinical Assistant Professor of Surgery, University of Illinois
    College of Medicine
Tactical Physician, Special Tactical Assistance Trauma
    Team (STATT)
Auxiliary Deputy Sheriff, Peoria County Sheriff's Office
Peoria, Illinois

Neil Jones
Firearms Instructor
Tactical Firearms Unit
Sussex Police
Lewes, Sussex, United Kingdom

Sean Johnston, EMT-P, Tactical Paramedic
Patrol Officer
Peoria Police Department
Peoria, Illinois

Thomas M. Kamplain, Jr, MS, NREMT-P, Tactical Paramedic
Director, EMS/Fire Science
DeKalb Technical College
Covington, Georgia

Shane Knox, MSc HDip-EMT
Advanced Paramedic
Training and Development Officer
HSE-National Ambulance Service College
Ballinasloe, County Galway, Ireland

Terry G. Kaufman
Tactical Medic, Lafayette Police Department
Manager, Flight Safety, Petroleum Helicopters, Inc.
Lafayette, Louisiana

Jacqueline E. Krajecki, RN, BSN, MSNA, EMT-LP, CEN, CCRN, CFRN, CRNA
Certified Registered Nurse Anesthetist
The Anesthesia Group of Sarasota
Sarasota, Florida

Gordon L. Larsen, MD, FACEP
Medical Advisor, Technical Rescue/Zion National Park Search and Rescue Team
Attending Emergency Physician, Southwest Emergency Physicians, Dixie Regional Medical Center
St. George, Utah

Christopher J. Loscar, NREMT-P
St. Clare's Hospital MICU
Dover, New Jersey

Mark A. Lorenz, MD, AAOS
Orthopedic Surgeon, Hinsdale Orthopaedics
Clinical Associate Professor, Loyola University Medical Center
Hinsdale, Illinois

David Q. McArdle, MD
Attending Emergency Physician, Georgia Emergency Associates, South East Georgia Medical Center, Brunswick, Georgia
Occupational Medicine Physician, Defense Support Systems LCC
Federal Law Enforcement Training Center, Glynco, Georgia
Reserve Officer/Tactical Physician, University of Colorado Police at Boulder, Colorado
Affiliate Faculty Department of Criminology & Homeland Security, Regis University, Denver, Colorado
President, TacMedMD LLC
Medical Director, ColoradoSTAR
Centennial, Colorado

Kevin J. McCollin, MBA/HCM, NREMT-P
Director of Emergency Medical Services
Dugway Emergency Medical Services
Dugway, Utah

Lt. Craig McElhaney, NREMT-P
SWAT Medic
Miramar Fire-Rescue
Miramar, Florida

Tom McGarey, MA Ed, BSc
Paramedic Tutor
Regional Ambulance Education Centre
Northern Ireland Ambulance Service
Belfast, County Antrim, Northern Ireland

Sean D. McKay, EMT-P, Tactical Paramedic
Instructor, Tactical Medicine
Operational Rescue
Associate, Asymmetric Combat Institute
Taylors, South Carolina

Michael R. Meoli, Firefighter, EMT-P, Tactical Paramedic, SOC (SEAL)
Tactical Paramedic Firefighter, Special Trauma and Rescue (STAR) Team
Mobile Medical Strike Team, Paramedic Field Training Officer/Preceptor
San Diego Fire and Rescue Department
Special Warfare Operator Chief (SEAL)
Special Operations Command (SOCOM) Advanced Tactical Practitioner (ATP)
Casualty Assistance Calls Officer (CACO)
Tactical Combat Casualty Care (TCCC) Instructor/Trainer
Command Fitness Leader (CFL), US Navy Reserve SEAL Team 17
Coronado, California

Rick F. Miller, MD, FACEP
Director, Pediatric Emergency Medical Services, OSF Saint Francis Medical Center
Clinical Associate Professor of Surgery, University of Illinois College of Medicine
Tactical Physician, Special Tactical Assistance Trauma Team (STATT)
Auxiliary Deputy Sheriff, Peoria County Sheriff's Office
Peoria, Illinois

Alan Moore
Paramedic and Registered Nurse
London, England, United Kingdom

Wren Nealy, Jr, EMT-P, Tactical Paramedic
Director of Special Operations, Cypress Creek Emergency Medical Services
Lead Instructor, Tactical Medical Operational Support Course
Houston, Texas
Deputy Sheriff and SWAT Assistant Team Leader, Waller County Sheriff's Office
Hempstead, Texas

Bohdan (Dan) T. Olesnicky, MD, ABEM, ABIM
Director of EMS, Eisenhower Medical Center
Instructor, International School of Tactical Medicine
SWAT Physician, Palm Springs Police Department SWAT
Palm Springs, California

Kevin Olver
Police Tactical Firearms Trainer
Cleveland and Durham Police Tactical Training Centre
Stockton-on-Tees, Cleveland, United Kingdom

Brian P. Pasquale, MPH, NREMT-P
SSG (ret), 68W_W1, USSOCOM-SOF-Paramedic
Co-founder
Tac-Med LLC
Collegeville, Pennsylvania

William F. Pfeifer, MD, FACS
Clinical Professor of Surgery, Rocky Vista University College
  of Osteopathic Medicine
Associate Clinical Professor of Surgery, University of
  Colorado Health Sciences
Mile High Surgical Specialists
Denver, Colorado

Jason R. Pickett, MD, EMT-P/T
Assistant Professor, Division of Tactical Emergency
  Medicine
Department of Emergency Medicine, Boonshoft School
  of Medicine
Wright State University
Major, USAR Medical Corp
Kettering, Ohio

Scott Plantz, MD, FAAEM
Associate Clinical Professor
Mount Sinai Hospital, Department of Emergency Medicine
Chicago, Illinois

Guadalupe (Wally) Quintanilla, EMT-P, AAS
TEMS Team Leader, South Suburban Emergency
  Response Team
Corporal, Posen Illinois Police Department
Posen, Illinois
Engineer/Paramedic, Orland, Illinois Fire Protection District
Orland Park, Illinois

Colleen S. Ragon, RN, MSN, CEN, CFRN
Tactical Nurse, Special Tactical Assistance Trauma
  Team (STATT)
Central Illinois Emergency Response Team (CIERT)
Peoria Police Special Response Team (SRT)
Illinois Law Enforcement Alarm System (ILEAS)
  Region 6 Team
Auxiliary Deputy Sheriff, Peoria County Sheriff's Office
Flight Nurse Specialist, Life Flight, OSF Saint Francis
  Medical Center
Peoria, Illinois

David Rathbun, EMT-P
Los Angeles County Sheriff, Special Enforcement
  Bureau (ret)
Tactical EMS Chair, National Tactical Officers Association
La Canada, California

John Rigione, EMT-P
President
Emergency Medical Solutions, Inc.
Bangor, Pennsylvania

Hector Roman, AS, EMT-P, Tactical Paramedic
Hospital Corpsman 1st class (FMF)
Advanced Tactical Training, Inc.
Coral Springs, Florida

Malcolm Q. Russell, MBChB, DCH, DRCOG, MRCGP, FIMC RCS(Ed)
Managing Director
Prometheus Medical Ltd.
Hope-under-Dinmore, Herefordshire, United Kingdom

Navin Sharma, RN, BSN, CEN, EMT-P, Tactical Paramedic
Police Officer (ret)/Tactical Paramedic-RN
Instructor, Tactical Emergency Medicine
Vancouver, Washington

Daniel Smiley, EMT-P
Chief Deputy Director
State of California Emergency Medical Services Authority
Sacramento, California

Andrew Smith
Medical Emergency Response Team Paramedic
Royal Air Force
Chippenham, Wiltshire, United Kingdom

William Smock, MS, MD, FACEP, FAAEM
Professor, Department of Emergency Medicine
University of Louisville School of Medicine
Police Surgeon, Louisville Metro Police Department
Tactical Physician, Floyd County, Indiana Sheriff
  Department
Tactical Physician, United States Marshals Service, Western
  District, Kentucky
Medical Advisor, Louisville, Kentucky Division of the Federal
  Bureau of Investigation
Louisville, Kentucky

Chuck Soltys
Special Agent/EMT-B
Drug Enforcement Administration (DEA)
Chicago, Illinois

Brian L. Springer, MD, FACEP
Assistant Professor and Director, Division of Tactical
  Emergency Medicine
Department of Emergency Medicine, Boonshoft School
  of Medicine
Wright State University
Dayton, Ohio

Kent Spitler, RN, NREMT-P, BS, MSEd, CPP
Director, Department for EMS Education
Gaston College
Dallas, North Carolina

Clint Steerman, NREMT-P, Tactical Paramedic
Chief Executive Officer
Metro One Ambulance
Martinez, Georgia

Hugh E. Stephenson, Jr, MD, FACS
University of Missouri System Curator Emeritus
John Growden Distinguished Professor of Surgery Emeritus
Missouri University School of Medicine
Columbia, Missouri

Matthew D. Sztajnkrycer, MD, PhD
Medical Director, Rochester Police Department
Medical Director and Tactical Physician, Rochester Police
  Department/Olmsted County Sheriffs Office Emergency
  Response Unit
Associate Professor and Chair, Division of Emergency
  Medicine Research
Department of Emergency Medicine
  Mayo Clinic
Rochester, Minnesota

David H. Tang, MD, FAAEM
SWAT Team Physician and Reserve Police Officer, Palm
  Springs Police Department, Palm Springs, California
Attending Physician, Eisenhower Medical Center
Forensic Medical Director, Barbara Sinatra Children's Center
Rancho Mirage, California

xxvi Acknowledgments

Nelson Tang, MD, FACEP
Chief Medical Officer, Center for Law Enforcement Medicine
The Johns Hopkins University Director of Special
Operations, Department of Emergency Medicine
The Johns Hopkins Medical Institutions
Baltimore, Maryland

Nicholas R. Taylor, EMT-Tactical
Special Agent, United States Army Criminal Investigation
    Division
EMT-Tactical, Patrol Officer, Pontiac Police Department
Pontiac, Illinois

Richard Tovar, MD, FACEP, FACMT
Attending Emergency Physician, Medical College of
    Wisconsin
Tactical Physician, New Berlin Police Department
New Berlin, Wisconsin

Mark Tutila, NREMT-P, Tactical Paramedic
Instructor, Tactical Paramedic
Chicago, Illinois

Sydney Vail, MD, FACS
Medical Director, Trauma Surgery Program, Department
    of Surgery
Division of Burns, Trauma, and Surgical Critical Care
The Trauma Center at Maricopa Medical Center
Phoenix, Arizona
Medical Director of Tactical Medicine Programs and Tactical
    Physician, Arizona Department of Public Safety, State
    Police SWAT
Medical Director of Tactical Medicine Programs and Tactical
    Physician Tactical, Maricopa County Sheriff's Office
    SWAT Team
Phoenix, Arizona
Instructor, International School of Tactical Medicine
Palm Springs, California

Joshua S. Vayer, CSA
Division Director, Uniformed Operations
Federal Protective Service
US Department of Homeland Security
Washington, District of Columbia

Michael D. Volling, EMT-P
Chief of Police, Village of Glencoe
Tactical Commander, Northern Illinois Police Alarm System
    (NIPAS) Emergency Services Team
Village of Glencoe, Illinois

Rease E. Watson, EMT-P, Tactical Paramedic
Captain, Special Operations Division
Hazardous Materials/Weapons of Mass Destruction/
    Technical Rescue
City of Peoria Fire Department
Auxiliary Deputy Sheriff, Peoria County Sheriff's Office
Tactical Paramedic, Central Illinois Emergency Response
    Team (CIERT)
Peoria Police Department Special Response Team (SRT)
Illinois Law Enforcement Alarm System (ILEAS)
    Region 6 Team
Peoria, Illinois

Kenneth Whitman
Senior Law Enforcement Consultant, California Commission
    on Police Officer Standards and Training
Project Manager, POST Tactical Medicine Core
Competencies Program, Sacramento, California
Lieutenant, Rocklin Fire Department
Rocklin, California

John M. Wightman, EMT-P, Tactical Paramedic, MD, MA
Professor and Director for Academics
Division of Tactical Emergency Medicine
Department of Emergency Medicine
Boonshoft School of Medicine
Wright State University
Dayton, Ohio

Mark T. Wold, EMT-P, Tactical Paramedic
Public Safety Officer, Tactical Paramedic, Evidence
Technician, Juvenile Officer
Glencoe Police Department
Village of Glencoe, Illinois

Matt Zukosky, MA, NREMT-P, CIC
Emergency Medical Care Program Coordinator, Suffolk
    County Community College
Selden, New York
Tactical Paramedic, Southhampton Village Police
    Department
Southampton, New York

The authors would also like to thank:
Sheriff Michael McCoy, Chief Steve Settingsgaard, Captain Michael
Scally, Chief Deputy Joseph Needham, Lieutenant Jim Pearson,
Deputy Michael Ealey, Lieutenant Mike White, Lieutenant R. Scott
Cook, Lieutenant Mike Mushinsky, Lieutenant Doug Theobald,
Lieutenant Doug Gaa, Lieutenant Joe Hartwig, Lieutenant John
Ghidina, Lieutenant Ed Meister, Lieutenant David Rogers, Officer
Jeff Stolz, Officer Chad Hazelwood, Officer Rory Poynter, Deputy
United States Marshall Greg Sims, Bob and Carol Heinz, Pete
Fandel, Andrew Rand, Rex Comerford, Doctor Tom Trent, Doctor
Wade Richey, Doctor Justin Johnson, Doctor Nathan Jones, Doctor
A.J. Cummings, Doctor Greg Tudor, Doctor Jim Ellis, Doctor Bob
Tillotson, Doctor Tim Wheeler, Claire Merrick, Tim Murray, Doctor
Todd Nelson, John Gilman, Doug Wipfler, Jim Etzin, Shannon
Benko, Wes Smith, Mike Adams, Patrick Merfeld, J.T. Thomas,
Steve Slawinski, Rick Brown, Mike Marquis, Tony Centimano, Ross
Johnson, Alexis Ferraro, Jack Wipfler, Shirley Wipfler, Michelle
McDonough, Doctor Corey Massey, Henk Iverson, Doctor Jeff
Juhala, Doctor Moses Lee, Diane Wipfler, Rebecca Wipfler, Maria
Wipfler, Matt Wipfler, Seth Barker, Sean Johnston, Kevin Mowery,
Jim Mulay, Terry Kaufman, Ricky Wolfe, Garry Grugan, Ryan Beck,
Chuck Fugitt, James Bender, Doctor Jane Billeter, Doctor Bernard
Heiliczer, Doctor Bruce Sands, Doctor Mark Sloan, Leslie Stein-
Spencer, Sharon White, Rob Chiapano, Steve Slawinski, Randolph
Christianson, Andrew Hamilton, Steve Knickrehm, David Lis, Doctor
Josh Vayer Robert Raica, John Stoeber, John R. Allen II, Doctor
Jonathan Allen, Joseph Collins, Doctor Winn Curran, Christian
Davis, Don Dougherty, Steve Drewniany, Doctor Anthony R. DuBose,
Ken Elmore, Don Fallon, Kelly Fieux, Nathan Gunkel, Steve Harris,
Rick Leska, Chuck Menley, Andrea Michell, Doctor James Munis,
Doctor Robert L. Norris, Doctor Keith Rose, Gary Sommers, Kyle
Stjerne, Doctor Lynn Welling, Matt Willette, Gerald Smith, Steve
Simpson, Rick Smith, Command Sergeant Major Alex Cabassa,
Steve Simpson, Denise Louthain, Doctor Wade Richey, Major James
Ayer, and Claire Merrick.

*Special thanks to the excellent men and women, and
administrative support of:* Palm Springs Police Department,
California EMSA, California Police Officer and Standards Advanced
Medical Transport of Central Illinois, Peoria Police Department,
Peoria County Sheriff's Office, Central Illinois Police Alarm System
Region 6 team, Palm Springs Police Department, U.S. Marshals
Service, U.S. Secret Service, Illinois State Police Tactical Response
Team, Sisters of the 3rd Order of Saint Francis in Peoria, Illinois,
OSF Saint Francis Medical Center, Life Flight/OSF Saint Francis
Medical Center, Department of Emergency Medicine, Sister Judith
Ann Duvall, Keith Steffen (CEO) and administrative officers, OSF
Saint Francis Medical Center.

FOREWORD

During this 20th Anniversary of Tactical Emergency Medical Service (TEMS), it is a privilege and an honor to be able to address my special operations colleagues who provide TEMS care in the United States and globally. We have come a long way since the late Commander Dave Rasumoff, MD and I presented the first formal TEMS course in Los Angeles in 1989. Under the continued leadership and vision of Captain John Kolman (ret) and the National Tactical Officers Association (NTOA), we presented a second TEMS course in Tucson, Arizona, in 1990, co-sponsored by my department, the Pima County Sheriff's Department. We appreciated phenomenal success as measured by the continued demand for more information and training.

With a dedicated team, we initiated a special TEMS column, "Inside the Perimeter" in the NTOA publication, *Tactical Edge*. In one of our first articles in 1990, we coined the term "TEMS." Over the course of the next 20 years, many professionals, including the co-authors of this text, have contributed to the development of tactical medicine.

In the early 1990s, several formal training programs began with the goal of teaching tactical medicine. I was fortunate to work with many dedicated professionals, both civilian and military, to develop and instruct at the Counter Narcotics Tactical Operations Medical Support (CONTOMS) course.

Other successful programs ensued, such as the Heckler and Koch sponsored course, which is now known as the International School of Tactical Medicine, as well as other programs generated individually and by organizations.

Over the years, tactical medical providers (TMPs) have increasingly brought added value to tactical units nationally and internationally. Tactical medicine enhances the ability to succeed in each SWAT/special operations mission in many ways, including preventive medicine, monitoring, and improving tactical officers' health, and when needed, caring for those in need under austere conditions.

Tactical medicine is based on a military model that I first learned as a United States Army Special Forces Medic and Weapons Specialist. Like so much of our knowledge in emergency medical care and systems, the best practices often emanate from military battlefield experience.

As our body of knowledge has expanded and been scrutinized by appropriate peer review, the group of four co-authors of this text worked with many colleagues to write a book that comprehensively addresses the essentials of tactical medicine. Dr. John Wipfler, Dr. Lawrence Heiskell, Chief Jim Smith, and Dr. John Campbell have managed to capture the evolution of decades of experience and emerging science and apply it to TEMS through their new publication, *Tactical Medicine Essentials*. This textbook provides invaluable guidance to tactical commanders, operators, and medics from the novice to the most senior personnel. Use it wisely to optimize your team's health and for the best practices for care as needed.

VADM Richard Carmona (ret)
17th Surgeon General of the United States
Deputy Sheriff, Pima County, Arizona
Sheriff's Department
Tucson, Arizona

PREFACE

During the 1980s, the world saw the development of a trauma medical care education program that has since been adopted worldwide. This program was developed by Dr. John E. Campbell and was originally known as *Basic Trauma Life Support* (BTLS). Today it is known as *International Trauma Life Support* (ITLS) with Dr. Campbell continuing to serve as the editor of the textbook. Years ago, Dr. Campbell identified the need for additional education in several areas of EMS. He was particularly concerned about the global lack of knowledge and skill sets within EMS as they pertained to weapons of mass destruction (WMD) and tactical medicine. At that time, the majority of EMS professionals were not fully prepared or trained to respond to these critical incidents.

In 2000, a colleague of Dr. Campbell, Chief Jim Smith, a veteran police officer, college educator, and paramedic, developed a course outline and curriculum for these two areas. After first working together with colleagues on a WMD program, the need for tactical medicine program was further identified. As friends, Dr. Campbell and Dr. John Wipfler worked together and had previously discussed collaborating on a tactical medicine project. With over 17 years as an emergency physician and associate professor instructing at a Level I trauma center, tactical physician, flight physician, disaster physician, and a Major (ret) in the United States Army Medical Corps, Dr. Wipfler had developed a unique knowledge base and skill set. Rounding out the team of authors was Dr. Lawrence Heiskell, an emergency physician and reserve police officer who has pioneered, directed, and taught tactical medicine for over 16 years. With special editing contributions by Dr. Marty Greenberg, Dr. Glenn Bollard, and Navy SEAL Chief Mike Meoli, this team has labored over the past 5 years to create a training program for the providers of tactical medicine.

During the development process, Kenneth Whitman of the California Commission on Peace Officer Standards and Training (POST) and Dan Smiley of the California Emergency Medical Authority (EMSA) requested that Dr. Heiskell and Dr. Wipfler participate on an 18-agency member committee to develop the first state-wide Tactical Medicine Core Competencies and Standardized Training Recommendations for the state of California. The result was a first-of-its-kind milestone in statewide-standardized tactical medicine training. This textbook incorporates these recommendations and guidelines, which were finalized in March of 2010.

The authors greatly appreciate the support of the American College of Emergency Physicians (ACEP) and over 340 members of its Tactical Medicine Section. The chapters in this textbook were extensively reviewed and edited by numerous volunteer ACEP members, resulting in an even better educational resource.

The authors extend their sincere gratitude to the many excellent editors, reviewers, colleagues, and friends from diverse backgrounds who have all contributed to this textbook. The authors thank the excellent editorial and production staff at Jones & Bartlett Learning, especially Christine Emerton, Laura Burns, Jennifer Deforge-Kling, and Susan Schultz. In particular, we wish to thank our spouses and families for their patience and support as the hours and hours ticked by being spent producing an educational resource that hopefully will benefit many and save lives. The goal was, and remains to this day, to better enable tactical medical providers to safely, skillfully, competently, and confidently conduct tactical medicine support for special weapons and tactics (SWAT) and special operations teams.

INTRODUCTION

The concept of emergency medical support has evolved into the dynamic field of what is now know as tactical medicine. The absolute necessity of medical support is apparent and important now more than ever in the history of SWAT and law enforcement special operations. This textbook will be a great resource for you, the tactical medicine provider, in improving your knowledge and skill sets. The authors have provided you with decades of real world experience.

All aspects of tactical medicine is explained in detail. The book has information on how to handle everything from routine medical problems to more complex and serious injuries and illnesses that can occur in the tactical environment.

Saving lives and reducing liability are goals of every law enforcement agency. This book teaches and shows you how to accomplish this. It will be valuable tool for any tactical medicine provider who works with law enforcement agencies, their special operations teams/ SWAT, mobile field teams, bomb squads, K-9 units, and other elements with unique deployment circumstances that can benefit from close-up medical support.

Ron McCarthy
Los Angeles California Police Department Special
Operations Team (LAPD SWAT) (ret)
Los Angeles, California

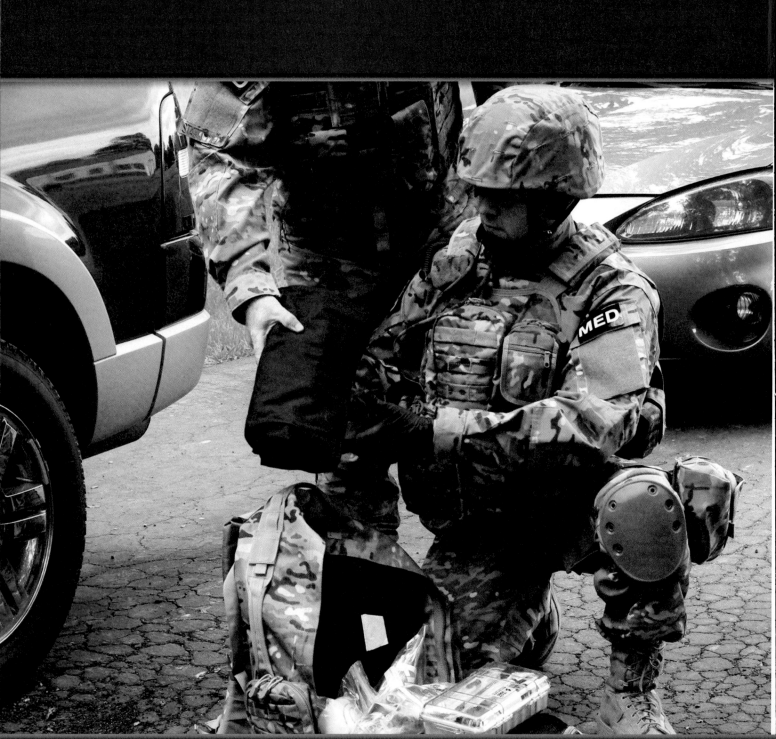

Elements of Tactical Medicine

CHAPTERS

History and Role of the Tactical Medical Provider

OBJECTIVES

- Define tactical medicine.
- Define tactical emergency medical support (TEMS).
- Discuss the history and evolution of TEMS.
- Describe the civilian emergency medical system.
- Describe the organization of and roles in law enforcement.
- Discuss the history of Special Weapons and Tactics (SWAT) units.
- Discuss the roles within the SWAT units.
- List the roles and responsibilities of the tactical medical provider (TMP) before, during, and after a callout.
- Define bilateral command.
- Describe the elements of TMP training.

Introduction

Special Weapons and Tactics (SWAT) units are specialized law enforcement units that deal with a variety of critical (or high-risk) incidents including barricaded felony suspects, hostage rescue scenarios, perpetrators armed with military-style weapons, organized crime, methamphetamine laboratories with chemical and explosive threats, terrorist acts, bomb threats, dignitary protection, riots, and other hazards **Figure 1-1**.

Tactical medicine is the services and emergency medical support needed to preserve the safety, health, and overall well-being of SWAT unit personnel.

Tactical emergency medical support (TEMS) is the prehospital emergency care provided during SWAT unit training and callouts (critical incidents). During training and during a callout, SWAT unit personnel are accompanied by personnel trained in TEMS—known as **tactical medical providers (TMPs)**.

The mission of the TMP is to support the wellness of the SWAT unit and perform emergency medical care in the tactical environment for any person in need, from SWAT unit personnel to suspect.

Training to become a TMP is challenging. The TMP often acts as the bridge between law enforcement and emergency medical services. You will be challenged, both physically and mentally, during this course. You must keep your body in excellent condition so you can master the skills needed to survive and provide medical care in a tactical environment. You must also remain mentally alert to cope with the various conditions and stresses you will encounter.

This chapter discusses the history of tactical emergency medical support, the modern emergency care system, the roles in a SWAT unit, the roles and responsibilities of a TMP, and the concept of bilateral command.

At the Scene

SWAT units are sometimes called by other names. Depending upon the local mission and other factors, SWAT units are sometimes assigned more general names such as special response team (SRT) or emergency response team (ERT). SWAT unit personnel are referred to as SWAT officers or tactical officers.

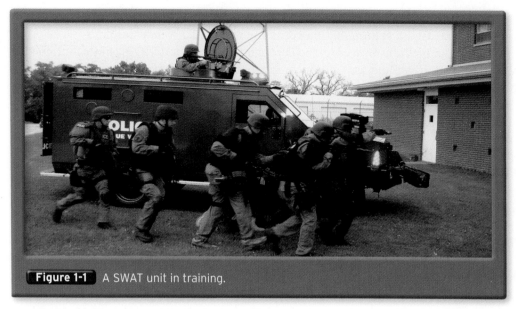

Figure 1-1 A SWAT unit in training.

The History of Tactical Emergency Medical Support

Napoleon Bonaparte and his surgeon, Dominique Jean Larrey, are recognized as having the first modern field medical evacuation system integrated into combat units. Those wounded in Napoleon's army were treated and evacuated by dedicated horse-drawn wagons and medical personnel during battle. The availability and provision of battlefield medical care undoubtedly contributed to his army's initial success.

Later, during the American Civil War, Clara Barton helped show the benefits of providing medical stabilization of wounded soldiers before and during transport from the battlefield. Her philosophy of treating soldiers as soon as possible was another step in the evolution of the present day military and civilian prehospital emergency care systems.

World Wars I and II saw the development of ambulance corps to rapidly care for and remove injured persons from the battlefield to take them to hospitals far from the front. But, during the 1950s and the Korean War, military medical researchers recognized that bringing the hospital closer to the field would give patients a better chance of surviving **Figure 1-2**. Helicopters, another new technology, brought patients to Mobile Army Surgical Hospitals (M*A*S*H units) that helped thousands survive.

Over the years, US Special Forces teams such as Delta Force or SEAL, as well as international military and police special operations teams such as

the German GSG9 or the Russian Spetsnaz, have integrated personnel who were specifically trained and equipped for special medical support during missions. Medical support has often contributed to the success of these missions. Over time, the evolution of other special operations military teams occurred, and a majority of these included their own medical assets. A key principle was found to be true: If a team cannot take care of injuries and illness, it is not a truly mobile, self-sufficient unit.

Unfortunately, emergency care of the injured and ill for civilians did not progress to a similar level. As late as the early 1960s, emergency ambulance service and care across the United States varied widely. In some places, it was provided by well-trained advanced first aid personnel who had well-equipped, modern ambulances. In a few urban areas, it was provided by hospital-based ambulance services that were staffed with interns and early forms of prehospital care providers. In many areas, the only emergency care and ambulance service was provided by the local funeral home using a

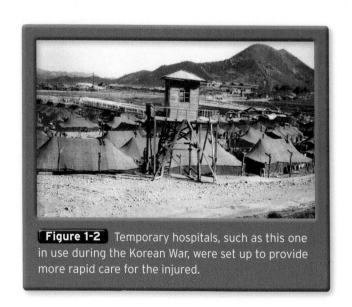

Figure 1-2 Temporary hospitals, such as this one in use during the Korean War, were set up to provide more rapid care for the injured.

hearse that could be converted to carry a cot. In other places, the police or fire department used a station wagon that carried a cot and a first aid kit. In most cases, these vehicles were staffed by a driver and an attendant who had some basic first aid training. In the few areas where a commercial ambulance was available to transport the ill, it was usually similarly staffed and served primarily as a means to transport the patient to the hospital.

Many communities had no formal provision for prehospital emergency care or transportation. Injured persons were given basic first aid by police or fire personnel at the scene and were transported to the hospital in a police or fire officer's car. Sick patients were transported to the hospital by a relative or neighbor and were met by their family physician or an on-call hospital physician who assessed them and then summoned any specialists and operating room staff that were needed. Except in large urban centers, most hospitals did not have the same emergency department staff available today.

The emergency medical services (EMS) system as we know it today had its origin in 1966 with the publication of *Accidental Death and Disability: The Neglected Disease of Modern Society*, known more commonly as "The White Paper." This report, prepared jointly by the Committees on Trauma and Shock of the National Academy of Sciences/National Research Council, revealed to the public and Congress the serious inadequacy of prehospital emergency care and transportation in many areas. As a result, Congress mandated that two federal agencies address these issues. Funding sources and programs were created to develop improved systems of prehospital emergency care.

In 1969, Dr Eugene Nagel began training fire fighters from the Miami Fire Department with advanced emergency skills such as cardiac monitoring and IV therapy. Dr Nagel also developed a telemetry system that enabled fire fighters to transmit a patient's electrocardiogram to physicians at Jackson Memorial Hospital and to receive radio instructions from the physicians regarding what measures to take.

In 1973, the Emergency Medical Services System Act defined the required components of an EMS system, with emphasis on regional development and trauma care. The act provided a structure and uniformity to the EMS system that came out of pioneering programs in Miami, Seattle, and Pittsburgh, and the Illinois Trauma System.

Many cities set up individual advanced EMS training, and regions added their own spin to what they thought was the essential standard of care. In 1977, the first National Standard Curriculum for paramedics

was developed by the US Department of Transportation, based on the work of Dr Nancy Caroline.

Through the 1980s and 1990s, EMS continued to evolve and the number of trained personnel grew. Federal funding and staff were reduced, and the responsibility for funding EMS was transferred to the states. The National Highway Traffic Safety Administration (NHTSA) developed "10 System Elements" in an effort to sustain EMS systems. The rapid advancement slowed greatly after this change in responsibility, primarily because of funding issues. Although it was made clear that the federal funding being provided was just "seed money" and that long-term local funding strategies needed to be developed, many states believed that the federal dollars would not go away. Unfortunately, federal funding of EMS did become obsolete.

Civilian Emergency Medical Services

The **emergency medical services (EMS)** system of today consists of a team of health care professionals who, in each area or jurisdiction, are responsible for and provide emergency care and transportation to the sick and injured. Each emergency medical service is part of a local or regional EMS system that provides the many prehospital and hospital components required for the delivery of proper emergency medical care. The standards for prehospital emergency care and the individuals who provide it are governed by the laws in each state and are typically regulated by a state office of EMS.

In most states, individuals who work on an ambulance are categorized into four training and licensure levels: **emergency medical responder (EMR)**, **emergency medical technician (EMT)**, **advanced EMT (AEMT)**, and **paramedic**. An EMR has very basic training and provides care before the ambulance arrives. EMRs may also perform in an assistant role within the ambulance. An EMT has training in basic life support, including automated external defibrillation, use of airway adjuncts, and assisting patients with certain medications. An AEMT has training in specific aspects of **advanced life support (ALS)**, such as **intravenous (IV) therapy** and the administration of certain emergency medications. A paramedic has extensive training in ALS, including endotracheal intubation, emergency pharmacology, cardiac monitoring, and other advanced assessment and treatment skills.

Each EMS system has a physician **medical director** who authorizes the emergency medical provider in the service to provide medical care in the field. The appropriate care for each injury, condition, or illness that the emergency medical provider encounters in the field is determined by the medical director and is described in a set of written standing orders and protocols. Protocols are a comprehensive guide delineating the emergency medical provider's scope of practice. Standing orders are part of protocols and designate what the EMT is required to do for a specific complaint or condition.

The medical director provides the ongoing working liaison between the medical community, hospitals, and the emergency medical providers in the service. If treatment problems arise or different procedures should be considered, these are referred to the medical director for his or her decision and action. To ensure the proper training standards are met, the medical director determines and approves the continuing education and training that are required of each emergency medical provider in the service.

Law Enforcement Overview

Law enforcement officers—from police officers to SWAT officers—are empowered to enforce the law and preserve order. Law enforcement officers are armed and authorized to use negotiation and physical force under certain conditions when carrying out their duties to prevent, protect against, detect, investigate, and prosecute criminal behavior. Law enforcement organizations consist of many levels (ranks) and positions. The names of these positions may vary throughout the United States, but the basic job description still applies. Positions in law enforcement include:

- **Patrol officers.** Patrol officers are the "eyes and ears" of law enforcement and are the largest component of a department. Patrol officers usually patrol within assigned areas while in uniform as they tend to the immediate needs of the community. They are usually the first responders on the scene.
- **Detectives (investigators).** These officers have been promoted from patrol and conduct detailed follow-up investigations of assigned cases (such as arson, rape, child abuse, homicide) with the goal of developing a case suitable for prosecution by the legal system of the criminal offender.
- **Supervisors (sergeant, lieutenant).** These officers coordinate and manage a group of personnel, such as patrol officers or detectives.

- **Chief executive officer (sheriff, chief of police, commissioner, marshal).** This officer leads, coordinates, guides, and manages all units and all personnel within the agency on a daily basis.
- **specialized units.** These law enforcement units are made up of officers with specialized training, including SWAT, internal affairs, training, and detention.

The History of SWAT Units

Before 1966, few law enforcement agencies utilized SWAT units for calls involving high-risk conditions, such as barricaded suspects carrying weapons. Regular patrol officers, who were often inadequately prepared, trained, and equipped, usually responded to these dangerous assignments and resolved them with what they had on hand.

A series of significant historic events led to an increased interest in specially trained units for law enforcement agencies in the United States. In 1965, the Los Angeles Watts Riots left over 1,000 wounded and 34 dead. The University of Texas clock tower shooting occurred when an ex-soldier used several guns to kill 14 people and wound 32 others on August 1, 1966. Civil unrest and multiple riots in the mid-1960s shook law enforcement agencies nationwide and forced them to consider how they would react to these violent acts in their own jurisdictions.

In 1967, the Los Angeles Police Department (LAPD) was among the first to organize full-time SWAT units specifically trained to handle high-risk incidents and has deployed paramedics with the SWAT unit since its inception. Over the past few decades, an increasing number of SWAT units have incorporated the TEMS philosophy. In addition, the Federal Bureau of Investigation (FBI) Hostage Rescue Team (HRT) and other government special operations teams routinely deploy with a TEMS component.

The Beginnings of TEMS Units

Law enforcement agencies in the United States have become increasingly aware of the value and benefits of a TEMS program. On a national level, there were meetings in 1989 and 1990 that further explored ideas and concepts of providing emergency medical support to SWAT units. In 1991, the first abstract and presentation speaking to this issue was delivered at the National Association of Emergency Medical Services Physicians meeting. In January 1993, a Subcommittee on Tactical Emergency Medicine was formed within the California Chapter of the American College of Emergency Medicine. The first National SWAT Physicians Conference took place in March of 1993. Several tactical medicine training programs also began in the early 1990s.

Today, training courses and tactical medicine conferences occur with increasing frequency. TEMS is an evolving specialty that is increasingly utilized by law enforcement agencies to save lives and ensure that SWAT units have the ability to resolve critical incidents as safely as possible.

Roles Within the SWAT Unit

SWAT units around the world have a similar organization of duties. Each SWAT unit member has a special area of expertise, such as assault, arrest, rescue, negotiations, and/or TEMS. Many SWAT officers are cross-trained and are able to fill in for several positions outside their specialties if needed. During a callout (or mission), each SWAT officer is assigned a specific role or position **Figure 1-3**.

The following SWAT unit positions are usually deployed during a callout:

- **Incident commander**. Typically an upper-level law enforcement administrator who supervises the entire operation from the **incident command center**.

- **Tactical operations leader**. Usually assumed by a mid-level law enforcement lieutenant who has extensive tactical experience. The tactical operations leader directs the details of the callout from either the incident command center or from a separate but nearby **tactical operations center (TOC)**.

- **Team leader**. Directs the SWAT unit personally when entering buildings and is often located in the middle of the entry team line.

- **Immediate reaction team**. A group of five to seven SWAT officers and at least two TMPs who stand ready to immediately respond while detailed tactical plans involving the entire SWAT unit are being created.

- **Marksmen (snipers)**. Located in a hidden position close to the criminal suspects, usually two or more marksmen observe and provide information, security, and precision long-range threat neutralization **Figure 1-4**.

- **Observer**. Deploys with the marksmen to assist and provide area security.

- **Point man**. Guides the entry team to the deployment area and enters the building or other structure first, equivalent to the point of a spear.

- **Breacher**. Carries a heavy metal **battering ram** and other tools (eg, crowbars, explosive entry devices, and hydraulic rams) to force open doors or walls **Figure 1-5**.

- **Entry team**. Usually four to eight SWAT officers are part of an entry team. The entry team is

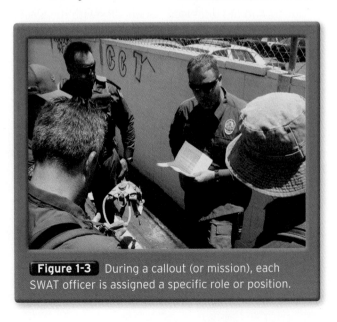

Figure 1-3 During a callout (or mission), each SWAT officer is assigned a specific role or position.

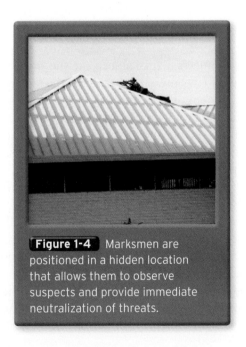

Figure 1-4 Marksmen are positioned in a hidden location that allows them to observe suspects and provide immediate neutralization of threats.

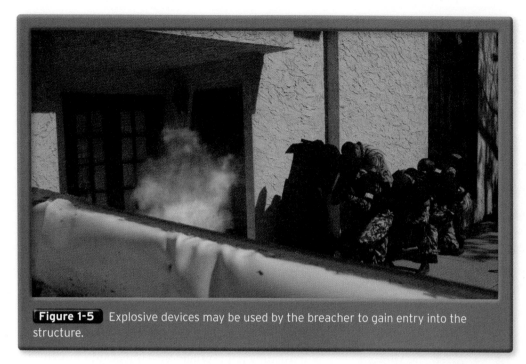

Figure 1-5 Explosive devices may be used by the breacher to gain entry into the structure.

responsible for finding and arresting criminal suspects and clearing the building. Depending upon the callout, the entry team may be responsible for rescuing hostages or clearing and securing specific rooms.

- **Gasman**. If the situation calls for it, the gasman may shoot or throw chemical agents into a building with the goal of forcing the criminal suspect(s) to leave the building.
- **Rear guard**. Provides rear security for the entry team.
- **Tactical medical providers**. TMPs provide medical support before, during, and after SWAT callouts. They may be organized as a sub-unit within a SWAT unit in order to provide comprehensive coverage. Tactical emergency medical care can also be provided by designated SWAT officers with ALS training.

In addition to the previously mentioned positions, there are several additional personnel who may play a significant role in a SWAT callout, depending upon the callout. The following positions are deployed on a case-by-case basis, and are not common among all SWAT units:

- **Negotiations team**. A group of law enforcement officers with special training in crisis negotiations and psychology. The negotiations teams help resolve a large percentage of SWAT incidents and are an integral part of SWAT units.

- **K-9 officer**. A law enforcement officer who trains and deploys dogs used to search a building, apprehend a fleeing subject, and sniff for drugs and explosives.
- **Rescue team**. A backup team of SWAT officers that is designated to stand by, ready to come to the aid of or supplement the primary entry team. It will ideally contain TMPs.
- **Perimeter security team**. Composed of additional, uniformed patrol officers and undercover patrol officers who are usually needed to provide an outer-perimeter security ring, to help ensure that no criminal suspects leave the callout site, and to prevent bystanders from entering the dangerous inner perimeter.
- **Bomb squad**. Composed of specially trained law enforcement officers and specialists who have unique equipment and protective gear to assist in recognition and inactivation or neutralization of explosive threats.

Roles and Responsibilities of the Tactical Medical Provider

The specific responsibilities of the TMP vary depending upon the type of callout and the level of care that the TMP is authorized to provide, from BLS (EMR and EMT levels) to ALS (AEMT and paramedic levels) **Figure 1-6**. The primary responsibility of the TMP is to provide emergency care inside or near the inner perimeter. The secondary responsibility is to optimize the health and safety of the SWAT unit.

Before a callout, the TEMS unit is responsible for:

- Attending SWAT unit training sessions
- Providing preventive medicine, health maintenance, and injury control measures
- Providing medical care to SWAT officers who become injured or ill at training

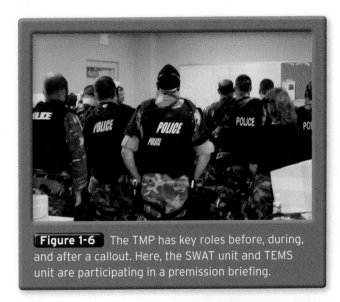

Figure 1-6 The TMP has key roles before, during, and after a callout. Here, the SWAT unit and TEMS unit are participating in a premission briefing.

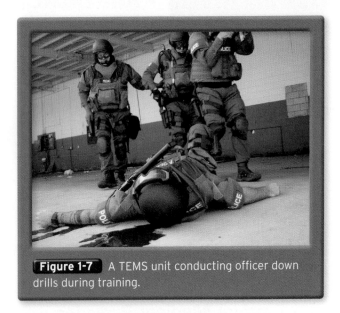

Figure 1-7 A TEMS unit conducting officer down drills during training.

- Preparing to deal with pertinent medical threats and hazards expected at a SWAT unit training event and during callouts
- Providing education in first aid and combat casualty care to SWAT officers, including:
  - Instruction in CPR, combat first aid, ballistics, field medicine, and other medically related topics that pertain to the tactical environment
  - Practicing "officer down" immediate action drills, extractions, and other scenarios **Figure 1-7**
- Identifying and preparing for any preexisting medical conditions of SWAT officers
- Making recommendations to optimize internal policies related to TEMS and general law enforcement health issues

- Serving as a resource for any medical concerns that affect the law enforcement agency

During a callout, the TEMS unit is responsible for:

- Remaining available to provide emergency medical care for those in need (ideally remaining close enough to respond within a 30-second response time for all injured SWAT officers)
- Participating in mission planning, preparing an assessment of medical threats, and providing appropriate advice while keeping the mission appropriately confidential to avoid any information leaks that would jeopardize the SWAT unit
- Preplanning and arranging emergency medical evacuation and transportation pertinent to the mission, including methods of transport, appropriate selection and notification of hospitals, and route planning
- Providing appropriate preventive and immediate medical care to SWAT officers, other law enforcement officers, and public safety personnel
- Providing secondary emergency care and triage for those in need, including bystanders, suspects, or others on site at the discretion of the SWAT unit leaders
- Providing "assessment and clearing" of suspects prior to incarceration as directed by the SWAT unit leader or commander
- Advising the command staff of developing medical concerns, and remaining available for medical consultation to the SWAT unit leadership
- Performing remote assessment of any downed victims in exposed areas and then advising the incident commander about the likely viability of the victims (their chances for survival)
- Improving SWAT unit performance and morale by the presence of immediate medical support, which has positive psychological benefits
- Functioning as a liaison with the local EMS system, hospitals, and officials from other public safety and law enforcement agencies

After a mission, the TEMS unit is responsible for:

- Participating in post-incident debriefing and review, assisting command staff with analysis of the operation/training event and any medical care delivered, and making improvements to the TEMS unit, policies, and procedures as needed
- Reviewing and documenting all medical treatment and records relevant to operational or training missions

- Appropriately optimizing treatment, rehabilitation, and mental health for injured SWAT officers through involvement with hospitals, physicians, family, and police department officials, while maintaining HIPAA/patient confidentiality regulations
- Incorporating "lessons learned" into future unit training and preparedness, thus assisting with preventive medicine efforts and the improvement of care

Bilateral Command

Typically, TMPs operate under the daily direction of the EMS medical director. During a tactical operation, however, the involved law enforcement agency is usually in charge of the overall scene. In situations where the TEMS unit is made up of emergency medical care providers from both law enforcement and civilian public safety agencies, a bilateral command exists. It is important to determine who is actually in control of the TEMS unit before training and callout missions.

In most circumstances, TMPs report directly to the law enforcement tactical operations leader (usually the lieutenant of the SWAT unit) during a mission. However, the protocol and procedures surrounding medical care and medical decision making are ultimately left to the EMS medical director. Therefore, this **bilateral command structure**, where law enforcement assumes command in the field while medical direction is given remotely, exists in most tactical environments. If a TMP is employed by the fire department and is essentially on loan to the police department, then the leadership structure and chain of command will be worked out by the involved agencies, but in most cases the mission priorities of the law enforcement leadership involved will have priority.

> ### At the Scene
>
> If a group of medical providers (such as TMPs in a TEMS unit) enters into a **mutual aid agreement** or contract to provide medical support for another public safety entity or government organization in a certain state, then that medical unit must function under the rules and regulations of the state EMS regulatory system.

TMPs rarely encounter discrepancies between on-scene command and medical direction because they should be trained in specific tactical medical protocols taking into consideration each approach to the patient in the tactical environment. Furthermore, direct online communication with **medical control** is often not possible or practical in the tactical environment. Thorough medical care is sometimes tactically inadvisable; therefore, in the chaotic tactical environment, the effective leadership by SWAT incident commanders should be followed to maximize unit safety. Medical procedures and patient assessment will be done only after the tactical environment has been appropriately stabilized. Therefore, the bilateral command issue is more theoretical in practical application.

Online medical direction, communicated face-to-face, by radio, by cell phone, or by another device, should be sought whenever there is a question about the most appropriate medical treatment option for a patient, or to receive advice in uncertain situations. For TMPs who function as part of a regional, statewide, or nationwide SWAT unit, and whose callout territory may take them outside of their own EMS region, the command structure differs. In this case, the medical direction should be arranged and provided to the TEMS unit by an EMS physician with wider jurisdiction. Ideally, the provision of medical direction consists of pre-established protocols and policies modified specifically

> ### At the Scene
>
> In most agencies, the EMS medical director has ultimate control and authority over the TEMS unit. In some agencies, an additional physician may assume the medical direction for the TEMS unit, providing off-line direction via procedures and protocols and providing online direction in person or over the radio. This additional physician may also assist with maintaining the health of the TEMS and SWAT units.

> ### At the Scene
>
> In nearly all circumstances, TMPs are required to comply with the state-mandated EMS rules and regulations, which may be diverse and complex. In addition, unique medical **tactics, techniques, and procedures (TTP)** may be specially permitted for the TEMS unit after appropriate EMS application and approval is given on an individual unit basis by the state EMS agency.

for the tactical environment. Follow the protocols and policies of your agency.

Command Systems: LIMS and NIMS

The Law Enforcement Incident Management System (LIMS) is based upon the **National Incident Management System (NIMS)**. NIMS is the standardized incident management protocol used throughout the United States, which is now required in all law enforcement operations. Under the LIMS system, there is a law enforcement incident commander (IC) who serves as command in most callouts **Figure 1-8**.

As in NIMS, under LIMS each law enforcement agency uses a similar scaleable incident management system but may elect to add or remove various components, such as the operations or planning sections. If the incident is large and involves multiple agencies, this framework may be included within a unified command with representatives from various agencies such as law enforcement, EMS, fire service, public works, and elected officials serving as the commanders in a unified command structure. However, only law enforcement managers command and direct law enforcement agency assets and operations.

Under LIMS, the safety officer and/or the TEMS unit can observe and report directly to the law enforcement IC any safety concerns, and can halt operations if a substantial hazard is discovered that will endanger personnel and the success of the mission. The planning section reports to the law enforcement IC and assists in providing viable plans to resolve the incident and intelligence on the suspects involved. The logistics and finance/administration sections secure the needed personnel and material items to support the operation. Logistics is also responsible for the staging of law enforcement, EMS, and other assets. The operations manager directly supervises tactical operations. Usually the entry team, tactical marksmen, and the TEMS unit report to the operations manager, and it is usually necessary for the TMP to interface through the external EMS system.

Tactical Medical Provider Training

Tactical Medicine Curriculum

There is currently no national standard TMP curriculum. There is a consensus among SWAT unit leaders, however, about the major areas that should be learned and practiced by TMPs. These include specific SWAT unit tactics, weapons training, and immediate action drills, as well as training in hazardous materials and bloodborne pathogen management.

In addition to completing a training program covering the essential knowledge and skills of tactical emergency medicine, you must also gain experience through routine training with the SWAT unit. Through ongoing SWAT unit trainings, you will learn about your specific unit's abilities, weapons, and tactics. Mastery of the specific SWAT unit tactics, weapons, immediate action drills, and many other important topics will come after multiple cooperative training exercises and real-world callouts. These experiences will enable you to gain the remainder of the knowledge and skills that will enable you to provide rapid, safe, and effective medical care in the tactical environment **Figure 1-9**.

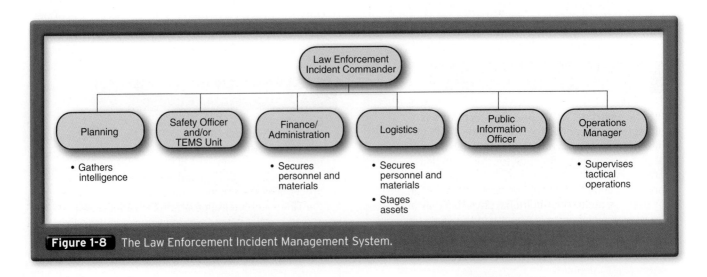

Figure 1-8 The Law Enforcement Incident Management System.

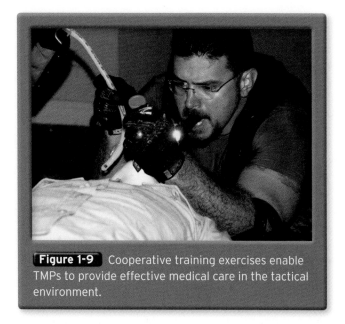

Figure 1-9 Cooperative training exercises enable TMPs to provide effective medical care in the tactical environment.

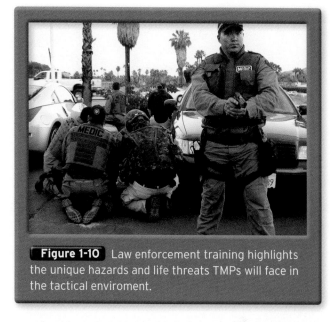

Figure 1-10 Law enforcement training highlights the unique hazards and life threats TMPs will face in the tactical enviroment.

Law Enforcement Training for Tactical Medical Providers

The law enforcement status and training required for tactical medical personnel is a joint decision of the leadership of each law enforcement agency, local EMS organization, and municipality associated with a TEMS unit. The options may vary between using fully trained and sworn law enforcement officers to provide medical support, as contrasted with using civilian medical personnel who have received baseline law enforcement and tactical training by working with the SWAT unit on an informal basis. In between these two options may be reserve police officer training, auxiliary deputy status, and other law enforcement positions.

There are several ways for TEMS unit personnel to acquire law enforcement training and possible certification, and the involved agencies should come to an agreement upon what will work best given the regional policies and political situations. A common approach is to have TMPs attend a reasonable amount of law enforcement training that they and their designated law enforcement agency mutually agree upon, within their time constraints, funding, and local policies. Law enforcement training will highlight the unique hazards and life threats faced by anyone entering the tactical environment **Figure 1-10**.

The bottom line is that you must have a baseline understanding of law enforcement and the operational aspects of the SWAT unit. In every unit, the primary role of the TMP is medical support, but, as in any uncontrolled environment, the unexpected sometimes occurs. You must be prepared to make a split-second

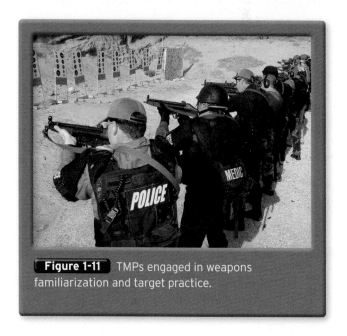

Figure 1-11 TMPs engaged in weapons familiarization and target practice.

decision when faced with an armed and highly dangerous criminal suspect. There will be times when a SWAT officer may not be immediately present to assist in resolving the situation. You should learn and know use of force, self-defense laws, arrest and control techniques, and combat skills. Additional skills necessary in the tactical environment might include crowd control, weapon retention, and use of less-lethal weapons **Figure 1-11**.

If the TEMS unit is authorized to carry self-defense weapons, you must complete initial training and qualification, and ongoing requalification weapons requirements. Most armed units require completion of

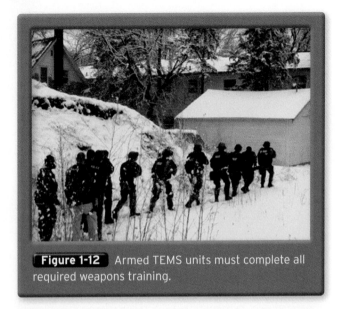

Figure 1-12 Armed TEMS units must complete all required weapons training.

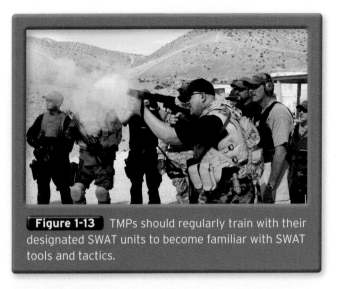

Figure 1-13 TMPs should regularly train with their designated SWAT units to become familiar with SWAT tools and tactics.

training held to the same standard as a law enforcement officer in basic police academy **Figure 1-12**.

Regardless of whether or not the medical personnel are armed, at a minimum all TMPs should learn and maintain skills in safe weapons handling and unloading, as well as techniques for rendering weapons safe. Participation in routine marksmanship training is desirable, and medical personnel should be familiar with all types of weapons used by the SWAT unit.

Unit Training

You will receive perhaps your most valuable education as you routinely participate with your own SWAT unit on a monthly basis. Most SWAT units are part-time and practice once or twice a month for about 8 to 16 hours per month. Larger US cities may have a full-time SWAT unit (eg, Los Angeles and New York City) who train and participate in high-risk warrant service and tactical callouts essentially every day. Tactical training sessions offer a good opportunity to learn about and practice the unit's tactics and tools.

Safety

Weapons training for TMPs must stress that, in the tactical environment, weapons should not be "fired and forgotten." TMPs should maintain weapons-handling skills and always seek to improve on their education.

More importantly, training offers opportunities to practice downed officer immediate action drills and other skills in order to perfect and maintain your own tactical medical knowledge and skills.

Two components are necessary for effective routine TEMS training: TEMS unit and SWAT unit involvement. TEMS training should be well-coordinated with routine SWAT training in order to ensure that all personnel (medical and nonmedical) are familiarized with each other's tools, techniques, and skills **Figure 1-13**. Routine training for SWAT and TEMS personnel should include tactical law enforcement training for TMPs, combat first aid training for SWAT officers, and training specific to unique hazards of the tactical environment (eg, hazardous materials and bloodborne pathogens). Cross-training within the SWAT unit as well as with other agencies involved in responses is an important consideration.

Hazardous Materials Training

Due to the ever-present and increasing risk of exposure to caustic chemicals, radioactive terrorism, biologic and chemical warfare agents, nerve agents, poisons, booby traps, and clandestine drug laboratory hazards, you must be able to prevent self-exposure and contamination. You must also be able to identify, decontaminate, and treat other officers exposed to hazardous materials (hazmat). You must be properly equipped and trained to deal with hazmat contingencies, as well as prepare nonmedical personnel in preventive medicine and decontamination training. TEMS units should know how to perform hasty field expedient decontamination as well as participate in full-scale fire department-based hazmat team decontamination. Additional hazmat training can

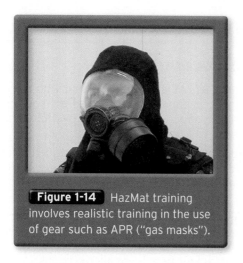

Figure 1-14 HazMat training involves realistic training in the use of gear such as APR ("gas masks").

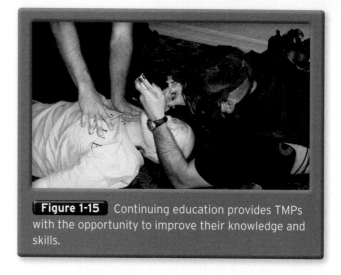

Figure 1-15 Continuing education provides TMPs with the opportunity to improve their knowledge and skills.

be sought through regional fire academies and training companies **Figure 1-14** .

Bloodborne Pathogens Training

The potential for exposure to **bloodborne pathogens** is a very real threat in the EMS and tactical environments. Exposure to **hepatitis**, **human immunodeficiency virus (HIV)** (which causes acquired immunodeficiency syndrome [AIDS]), and other viral diseases is largely preventable. Through personal protective equipment, the risk can be minimized. The use of **standard precautions** should always be ensured, as well as maintenance of accurate medical records that document the proper hepatitis B vaccination and other vaccines for SWAT officers. Tetanus prophylaxis, annual TB monitoring, and other occupational health matters should be appropriately recommended, supported, and documented.

Continuing Medical Education

As with any profession, in tactical medicine there will always be improvements to the system—new ideas, new equipment, and new techniques to learn about and adapt to. Medical professionals are held to a certain level of performance regarding continuing medical education. Much of this education is related to their continued job-specific medical career. You should continue your education and keep your skills sharp by attending advanced tactical medical training, attending conferences, and using other methods to improve your knowledge and skills **Figure 1-15** . Documentation of initial and continuing TEMS education is also important in order to prove you have successfully completed training and certification requirements.

Ready for Review

- Special Weapons and Tactics (SWAT) units are specialized law enforcement units who deal with a variety of critical incidents where the risk of violence is very high.

- Tactical emergency medical support (TEMS) units and tactical medical providers (TMPs) provide medical support to SWAT units in the tactical environment and during training.

- The experiences of special military forces has shown that if a team cannot take care of the injuries and illness of its unit in the field, then it is not a truly mobile, self-sufficient unit.

- The civilian emergency medical services (EMS) system consists of emergency medical responders (EMRs), emergency medical technicians (EMTs), advanced EMTs (AEMTs), and paramedics under the direction of the medical director.

- The personnel in law enforcement agencies includes patrol officers, detectives, supervisors, a chief executive officer, and specialized units, such as SWAT units.

- Violent events of the 1960s led to the creation by law enforcement of specialized units trained to handle high-risk incidents.

- Each SWAT unit member has a special area of expertise, such as assault, arrest, rescue, negotiations, and/or TEMS. Many SWAT officers are cross-trained and are able to fill in for several positions outside their specialties if needed.

- The specific responsibilities of the TMP vary depending upon the type of callout and the level of care that the TMP is authorized to provide. The primary responsibility of the TMP is to provide emergency care inside or near the inner perimeter. The secondary responsibility is to optimize the health and safety of the SWAT unit.

- Typically, TMPs operate under the daily direction of the EMS medical director. During a tactical operation, however, the involved law enforcement agency is usually in charge of the overall scene.

- Always seek to improve your skills by continuing your education and keeping your skills sharp by attending advanced tactical medical training, attending conferences, and using other methods to improve your knowledge and skills.

Vital Vocabulary

advanced EMT (AEMT) An individual who has training in specific aspects of advanced life support, such as intravenous therapy and the administration of certain emergency medications.

advanced life support (ALS) Advanced lifesaving procedures, such as cardiac monitoring, administration of IV fluids and medications, and use of advanced airway adjuncts.

battering ram A tool made of hardened steel with handles on the sides used to force open doors and to breach walls. Larger versions may be used by as many as four people; smaller versions are made for one or two people.

bilateral command structure A command structure for a TEMS unit that has law enforcement assume command in the field, while medical direction is given remotely during a mission.

bloodborne pathogens Pathogenic microorganisms that are present in human blood and can cause disease in humans. These pathogens include, but are not limited to, hepatitis B virus and human immunodeficiency virus (HIV).

bomb squad Specially trained police officers and specialists with unique equipment and protective gear to assist in the recognition and inactivation or neutralization of explosive threats.

breacher SWAT officer who carries a heavy metal battering ram and other tools to force open doors or walls.

emergency medical responder (EMR) The first trained individual, such as a police officer, fire fighter, lifeguard, or other rescuer, to arrive at the scene of an emergency to provide initial medical assistance.

emergency medical services (EMS) A multidisciplinary system that represents the combined efforts of several professionals and agencies to provide prehospital emergency care to the sick and injured.

emergency medical technician (EMT) An individual who has training in basic life support, including automated external defibrillation, use of a definitive airway adjunct, and assisting patients with certain medications.

entry team Four to eight SWAT officers who are primarily responsible for finding and arresting suspects and clearing the building.

gasman SWAT officer who may shoot or throw chemical agents into a building to force suspects to leave the building.

hepatitis Inflammation of the liver, usually caused by a viral infection, that causes fever, loss of appetite, jaundice, fatigue, and altered liver function.

human immunodeficiency virus (HIV) Acquired immunodeficiency syndrome (AIDS) is caused by HIV, which damages the cells in the body's immune system so that the body is unable to fight infection or certain cancers.

immediate reaction team A group of five to seven SWAT officers and at least two TMPs who stand ready to immediately respond to the incident while detailed tactical plans involving the entire SWAT unit are being created.

incident command center The location at the scene of an emergency where incident command is located and where command, coordination, control, and communications are centralized.

incident commander An upper-level law enforcement officer who supervises the entire tactical operation from the incident command center.

intravenous (IV) therapy The delivery of medication directly into a vein.

K-9 officer Law enforcement officer who trains and deploys police dogs.

law enforcement officers Personnel who are armed and authorized to use negotiation and physical force under certain conditions when carrying out their duties to prevent, protect against, detect, investigate, and prosecute criminal behavior.

marksmen (snipers) SWAT officers trained in precision long-range threat neutralization.

medical control Physician instructions that are given directly by radio or cell phone (online/direct) or indirectly by protocol/guidelines (off-line/indirect), as authorized by the medical director of the service program.

medical director The physician who authorizes or delegates to the TMP the authority to provide medical care in the tactical environment.

mutual aid agreement A contract entered into by a group of medical providers (eg, a TEMS unit) to provide medical support for another public safety entity or government organization.

National Incident Management System (NIMS) A Department of Homeland Security system designed to enable federal, state, and local governments and private-sector and nongovernmental organizations to effectively and efficiently prepare for, prevent, respond to, and recover from domestic incidents, regardless of cause, size, or complexity.

negotiations team Law enforcement officers with special training in crisis negotiations and psychology.

observer SWAT officer who assists marksmen and provides area security.

paramedic An individual who has extensive training in advanced life support, including endotracheal intubation, emergency pharmacology, cardiac monitoring, and other advanced assessment and treatment skills.

perimeter security team Uniformed patrol officers and undercover officers who provide outer-perimeter security to ensure no suspects leave and no bystanders enter the callout site.

point man SWAT officer who guides the entry team to the deployment area and enters the building or other structure first.

rear guard SWAT officer who provides rear security for the entry team.

rescue team Team of tactical officers who stand by, ready to come to the aid of or supplement the primary entry team.

Special Weapons and Tactics (SWAT) unit Specialized law enforcement units who deal with a variety of critical incidents including barricaded felony suspects, hostage rescue scenarios, perpetrators armed with military-style weapons, organized crime, methamphetamine laboratories with chemical and explosive threats, terrorist acts, bomb threats, dignitary protection, riots, and other hazards.

standard precautions An infection control concept and practice that assumes that all body fluids are potentially infectious.

tactical emergency medical support (TEMS) Prehospital emergency care during special weapons and tactics training and tactical missions.

tactical medical providers (TMPs) Medically trained persons whose mission it is to support the wellness of the SWAT officers and perform emergency medical care in the tactical environment for anyone in need.

tactical medicine The services and emergency medical support needed to preserve the safety, health, and overall well-being of SWAT officers.

tactical operations center (TOC) Location at the scene of a critical incident involving the SWAT unit, which is where the SWAT officers and SWAT unit leaders meet and make plans and preparations.

tactical operations leader Directs the details of the callout from either the incident command center or from a tactical operations center.

tactics, techniques, and procedures (TTP) Unique methods, tools, and description of medical and other types of procedures that are utilized by TMPs and SWAT officers to complete a mission.

team leader Directs the SWAT officers personally as a member of the entry team when entering buildings, often located in the middle of the entry team line.

Safety and Wellness of the Tactical Medical Provider

OBJECTIVES

- Describe the key components of a healthy lifestyle, including exercise, nutrition, personal hygiene, and sleep.

- Describe the key components of stress management, including quiet downtime, hobbies, and maintenance of lasting personal relationships.

- Discuss the critical incident stress management (CISM) process and how SWAT units can engage in this process through routine post-incident analyses, critical incident stress debriefings (CISDs), and defusing sessions, while monitoring for any SWAT officer's need for additional assistance.

- Discuss the Health Insurance Portability and Accountability Act (HIPAA) and its impact on the tactical medical provider (TMP).

Introduction

Most public safety professionals, including tactical medical providers (TMPs), are motivated by the challenges associated with helping and saving the lives of fellow citizens. Public safety professionals are often called to scenes of significant human tragedy and conflict such as horrific automobile wrecks and crimes that leave innocent citizens devastated. The cumulative effect of these stressful events can affect the public safety professional both mentally and physically. There are many strategies that you can use to effectively deal with the stress associated with the job. This chapter will provide suggestions about how to stay in top physical, mental, and emotional shape.

You must understand and recognize the unique physical and psychological stressors and risks that working with law enforcement brings. With this awareness, you can then watch for, identify, and assist yourself and Special Weapons and Tactics (SWAT) officers in facing and dealing with the unique stressors of law enforcement. Human beings have defense mechanisms that may be either healthy or unhealthy ways of dealing with the stress of the job. Appropriate support from TMPs, fellow SWAT officers, department counseling, and/or referral to psychiatric services may be indicated depending upon the nature and degree of mental health disturbances. A daily focus on personal wellness can prepare you and your fellow SWAT officers for success in the field.

Maintaining a healthy body, getting adequate sleep, eating nutritious food, creating a daily schedule that allows the highest priorities to be given proper attention, taking time for self-reflection, and arranging for proper mental health support when needed are all steps of being well. Achieving and keeping a balance of the important things in life is a worthy thing to do, but it takes planning and energy to accomplish this balance.

Health and Wellness

Preventive Medicine Principles

The use of preventive medicine principles is an essential task. Preventive medicine is using common sense and vigilance to look for signs of stress, illness, and physiological and psychological abnormalities in order to intervene and prevent illness and injury from occurring or becoming worse. It includes knowing each SWAT officer's medical history, analyzing potential or actual threats, gathering important additional information at the scene of training or actual callout, and suggesting specific preventive measures to SWAT officers and commanders in an appropriate and timely fashion.

Wellness for the SWAT Unit and TEMS Unit

The key to longevity in law enforcement is the maintenance of physical, mental, emotional, and spiritual health. The decision to make healthy choices, such as quitting smoking or starting and maintaining a regular exercise program, begins with a choice and ends with the change. Changing bad habits and implementing good ones is difficult. It may seem impossible at first, but the rewards of new good exercise and healthy eating habits bring a sense of energy and physical fitness, and more importantly a sense of control to your life **Figure 2-1**.

SWAT and TEMS units are increasingly recognizing the relationship between personal and professional wellness. Many have begun to realize that a challenging and exciting career in public safety also places stress on their bodies, minds, and relationships. Only through an integration of personal and professional wellness can SWAT and TEMS officers have long, effective, and satisfying careers.

Diet and Nutrition

Good nutrition is essential to a healthy body. The diet of too many emergency care professionals and law enforcement officers is unfortunately not ideal. Fast food, fast-paced work schedules, understaffing, overtime, and other constraints lead many professionals to buy unhealthy foods and drinks, which leads to a poor diet. Due to the physical and mental demands placed on tactical medical providers, physical fitness and good nutrition is critical. Being overweight is a liability in this profession.

In the last 10 years, research has demonstrated that a low-fat, high-complex carbohydrate diet is the best way to improve health and to increase life span. A moderate amount of protein and essential fatty acids is needed to maintain muscle mass and a healthy brain. The National Research Council recommends a total fat intake of 30% or less of the total calories consumed, saturated fat intake of less than 10%, and a total cholesterol intake of less than 300 mg daily. The Council also recommends an increased intake of complex carbohydrates, moderate protein intake, moderated alcohol intake, and less than 6 grams per day of salt, along with maintenance of adequate calcium and fluoride. Also advised is the recommended daily allowance (RDA) of supplemental vitamins and minerals.

Other important considerations in planning a healthy diet are food moderation and variety. Consuming a variety of foods provides a better balance of nutrients. A moderate diet provides limited salt and simple sugars without adding excess calories. The four food groups popular 20 years ago have been replaced by a new classification system called the food pyramid. An excellent website is www.mypyramid.gov, developed by the US Department of Agriculture, which explains this in detail and has good recommendations for a healthy diet **Figure 2-2**. The emphasis is placed on carbohydrates, fruits, and vegetables, and it represents a big reduction in the recommendations concerning the consumption of animal products.

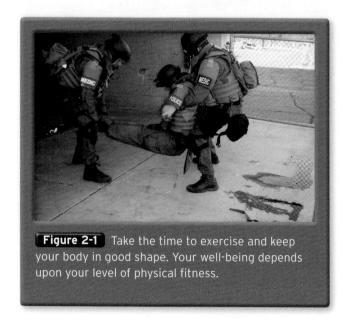

Figure 2-1 Take the time to exercise and keep your body in good shape. Your well-being depends upon your level of physical fitness.

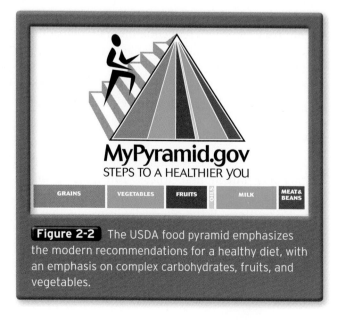

Figure 2-2 The USDA food pyramid emphasizes the modern recommendations for a healthy diet, with an emphasis on complex carbohydrates, fruits, and vegetables.

Safety

Alcohol is a substance to avoid. Alcohol is a mood-altering substance that can be abused. Excessive alcohol use can damage the body and affect performance. SWAT officers or TEMS providers who have consumed alcohol must not be permitted to engage in emergency operations.

Drug use has absolutely no place in public safety. Many law enforcement departments have drug-testing programs to ensure that personnel do not use or abuse drugs. The illegal use of drugs endangers your life, the lives of your unit, and the public you serve.

Work is usually busy and stressful, which sometimes results in quick meals at fast food restaurants. Do not use food as a stress reducer. Make time for adequate meal breaks during the shift. Bring some fruit, low-fat muffins, and high-fiber snacks to eat between meals.

Carry water bottles with you to help maintain a good hydration level. If you only drink when thirsty, you will not be able to maintain a good hydration level. Sip water often throughout the day. The human body sometimes confuses thirst with hunger, which can result in excess food intake. Some beverages actually increase hunger and overeating. For example, sodas do not contain ingredients to satisfy the body's nutritional needs.

If you wish to pursue weight loss or improved weight control, exercise more, consume fewer calories, and follow a diet of nutritious foods. This is much easier said than actually done. There are a wide variety of gimmick or crash weight-loss programs that are advertised, and although some are quite popular, they almost never work in the long term. The vast majority of the participants eventually gain more than their original weight back. A weight reduction program that actually works in the long term must include dietary changes and habits that you can live with for the rest of your life. Choose wisely. Consult the advice and support of your physician for healthy and effective weight-loss programs.

Exercise

Being in a SWAT or TEMS unit requires a high degree of physical and mental fitness. You need to be an athlete warrior. Proper physical fitness requires planned exercise routines. Being physically fit means that you will be prepared for duty in addition to looking and feeling better. Exercise will also help you to maintain an appropriate weight and a healthy body. It will also

aid you in critical self-defense skills, and may be the life-or-death deciding factor if you are ever engaged in close quarters confrontations. Your degree of fitness can literally save your life.

Cardiovascular health is essential. A strong heart will enable you to perform in the stressful tactical environment. Aerobic exercise is an important component

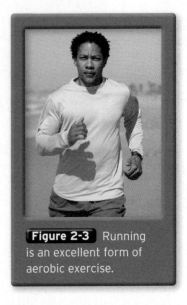

Figure 2-3 Running is an excellent form of aerobic exercise.

in cardiovascular health. Aerobic exercise essentially involves the repetitive use of the large muscle groups over a period of time **Figure 2-3** . According to the Centers for Disease Control and Prevention (CDC), a healthy adult needs to perform at least 150 minutes of vigorous-intensity aerobic activity a week. This could translate into running for 30 minutes or more, five times a week. You will know that you are exercising vigorously when you need to take a breath after speaking a few words.

Weight training is an additional component to a healthy exercise routine **Figure 2-4** . Regular weight training helps to build and maintain muscle mass, which can reduce with age. A well-rounded exercise program includes both aerobic and weight training. Seek

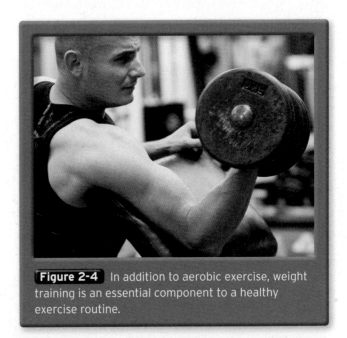

Figure 2-4 In addition to aerobic exercise, weight training is an essential component to a healthy exercise routine.

Safety

It is best to begin at a slower pace and then progressively increase the duration and intensity of a workout regimen.

out programs or machines that appeal to you. Exercise should not be boring or feel like a waste of time.

When planning your weekly schedule, set aside time to properly exercise. Some people find that exercising when they first arise in the morning is convenient and it seems to provide them with extra energy throughout the day. Others find that exercising after work is an excellent way to unwind and to relieve stress. Exercising late in the day can interfere with sleep patterns, so experiment and develop a schedule that works well for you.

Try to squeeze in small bits of exercise throughout the day by doing things like climbing stairs instead of using the elevators. Once a daily exercise routine is established, add variety and incentives to maintain your interest in the program. These incentives include working out with a fellow personnel or friend, goal setting, watching a variety of movies or sports programs during workouts, or keeping a log of workout accomplishments and goals to reach.

Exercise is also an essential part of any weight loss program. Merely reducing caloric intake by itself will reduce both muscle mass and fat tissue. The combination of decreased caloric intake and increased exercise will maintain muscle mass and reduce excess fat tissue. The overconsumption of food is a major problem. People often do not recognize the sensation of satiety and therefore do not know when to stop eating. Ideally, you should only eat when you are moderately hungry and you should stop when you are satisfied. Eating slowly is important so that the body has time to readily evaluate your satiety. This is often difficult during tactical operations.

At the Scene

Optimal fitness is essential for all SWAT personnel, including TMPs. Not only will regular cardiovascular workouts increase your endurance in the field, but exercise is an excellent means of relieving job-related stress. Exercising as a unit can also encourage teamwork between SWAT and TEMS units.

Safety

It may be tempting to use artificial chemicals and hormones such as anabolic steroids in order to increase muscle mass. The short-term benefits of steroid use are overwhelmed by the negative effects of smaller testicles, erectile dysfunction, growth of male breasts, and psychological changes, as well as liver and cardiovascular damage. Women who use steroids suffer from liver damage, hair loss, acne, male pattern baldness, deeper voice, increased facial hair growth, and breast atrophy. Many of these effects are irreversible.

Personal Hygiene Considerations

Personal habits related to maintaining a healthy body are highly important, yet not everyone has learned how to do it correctly. It is important to go to the dentist at least every 6 months for teeth cleaning and inspection. Brush your teeth at least two times per day, if possible after every meal. Chew sugarless gum between meals to prevent cavities. Floss your teeth at least once a day to reduce plaque and food debris between teeth and keep gums healthy and strong. Dental infections are often painful and can lead to lost time from work.

Cleanliness of your body is also important. A daily shower plus scrubbing of your arms, legs, and torso will slough off dead, dry skin and help your skin stay healthy. It is important to wash your hands before meals, before preparing food, and after restroom use. After washing your hands, use a paper towel to dry them and then use that towel to turn off the water faucet and open the door, in order to keep your hands as clean as possible.

When sneezing or coughing in order to avoid spreading germs, it is better to cough into the crook of your elbow while turning away from nearby people. If you use a tissue or handkerchief, wash your hands soon after or use antibacterial lotion or wipes. Never eat any food with your bare hands unless you have washed and cleansed them properly. Consider keeping several alcohol-based hand wipe mini-towels with you at all times in order to cleanse your hands and work surfaces and thus kill any germs before they cause you illness. This includes using the alcohol-based towels after using the serving spoons in a buffet food line. Use common sense to take good care of your body. Avoiding germs is a key essential of staying healthy.

Although the incidence of serious disease and illness is fairly rare for young, healthy persons, it is very important to establish and maintain annual attendance at a primary care physician's office. In addition, women should see an OB/GYN physician on an annual basis for important routine tests and exams. Depending upon family and personal history, there may be routine diagnostic medical testing that is indicated for those in their 30s, 40s, and older. Everyone dreads being told bad news by a doctor, and some are simply afraid of needles and shots and thus refrain from routine visits. However, being successful in the tactical environment means that you have to keep your body healthy and this requires preventive yearly physicals.

Sleeping Habits

Being alert is of the utmost importance. The major determinants of alertness include the total sleep time the night before, the quality of sleep, and a regular sleep and work schedule. The healthy habits of exercise and proper eating are important factors in obtaining a period of quality and rejuvenating sleep. Maintaining regular meals during the waking period aids in general mental alertness and aids in sleep. Avoid caffeine and alcohol within 6 to 8 hours of bedtime.

Try to develop and practice a regular sleep ritual. If you find that you cannot fall asleep in 30 minutes, then arise and perform an activity conducive to sleep such as watching television or reading. Carefully plan and make it a high priority to allow your body adequate, restful sleep, especially taking into consideration the challenges of shift work. Sleep scheduling considerations include shift rotation and power napping.

Shift Work

Shift work is common in emergency medical services and law enforcement because the work hours of public safety are 24 hours a day, 7 days a week, and 365 days a year. Continuous shift coverage is required to serve our communities around the clock. Shift workers have a rotating schedule of working day, evening, and night shifts over a variable period of time **Figure 2-5**. Shift workers with shifts that rotate in less than 3-week cycles sleep an average of only 5 hours. This is not enough sleep for the body to function properly and leads to chronic sleep deprivation.

Chronic sleep deprivation may be one factor explaining why the average life span of shift workers is shortened by 5 years and may be as damaging as smoking a pack of cigarettes a day. Shift workers also have eight times the risk of developing stomach ulcers. Mood swings and depression are up to 15 times more likely. In addition,

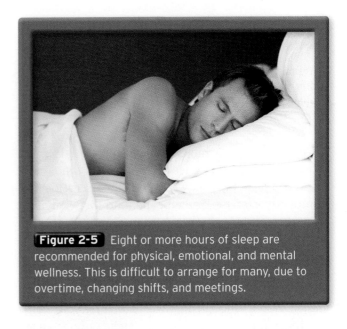

Figure 2-5 Eight or more hours of sleep are recommended for physical, emotional, and mental wellness. This is difficult to arrange for many, due to overtime, changing shifts, and meetings.

higher rates of alcohol abuse, high blood pressure, divorce, decreased fertility in women, and work-related accidents are seen in rotating shift workers. The good news is that knowledge and proactive measures can improve the health and lives of shift workers greatly. If the shift rotation cycle is longer than 3 weeks, the extra time allows the shift worker's body a chance to adjust to a new schedule.

Anchor sleep is a tool that can assist shift workers in obtaining 8 hours of sleep and maintaining a consistent schedule for the body. **Anchor sleep** is a scheduled period of rest, at least 4 hours in length, that is consistently maintained. For example, if you are on the third shift (night shift) from 10:00 PM to 7:00 AM, the anchor sleep period could be from 8:00 AM to 12:00 PM.

Safety

Mental performance varies with the time of day. Most performance curves can be brought into line with the 24-hour body temperature curves. Those who like to go to bed and rise early to accomplish tasks (morning people) have their temperature peak usually before noon. People who like to complete tasks at night and sleep late into the morning (evening people), experience their temperature peak later in the day. A relationship exists between speed, accuracy, reaction time, and body temperature. People generally do their best at times when their temperature is highest, usually in the middle of the wakeful period, with poorer performance earlier or later in their personal day.

Safety

Those working evening (second shift) or night shifts (third shift) should try to maintain the same sleep period all week, even during nights off, to prevent disruption of the biological clock. Many unfortunately ignore this reality because it too often will interfere with daytime social and family functions. A compromise is to at least arrange your sleep schedule to allow for a consistent block of 4-hour anchor sleep each day.

On work nights, the full 8 hours of sleep may be from 8:00 AM to 4:00 PM. On days off, sleep could occur from 4:00 AM to 12:00 PM, thus leaving more free time during the day. The body's schedule is anchored by dedicating the same 4 hours each day to sleep while allowing greater flexibility for the remaining required 4 hours of sleep. Most people have family responsibilities, friends, hobbies, and other commitments during the day. As a result, sleeping until noon is preferable to sleeping through later daytime hours.

Power Naps

A short period of sleep, a nap, is good for your mind and body. Napping is thought by most experts to be useful in promoting mental alertness. However, there are right and wrong ways to nap. If you take a nap, wake up at least 20 minutes before starting your shift to eliminate sleep inertia. Incorporating 30- to 45-minute power naps into your daily schedule can be helpful for remaining alert on the job. However, napping for longer than 2 hours can negatively impact sleep the following night and should be avoided.

If you work a double shift or have an extended SWAT callout on top of a long shift, then this may lead to a very long day with considerable **sleep deficit**. A sleep deficit occurs when several days go by with a person only getting 4 to 6 hours of sleep per night. This leads to increased irritability and moodiness, short temper, difficulty thinking, slowed reaction time, difficulty with memory, and other issues. Chronic sleep deprivation due to a sleep deficit is a real phenomenon that can lead to fatigue and negative effects. The sleep deficit can be partially reversed if you are able to sleep for 12 or more hours straight.

Exposure to Light

In a 1964 study by Wilse B. Webb and Harlow Ades, shift workers who worked under exposure to bright, daylight-type, 1,000-lux ambient light were significantly more alert and exhibited better cognitive performance during their 8-hour shift than those operating in a low-light environment. At the end of the night shift, try to avoid bright light before daytime sleep. Upon awakening after a solid 8 hours of sleep, try to spend 1 to 2 hours outside in bright sunlight or use bright lamps to increase ambient light.

Stress Management

A career in public safety is stressful. The baseline stress level from daily activities is high. Understanding the causes of stress and knowing how to deal with them are critical to job performance, health, and interpersonal relationships. To prevent stress from affecting your life negatively, you need to understand what stress is, its physiologic effects, what you can do to minimize these effects, and how to deal with stress on an emotional level.

Stress is the impact of stressors on your physical and mental well-being. Stressors include emotional, physical, and environmental situations or conditions that may cause a variety of physiologic, physical, and psychological responses. The body's response to stress begins with an alarm response, followed by a stage of reaction and resistance, and then recovery or, if the stress is prolonged, exhaustion.

Stress can have physical symptoms such as fatigue, changes in appetite, gastrointestinal problems, or headaches. It may cause insomnia, irritability, inability to concentrate, and hyperactivity. Additionally, it may present with psychological reactions such as fear, depression, guilt, oversensitivity, anger, irritability, and frustration. Often, today's fast-paced lifestyles compound these effects by not allowing a person to rest and recover after periods of stress. Prolonged or excessive stress has been proven to be a strong contributor to heart disease, hypertension, cancer, alcoholism, and depression.

There are many methods of handling stress. Some are positive and healthy; others are harmful and destructive. The term "stress management" refers to the tactics that have been shown to alleviate or eliminate stress reactions. Downtime, personal beliefs, hobbies, and personal relationships are all positive tools in managing stress.

Downtime

Taking time for personal reflection, time to be alone and think about and reflect on a day's events, is important for nearly all humans. This allows time to sort through things, to decide the pros and cons of decisions that need to be made, and to clarify past events and take time to make plans for the future. Arrange for a "cave room" or other private space and time to be alone to reflect on your life and events. Despite the incredible demands of the job, it is important to set aside time for personal reflection.

Spirituality

Spirituality is a powerful factor that plays a prominent role in the lives of many public safety professionals. Facing the many tragedies and difficult situations encountered by public safety professionals can be eased by spiritual beliefs. Many law enforcement officers, EMS providers, and fire fighters describe a rich sense of their own spirituality that keeps their lives in proper perspective, including their views of mortality.

Hobbies and Interests

Another area of importance that will help maintain a balanced lifestyle is taking time to seek some non-work-related hobbies and interests. Whether it is stamp collecting, woodworking in a shop, rebuilding an old sports car, or going bowling with friends, it is important to develop something fun and enjoyable to do that is away from and not related to work. These things will all increase the variety and enjoyment of life. Set time aside for downtime. Some choose to go hunting in the woods, others sit in front of a TV and watch sports, and others go for a long hike or jog alone **Figure 2-6** .

Maintenance of Lasting Personal Relationships

Personal relationships are essential for wellness **Figure 2-7** . We are all human and need a certain amount of closeness with others. We also have a need to feel accepted. A healthy life is characterized by enduring relationships of personal significance. These relationships nurture us, but at the same time they also require that we afford ourselves time to maintain them. Relationships should be a high priority on your list of goals.

For many, one of the most important relationships is with a spouse or partner. The impact of the stress of the job on a spouse or significant other can be great. Often relationship problems involve conflicting communication styles, misperceptions of problems, and differing needs for intimacy. Spending at least 15 minutes (or longer) each day discussing feelings and emotions with your significant other is an important part of a healthy relationship. Frequent discussions should take place regarding the demands of family life, work, and the impact of rotating shifts. Shift work interferes with evenings, weekends, and holidays and often requires silence and darkness during the day for sleep. This is difficult to explain to young children. The disruption of sleep can cause mood swings and chronic fatigue.

Unpleasant work situations may spill over into interactions at home. Family members may fear that their loved one will be injured or even killed at work by violence and thus worry constantly. It is important to take steps to reassure family members that although the job does have risks, the statistical chance of being killed at work is actually quite low. If family members are worried about their own security, then steps can be taken to increase family safety and provide reassurance.

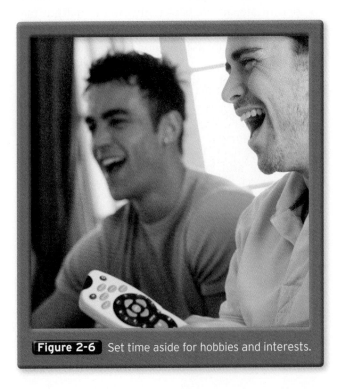

Figure 2-6 Set time aside for hobbies and interests.

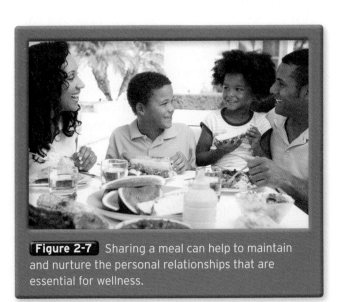

Figure 2-7 Sharing a meal can help to maintain and nurture the personal relationships that are essential for wellness.

A wise person will choose to have friends who are associated with work, as well as selecting friends who are outside of work. This may be difficult for emergency care providers and law enforcement officers due to the nature of their work and confidentiality issues. Often the brothers and sisters of public safety find themselves to be somewhat of an isolated society, and thus mainly seem to gather in groups with each other. That being said, it is still a choice to branch out of the circle of public safety and seek out quality friends who are in other careers.

Critical Incident Stress Management

TEMS and SWAT units routinely operate under circumstances that exceed the demands of the typical workplace. A **critical incident** is any situation faced by an emergency services worker that generates an unusually strong internal and/or external emotional response that overwhelms the ability to cope with the experience, either at the scene or later. Depending on the individual, a critical incident may provoke minimal or no reaction from the involved person. For others, it may cause a major emotional upheaval, having lasting negative effects.

An atypical threat level and the presence of imminent danger make critical incidents emotionally loaded and highly unpleasant events to take part in or observe. The duration of such an incident may last only a few seconds (eg, a shooting), or it can extend for several hours or days (eg, a tactical or rescue operation). Critical incidents include the following examples:

- The serious injury or death of a law enforcement officer or other public safety professional, in the line of duty or off-duty
- The unintentional injury or death of a bystander during an emergency services operation
- Multiple deaths or serious injuries due to disaster, a large car wreck scene, or an active-shooter scenario
- Serious injury or death of a child, infant, newborn, unborn child, or pregnant female
- Any situation that attracts an unusual amount of attention from the media; this might be a situation where accusations of wrongdoing arise from people in the community
- Any loss of life after extraordinary and/or prolonged search-and-rescue efforts
- Any situation that causes an intense emotional response beyond the normal coping mechanisms

of emergency services workers; some feelings that are particularly difficult to deal with include powerlessness, helplessness, and hopelessness

Critical Incident Stress Management Team

Throughout the United States, trained **critical incident stress management (CISM)** teams of peers and mental health professionals may provide counseling resources in assisting emergency medical personnel, fire fighters, and law enforcement officers in coping with stressful experiences. CISM teams are specially trained in the provision of preincident education, specialty briefings, on-scene support, defusing following a critical incident, demobilization of responders at the incident scene, formal post-incident debriefing meetings, one-on-one critical incident debriefings, and follow-up stress management services. Their goal is to allow a process to occur that will hopefully help the emergency services personnel to recover from the emotionally disturbing incident and continue to lead a productive career instead of being harmed and disabled mentally.

Statistically, 95% of SWAT unit callouts are resolved without any serious injuries or death. However, 5% of incidents do result in death or serious injury to either the perpetrators or law enforcement. This increases the risks for serious psychological trauma among SWAT and TEMS units. Fortunately, less than 5% of emergency services personnel will develop long-term **post-traumatic stress disorder (PTSD)**.

Law enforcement and EMS agencies should have established protocols and procedures for initiating the CISM process. You may be able to contact a CISM team directly by calling telephone directory assistance in your area and asking for CISM. CISM teams may also be requested through command staff and unit leaders. The International Critical Incident Stress Foundation, Inc is a company dedicated to limiting the effects of stress on emergency services providers through education and support services. For more information, go to the foundation's website at *www.icisf.org*.

There are certain types of emergencies that may have a serious effect on SWAT personnel. Any of these personnel or other emergency services workers who are involved in an unusually stressful incident are encouraged to get counseling. As a TMP, you should watch for SWAT officers who were closely involved or affected by the incident and strongly encourage those individuals to become involved with CISM. It is best if the SWAT officer knows about the services

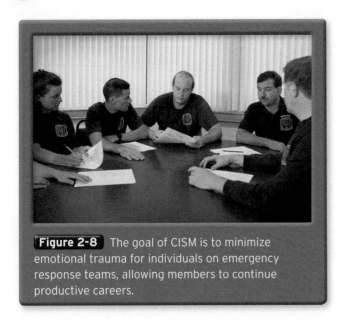

Figure 2-8 The goal of CISM is to minimize emotional trauma for individuals on emergency response teams, allowing members to continue productive careers.

and advantages of CISM ahead of time, and if needed, the SWAT officer can and should choose to attend voluntarily. However, some choose to not attend for a variety of reasons ("I don't need it," "No time," "I'm fine," etc). Ideally, the law enforcement agency will have the wisdom, authority, and protocols for administrative officers to order those SWAT officers affected to attend these debriefings and counseling sessions for callouts where significant issues or poor outcomes occurred **Figure 2-8**. The SWAT unit should be familiar with the CISM resources available to them in their area prior to any need for such services.

Debriefings are usually held within 24 to 72 hours after a major incident. The CISM coordinator for the region should be contacted after discussion with law enforcement agency leaders, and the CISM sessions should be efficiently and rapidly scheduled to allow maximal benefit within the 72-hour window. There are several types of CISM counseling sessions that can be utilized depending upon the situation and the personnel involved in the incident.

Debriefings

There are several types of debriefings that a SWAT officer may participate in. Typically a SWAT unit will arrange for a normal **post-incident analysis**. This type of debriefing is a routine critique following an incident

when information surrounding the response is reviewed and discussed in an effort to learn lessons to improve future responses. The debriefing for critical incidents is a separate, additional meeting.

A **critical incident stress debriefing (CISD)** is a confidential peer group discussion in which specially trained teams work with emergency personnel who have been involved in traumatic calls or other painful incidents. CISDs usually occur within 24 to 72 hours of the incident. All personnel who were involved in the incident, including TMPs, are invited to attend. Strict confidentiality is expected of all who participate. These debriefing sessions help to reduce stress and teach participants how to control the normal reactions to critical incidents. These debriefings can be a group setting with the entire unit, part of the unit, or with a single person. These are typically semistructured conversations with the purpose of informing the group about the details of what happened, the individual reactions to the incident, and allow an opportunity for the individual to talk about it. This is an effective strategy that is aimed to improve the mental health of the involved personnel and decrease the negative effects of the traumatic situation that the unit was exposed to.

Defusing Sessions

The defusing session is a shortened version of a CISD and is done as early as possible after the incident. It is a small group process instituted after any event powerful enough to trigger stress reactions. Proper use of defusing can either eliminate the need for a full debriefing or enhance the debriefing if one is necessary. A defusing renders something harmless before it can do damage.

Follow-up Stress Management Services

The CISM team leaders who met with the SWAT unit will gather the facts and discuss the conversations that occurred during the debriefing and other meetings. They will use their training and expertise to decide how best to support the team in the near future and may suggest additional meetings and further counseling for select tactical officers or TMPs who seemed to be especially in need of future support. They will suggest other follow-up services depending upon the predicted need.

At some point in time, a person in emotional distress may realize he or she needs assistance. There are multiple symptoms that should prompt SWAT officers, TMPs, or other emergency services professionals to seek professional counseling and assistance. These symptoms include intense feelings of social discomfort, suicidal thoughts or plans, self-destructive acting out (alcohol binges, inappropriate sexual behavior, aggressive behavior, or substance abuse), intense family conflict, a feeling of losing control over impulses, and significant sleep disturbance.

The decision to "get help" is a very hard step to take. For public safety professionals who are used to always taking charge and who are expected to "have their act together," seeking help is highly unnatural and is something that many find difficult. If they are fortunate enough, they will take the steps and seek the assistance and counseling that is needed. Sometimes conditions may deteriorate to the point where a commanding officer will need to become involved and order the professional to get appropriate help. Other times it may be a friend or respected coworker who notices something different and makes the suggestion to seek help. Unfortunately, too many times the behavior changes go unnoticed or coworkers are too busy or hesitant to stop and help, and eventually things deteriorate until job performance is affected. To avoid this:

- **Recognize that there is a problem.** This may be determined by the individual or by friends, or through contact with personnel within the department or agency. Make a decision to act on it.
- **Contact and meet with available, respected, and confidential resources.** This may be a psychologist or mental health worker who is associated with the law enforcement agency or it may be a resource independent of the employer.
- **Research helpful sources of information for dealing with the situation.** Go to your local library, or search the Internet for further information on sources of additional assistance, such as the International Critical Incident Stress Foundation. The website www.policepsych.com is another resource offering a wide range of articles and supportive information.

Patient Confidentiality

TEMS units must take proactive steps to ensure the confidentiality of patient information. TEMS units have access to important and personal information. Steps must be taken to safeguard medical information as effectively as possible. While the TEMS may not be strictly bound by the **Health Insurance Portability and Accountability Act (HIPAA)**, the act does provide guidance on the types of information that should be kept in confidence (eg, regarding patient diagnosis, medical care, and prognosis).

Generally, the patient's personal information should only be shared with those medical providers who have a direct responsibility for a patient's medical care. However, there are circumstances under which patient confidentiality may be violated by TEMS units. If done properly, the sharing of select patient information will be beneficial by possibly preventing further harm by criminal suspects. TEMS leaders should outline the policy for breach of patient confidentiality during routine training, so that everyone is aware of how and when it should be done. In addition, make sure you are aware of the policies and procedures governing your particular agency.

During patient confidentiality training, several circumstances may be discussed. One exception allowing for a breach in patient confidentiality might be if a suspect or SWAT officer's medical situation poses a threat to other team members or bystanders. Another exception could occur in situations where the SWAT officer is suffering from a mental condition or physical injury that may potentially interfere with that SWAT officer's performance. All medical issues that have the potential to compromise a SWAT officer's performance should be reported as soon as possible to the appropriate leadership of the tactical unit.

To ensure that you are protecting the patient's confidentiality, do not give any information to anyone other than those directly involved in the care of the patient. Do not share confidential patient information with the patient's relatives or friends. Do not discuss the patient or the incident with your family or friends. Information discussed during SWAT unit debriefings, charts related to specific

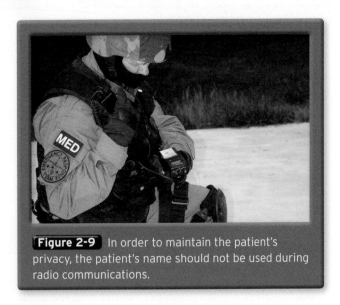

Figure 2-9 In order to maintain the patient's privacy, the patient's name should not be used during radio communications.

cases, and patient case reviews is considered private and confidential.

Radio Reporting

While communicating by radio during a response, the patient's name should not be used **Figure 2-9**. This is important to remember, as home radio scanners are able to pick up transmissions from TMP radio communications. In major cities there are literally thousands of citizens who listen in on police, EMS, and fire radio frequencies. If the patient's name must be used in communications, then attempts should be reasonably made to use cellular phone or landline communications, which are more secure.

Ready for Review

- By maintaining a healthy lifestyle through diet, exercise, and proper sleep habits, you can stay healthy both mentally and physically.

- Take an active role in maintaining low stress levels through downtime, personal beliefs, hobbies, and personal relationships.

- CISM is designed to provide the SWAT and TEMS units with a process and counseling whereby stressful critical incidents can be discussed and dealt with in a helpful and therapeutic manner.

- Tactical medical providers can assist with many mental health–related issues when providing support for SWAT units.

Vital Vocabulary

anchor sleep A specific period of time at least 4 hours long, during which a responder sleeps every day, both on-duty and off-duty, while on a particular shift rotation.

critical incident Any situation faced by an emergency services worker that generates an unusually strong emotional response (internal and/or external), which overwhelms the ability to cope with the experience, either at the scene or later.

critical incident stress debriefing (CISD) A confidential peer group discussion in which specially trained teams work with emergency personnel who have been involved in traumatic calls or other painful incidents; CISDs usually occur within 24 to 72 hours of the incident.

critical incident stress management (CISM) A process that confronts the responses to critical incidents and defuses them, directing the emergency services personnel toward physical and emotional equilibrium.

Health Insurance Portability and Accountability Act (HIPAA) Federal legislation passed in 1996. Its main effect in EMS is in limiting availability of patients' health care information and penalizing violations of patient privacy.

post-incident analysis A routine critique following an incident when information surrounding the response is reviewed and discussed in an effort to learn lessons to improve future responses.

post-traumatic stress disorder (PTSD) A delayed stress reaction to a prior incident. This delayed reaction is often the result of one or more unresolved issues concerning the incident, which if untreated, can lead to short-term and long-term difficulties with job performance and family life.

sleep deficit The result of several days going by with a responder only getting 4 to 6 hours of sleep per night. Sleep deficit leads to decreased performance and increased risks of multiple hazards such as falling asleep at the wheel while driving, memory deficits, increased risks of infections and poor health, and sleep disturbances.

SWAT Unit Essentials

OBJECTIVES

- Describe the primary mission of the Special Weapons and Tactics (SWAT) unit.

- Name the various types of missions and indications for SWAT unit callouts.

- Describe forcible entry tools used by SWAT units.

- Describe less-lethal weapons used by SWAT units.

- Describe close-range impact weapons used by SWAT units.

- Describe electronic control devices (ECDs) used by SWAT units.

- Describe compressed-air technology used by SWAT units.

- Describe the types of extended-range impact projectiles used by SWAT units.

- Describe noise-flash distraction devices (NFDDs) used by SWAT units.

- Describe the primary types of chemical and smoke agents used by SWAT units.

Introduction

A SWAT unit is composed of highly trained, athletic law enforcement officers **Figure 3-1**. SWAT officers are able to apply their expertise to very adeptly assume a number of different emergency response duties. The SWAT unit is equipped with sophisticated equipment and weapons, and their training allows them to assume full control of specific high-risk situations that must be dealt with and resolved by civilian law enforcement agencies.

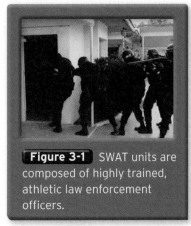

Figure 3-1 SWAT units are composed of highly trained, athletic law enforcement officers.

These tactical situations are usually considered too complicated or too high-risk for non-SWAT patrol police officers and sheriff's deputies. A SWAT unit is organized to function as both a crisis-intervention and rescue unit. Positions within the unit are designated to give SWAT units the ability to conduct negotiations as well as assault operations.

Mission Goals

A SWAT unit's primary mission is to plan and execute high-risk law enforcement operations that include, but are not limited to, high-risk warrant service, felony arrests, barricaded suspects and subjects, hostage rescue, **dignitary protection**, and terrorist incidents. Prospective SWAT officers usually are required to have at least 2 or more years of full-time law enforcement experience and complete a screening process before attending a recognized basic tactical operations course.

The goal of a SWAT unit is to accomplish its mission without needless injury or death resulting from the unit's intervention. Most of the time, the purpose of the mission is to end the threat posed by a criminal(s) and to arrest the criminal(s) without anyone being harmed. The main focus during all SWAT unit interventions is to preserve the life and safety of victims, bystanders, hostages, and team members. SWAT units are able to accomplish this. In fact, 95% of SWAT callout incidents are resolved peacefully, without any injuries to suspects, bystanders, or SWAT officers.

Types of Incidents Requiring Activation

A SWAT unit is primarily activated to assist with a high-risk incident or arrest-warrant service for which the threat is felt to be too high for typical patrol officers or detectives to resolve. Additional types of incidents include:

- **High-risk search warrants**. These include searches for drugs, weapons, or other hazardous items.
- **High-risk arrest warrants**. These include arrest warrants for felony suspects likely to engage in a gun battle or put up other significant resistance when arrested.
- **Armed, dangerous, criminal, barricaded suspects**. According to the Anne Arundel County (Maryland) Police Department, these are criminal suspects who have taken a position in a physical location, most often a structure or vehicle, fortified or not, that does not allow immediate police access and who are refusing police orders to exit. Barricaded suspects may be known to be armed, thought to be armed, have access to weapons in the location, or be in an unknown weapons status.
- **Barricaded subjects**. According to the Anne Arundel County Police Department, these subjects are persons who are not suspected of committing a crime, but are the focus of a legitimate law enforcement intervention effort, most often involving threats of suicide and/or witnessed self-destructive behavior. These situations most often

involve persons with mental illness. Many do not possess weapons, but it is uncertain who does, and therefore all are potentially extremely dangerous for responding SWAT units and TEMS units.

- **Hostage situations**. These occur when a suspect holds innocent bystanders captive to act as a point of leverage against law enforcement—for example, a bank robbery where the suspects force five employees and two customers into the bank vault and hold them captive until authorities have "guaranteed" that their demands will be met.
- **Suicidal individual(s) with explosives or guns**. It is unfortunate but fairly common for emotionally disturbed persons to threaten suicide with a firearm or explosive and then point a gun at law enforcement or threaten to detonate an explosive, thus requiring an appropriate use-of-force response by law enforcement.
- **Active-shooter scenarios**. These include office, workplace, or school shootings, where a suspect is actively shooting innocent bystanders with a firearm, which requires immediate response by law enforcement.
- **Riots or other civil disturbances**. Riots occur when a large crowd of people gather to protest a certain act or demonstrate for or against a cause, resulting in a civil disturbance, such as the 1992 riots in Los Angeles after the Rodney King verdict **Figure 3-2** .
- **Mass gatherings**. Political conventions, sports events, or demonstrations are considered to be

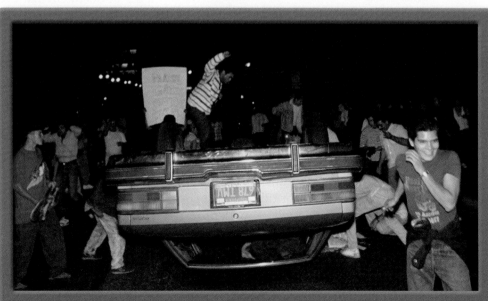

Figure 3-2 The civil unrest caused by riots calls for the presence of SWAT officers to help restore order.

mass gatherings and have potential for a loss of civility and control.

- **Dignitary protection and/or executive protection.** A SWAT unit may provide motorcade and other protection of very important people (VIPs), such as elected officials (eg, president of the United States, prime ministers), wealthy business executives, well-known entertainers, and other wealthy individuals.

- **Clandestine laboratory raids.** Methamphetamine (meth) labs continue to increase in parts of the country. These illegal labs contain raw materials and toxic by-products that are carcinogenic.

- **Escaped-convict searches.** Prisoners may escape from incarceration or from law enforcement custody. These searches may take place in urban or remote wooded environments, and are often considered very high risk due to the fugitive criminal(s) at large.

- **Bomb threats.** These include packages left in a crowded location that may potentially be a bomb, thus requiring neutralization by a police bomb squad; improvised explosive devices (IEDs); or a search of a building after a phoned-in bomb threat.

- **National security incidents.** These include a direct threat on federal or state officials; release of chemical, biological, or nuclear agents; or simultaneous attacks by multiple terrorists.

- **Terrorist-initiated events.** Including a single active shooting or multiple attackers who may take hostages with the intent of exploding bombs and using machine guns to kill as many as possible at an opportune time when the press are present to document and spread the news of the terrorists' attacks.

Weapons and Tools

To ensure safety against threats posed by the high-risk tactical environment, most SWAT units carry pistols, long guns (eg, carbines, shotguns, or rifles), and less-lethal weapons (eg, impact weapons, shotgun beanbag-type rounds, TASERs). Most SWAT officers also carry at least one knife and some will carry backup weapons. Additionally, chemical munitions are useful and may be deployed to safely resolve a critical situation.

You must become and remain familiar with your unit's firearms and weapons systems, and acquire the ability to render them safe. Commonly used by the entry team is the M-4 style carbine-length M-16/AR-15 rifle that fires the .223-caliber (cal)/5.56-mm NATO cartridge, 40 S+W, and 9-mm. Another commonly used

weapon is the Heckler and Koch MP-5 submachine 9-mm gun. Marksmen use bolt-action or semiautomatic rifles chambered in .223 cal, .308 cal, and others. Many SWAT units utilize four to six different types of long guns and eight to twelve different types of pistols. At a minimum, you should be familiar with how to make these weapons "safe" by manipulating the safety and magazine release, and ideally know how to fire these weapons under duress should the need arise. This is especially true if you are not a law enforcement officer and have had no formal law enforcement education. Chapter 5, "Firearm Safety and Marksmanship," covers securing a firearm safely in detail.

Forcible Entry Tools

Different SWAT units carry a variety of forcible entry tools, protective gear, and surveillance tools **Figure 3-3** . A detailed review of all these devices is not listed in this textbook due to operational security concerns but, over time, you will learn about and further understand the wide variety of tools and tactics utilized to accomplish the mission. These devices are valuable tools; however, these tools can also cause injuries to the SWAT officers and suspects. The assessment and treatment of these injuries is discussed in Section 2 of this book, "Assessment and Management of Injuries."

Forcible entry tools may vary from simple heavy metal rams to breach a door, shotgun powdered metal ammunition rounds to shoot out locks and hinges, or explosive breaching devices. Power tools, such as a gas-powered circular breaching saw, can be used. If necessary, a cutting torch can be used to cut through and melt metal in order to breach an entryway **Figure 3-4** .

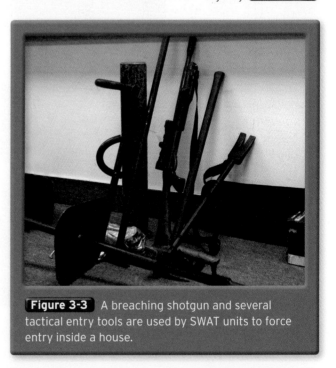

Figure 3-3 A breaching shotgun and several tactical entry tools are used by SWAT units to force entry inside a house.

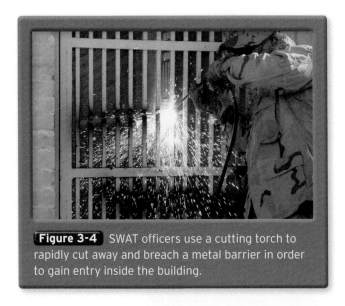

Figure 3-4 SWAT officers use a cutting torch to rapidly cut away and breach a metal barrier in order to gain entry inside the building.

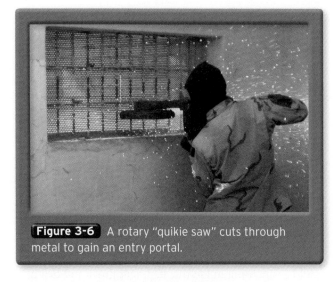

Figure 3-6 A rotary "quikie saw" cuts through metal to gain an entry portal.

Door rams use weight and force to breach a door. These heavy tools can also produce musculoskeletal strain injuries when used improperly **Figure 3-5**. Shotgun breaching rounds have the propensity to produce minor missile wounds along with eye injuries,

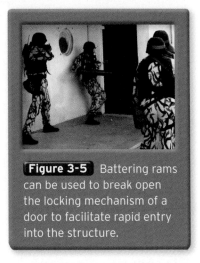

Figure 3-5 Battering rams can be used to break open the locking mechanism of a door to facilitate rapid entry into the structure.

making eye protection essential. Explosive breaching can produce shrapnel-type injuries and rare blast injures. Hot metal from rotary "quickie saws" can cause burns and flying sparks, and high-speed particles can cause ocular injury **Figure 3-6**. Eye and ear protection is essential when these types of breachings are used.

Ground-level windows are often opened using a large metal tool, and the glass is broken and the rim of remaining glass is raked away to make the entry safer when gaining access. This is referred to as "break and rake." Lacerations and eye injuries may result from this, but use of full-arm leather welding gloves and eye protection helps protect the SWAT and TEMS units.

SWAT Explosive Breaching Considerations

SWAT unit entry teams may employ explosive materials for breaching (blasting to create an entry, gun port,

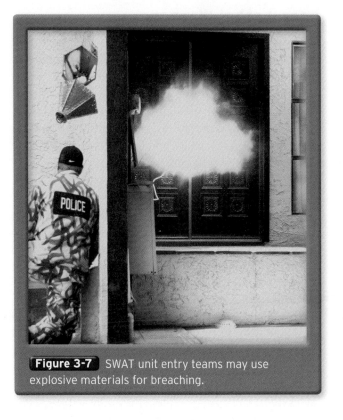

Figure 3-7 SWAT unit entry teams may use explosive materials for breaching.

or observation hole) so that the entry team can enter or visualize the interior of the building via a door or structural wall **Figure 3-7**. The use of explosives to open or breach a locked door or create a hole in a wall has the advantage of allowing SWAT officers to temporarily stun suspects, which allows time for the SWAT unit to rush inside to rescue hostages and quickly arrest or neutralize high-risk suspects.

The explosive devices include blasting caps, detonation cord (det-cord), various types of high explosives, and the use of a variety of metal or water-based devices that are used to strategically place explosives at the point of entry. A remote-control device (air, flash-tube, or electrical) is typically used to detonate the explosive at the exact time needed in order to maximize surprise and enhance the ability of the entry team to accomplish the mission successfully.

Injury can occur to nearby SWAT officers or to anyone who is too close to the explosive breach or entry. Blast injuries from explosive devices primarily affect air-filled structures, possibly causing ruptured ear drums, pulmonary contusions, and abdominal hemorrhage or perforation. They can also cause crush injuries, injuries from flying debris or fragments, burns, or eye injuries. They can also expose the individual to toxic inhalations. The explosives utilized by a modern SWAT unit are quite dangerous and could easily result in life-threatening injuries and death.

Less-Lethal Weapons

Less-lethal weapons are designed to incapacitate a person while limiting the exposure of SWAT officers to undesirable situations. During normal use, these types of weapons do not penetrate the body, with the exception of the small fish-hook-like probes of the TASER. Less-lethal weapons are increasingly used by law enforcement agencies, and improvements and new devices are continually produced. Initially utilized only by SWAT units to help resolve difficult situations, these devices are now routinely used by patrol officers as well.

It is standard for SWAT units to incorporate some type of less-lethal weapon option into their approach to resolving critical incidents. These weapons have saved the lives of many citizens and resulted in fewer lethal encounters and injuries to SWAT officers and suspects.

Without less-lethal weapon options, law enforcement officers would be forced to use more aggressive means of resolving critical incidents, such as deadly force with a firearm. The term "less-lethal" is used because although these weapons are designed to neutralize or control criminal suspects without significant harm, in rare circumstances the use of these devices may result in the death of the suspect.

You should be knowledgeable in the recognition and management of injuries that are caused by less-lethal weapons. All treatment should be preceded by a full patient assessment. Transportation to a hospital or alternate receiving facility should be done on a case-by-case basis. Chapter 17, "Ballistic, Blast, and Less-Lethal Weapons," discusses the assessment and treatment of these injuries in detail.

Close-Range Impact Weapons

The modern law enforcement officer maintains a variety of weapon options in order to assist with gaining compliance. The simplest impact weapon is the fist or heel of the hand, which can be used to strike the suspect. Elbow, knee, and head-butt strikes are also blows that may be used. Some law enforcement agencies continue to authorize lead-impregnated gloves, lead-filled leather sticks called *saps*, and other devices. When a law enforcement officer is carrying a handgun or backup weapon, there is never really an "unarmed" fight; however, the fight could turn into a lethal confrontation if the suspect grabs the weapon away from the law enforcement officer.

The most commonly carried impact weapon is the **expandable baton**, commonly known as the ASP (Armament Systems and Procedures). This device is carried on the duty belt and is usually arranged so the law enforcement officer can immediately access it with a simple, rapid flick of the wrist. This motion and sound will often cause suspects to stop what they are doing and begin obeying commands **Figure 3-8**.

There is also fairly common use of a simple wooden **nightstick**, and a more modern nightstick called the Monadnock Side Handle (PR-24), which is about 2-feet long with a handle positioned at a 90-degree angle to the stick, toward one end. There are many uses for this device. Proper training and certification are required before law enforcement officers or TMPs are allowed to carry and use these and other weapons. If you are permitted and choose to carry this weapon, you must learn the proper striking points and areas to *avoid,* including the head, neck, and groin. Impact weapons can be used in defense, to strike suspects, and as leverage when gaining compliance via holds and joint locks.

Electronic Control Devices (ECDs): The TASER® ECD

One of the more commonly used, less-lethal devices is the TASER, which uses a discreet electrical signal that overrides the command and control systems of

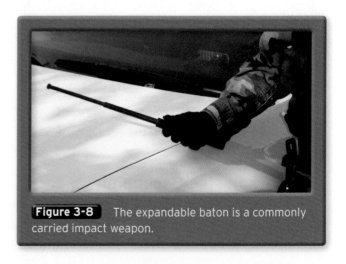

Figure 3-8   The expandable baton is a commonly carried impact weapon.

the body to impair muscular control by *neuromuscular incapacitation*. ECDs may be deployed by direct contact with the handheld electrode unit known as a drive-stun or as probes that are launched from a pistol-like device up to 35 feet away by compressed nitrogen. These probes attach to clothing or skin, and each remains attached to the TASER unit by insulated wire through which a low-amperage high-voltage electrical shock is conducted. TASER is the most commercially recognized brand of ECDs and is produced by TASER International. TASER ECDs deliver approximately 80 to 125 microcoulombs that last 5 seconds per cycle (one squeeze of the trigger automatically delivers a 5-second cycle). It stimulates motor nerves causing uncontrollable muscle contractions that inhibit the subject from being able to perform coordinated movement. While the effects can be painful, the system does not work on pain compliance and the suspect tends to fall forward to the ground **Figure 3-9**.

Compressed-Air Technology

The use of paintball or **compressed-air technology** has increased significantly over the past 20 years. Increasingly, SWAT units use .68 caliber paintballs and Simunitions—plastic bullets with paint-colored fluid that marks where the SWAT officers were struck—in force-on-force realistic tactical training. Recently, several manufacturers have designed ammunition that has applications for law enforcement. One such device is the "glass ball" which can be used to break windows and distract suspects who are barricaded inside a building.

Another less-lethal device is a plastic-coated .68 caliber projectile filled with either **oleoresin capsicum (OC)** (pepper spray) or the newer **pelargonyl vanillyamide (PAVA) capsaicin II**, both of which are very hot and irritating to mucous membranes, eyes, and skin. This is the same type of OC that law enforcement officers carry on their belts in canisters. Riot police, patrol, SWAT, and corrections officers can utilize these "pepperballs" to gain compliance and stop inappropriate behavior. They are fired from semiautomatic, high-pressure air launchers, similar to the common paintball systems used by citizen paintball markers or guns. The plastic sphere bursts upon impact, releasing the OC powder or liquid on and around the intended target, causing irritation of the eyes, nose, mouth, and hopefully forcing suspects to comply.

Extended-Range Impact Projectiles

Less-lethal projectiles are normally lead shot–filled bags, referred to as **shotgun beanbag rounds Figure 3-10**, or rubber or wooden projectiles. Most are launched from a shotgun or from a 39- or 40-mm, grenade-type launcher that is designed as an extended-range weapon. Initial beanbag rounds were typically squares of fabric with #9 lead shot sewn inside, but new and more accurate rounds look like a miniature sock filled with lead shot and a small cloth tail that stabilizes the device and leads to increased accuracy.

The rationale behind beanbag usage is that the firearm delivery affords standoff distance and is safer for the suspect than use of a conventional firearm. Beanbags carry a good deal of energy, but that energy is dispersed over a larger area, usually preventing serious penetrating injury. The impact produces pain and in most cases causes the suspect to comply without resistance. The manufacturers

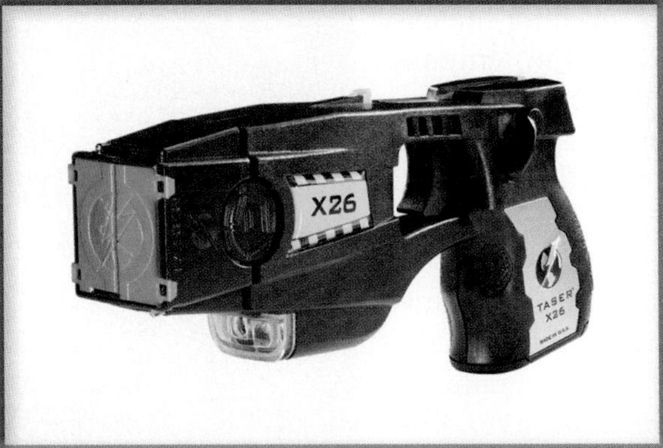

Figure 3-9 The TASER® ECD.
Source: TASER® X26™ photo courtesy of TASER International, Scottsdale, AZ-USA.

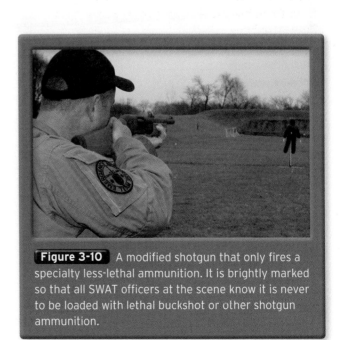

Figure 3-10 A modified shotgun that only fires a specialty less-lethal ammunition. It is brightly marked so that all SWAT officers at the scene know it is never to be loaded with lethal buckshot or other shotgun ammunition.

of beanbag–type rounds encourage shots that avoid the head, neck, and pelvis, and instead target the torso.

Noise-Flash Distraction Devices

Noise-flash distraction devices (NFDD)s use a flash powder charge to produce a bright flash and extremely loud explosion, which stuns, distracts, and disorients suspects. These are also sometimes called "flash-bangs" or flash-sound diversionary devices (FSDDs). It is incorrect to refer to these devices as "concussion grenades" as they do not cause concussions when used correctly. NFDDs are used to stun suspects for several seconds allowing more entry team members to safely enter the room to contain and deal with any threats **Figure 3-11**. The Defense Technology (Def-Tec) #25 is an example of a commonly used FSDD and produces approximately 1 million candela of light and 175 decibels of sound.

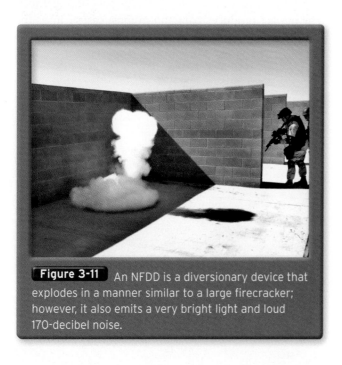

Figure 3-11 An NFDD is a diversionary device that explodes in a manner similar to a large firecracker; however, it also emits a very bright light and loud 170-decibel noise.

Less-Lethal Chemical Agents

Less-lethal chemical and/or gas munitions are commonly employed in the tactical environment. The purpose of chemical munitions is to incapacitate suspects in a less-lethal manner. They may be used in crowd control, for motivating barricaded subjects to surrender, to immobilize aggressive subjects, or for concealment (smoke). Chemical munitions may be delivered through multiple mechanisms, including handheld sprays or foggers to cover larger areas, grenades, paintball projectiles, 12-gauge shotgun rounds, or 39- or 40-mm projectiles.

Potential deflection of projectiles, wind direction, known health problems of suspects, and subsequent movement of individuals or crowds should all be considered prior to deployment of these munitions. If the criminal suspect is educated and well-prepared, he or she may take steps to limit chemical exposure and negate its effect, such as covering the face with wet towels, using a gas mask, etc. Lethal results may occur with chemical agents if toxic concentrations are reached or enough room oxygen is displaced. Common agents utilized include oleoresin capsicum, 2-chlorobenzalmalononitrile (CS), phenacyl chloride (CN), and hexachloroethane (HC).

Oleoresin capsicum (OC) spray is a derivative of cayenne pepper. It has been available since 1973 and is classified as an inflammatory agent. It is a tool that is not 100% reliable, but often is successful when used for stopping a physical attack or improving suspect compliance to commands. A small percentage of humans and dogs are not affected at all by OC spray. Also, some emotionally disturbed persons are essentially immune to it.

OC is standard issue to many law enforcement officers and is the most common chemical agent currently in use **Figure 3-12**. Its effects include immediate tearing, involuntary eyelid closing, airway swelling, mucus production, intense facial burning sensations, and possible loss of coordination. OC may have an increased effect on freshly shaved, fair-skinned, or sunburned individuals. The effects gradually diminish over the following 30 minutes,

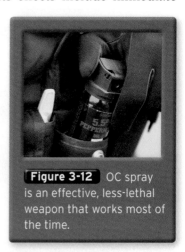

Figure 3-12 OC spray is an effective, less-lethal weapon that works most of the time.

and usually have no long-term effects. There is no lethal effect except in the extremely rare allergic reaction or in persons with severe asthma.

Some OC dispensers have a special marker dye incorporated that allows accurate identification of the suspect. Some have an alcohol base, and it is possible that the spray could result in a fire on the suspect's clothing and involved skin. Avoid alcohol-based OC spray whenever flames are nearby or if a TASER or other electronic device is used.

OC is delivered as a fogger, a liquid spray, or a foam. Because of its rapid action, OC may be inappropriate for crowd control as individuals may fall down to the ground rather than disperse. OC may be mixed with tear gas.

Phenacyl chloride (CN) tear gas is a type of tear gas that has an aerosol delivery and is used in grenades and projectiles. It causes nasal irritation, tearing, burning skin sensation, and involuntary eye closure. It is rarely used because of potential allergic reactions (1 in 1,000). **2-chlorobenzalmalononitrile (CS) tear gas** is a powerful tearing and/or irritant agent. It is a fine yellow powder that has a pungent, pepper-like odor. It causes immediate nasal irritation, tearing, involuntary eye closing, and profuse mucus production. Heavy salivation, chest tightness, and a sense of panic may occur.

Hexachloroethane (HC), also referred to as a **smoke grenade**, is a solid that may be chemically colored in a variety of ways. It smells like smoke and is used to provide cover **Figure 3-13**. Smoke grenades and other smoke agents may be used in a tactical environment to block the view of the suspect while an entry team approaches, for distraction, or other tactical uses. HC

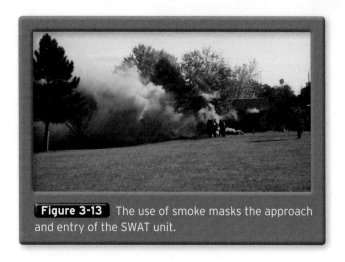

Figure 3-13 The use of smoke masks the approach and entry of the SWAT unit.

may also be deployed with other less-lethal chemical agents.

Smoke grenades and similar chemical weapons devices work by burning a solid ingredient, and may start fires or cause burns, as the normal dispersion method is by burning this solid within a grenade. These grenades become very hot and may disperse sparks or flames, which may result in fire. To avoid burns, SWAT officers should not handle the expended grenades while they are still hot. Inhalation of smoke from grenades, particularly military grenades, may produce pulmonary edema, a dangerous condition where fluid builds up in the lungs and can lead to heart failure.

The gases produced are acidic in nature. Avoid the inhalation of this smoke. Burning smoke grenades should never be used indoors due to their fire and inhalation hazards, and the fact that the smoke may displace oxygen.

Ready for Review

- A modern SWAT unit is composed of highly trained athletic law enforcement officers who are called out to respond to situations that are too complex or hazardous for law enforcement officers with only conventional training.

- The goal of any SWAT unit is to accomplish special operations missions without unnecessary loss of life or injury, and with the objective of maintaining the safety of the unit, hostages, bystanders, and victims at the incident. Over 95% of SWAT callout incidents are resolved peacefully, without injuries to suspects or officers.

- Types of missions and indications for SWAT callout include high-risk search and arrest warrants, barricaded suspects or subjects, hostage situations, suicidal suspects, active-shooter scenarios, riots, mass gatherings, dignitary protection, motorcade protection, clandestine laboratory raids, escaped-convict searches, bomb threats, national security incidents, terrorist-initiated events, and other critical incidents.

- Forcible entry tools, protective gear, and surveillance tools allow SWAT units to rapidly breach barriers to gain entry into a building or structure.

- Less-lethal weapons are designed to incapacitate a person while limiting the exposure of SWAT officers to undesirable situations.

- The sap, ASP, PR-24, and simple wooden nightstick are close-range impact weapons used to gain compliance.

- Electronic control devices, such as the TASER, use high-voltage electrical energy to interrupt voluntary muscular control.

- Compressed-air technology incorporates less-lethal ammunition such as "glass balls" to cause distractions and chemical irritants such as "pepper spray" with semiautomatic, high-pressure air launchers.

- Extended-range impact projectiles are less-lethal projectiles, such as lead shot–filled bags, that are launched from a shotgun or grenade-type launcher.

- Flash-sound diversionary devices (FSDDs) are capable of a loud, 170-decibel blast and a brilliant white flash that serves to distract and confuse suspects.

- Less-lethal chemical agents are irritants used to temporarily incapacitate crowds or suspects. These chemicals can cause serious side effects.

- Smoke agents are used to cover and conceal. These agents can cause burns as well as inhalation injuries.

Vital Vocabulary

2-chlorobenzalmalononitrile (CS) tear gas A tearing and/or irritant chemical agent; a fine yellow powder that has a pungent, pepper-like odor.

barricaded subjects People who are not suspected of committing a crime but are the focus of a legitimate police intervention effort, most often involving threats of suicide and/or self-destructive behavior involving the mentally ill.

barricaded suspects Criminal suspects who have taken a position in a physical location, most often a structure or vehicle, fortified or not, that does not allow immediate police access and who are refusing police orders to exit; may be known to be armed, thought to be armed, have access to weapons in the location, or be in an unknown weapons status.

compressed-air technology Use of a paintball marker firearm (.68-caliber) to shoot small projectiles of variable contents, but most involve use of oleoresin capsicum (OC), which is a powder or liquid irritant that will cause suspects to stop their actions and retreat.

dignitary protection Providing personal protective services to very important persons (VIPs).

expandable baton Commonly known as the ASP; a less-lethal, handheld device.

less-lethal weapons Weapons designed to incapacitate a person while limiting the exposure of officers to undesirable situations. During normal use, these types of weapons do not penetrate the body, with the exception of small, TASER fish-hook-like probes.

nightstick A plastic or wood baton or stick that is used by law enforcement to force the compliance of a suspect.

noise-flash distraction devices (NFDDs) Devices that use a flash powder charge to produce a bright flash and extremely loud explosion to stun, distract, and disorient suspects, allowing entry team members to safely enter the room to contain and deal with any threats; sometimes called "flash-bangs" or flash-sound diversionary devices (FSDDs).

oleoresin capsicum (OC) spray A derivative of cayenne pepper; classified as an inflammatory agent. It is used to force compliance with instructions.

pelargonyl vanillyamide (PAVA) capsaicin II A powder irritant used by law enforcement to force compliance with instructions.

phenacyl chloride (CN) tear gas A type of tear gas that is used in grenades and projectiles for aerosol delivery. It is reliable and offers many advantages when faced with a noncompliant suspect(s).

shotgun beanbag rounds Small sacks of lead pellets designed to be shot at noncompliant suspects, causing pain and bruising, enabling the law enforcement officers to arrest and manage a difficult situation.

smoke grenade A device that emits hexachloroethane (HC), which is a solid that may be chemically colored in a variety of ways. It smells like smoke and is used to provide cover during tactical movement.

Equipment of the Tactical Medical Provider

Introduction

When engaged in tactical special operations, all Special Weapons and Tactics (SWAT) and tactical emergency medical support (TEMS) units must be properly equipped to succeed in the mission. Each member of the SWAT and TEMS unit must be prepared and ready to perform his or her role as expected. As the TMP, you will need to bring a fairly substantial variety of medical equipment and gear to save lives. This chapter discusses the medical equipment and gear you will be carrying into the tactical environment.

The Tactical Medical Provider Uniform

Generally, SWAT and TEMS uniforms are composed of a poly-cotton blended, durable ripstop cloth material that may be selected as appropriate for the regional weather. Thin, permeable, summer-weight, as well as thicker, winter-weight battle dress uniform (BDU) pants and shirts are available. Most SWAT and TEMS units wear a black or dark-colored T-shirt or undergarment underneath the BDU shirt. This undergarment should be made of insulating wicking material (eg, polypropylene or Thermax) that rapidly draws sweat away from the body to prevent heat and cold injuries. Avoid cotton. Some SWAT units utilize outer and inner fire-resistant Nomex coveralls or clothing to help minimize burns in the event of fire or explosion.

Most SWAT units have their TMPs wear the same color and style of uniform as they do. This minimizes recognition errors during high-risk operations, prevents terrorists or criminals from specifically targeting TMPs, and encourages a sense of camaraderie. Some SWAT units mark the exterior uniform and helmet with a small and subtle camouflaged

At the Scene

Depending upon the SWAT unit's preference, there may be a need for one or two uniforms per officer. Many SWAT units ask that tactical officers and TMPs make use of two uniforms, including a designated training uniform and a second uniform for actual callouts.

medical marking (eg, a subdued Star of Life, green cross, or caduceus) that allows others at the scene, at close range, to identify the TMP. These patches can be attached with Velcro in order to allow for their quick removal in certain circumstances. Other SWAT units choose not to identify their medical personnel for security reasons. If used, the medical insignia and identifying patches should be similar to the SWAT officers', and should also potentially include a small, camouflaged medical insignia identifying the TMP as medical personnel **Figure 4-1**. Bright red crosses or other noncamouflaged patterns causing the TMP to stand out in the field are considered by some experts to be inappropriate in the tactical environment.

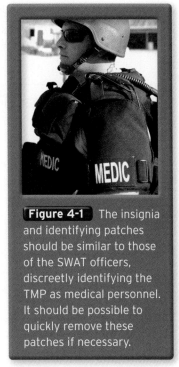

Figure 4-1 The insignia and identifying patches should be similar to those of the SWAT officers, discreetly identifying the TMP as medical personnel. It should be possible to quickly remove these patches if necessary.

Additional Insignia

Law enforcement insignia patches are nearly always worn on the TMP uniform. They should accurately and easily describe the unit a member is associated with; this is especially important in regions where multiple jurisdictions may be involved at a scene. Insignia patches are commonly found on the shoulders of the TMP uniform, and are often also located on the front and back of the outer material covering the ballistic vest. Additional patches including nameplates are located elsewhere on the uniform. Each TMP should be personally known to each of the tactical officers; therefore, nameplates are not generally useful on the outermost layer of the uniform during actual callouts.

The outer medical vest may also have markings designating an individual as a MEDIC (TMP), MED (tactical physician), or other health care provider in the tactical environment. For TEMS units that support more than one SWAT unit, at least one separate and unique uniform should be worn for each SWAT unit. Otherwise, removable Velcro patches are effective for allowing TEMS units to switch insignias and/or identification when working with multiple SWAT units.

Extreme Weather Garments

As a TMP, you should have several uniforms that appropriately match the environmental conditions you expect to face in the tactical environment. Proper clothing will enable you to function comfortably and safely. Uniform considerations for damp or rainy weather, for instance, include camouflaged rain ponchos or outer coverings, backpack rain covers, and waterproof hats. Extreme weather garments include:

- **Footwear**. Waterproof, quiet boots, providing good ankle support and all-around traction for use inside buildings and outdoors. A hardened front boot style should be considered, to prevent toe injuries.
- **Socks**. Two layers: an inner, thin, wicking, liner sock and an outer, thick sock.
- **Underwear**. Cotton briefs are acceptable, but other cotton clothing should be avoided. All other underclothing should be a modern synthetic style with wicking ability.
- **Cold weather gear**. Includes appropriate insulated hats, gloves, neck gaiters, insulated clothing, parkas, boots, and a four-layer system that allows clothing layers to be removed or added to match the weather conditions.
- **Wet weather gear**. Waterproof uniform, consisting of either a poncho or raincoat and rain pants. Waterproof bags should be considered for protection of medical gear and backpacks. All medical supplies (eg, tourniquets and bandages) inside medical packs should be sealed in waterproof bags or cases.
- **Hot weather gear**. Lightweight, nonabsorbing, rapidly evaporating clothing material for shirts and pants will enhance cooling if hot, humid weather is present. Ribbed liner shirts should be worn under ballistic vests. Hats will help block radiation from the sun.

Cold Weather Gear

A cold weather uniform should include a wind- and waterproof four-level system. Using a multiple-layer system of clothing provides you with a means of adapting to changes in climate and other environmental conditions. The suggested four-layer system includes:

1. A first inner liner layer of long underwear made of sweat-wicking synthetic material
2. A second layer of a thicker "pile" synthetic jacket and pants
3. A third layer of insulated goose down or modern equivalent (parka and pants providing an air-space layer for insulation) in extreme cold
4. A fourth outer layer of a wind- and waterproof jacket and pants

Insulated hats that fit under a helmet are important, as well as clothing that can be worn over the neck (eg, a neck gaiter), face (eg, a face mask), or clothing to cover the entire head and neck with only the nose and eyes showing (eg, a **balaclava**). Insulated, waterproof gloves and footwear are especially important. Electric or air-activated heat packs may provide additional warmth to feet and hands in severely cold weather. You need to maintain normal sensation and functioning of your hands at all times; a hot pack stored in your pocket will help to keep your hands and fingers warm and ready to use.

Warm Weather Gear

Appropriate clothing should be worn in hot weather. This includes breathable, light-colored clothing; ventilated, ribbed inner liners worn under ballistic vests (to increase air circulation and evaporation of sweat); and other special shirts to be worn under ballistic vests that promote cooling of the body.

Safety

Cotton is comfortable, but should be avoided in cold and hot climates. "Cotton kills" is a phrase that refers to the heavy sweat absorption by cotton clothing during physical exertion. In the winter, sitting or standing for hours in a wet shirt can lead to hypothermia. In hot weather, evaporation under ballistic vests and uniforms is ineffective and will lead to overheating and potentially heatstroke. Modern, synthetic, sweat-wicking undergarment clothing should be used year-round.

Such shirts are made of modern fabrics that help to absorb sweat and increase its evaporation rate, thus enhancing cooling rates and decreasing heat injuries.

Tactical Personal Protective Equipment

Tactical personal protective equipment (TPPE) is designed to protect you from both medical threats and violent threats in the tactical environment Figure 4-2 . It includes gear from ballistic helmets to protect the head from trauma to nitrile gloves to protect the body from bloodborne pathogens. It is critical to wear TPPE during both training and actual callouts because individuals tend to perform as they have trained. In other words, if you use TPPE during training, when a true callout occurs you will be prepared to properly utilize this protective gear.

During training and callouts, always wear TPPE that protects your body against physical harm, takes appropriate standard precautions, and ensures respiratory protection. Table 4-1 is an inventory of standard TPPE. Chapter 25, "Hazardous Materials and Clandestine Drug Labs," covers

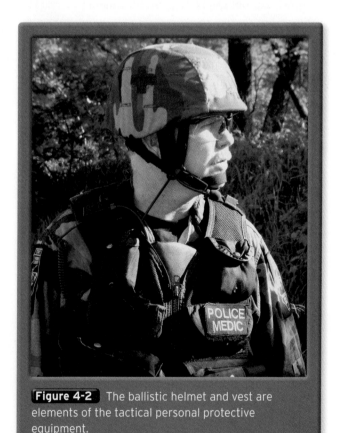

Figure 4-2 The ballistic helmet and vest are elements of the tactical personal protective equipment.

Table 4-1	Tactical Personal Protective Equipment Inventory

- Ballistic vest with shoulder protection
- Ballistic helmet
- Black balaclava
- Eye protection
- Ear protection
- Inner gloves
- Outer gloves
- Medical protective gear
- Kneepads
- Air-purifying respirator (APR)
- Canteen or hydration system
- Flashlight

Modified from Wipfler III J and Greenberg M. Building a TEMS Team. *The ITAO News.* 2005; 1(4):6-9. Reproduced with permission of the Illinois Tactical Officers Association.

the specific protective gear to wear during callouts involving hazardous materials.

The Ballistic Vest

The **ballistic vest** is constructed of materials that are designed to defend against small arms projectiles and shrapnel. The design and size used is normally dictated by the expected threat (eg, caliber of weapon) and whether the vest is to be worn open as an outer level, worn under normal clothing, or concealed. Some civilian EMS and fire service personnel routinely wear ballistic vests for protection against gunshot wounds as they respond to calls in dangerous areas with high crime threats. The use of ballistic vests by law enforcement officers is nearly universal and is mandatory by most agencies.

Soft body armor, a ballistic-resistant fabric worn concealed under the uniform or over the uniform, is made from polyethylene fiber. Examples of soft body armor include Spectra, made by Allied-Signal, Inc; Kevlar, made by DuPont; and Twaron, made by AkzoNobel.

The National Institute of Justice (NIJ) has tested, defined, and rated ballistic vest threat levels (from the lower Type IIA to the highest Type IV vest), which are designed to defeat specific projectiles fired from specific types of weapons. The following threat protection levels are available for soft armor:

- **Type IIA.** Type IIA armor can usually stop a 9-mm full-metal-jacketed bullet fired from a 4-inch barrel, as well as a .357 Magnum, semijacketed, soft-point bullet fired from a 4-inch barrel. Other nonmandated rounds that this threat level may stop include most non-full-metal jacketed

9-mm rounds, several .44 Magnum rounds, and 12-grain, 00 buckshot.
- **Type II.** Threat protection Type II is stronger than IIA and will stop the mandated 9-mm full-metal-jacketed bullet fired from a 5-inch barrel, as well as the .357 Magnum, semijacketed, soft-point bullet fired from a 6-inch barrel. This vest will likely stop nonmandated rounds such as 12-grain shotgun slugs and a variety of 9-mm full-metal-jacketed bullet rounds.
- **Type IIIA.** Threat protection Type IIIA stops the mandated 9-mm full-metal-jacketed bullet fired from a 16-inch-barreled carbine, as well as the .44 Magnum fired from a 6-inch barrel.

Some tactical officers may use **hard body armor inserts**. These rigid inserts are usually made of steel, ceramics, aluminum, or titanium and are used for added frontal-torso protection in addition to soft body armor. Hard body armor is available in the following threat protection levels:

- **Type III.** Threat protection Type III with a hard insert is designed to protect against the common M-4/AR-15 rifle round and also the center-fire rifle rounds.
- **Type IV.** Threat protection Type IV is the highest and thickest level of protection, and it protects against the armor-piercing (AP) round as usually fired from a hunting rifle, M-1 Garand, or other rifle.

Type III and Type IV armor require rigid metal and/or ceramic plates to be effective against rifles and some very fast pistol rounds, and are quite heavy. Many of the older styles of Type IV hard body armor are not used routinely due to their heavy weight (over 40 lb total vest weight). Newer vests and plates continue to improve and lighten as companies improve upon the technology. Some of the newer Type IV vests weigh 17.5 lb and have proven effective in Iraq against multiple hits from automatic weapons including the commonly available AK-47 or SKS rifles.

Another type of protective vest is the **stab-resistant ballistic vest**, which is made primarily for prison guards. It is designed to be resistant against puncture from knives, improvised edged-weapons (shanks), and other pointed or edged weapons (screwdriver). The NIJ Standard–0115.00, *Stab Resistance of Personal Body Armor*, categorizes stab-resistant body armor as "edged blade" or "spike class." Edged-blade class body armor protects the wearer against high-quality or engineered blades, including kitchen and sporting knives. This threat is more frequently encountered on the street. Spike class body armor protects the wearer against

Safety

Some bullet-resistant vests will not stop knives from being thrust through the ballistic material. Be aware of the capabilities and limitations of your unit's body armor.

improvised weapons, such as those commonly used by correctional facility inmates. Most ballistic vests are not knife resistant unless specified.

For your safety, you should wear a ballistic vest. Federal Bureau of Investigation (FBI) statistics show that the odds of surviving a shootout are 14 times higher if body armor is worn. The minimal protection level recommended for general law enforcement officers is Type II body armor—rated against most pistols, shotguns, and some automatic weapons (including the Maschinenpistole 5 [MP-5] submachine gun commonly used by SWAT units). As a TMP, you should wear nothing less than Level II body armor. SWAT and many TEMS units utilize the heavier but more bullet-resistant Type III vests, with some units utilizing ceramic or other plates (Type IV) to defeat rifle rounds.

The Ballistic Helmet

Ballistic helmets are worn to help protect the scalp, skull, and brain from trauma Figure 4-3 . The helmet is used in many occupations and works quite well in protecting the wearer from small bumps and scrapes when working in confined spaces or structures with low overhead (such as an armored vehicle doorway). Certainly one of the most dangerous threats is a fired bullet, and the Type III helmet is able to effectively stop or deflect all but the most powerful rifle bullets. The Type III helmet protects against explosions with accompanying shrapnel, as well as possible blows from sticks, knives, or other weapons.

The weight and bulk of a helmet may be an inconvenience. Newer materials and suspension systems, however, have resulted in lighter and more comfortable helmet styles. The suspension system is important because it holds the outer helmet securely in the proper position and separates the skull from the helmet. A bullet striking the helmet will often bounce off but, in doing so, may deform the helmet inward. This may result in significant head injury (eg, significant concussion, skull fracture, or worse) if there is insufficient gap between the skull and the inner helmet.

In a tactical environment you can usually position yourself behind hard cover for safety, but you may need to occasionally glance around corners or edges of trees, resulting in exposing part of your head. In addition, many head injuries might occur while getting into or out of armored vehicles. These and other head injuries may be prevented through the use of ballistic helmets. An ideal helmet is bullet resistant and lightweight, allows access to the ears so that a stethoscope and radio can be used, and has a secure and comfortable four-point helmet harness system, with a ballistic face shield. The ballistic face shield is mounted to the front of the helmet and is designed to protect the face from rocks and debris.

The Balaclava

Many authorities recommend the use of a balaclava for protection of the face, head, and neck Figure 4-4 .

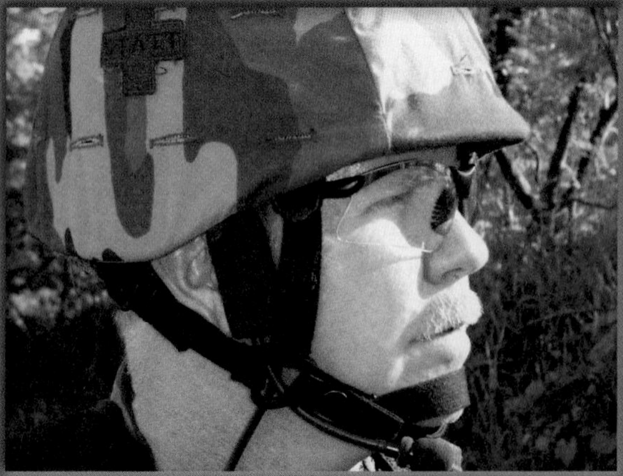

Figure 4-3   The ballistic helmet protects the head from traumatic injuries caused by bullets, blows, or shrapnel.

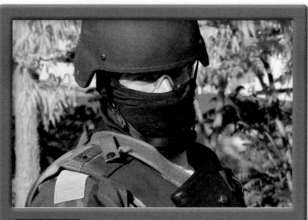

Figure 4-4   The balaclava protects the face, head, and neck from the elements, in addition to protecting the identity of the wearer.

There are three reasons to use this device. The first is to provide protection against fire and explosions in the event of a methamphetamine laboratory or chemical fire (especially if the balaclava is made of Nomex, a fire-resistant cloth material). The second is to provide some warmth and protection against cold elements. The third is to conceal the identity of SWAT and TEMS unit personnel from suspects and the news media. If suspects can identify exactly who was at the scene, they may threaten revenge in the form of future violence. Although most callouts end with no serious injuries, if the suspect is highly prone toward violence, it may be prudent to protect the identity of all involved in the tactical operation.

Eye Protection

Eye protection is extremely important in the tactical environment. Acuity of vision is critical when shooting or performing medical tasks. The loss of an eye or impaired vision will result in disability and an individual's removal from the SWAT unit due to visual limitations. If dust, other materials, or traumatic injury causes pain and/or loss of vision in the midst of a mission, a SWAT or TEMS unit personnel may be rendered useless. This may result in unnecessary injury or death. Therefore, it is extremely important to not neglect this important asset. Eye goggles or glasses with shatter-resistant polycarbonate lenses are essential to protect eyes from flying debris, dust, bullet fragments, direct trauma, and many other hazards. For the TMP, eye protection should also block any blood or body fluids that may be coughed or splashed into the face while providing medical care.

There are basically two ways to protect the eyes: minimize threats from trauma by maintaining vigilance against threats to the eyes and taking evasive action, and wearing impact-resistant eyewear or goggles. The best goggles are devices that protect the eyes from flying debris and objects coming from all directions, including the sides. A wrap-around design is effective to this end,

Safety

The reflection of sunlight or bright lights off of goggles and other protective eyewear can potentially reveal a SWAT unit's position to suspects. You can minimize this effect by using semicurved lenses that wrap around the eyes and onto the lateral aspect of the cheek, and also by choosing goggles that are coated with nonreflective material on the frame and also over the shiny lenses.

Safety

An extra pair of goggles or protective glasses should be kept close by in case the first pair is broken or misplaced.

though it does create distortion of vision around the edges of the lens. Protective goggles should be tight enough to seal out dust particles and flying empty brass casings (from a SWAT officer's weapon). Protective eyewear should be fitted appropriately in order to stay on during high-performance operations (eg, rappelling, parachuting, windblast incidents). Protective eyewear should also be large enough to ensure a clear view of the surroundings.

The color of the lenses should be chosen to suit the environment. Yellow- or amber-colored lenses improve night vision and resolution, while dark lenses improve vision on bright, sunny days. Dark lenses can also provide protection against less-lethal light-emitting diode (LED) disorientation devices. If the callout scenario may involve going into the shade, a forest, or inside a building, then dark lenses should be avoided because the dark color will hinder clear vision. Clear lenses are often the best overall color because they allow true vision without color disturbance or excessive darkness of vision.

Most of the newer tactical goggles have polycarbonate or "impact-resistant" lenses that provide a shatter-resistant shield against most low- and intermediate-speed projectiles. Some crowd-control or riot gear will have large polycarbonate face shields that attach to helmets, allowing ballistic protection against smaller-caliber handgun bullets and explosive shrapnel. You will be best served by wearing comfortable eye protection with polycarbonate lenses that allow clear vision.

One dangerous problem with some goggles and glasses is that they can obstruct vision when they become fogged up with moisture. Test all equipment, including eye protection, under realistic training conditions. Use antifog ointment and/or spray and work with your eye protection to make sure it functions well during different types of scenarios. If fogging continues, then better eye protection with increased ventilation should be utilized.

Safety

If corrective lenses are needed, then prescription protective glasses are available.

Hearing and Ear Protection

As a TMP, you will have repeated exposure to high-decibel noise in the form of gunfire; noise-flash distraction devices (NFDDs) or "flash-bangs;" explosive breaching; and other loud sources. For example, most SWAT units are now using 5.56-mm caliber rifles with Messier 4 (M-4)-style, the Armalite model 15 (AR-15), or M-16 rifles that have a harsh muzzle blast. This can immediately cause a lasting ear-ringing and decreased hearing for several minutes, with inevitable long-term hearing damage. Without sound suppressors, the tactical officer and the TMP are suddenly exposed to 160 to 170 decibels of noise during rifle fire. This effect is even more intense when rifles or pistols are fired within the often small confines of a building.

Repetitive exposure to loud noise can cause hearing loss, which becomes worse with every loud noise encountered. Hearing damage is not usually repairable by the body, and so the result of repeated loud noise exposure is accumulative hearing loss. The damage may eventually require early retirement. The ability to hear surrounding threats in the tactical environment is critical, as is the ability to listen in on radio or other communication channels. Therefore, it is very important to take all practical measures to properly protect hearing during training and callouts.

Several methods of hearing protection may be utilized. Small foam earplugs are simply rolled between the fingertips to compress, inserted into each ear, and then allowed to expand and seal the ear canal to help block loud noise. Even better protection can be obtained with custom, ear-molded earplugs that provide a tight seal and block noise significantly. With custom, ear-molded earplugs, plastic material is inserted into the ear canal and outer ear and allowed to harden into a set of reusable plugs. The other primary method of

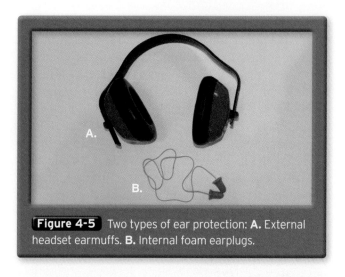

Figure 4-5 Two types of ear protection: **A.** External headset earmuffs. **B.** Internal foam earplugs.

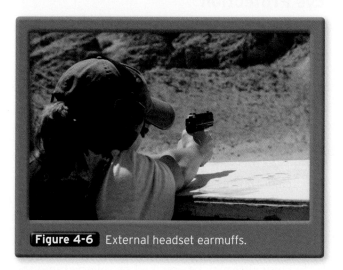

Figure 4-6 External headset earmuffs.

hearing protection is the use of external headset earmuffs **Figure 4-5**. These may be simple or electronic, and may reduce the sound intensity by 15 to 35 decibels **Figure 4-6**.

Commercial earplugs and earmuffs are available that have electronic "cut-off" switches that block loud noise within a few milliseconds. They allow for normal or amplified hearing and are able to shut off during gunfire or loud noise signatures.

Many units train with ear protection, but then deploy on actual callouts without any ear protection. This is not ideal, and there are increasingly better options to protect hearing and operationally deploy with systems that allow tactical hearing while protecting the ears. Some electronic headset earmuffs have internal radios and headset microphones built in **Figure 4-7**. These electronic headset earmuffs may also have the ability to plug into the unit's radios, allowing for simultaneous ear protection, external electronic noise detection, and radio communication. The electronic headset earmuffs should

Safety

Hearing loss has affected many veterans returning from Iraq and Afghanistan. Exposure to excessive noise levels is a common threat in the tactical environment, and steps should be taken to protect your hearing and the hearing of your fellow SWAT and TEMS personnel. The Occupational Safety and Health Association (OSHA) standard CFR 1910.95, *Occupational Noise Exposure*, mandates that employers provide hearing conservation programs.

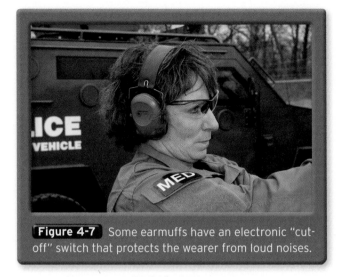

Figure 4-7 Some earmuffs have an electronic "cut-off" switch that protects the wearer from loud noises.

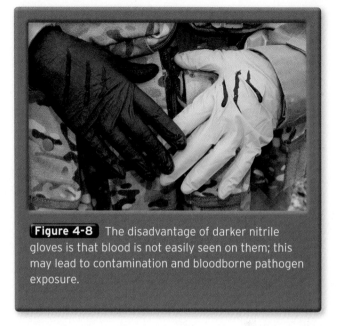

Figure 4-8 The disadvantage of darker nitrile gloves is that blood is not easily seen on them; this may lead to contamination and bloodborne pathogen exposure.

Safety

You should receive training in hand and arm signals, in the event that radio communication is cut off or unavailable.

be compatible with the helmets and communication equipment. Although more expensive, these devices work very well and are increasingly utilized by SWAT units.

Gloves

The use of gloves is critical for protection against bloodborne pathogens. Depending upon the weather conditions, you will typically wear **nitrile gloves** for protection against bloodborne pathogens during a mission **Figure 4-8**. Nitrile gloves tend to be utilized by TMPs more often as they are more durable and chemical-resistant, and also come in dark colors to aid with camouflage. Over the top of these gloves you may choose to wear leather, Nomex, or perhaps puncture-resistant Kevlar-based gloves. The advantages of having two layers of gloves is that the more delicate inner glove may be protected during patient or downed-officer searches and weapons removal, removal of outer clothing, and normal wear-and-tear during tactical operations. When delicate hand sensation is required (eg, for starting an intravenous [IV] line or performing some other medical procedure), then the outer leather or other type gloves can rapidly be removed and the nitrile inner glove remains for protection against bloodborne pathogens.

During extremely cold weather, many TMPs utilize more bulky mitten-style gloves with air-activated heat packs inside to keep their hands warm. These air-activated heat packs are inexpensive and last for 4 to 6 hours, generating nontoxic heat. Obtain a large supply of these heat packs and distribute them to tactical officers before and during cold weather operations to help maintain warmth.

Medical Protective Gear

Before initiating medical care of victims, you must first protect yourself and then ensure the protection of your unit. This protection must include **personal protective equipment (PPE)** that will prevent accidental exposure to infectious diseases transmitted in the blood, sputum, vomit, or other body fluids. Standard precautions must be taken into consideration when deciding upon the PPE to don. Proper PPE includes effective head covering, eye protection, and a face mask that will prevent bodily fluids from contaminating your eyes, nose, or mouth. As mentioned previously, gloves should be used—ideally in a two-glove, double-layer system—to improve the barrier and allow you to change external gloves between patients or procedures while continuously wearing one pair of inner gloves.

If decontamination or a particularly bloody victim is involved, then a plastic or fluid-impermeable apron or coverall Tyvek uniform may be useful to prevent blood and chemicals from soaking through a cloth uniform to the underlying skin. Waterproof boots or shoe coverings should also be considered. Sturdy leather boots with a Gortex inner liner are more practical in the TEMS setting to prevent water, blood, and fluids from soaking through.

Any abrasion or open sore on your skin should be well covered and waterproofed before the mission in order to prevent communicable diseases from being introduced into that wound. Collodion is a clear ointment that covers abrasions well. Opsite IV clear covering or other clear membranes may be used as well. Common sense and proper preparation will go far in preventing exposure to serious infections such as tuberculosis, hepatitis, and human immunodeficiency virus (HIV).

Kneepads

Kneepads are worn to protect the knees, especially when crawling or kneeling on the ground is necessary for treating patients. Kneepads protect the knees from blood or sharp materials (eg, rocks or glass) on the ground. Rocks and broken glass increase the chance of injury and accidental exposure to bloodborne pathogens Figure 4-9 .

In addition to kneepads, many TEMS units also utilize elbow pads in the event that they need to crawl on their bellies, elbows, and knees to approach

or treat patients. It is important that knee and elbow pads be fitted and tested extensively prior to their use in the tactical environment. A broad elastic band as well as appropriate, conforming plastics and foam are important. Some newer model elbow- and kneepads have a hard exterior with a gel insert. At the very least, elbow and knee protectors should allow for a full range of motion, should not cut off circulation, should not cause pain with extended wear, and should remain in place.

Hydration Systems

Hydration systems are not really protective in terms of stopping or blocking a threat, but they are the only practical way to counter a common threat facing a SWAT unit Figure 4-10 . Those threats are dehydration and overheating due to strenuous exertion in time-pressured, stressful, and dangerous situations. Heavy uniforms and loads of gear decrease effective evaporative heat loss and increase risks for heat injury.

Dehydration quickly leads to fatigue, dulled thinking, weakness, and a significant decrease in performance. In rare circumstances, it may lead to more severe heat illness and possible heatstroke. A small percentage of heatstroke patients, even if healthy, young, and fit, will die from this underestimated environmental threat. Performance suffers even if there is mild dehydration. Many make the mistake of waiting until they are thirsty before seeking water or other fluids. This is too late. Subtle fatigue and slowed thinking can result from mild dehydration, and if SWAT and TEMS unit personnel know they will be exerting themselves, they should initiate early hydration efforts in order to prevent it. Guidance for management of dehydration and heatstroke in the tactical environment is provided in Chapter 22, "Environmental Injuries."

One of the common mistakes is simply not drinking enough. This is due to several factors, including trying to avoid urination, lack of planning, not having the capacity to carry

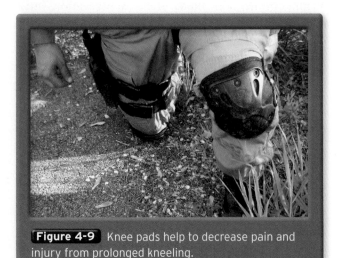

Figure 4-9 Knee pads help to decrease pain and injury from prolonged kneeling.

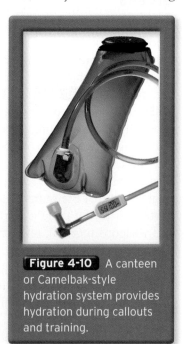

Figure 4-10 A canteen or Camelbak-style hydration system provides hydration during callouts and training.

fluids on the mission, and fear of exposure. The human body needs more fluids during a stress response, so during the high-stress situation of a callout it is especially critical to remain hydrated. Good choices of fluids include a mixture of water and orange juice or athletic fluid-replacement drinks with a good combination of electrolytes. If possible, caffeine should be avoided because it causes more fluid loss by causing increased urination. Cool liquids taste better and are more rapidly absorbed.

Prehydrate before a mission and continue to drink plenty of appropriate fluids during the mission in order to maintain hydration. During peak performance, it is suggested that each tactical officer drink about 1 liter of fluids or more per hour. One of the essential functions of TMPs in these circumstances is to assist the command staff and SWAT unit with ensuring easy access to water, along with appropriate fluids containing replenishing electrolytes in order to prevent heat injuries and dehydration. The backpack style or Camelbak hydration systems have become standard issue, and all TEMS units should use these routinely.

Gas Mask or Air-Purifying Respirator

The gas mask or **air-purifying respirator (APR)** is an essential piece of equipment that you must keep immediately available, remain comfortable with, and be operationally effective while using **Figure 4-11**. There are many chemicals and agents that the SWAT team may be exposed to such as booby-trap chemicals, toxic substances at a clandestine methamphetamine laboratory, riot control gas, and other law enforcement–related chemical agents.

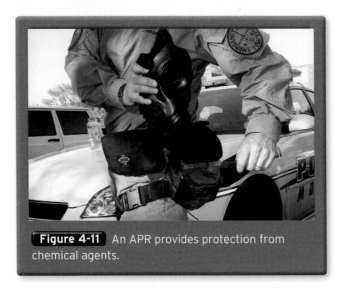

Figure 4-11 An APR provides protection from chemical agents.

If the SWAT unit introduces "gas" (ie, tear gas or another chemical) into the house where the suspect is located, then any suspect or tactical officer who enters the house will soon be contaminated with noxious chemicals. If any medical care is urgently needed for these individuals, you will quickly be overwhelmed and rendered ineffective by the severe pain, tearing, respiratory difficulty, and psychological effects if you are not wearing an APR.

Use of the APR requires proper training because it can cause mild claustrophobia, limit breathing, and hinder communications. If you are properly trained and comfortable with wearing a full-face APR with the appropriate filtration system, then medical care can be provided quickly and effectively in environments with hazardous atmospheres such as a chemical release from a tanker truck, intentional use of OC, or CS present at a scene with a downed officer.

Flashlights and Illumination Tools

Many tactical callouts occur at night or inside poorly lit buildings. To operate safely in the tactical environment, you must arm yourself with knowledge of the tools and equipment that allow you to perform well in low-light conditions. This is accomplished by use of flashlights or other illumination tools, and possibly the use of **night vision equipment** or thermal imaging equipment. There are several categories of lights and ways illumination is used. There are simple handheld lights, as well as lights that can be attached to the head or helmet by a strap system.

Before a light is turned on at night or in low-light environments, its use should be authorized by the SWAT incident commander or leader. The use of a light could reveal the position and advertise the location of anyone using that light. In the dark, the suspect may not realize that the SWAT unit is approaching, but a sudden accidental release of light from even a quarter-second flashlight beam can result in dire consequences. You must be certain of the circumstances and tactics before using a light source.

You should have several illumination tools, including at least two handheld and two head-mounted

Safety

Prescription lenses can be made and fitted into APR to ensure that vision is maintained.

flashlight systems. Weapon-mounted lights are a part of the weapon system and should never be used as a light source for TMPs or for procedures in the tactical environment. Discreet red or blue lenses should be used in at least one flashlight for low-light, stealth movement, which preserves night vision. SWAT and TEMS units should consider the use of night vision equipment and thermal imaging devices to aid tactical operations low-light environments.

Night Vision Equipment

There are several types of night vision equipment. Night vision devices may have some utility for the TMP because they can assist in patient evaluation and possibly remote assessment in areas where light cannot be used due to nearby threats. Night vision monoculars, night vision binoculars, and night vision goggles are other devices that enable SWAT units to see in the dark. These devices require some slight degree of infrared or ambient light. In fact, with just starlight, they can be used to readily identify objects and people in darkness up to several hundred yards away. The use of a monocular will allow you to simultaneously "see" in the dark to safely navigate and approach the patient, and utilize your other eye for up-close medical procedures such as intubation, starting IVs with very faint near lighting, and other procedures. Through the use of night vision devices, you can assess downed officers from a distance.

An **infrared flashlight**, which emits light invisible to the human eye, may be used to illuminate the area, allowing you to discern the presence of objects and humans more than 400 yards away.

Thermal Imaging Equipment

Thermal imaging devices cause objects (eg, human bodies and fire) that emit heat to appear whiter on a device screen. During law enforcement search-and-rescue operations or searches for escaped convicts, the use of thermal imaging devices can rapidly screen a section of woods or a field for warm human bodies. Fire departments routinely use **thermal imaging devices**

to search buildings for hot spots and to conduct rapid searches in smoke-filled rooms.

Recently technology has enabled these devices to be reduced in size so they can be easily held in one hand. The incredible sensitivity of this equipment allows the viewer to see very subtle temperature differences, making these devices ideal for search and rescue and identifying suspects in urban and woodland environments. They make nighttime missions much safer as suspects can be easily seen in most conditions. Both SWAT and TEMS unit personnel can utilize these devices to help identify where a suspect or a patient can be found.

Essential Emergency Medical Gear: A Four-Level System

Overall, there is wide variation in the type and amount of medical equipment that may be brought to provide emergency care, and the method with which these supplies are carried or transported to the scene varies with each TEMS unit. As always, follow the standards of your agency. Medical gear is dependent upon the level of training of the TMPs, their experience and preferences, tolerance of size of load or backpack, type of mission, predicted number of patients in a worst case scenario, backup medical support, likelihood of rapid extraction and transportation, and the potential need for extended medical care. An overloaded, bulky TMP with too much gear may quickly wear down and be less able to carry or drag a downed officer through a building. On the other hand, a minimally equipped TMP with a single small fanny pack who enters a large building with multiple victims will rapidly require more gear and medical supplies, especially if sustained gunfire delays extraction of victims from the building. Careful planning and realistic attitudes along with personal preferences will determine what type of gear is carried.

The following is a four-level system based on tactical combat casualty care (TCCC) principles (see Chapter 11) and is commonly used by TEMS units throughout the world:

- **Level 1.** Level 1 gear is used by both SWAT and TEMS unit personnel and is essentially a basic trauma kit composed of simple, practical items. Commonly, this includes a trauma bandage and a tourniquet. Additional items may include a **nasopharyngeal airway**, personal nitrile

---

Safety

Infrared markers can be useful for identifying SWAT officers in the dark, such as a small flashing infrared flashlight marker that clips to the shoulder or helmet.

gloves, and a **cardiopulmonary resuscitation (CPR) mask**. These items allow SWAT officers to provide self-aid and buddy-aid immediately, and are universally carried by all SWAT officers and TMPs in the same location on their load-bearing gear.

- **Level 2.** Level 2 gear is the TMP's medical vest/belt/ thigh pack that is attached to the body during the entire mission **Figure 4-12**.

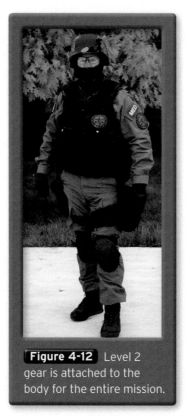

Figure 4-12 Level 2 gear is attached to the body for the entire mission.

- **Level 3.** Level 3 gear is the medical backpack. The backpack can remain with TMPs most of the time and is usually not carried on the back but set on the ground or just outside of the building during entries.
- **Level 4.** Level 4 gear is an advanced medical pack, which typically remains secured and is brought to the scene when callouts occur. It is a large and bulky item that is best maintained at the command center or in the SWAT vehicles for use with sustained in-field operations or more advanced on-site medical care.

Level 1

Each member of the SWAT and TEMS units should carry an **individual first aid kit (IFAK)** that contains a few simple but effective first aid devices and that is located in the same area of the body on each TMP. **Table 4-2** summarizes the typical contents of an IFAK.

Every SWAT officer and TMP should carry these items in an easy-to-access pouch that is attached to the front of their body where it can be reached and utilized within seconds. In fact, most SWAT officers already have one of the ideal kinds of first aid pouches, which is the double-magazine pouch. A 4-inch tactical compression

Controversy

What medical gear should be used for inner perimeter tactical missions? This is a controversial question because a wide range of opinions exist. One side of the thinking is that only the most simple and most efficient basic airway and hemorrhage control methods are needed for rapid stabilization and extraction. On the other side of the discussion is the opinion that a variety of medical gear and supplies should be carried for treating multiple patients for prolonged periods of time. In a setting where immediate extraction may not be tactically possible due to threats or lack of transportation, some feel that any advantage at the point of injury will increase the odds for a positive outcome. Another approach to gear selection and packing takes into consideration the equipment necessary for commonly performed as well as time-intensive procedures. Units that follow the third approach will create a suggested packing list during preplanning tailored to their particular tactical environments.

Table 4-2	Typical Contents of an IFAK

- 1 tactical tourniquet
- 1 tactical compression bandage
- #28 F nasopharyngeal tube
- Nitrile gloves (2 pairs)
- CPR mini-mask
- Band-Aids
- Acetaminophen (Tylenol)
- Ibuprofen
- Other minor first aid items

Modified from Wipfler III J and Greenberg M. Building a TEMS Team. *The ITAO News.* 2005; 1(4):6-9. Reproduced with permission of the Illinois Tactical Officers Association.

dressing, a tactical tourniquet, and a small waterproof bag with gloves and other small items can fit within this pouch **Figure 4-13**. **Tactical compression dressings** are gauze that is already attached to elastic wrapping with prerigged cinching and fastening devices. They should be vacuum-packed, sterile, lightweight, and easily deployed. **Tactical tourniquets** are lifesaving devices. Use of a tourniquet is discussed in more detail in this chapter. The same style of tactical tourniquet should be chosen and used by everyone on the unit. SWAT

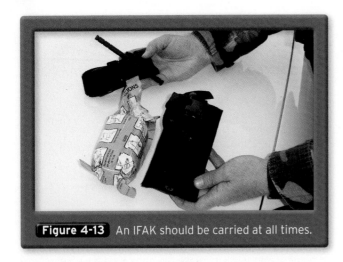

Figure 4-13 An IFAK should be carried at all times.

officers should attach their Level 1 IFAK gear in the same place so there is no delay when another person provides medical care. TMPs should carry identical Level 1 gear, as well as extra bandages and tourniquets in their other packs.

Level 2: Medical Vest With Utility Pouches, Belt, and Thigh Packs

Levels 2, 3, and 4 equipment are to be used only by the TMP. Level 2 medical gear is attached to the TEMS unit personnel at all times while operational. Note an important point: The Level 2 medical vest should be sized large enough to fit over or incorporate a Level III or IV ballistic vest. Some Level 2 medical equipment may be attached to a belt with thigh pouches so it can be picked up as a single unit, thus ensuring that it can be rapidly donned without forgetting any items. See **Table 4-3** for a list of Level 2 gear, which includes a vest, thigh pack, and belt.

Level 3: Tactical Medical Backpack

Level 3 gear is carried in a medium to large-sized backpack, and brought with the TMP when needed. It should be *close by at all times* during training and callouts. **Table 4-4** lists the Level 3 gear stored in a tactical medical backpack.

Level 4: Tactical Medical Advanced Life Support Kit

The Level 4 medical pack is kept locked in a controlled environment until the callout and then is taken out of storage and placed into the SWAT raid truck or van. This kit is to remain near or at the command center or tactical operations center (TOC). The contents may include narcotics and other controlled substances

that must be properly locked and controlled under federal DEA guidelines. In addition, exposure of these controlled medications to high heat or extreme cold should be prevented. It is important to protect oral and IV antibiotics, paralytics, and other sensitive medications.

Table 4-5 lists the equipment generally included in the Level 4 advanced medical supply kit.

Additional BLS Trauma Management Kit

Many SWAT units also keep a simple BLS trauma kit in the SWAT van or raid vehicle at all times. The purpose is to have available to the tactical officers a ready source of simple first aid materials and dressings that can be used by the SWAT officer if the TMPs are not available. This equipment is also a source of additional medical supplies should the mission require response to a mass-casualty incident.

A supplementary BLS kit contains simple medical supplies that can be used by anyone trained in simple first aid and TCCC, and may be expanded or contracted in size depending upon the expected length of the mission, number of people involved, and the expected types and number of casualties. This kit can contain any of a number of items including but not limited to medical dressings, trauma bandages, over-the-counter (OTC) medications for common medical complaints, backboards, litters, decontamination supplies, and other items. Each medical unit will need to discuss the possible types of missions and the limitations of the storage arrangements. The SWAT van may be subject to extreme heat or cold, and the exact contents will vary depending upon the local needs and preferences of the medical and tactical personnel.

Tactical Medical Supplies

The medical supplies used in a callout will vary depending upon the situation, types of patients involved, mechanism of injury or degree of illness, and location. The following section describes specific supplies that are commonly used in the tactical environment.

Tactical Compression Bandages

Tactical compression bandages are designed to be used anywhere on the body where a cut or other injury has resulted in skin damage with bleeding **Figure 4-14**. They are elastic, and thus can be used for the head, neck,

Table 4-3	Minimum Level 2 Tactical Medical Gear
Medical Vest With Utility Pouches	**Thigh Pack**

• 1 stethoscope
• Nitrile gloves (2 pairs)
• 1 face mask with clear eye shield
• Trauma scissors (1 pair)
• Medical tape (1 roll)
• 1 folding knife
• 2 tourniquets
• 2 combat compression dressings
• Minor wound medical kit: alcohol wipes, Virex wipes, Band-Aids, Steri-Strips, Benzoin, Bacitracin, and/or other antibiotic ointment
• OTC medications: acetaminophen (Tylenol), ibuprofen (Motrin or Advil), and antacid tablets (Tums) for minor complaints
• Eye protection: goggles, clear polycarbonate glasses
• Ear protection: foam earplugs, custom earplug inserts, or earmuffs (standard or electronic noise-canceling)
• Personal ID, law enforcement badge
• Cell phone, pager, portable radio with tactical headset
• Flashlights (× 2, lithium-battery powered): 1 handheld and 1 headlight
• Binoculars, night-vision monocular, and/or NVGs
• Pen and weatherproof pad of paper for notes
• Documentation: list of each tactical officer's abbreviated name, medical history, and allergies
• Digital camera (for evidence preservation, documentation, interesting cases, and future education)
• Personal dosimeter (in scenarios where the risks of radiation contamination are present)
• Handcuff keys and cutting device for plastic handcuffs
• Extra batteries in backpack
	• Airway management kits:
	  – Oral intubation gear: endotracheal (ET) tubes (6.5 and 7.5), 1 stylet, adult oropharyngeal airway, laryngoscope with #3 blade, 10 cc syringe to inflate the ET cuff, device to secure ET tube to the mouth or neck area, double-lumen airway tube (King airway or Combitube) along with appropriate syringes to inflate cuffs with air
	  – Bag-mask device or a mouth-to-mask ventilation system
	  – Surgical airway kit: Betadine solution, cricothyrotomy hook, scalpel, 6.5 ET tube or tracheostomy tube, 4-inch × 4-inch gauze strips, strap to secure to neck
	  – 4 Cook or 14-G, IV, 3.5-inch needles (for chest decompression)
	  – Additional compression trauma bandages
	  – Asherman Chest Seal (ACS) (× 4)
	
	Belt (may be attached to the bottom of the vest)
	
	• Multitool (with pliers, small saw, screwdrivers, other tools)
	• Handheld, vibratory metal detector
	• APR (with NBC filter properly sealed)
	• Handcuffs or flex cuffs, defensive pistol and holster, extra magazines, pistol light, expandable baton, and pepper foam (if issued and/or approved)

Modified from Wipfler III J and Greenberg M. Building a TEMS Team. *The ITAO News.* 2005; 1(4):6–9. Reproduced with permission of the Illinois Tactical Officers Association.

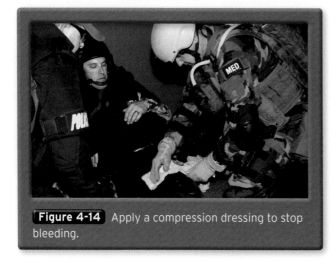

Figure 4-14 Apply a compression dressing to stop bleeding.

torso, and extremities. They are available in dark green and other colors that blend into the tactical environment.

There are several tactical bandages to choose from. Some of the more popular types include:

- Emergency Bandage (Israeli Combat Dressing)
- Olaes compression bandage
- Original H & H CINCH tight
- Bloodstopper

The compression bandage is effective and is an important part of the tactical medical gear. Although some of these bandages can be twisted with a built-in rigid 3- or 4-inch stick-like device to twist the bandage very tightly (windlass-type device) and thus turn into

Table 4-4   Minimum Level 3 Tactical Medical Gear

- A backup advanced airway management kit, which includes:
  - A second set of Level 2 airway supplies
  - Magill forceps (1 pair)
  - 1 laryngoscope with #1 and #3 blades (pediatric and adult sized)
  - Full size range of ET tubes (pediatric through adult sizes)
  - Curved hemostats
  - 1 scalpel
  - 1 cricothyrotomy hook
- An assortment of IV catheters (including 14, 16, 18, 20, and 22) and IV starting kits
- Two 1-liter IV fluid bags (one LR, one $D_5\frac{1}{2}NS$), 2 blood tubing IV lines with in-line hand pump, and 1 pressure bag for IV fluids
- Disposable hot and cold packs as well as air-activated hot packs
- Additional trauma dressings, tourniquets, gauze bandages, and chest seals
- 1 stretcher and/or litter (made of fabric, allowing one-man drag extraction)
- 2 SAM splints
- Additional standard protection supplies (gloves, masks, eye protection)
- 50 feet of 400-lb parachute cord
- Emergency thermal blankets, lightweight poncho
- Second backup headlight, handheld flashlight
- Sunblock lotion and insect repellant
- GPS unit for orienteering and calling in medevac/helicopter
- OTC medications: acetaminophen (Tylenol), ibuprofen (Motrin)
- Advanced cardiovascular life support (ACLS) medications (stored in a crush-proof box): atropine, epinephrine, lidocaine, nitroglycerine sublingual spray, baby aspirin 81-mg tabs
- 6 or more Mark 1 NAAK kits: high-dose atropine, Benadryl
- Consider narcotic and other advanced pain medications
- Antibiotics
- Large, full-size white bed sheet (for making mass-casualty emergency dressings, an improvised field table to keep track of gear during patient care, and slings)
- Medical waste bags and 1 disposable sharps hard plastic container

Modified from Wipfler III J and Greenberg M. Building a TEMS Team. *The ITAO News.* 2005; 1(4):6–9. Reproduced with permission of the Illinois Tactical Officers Association.

Table 4-5   Minimum Level 4 Tactical Medical Gear

- Assorted medications
- Assortment of syringes and needles, alcohol wipes
- Suture kits ($\times$ 2), skin glue, skin staplers ($\times$ 4), wound care supplies
- Gauze, basin, nitrile gloves, suture material, Betadine swabs
- Sterile saline (two 1-L bottles) for irrigation and/or cleaning of wounds
- Additional IV fluid (two 1-liter bags each 0.9% normal saline [NS], $D_5\frac{1}{2}NS$), IV lines, IV starting kits
- Dental kit: mirror, dental floss, clove oil, topical anesthesia, tongue blades, stoma wax, temporary filling material, cyanoacrylate glue ($\times$ 14)
- Additional trauma supplies: antiseptic towelettes, compression elastic bandage, trauma pads, eye

dressing, rigid eye shield, cotton swabs, SAM splints, triple antibiotic ointment, Band-Aids, tape, nonstick gauze, moleskin/blister kit, irrigation syringes and solution, Betadine scrub brushes, extra cold packs, heat packs, Cook pneumothorax kits, thermometer, extra stethoscope, trauma scissors
- Patient information tags, triage tags
- Two emergency thermal blankets
- Strobe light and smoke markers for designating a landing site
- Medical waste bags, disposable sharps hard plastic container
- SKED or other portable stretcher that can be kept in the raid/SWAT vans

Modified from Wipfler III J. Combat medicine: new things a tactical officer should know. *The ITAO News.* 2004; 17(4):36–39. Reproduced with permission of the Illinois Tactical Officers Association.

a makeshift tourniquet, these do not work as well as designated tourniquets.

Tactical Tourniquets

A tactical tourniquet is a medical device that is used to stop arterial and venous bleeding from the arms and legs (extremities). Tactical tourniquets compress the blood vessels so that no blood flows past the device, thus significantly slowing or stopping hemorrhage.

The number one cause of preventable death in combat is extremity hemorrhage. Remember that bleeding must be stopped as soon as possible. If you are close to an injured tactical officer and can rapidly and safely apply a compressive dressing to the extremity wound and effectively stop the bleeding, then a tourniquet may not be necessary.

However, if a SWAT officer is alone or separated from his or her unit and has a serious gunshot, knife wound, or other serious trauma to an arm or leg, then a tourniquet should be applied immediately after the suspect is neutralized. If the SWAT officer wrongly attempts to apply direct pressure or a standard compression dressing and serious bleeding continues, then the SWAT officer is at risk of becoming weak and unconscious and potentially bleeding to death. The main advantage of using a tourniquet is that when properly applied, the bleeding is stopped and management of the wound is completed for the short term.

Currently, it is highly recommended by experts that tourniquets be carried by every SWAT and TEMS unit personnel. You should carry several tourniquets. There are many different styles of tourniquets available including:

- Combat Application Tourniquet (CAT)
- Special Operations Forces Tactical Tourniquet (SOFTT)
- Mechanical Advantage Tourniquet (MAT)
- NATO, Delfi EMT tourniquet

It is important for each SWAT officer to have the knowledge, equipment, and skill to utilize a tactical tourniquet on his or her own leg or arm or on others nearby if it is indicated. If a formal tourniquet is not available but urgently needed, then improvised tourniquets from clothing or other material may work.

Clotting Agents, Hemostatic Bandages, and Hemorrhage Control

There are multiple agents and bandages that that are designed to stop or slow down serious blood flow from injury, including **hemostatic agents** and bandages. Hemostatic agents assist with controlling bleeding by

Controversy

Many hemostatic agents have yet to be thoroughly and scientifically investigated, and at the time of publication of this text, many are considered controversial **Figure 4-15**. However, there are first-hand accounts of some of these agents working; in theory and according to some animal studies, these agents do work to some degree. Medical directors and TEMS unit commanders should explore up-to-date research studies involving these agents and validate for themselves the usefulness and indications for using these hemorrhage control products. New agents will inevitably be developed, and only through careful, unbiased research will it be determined what actually works best in the tactical environment.

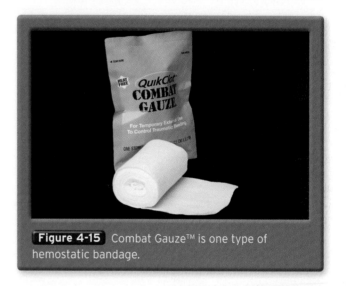

Figure 4-15 Combat Gauze™ is one type of hemostatic bandage.

enabling the formation of a blood clot. There is some controversy surrounding these items, so obtain the proper training if your agency uses these items and follow the protocols of your agency.

Occlusive Dressing With a Relief Valve (ACS or Equivalent)

Medical care for penetrating trauma to the chest often should include application of a one-way valve-type dressing such as the Asherman Chest Seal (ACS), Bolin Chest Seal, or an occlusive dressing taped or secured on three sides **Figure 4-16**. If a patient is sweating or bleeding from a wound, tincture of Benzoin may be needed to secure an ACS to the patient's skin. All of these dressings work by preventing air from entering the chest directly through the wound, but allow the escape of air pressure. Chapter 18, "Thoracic and Torso Injuries," covers penetrating trauma to the chest in detail.

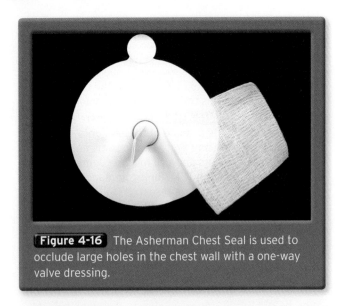

Figure 4-16 The Asherman Chest Seal is used to occlude large holes in the chest wall with a one-way valve dressing.

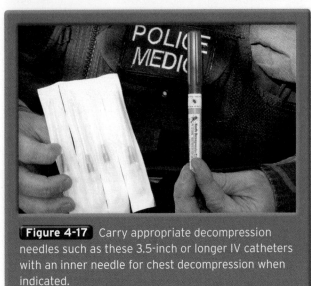

Figure 4-17 Carry appropriate decompression needles such as these 3.5-inch or longer IV catheters with an inner needle for chest decompression when indicated.

Chest Decompression Devices

The number two cause of preventable death from battlefield combat injuries is tension pneumothorax. Assessment and treatment of a tension pneumothorax is covered in detail in Chapter 18, "Thoracic and Torso Injuries." It is important for appropriately trained and certified personnel to carry several decompression needles to treat this condition **Figure 4-17**. The types of needles are discussed in detail in Chapter 18.

Airway Devices

The TEMS unit should carry a variety of airway devices. These devices range from simple oxygen masks to surgical airways. Unfortunately, it is common knowledge amongst criminals to shoot police officers where they

do not have protective armor, such as the face and neck. This and other factors result in SWAT officers being at high risk for a gunshot to the neck or face that may cause immediate airway obstruction. All TMPs should keep airway devices that will enhance their ability to obtain and maintain an airway in these settings.

Ideally, TMPs are certified and prepared to provide an immediate surgical airway by performing a surgical cricothyrotomy. The tools needed include:

- An airway tube (ET tube)
- A sharp knife/scalpel
- A cricothyrotomy hook
- Betadine or alcohol skin prep

You must also be proficient in the use of many other airway devices, including intubation and proper ET tube placement, and blind insertion airways such as the King airway and Combitube. These procedures and indications are described in Chapter 14, "Advanced Airway Management."

Automated External Defibrillator

The automated external defibrillator (AED) is a medical treatment device that has been proven to save lives **Figure 4-18**. If a person suddenly collapses and is noted to be unresponsive and without a pulse, it is likely that person is experiencing a lethal abnormal electrical rhythm or cardiac arrhythmia.

Unfortunately, over the years there have been multiple sudden deaths from cardiac arrhythmias during SWAT unit training, annual physical training, and SWAT unit tryouts. In some instances, tactical officers overexerted themselves and then suffered a cardiac arrest due to a sudden heart attack or lethal arrhythmia, and they likely died a preventable death due to lack of an AED at the location of training. All fire and police agencies are well advised to bring an AED whenever there is physical training or significant physical exertion. In addition, there are occasional circumstances at SWAT callouts where a bystander or other person suffers a heart attack and collapses due to the stress.

Statistically, if a bystander or TMP properly uses an AED on a collapsed victim with ventricular tachycardia or fibrillation, there is an 80% chance of survival if the patient is shocked within 2 minutes of collapse. If the AED is not nearby and its use is delayed until 8 minutes after cardiac arrest, that person has only a 20% survival rate. There is a big difference in survival between 2 and 8 minutes; therefore the AED should be kept immediately available. *Note that this is a state-law required piece of equipment for most EMS and TEMS agencies.* In addition, nearly all fire trucks and rescue trucks carry AEDs, and many police agencies now routinely carry these in the trunks of their squad cars.

The only disadvantage is that the average AED is heavy at 6 to 12 pounds in weight, and this weight and bulk prevent the routine carrying of this device. Smaller units are available that may fit into a backpack. Indeed, the actual need for an AED inside of the inner perimeter is quite rare, and some feel that the best location is to keep it in a secure location nearby at the command center or in the standby ambulance. The patient can be urgently brought to that location, or someone can run and obtain the AED if needed. Some newer AED units are less than 2 pounds and may be more practical to carry.

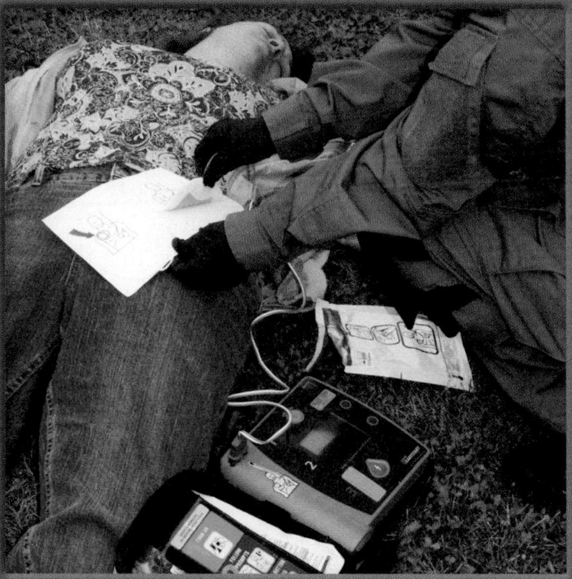

Oxygen Tanks

Most tactical medical emergencies can be handled without the use of oxygen. Tactical officers are generally very fit athletes, and if a gunshot wound occurs, the primary airway and breathing problems are mechanical, such as an obstructed airway or collapsed lung. Most of these patients can be ventilated with a 21% environmental oxygen level without any problems for the short duration of time it takes to reach a hospital or the ambulance. The risk-to-benefit ratio of bringing an oxygen tank inside of the outer perimeter is high, therefore it is usually not worth it.

A high-pressure oxygen tank is a risk for a lethal outcome as the pressure contained inside is often over 3,000 psi. This high pressure will cause a tremendous release of energy and, essentially, an explosion will occur if a bullet or metal explosion fragment strikes the tank and punctures it. The oxygen will also increase the risk of a flash fire with resultant burns.

The decision whether or not to carry oxygen into the tactical environment is dependent on the agency. The oxygen tank is usually kept at the command center or nearby ambulance and is not utilized in the tactical environment. If an elderly patient with chest pain or a severely asthmatic patient is encountered, the patient can either be moved to an ambulance or the oxygen can be brought to him or her in a safer location.

Stretchers and Extraction Gear

Extraction and rapid transportation of the critically injured tactical officer is one of the primary responsibilities

Figure 4-18 AEDs can save lives, and therefore all SWAT officers and TMPs must be familiar with their use. Keep an AED nearby for immediate use during all training activities and callouts.

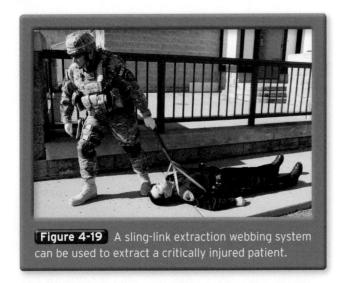

Figure 4-19 A sling-link extraction webbing system can be used to extract a critically injured patient.

of the TEMS unit **Figure 4-19**. After abolishing threats, the injured tactical officer may need to be rapidly moved out of harm's way to a point behind hard cover. There are many techniques and devices designed to extract and transport these patients. These include a simple body drag by grabbing the "drag handle" on the upper back of tactical vests; grabbing the downed tactical officer by an arm or foot and dragging him or her; using one-, two-, or four-man carries **Figure 4-20**; using webbing harness drags and carries; using stretchers (soft nylon, collapsible, semirigid, and rigid); and newer techniques such as attaching a short drag line to the TMP's belt

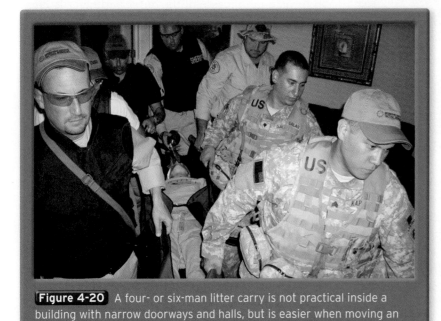

Figure 4-20 A four- or six-man litter carry is not practical inside a building with narrow doorways and halls, but is easier when moving an injured victim outside and across open terrain.

and attaching it to the downed tactical officer and dragging the tactical officer using the legs and lower body, allowing both hands to be free to provide armed response to any attackers. Having several gear options and techniques to use in extracting and transporting patients is ideal. Further discussion may be found in Chapter 16, "Extraction and Evacuation."

Field-Expedient Decontamination Equipment

TMPs should be prepared to perform emergency decontamination at all times. The unexpected booby trap of sulfuric acid spilled onto tactical officers or the accidentally discovered methamphetamine lab with caustic contamination may require rapid removal of the SWAT officer's gear and uniform followed by field expedient decontamination with plenty of water and possibly soap. A common garden hose and on-site arrangements for water and decontamination should be planned and prepared for in advance. Chapter 24, "Weapons of Mass Destruction," covers decontamination in detail.

Personal Dosimeters

Although statistically this might be considered an unlikely event, the threat of a radioactive material being placed next to a conventional explosion and scattering radioactive debris (a dirty bomb) in a large area is a modern reality. Tactical officers and TMPs may be able to detect many radioactive material threats by carrying a small (several inches) electronic, personal dosimeter on their load-bearing vest **Figure 4-21**. There are several varieties of these devices, and some of the more advanced units can actually "count" the amount of radiation that the wearer has been exposed to, thus indicating when a maximum recommended dose (exposure) has been reached. Those types of units are called personal dosimeters.

Another threat is the silent release or distribution of radioactive dust or other material in a large crowd, which would silently expose many to radiation. Use of a device such as the personal dosimeter may be the only way to notify authorities of the terrorist incident. A nuclear explosion would of course be devastating, and

TEMS units and other public safety officials would need to be able to detect and manage individuals who have radioactive dust particles contaminating their clothing, cars, and other personal items.

Additional Equipment to Consider

Surgical Equipment

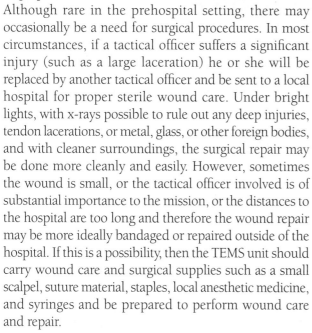

Figure 4-21 A personal dosimeter.

Although rare in the prehospital setting, there may occasionally be a need for surgical procedures. In most circumstances, if a tactical officer suffers a significant injury (such as a large laceration) he or she will be replaced by another tactical officer and be sent to a local hospital for proper sterile wound care. Under bright lights, with x-rays possible to rule out any deep injuries, tendon lacerations, or metal, glass, or other foreign bodies, and with cleaner surroundings, the surgical repair may be done more cleanly and easily. However, sometimes the wound is small, or the tactical officer involved is of substantial importance to the mission, or the distances to the hospital are too long and therefore the wound repair may be more ideally bandaged or repaired outside of the hospital. If this is a possibility, then the TEMS unit should carry wound care and surgical supplies such as a small scalpel, suture material, staples, local anesthetic medicine, and syringes and be prepared to perform wound care and repair.

Emergency Ultrasound

The modern, small, portable ultrasound machine can be used in many ways for emergency medical diagnosis and procedures. Portable ultrasound machines operate on battery and plug-in AC electrical current, and some models can be hooked up to a small laptop computer. Ultrasound is very safe to use, and can be used to detect intra-abdominal bleeding (ruptured spleen or liver, internal bleeding), cardiac tamponade, and congestive heart failure; evaluate for pulseless electrical activity (PEA), penetrating trauma, hemothorax, pneumothorax, foreign bodies, pregnancy complications, and deep vein blood clots; diagnose fractures; and assist with medical procedures (central IV lines, drainage of abscesses, joint aspiration), among many other uses.

Although the cost of a durable portable ultrasound unit is still in excess of $8,000, they are now less expensive than a standard EMS cardiac Lifepak 12 monitor and can be quite useful in assessing a patient with acute illness or injury. Increasingly, emergency medical professionals such as physicians, flight paramedics, and nurses use ultrasound in daily care. In large mass-casualty incidents (MCIs), emergency ultrasound has been used effectively and accurately to screen hundreds of people for severe trauma and triage in primitive prehospital conditions. The utility of this device in normal SWAT search warrants and simple incidents is limited due to the short transportation times, but for extended or remote operations, this device would be worthwhile to consider.

Metal Detector

The first priority of a tactical officer is to make the scene safe. When dealing with potential criminals, the suspect should be thoroughly searched for weapons before any medical care is initiated. The obvious knife or gun found in a front pocket is easy to identify and remove. What is more difficult to find is the small handcuff key or bobby pin sewn into the suspect's pant's posterior (the back surface of the body) beltline that is hidden and easily missed by a "pat-down" search, yet later may result in the death of a police officer transporting that suspect to jail. Even worse is the small hidden pistol that has been placed in the groin/crotch area of a male or female suspect—an area that some SWAT officers and TMPs may be hesitant to touch during the search due to social attitudes or stigmas. This is especially true when searching a suspect of the opposite gender. Allegations of sexual misconduct can stem from SWAT officers who search the groin area, and therefore proper technique and witnesses should be utilized to perform a thorough search.

Because of the wide variety of weapons, including keys, razor blades, hypodermic needles, bobby pins, and other threats, a handheld metal detector is a key piece of equipment that TMPs and tactical officers should utilize to thoroughly search suspects, hostages, or other persons who may represent a threat. The most optimal unit is a small, handheld, 9-volt battery-powered metal detector unit that does not "beep" or have a visible or auditory alarm. Instead, this vibratory metal detector wand is used by holding it about one-half inch away from the clothing of a suspect; when metal is detected, the device vibrates silently and gently **Figure 4-22**. This offers the tactical advantage of allowing the searching person to find objects, but does not inform the suspect that the object has been found.

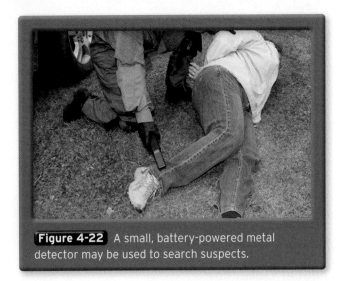

Figure 4-22 A small, battery-powered metal detector may be used to search suspects.

If a metal detector with an auditory alarm sounds, the suspect may realize that his or her weapon or "last-ditch" ability to escape has been detected. This may precipitate a violent struggle as the suspect attempts to obtain the gun, knife, or other weapon and escape. If a suspected weapon is detected silently, then the surrounding SWAT officers can quietly discuss this and use a safe tactic to appropriately remove the weapon.

Ready for Review

- The uniform and clothing worn by TMPs and tactical officers should be protective, comfortable during normal and extreme weather, and blend with the local environment. The proper selection of cold and hot weather clothing will enhance mission success.

- Insignia and individual identification may be used during training and for visualization during close conversation distance, but in general, should not be seen during a callout.

- Medical markings may increase the likelihood of being targeted and should be minimally visible.

- Extreme weather clothing and protective gear include a four-layer system of clothing during cold weather operations designed to wick away sweat and prevent unnecessary cooling and thus decrease cold injuries. Protective gloves, hats, gaiters, and balaclavas all have benefits and should be used when needed.

- Hot weather clothing is light, breathes easily, and also wicks away body perspiration.

- PPE carried by TMPs should be used appropriately for all patients. It is impossible to determine by external appearance which patients are carriers of bloodborne pathogens and which are not.

- Ballistic protective gear is essential for training and callouts, and includes body armor, helmets, face shields, and other equipment.

- The mission requirements and medical threats should guide the medical equipment and resources used. Medical gear should be attached or carried in a reliable, tactically quiet, secure method. This may include vest/belt/thigh pouches, backpacks, or a medical kit stored nearby for immediate access if needed.

- SWAT officers and TMPs should all have an IFAK on their person at all times.

Vital Vocabulary

air-purifying respirator (APR) A gas mask worn to filter particulates and contaminants from the air.

balaclava Black or camouflage-colored stocking-hat type of head cover that slips over the head and neck, covering the entire head except for the eyes, nose, and possibly mouth.

ballistic vest Designed to stop many types of bullets, help defeat shrapnel, and resist puncture by other projectiles; worn underneath other protective garments and gear.

cardiopulmonary resuscitation (CPR) mask A portable face mask used as a standard precaution to protect emergency care providers administering rescue breaths to a patient.

hard body armor inserts Rigid inserts made of steel, ceramics, aluminum, or titanium that are used for added frontal-torso protection in addition to soft body armor; available in threat protection Levels III and IV.

hemostatic agents Agents that assist with controlling bleeding by enabling the formation of a blood clot.

individual first aid kit (IFAK) A medical kit that contains the essential first aid supplies for a tactical officer or TMP, and is usually located on the vest or in a cargo pocket that is supposed to be carried in the same location.

infrared flashlight Device that emits infrared light, which is invisible to the human eye; may be used to illuminate an area, allowing SWAT and TEMS officers to discern the presence of objects and humans more than 400 yards away.

nasopharyngeal airway An airway adjunct inserted into the nostril of a casualty who is not able to maintain a viable airway.

night vision equipment Devices that enable humans to see in the dark, using infrared or ambient light to identify objects and people up to several hundred yards away.

nitrile gloves Inner gloves, made of synthetic latex. They are more durable and chemical-repellant than rubber gloves, and do not cause problems for officers or citizens with latex allergies.

personal protective equipment Protective equipment that OSHA requires to be made available to emergency medical providers. In the case of infection risk, PPE blocks entry of an organism into the body.

soft body armor A ballistic-resistant fabric worn concealed under the uniform or over the uniform, made from polyethylene fiber.

stab-resistant ballistic vest A vest designed to be resistant against puncture from knives, shanks, and other pointed or edged weapons.

tactical compression dressings Gauze that is already attached to elastic wrapping with prerigged cinching and fastening devices; should be vacuum-packed, sterile, lightweight, and easily deployed.

tactical personal protective equipment (TPPE) Personal protective equipment designed to protect TMPs from medical and violent threats in the tactical environment, including clear goggles, protective mask, nitrile gloves, and head and boot protection.

tactical tourniquet A medical device used to stop arterial and venous bleeding from the arms and legs (extremities) and compresses the blood vessels so that no blood flows distal to (past) the device, thus significantly slowing or stopping hemorrhage.

thermal imaging devices Electronic devices that detect differences in temperature based on infrared energy and then generate images based on those data; commonly used in obscured environments to locate victims and/or suspects.

Firearms Safety and Marksmanship

OBJECTIVES

- List the five rules of firearms safety.
- Describe the common types of handguns.
- Describe the characteristics of the pistol.
- Describe the characteristics of a long gun.
- Describe the common types of a long gun.
- List the four components of ammunition.
- Describe the common types of bullets.
- Describe the basics of firearm marksmanship.
- Describe how to secure a firearm from a downed SWAT officer or suspect.

Introduction

Tactical medical providers (TMPs) must be competent with firearms. You may already have significant proficiency from prior training and experience or you may be new to firearms. No matter what your level of experience is, as a TMP you must retain safe practices in weapons handling in order to be able to safely disarm downed officers and suspects when necessary. This chapter discusses the steps toward achievement of this goal.

Firearms safety training and familiarization first should be learned in the classroom by formal instruction, and then gradually learned and reinforced by hands-on, supervised instruction, followed by routine training and weapons use. At an appropriate time and place, advanced firearms skills incorporated into close quarters battle, scenario-based training can be learned and refined. During training and in the tactical environment, the five rules of firearms safety must always be adhered to.

1. Treat every weapon as though it is loaded. You must handle a gun in the same manner whether or not it is thought to be loaded.
2. Never touch the trigger unless you have decided to shoot.
3. Always keep the weapon pointed in a safe direction. Never point the gun at anything you do not want to destroy. Follow the "laser rule." Imagine that a laser beam is constantly projected down through the barrel. You should never allow that beam to point at any part of your body or at a person or an object that you do not want to shoot.
4. Always be certain of your target and the background behind the target.
5. Always maintain control of your firearm and prevent unauthorized persons from gaining access to the gun **Figure 5-1** .

The fifth rule cannot be stressed enough, as many accidents are caused when the owner of the firearm stores the gun in an unsecured location or indulges in a moment of carelessness that results in a tragedy. You must take steps to prevent unauthorized use, including choosing a secure snatch-resistant holster (for pistols); obeying the state laws and lawfully transporting and storing the weapon in an appropriate gun case; using a safe, child-resistant box with rapidly accessible combination lock; or securely locking the weapon in a gun safe either at the police station or at home. If all five rules are followed, with rare exception, unintentional injuries should be prevented.

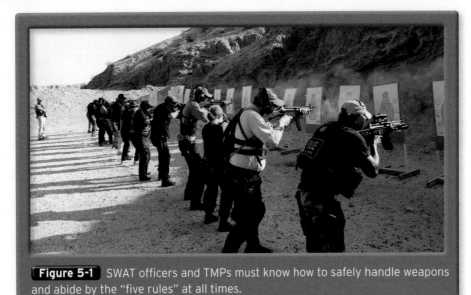

Figure 5-1 SWAT officers and TMPs must know how to safely handle weapons and abide by the "five rules" at all times.

Firearms Overview

The following sections briefly review the various types of firearms used by law enforcement, civilians, and criminals. In general, handguns are less powerful and less accurate than rifles, but they are more easily hidden (concealable) on the body. Handguns are used most often in officer-involved shootings, and are most likely the weapon you will face.

Safety

There are some powerful pistols that actually are nearly equivalent to rifles as they are designed for hunting and in fact shoot rifle-caliber ammunition.

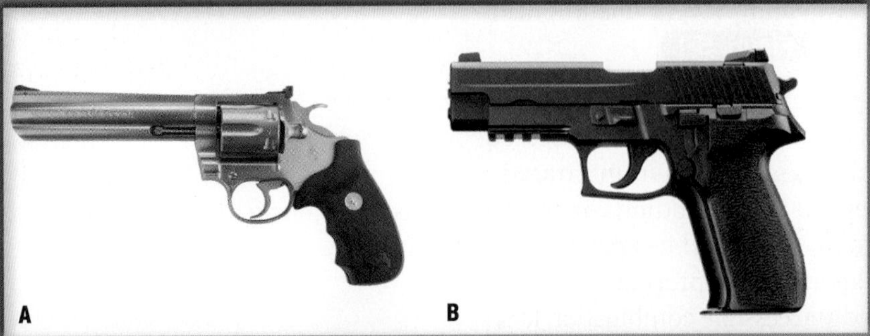

Figure 5-2 Two common types of handguns: (**A**) double-action revolver and (**B**) semiautomatic pistol.

Handguns

Handguns have short barrels and can be carried and fired with one hand. These firearms are usually easily concealable. The common forms are single- and double-action revolvers, semiautomatic pistols, and derringers **Figure 5-2**.

Revolvers have a cylinder that rotates and holds the rounds of ammunition. In a double-action revolver, the trigger may be pulled to first cock back the hammer; further pressure on the trigger will release the hammer, discharging the round of ammunition. Each pull of the double-action trigger will rotate the cylinder, allowing the next round of ammunition to be shot. It can also be fired in the same manner as a single-action revolver.

The single-action revolver ("cowboy handgun") may be cocked by using a thumb to pull back the hammer, which rotates the cylinder to bring a fresh round of ammunition in alignment with the barrel and cocks the gun **Figure 5-3**. The gun is now ready to fire and will discharge even with a slight squeeze of the trigger. The cylinder may rotate in either a clockwise or counterclockwise direction depending on the revolver's manufacturer. The single-action trigger pull is usually very consistent and light, and thus for most people it is more accurate than the double-action pistol.

Pistols are semiautomatic firearms and are the type most commonly used by law enforcement in the United States **Figure 5-4**. Pistols use either gas from a discharged round or recoil to extract and eject the spent case and to feed the next round into the chamber of the weapon. To chamber the initial round, the slide must be pulled back and then released, which strips off the top round of ammunition from the magazine and moves it forward into the chamber, ready to fire. Rounds of ammunition are fed from the magazine to the chamber. The magazine is usually a detachable part of the firearm that can be filled with rounds. Each time the gun is fired, it will eject the empty brass case, and then load the next

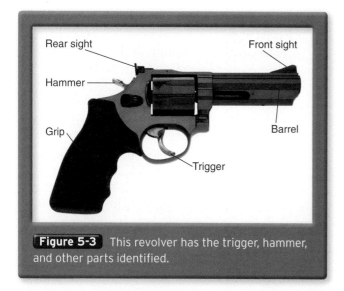

Figure 5-3 This revolver has the trigger, hammer, and other parts identified.

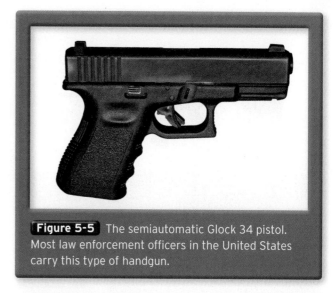

Figure 5-5 The semiautomatic Glock 34 pistol. Most law enforcement officers in the United States carry this type of handgun.

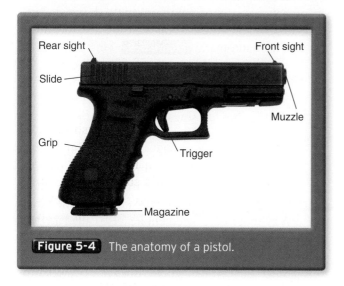

Figure 5-4 The anatomy of a pistol.

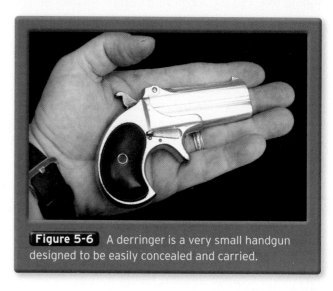

Figure 5-6 A derringer is a very small handgun designed to be easily concealed and carried.

live round of ammunition, making it ready to fire again. Pistols typically have removable magazines that can hold anywhere from 6 to 33 rounds of ammunition depending on the make, model, and caliber of the pistol. By comparison, revolvers store their ammunition in cylinders that only hold 5 to 10 rounds. Extended magazines are available for certain pistol weapon systems that can hold from 50 to 100 rounds of ammunition. An advantage of a pistol is the ability to reload the weapon with a full magazine in less than 2 seconds. Most police officers carry one magazine in the pistol plus two additional magazines on their utility belt **Figure 5-5**.

Derringers are very small handguns that traditionally have two barrels that are 1 to 4 inches in length **Figure 5-6**. The barrels are nearly parallel and are vertically adjacent. They are loaded at the breech end by "breaking-open" the gun at a hinge point. Each barrel

can be loaded with one round at a time, and a separate trigger pull is required to fire each round. These guns are not used by law enforcement officers as primary weapons but are sometimes carried as a backup or as an off-duty weapon. The ease with which these guns can be concealed makes them attractive to criminals and therefore dangerous to TMPs. A thorough search for weapons, even in suspects who have already been searched by others and are in restraints, is always a good idea prior to initiating medical care, if permitted by your law enforcement agency. Follow your local law enforcement protocols and procedures.

Long Guns

Long guns come in several forms. **Rifles** are long-barreled firearms that usually require two hands to operate, are

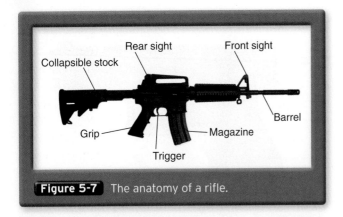

Figure 5-7   The anatomy of a rifle.

shoulder-fired, and have a barrel with rifling **Figure 5-7**. Rifling refers to the longitudinal spiral grooves on the inside of the barrel that are designed to impart spin to a bullet. This spin stabilizes the bullet during flight, thus increasing its accuracy. The rate of twist of the spiral rifling can vary and affect the bullet performance. Rifles come in a variety of styles, which differ in the way they feed ammunition into the chamber. They include single-shot, automatic, semiautomatic, lever-action, bolt-action, and pump-action rifles **Figure 5-8**. Rifles have the advantage of being more accurate and more powerful, and often will have a magazine that contains up to 30 rounds of ammunition. Certain models are capable of utilizing high capacity magazines that contain 20 to 100 rounds. They can be held with two hands and stabilized by placing the stock against the shoulder and the face or cheek near the officer's line of sight, allowing for a more accurate shooting platform.

- **Automatic rifles**. These shoot continuous rounds of ammunition "automatically" whenever the trigger is pressed and held down until the magazine runs out of ammunition. The number of rounds per minute varies. For example, the M-16 rifle on full auto will empty a 30-round magazine in less than 1.5 seconds. There is often a selector switch, usually the safety, which will allow the user to select safe, semiauto, 3-shot burst, or full auto. Fully automatic rifles and short rifles that shoot pistol-calibers known as submachine guns are usually used by law enforcement agencies and military forces. Most automatic rifles offer the option of mounting additional equipment such as night-vision sights, lasers, flashlights, bayonets, slings, and suppressors. Modern law enforcement agencies are increasingly buying and using automatic rifles as patrol rifles for patrol officers or for SWAT officers. It is possible for a

civilian to own an automatic rifle, but it requires a special license, a thorough background check, registration, finger printing, and license fees.

- **Semiautomatic sporting rifles**. These shoot one round each time the trigger is pressed but automatically reload the next round after each one is fired. The trigger must be released between firing rounds.
- **Carbines**. These are compact rifles with a shorter than normal barrel, usually less than 20 inches long. Carbines are often used by military forces that travel in tanks or other small vehicles. Carbines have the advantage of fairly reliable firepower in a compact weapon that is more easily carried than a full-size rifle.
- **Shotguns**. These are smooth-barreled long guns that fire a variety of ammunition and come in a variety of actions, including single-shot, side by side, over and under, bolt-action, pump-action, and semiautomatic **Figure 5-9**. Most shotgun barrels are removable and are smooth bored. There are also special rifled shotgun barrels for applications such as deer hunting with single-projectile shotgun slugs and sabot rounds.
  - The bore of a shotgun barrel is usually made with a constriction, or choke, toward the muzzle. The choke shapes the grouping of shot as the shot leaves the barrel and will narrow the spread of the shotgun pellets as they travel toward the target. A cylinder-bore-sized choke (also called an open choke) is actually no choke at all because the bore is the same diameter from breech to muzzle. Since the cylinder choke does not constrict the shot load at all, the shot scatters more than with any other choke.
  - The improved cylinder choke mildly constricts the shot group just before it leaves the barrel, producing a tighter (closer together) pattern of holes in the target. The modified or improved-modified chokes constrict the shot group even further, producing an even tighter target pattern.
  - The full or extra-full chokes keep the shot group tightly together as it leaves the barrel, producing the tightest (most narrow) target pattern. Some shotguns can be fitted with an adjustable choke or multiple choke sizes.

Firearm Caliber

The **caliber** of a firearm is the approximate diameter of the bullet used. Caliber is measured in inches and millimeters for rifles and pistols and in **gauge** for shotguns. When the barrel diameter is given in inches, the abbreviation

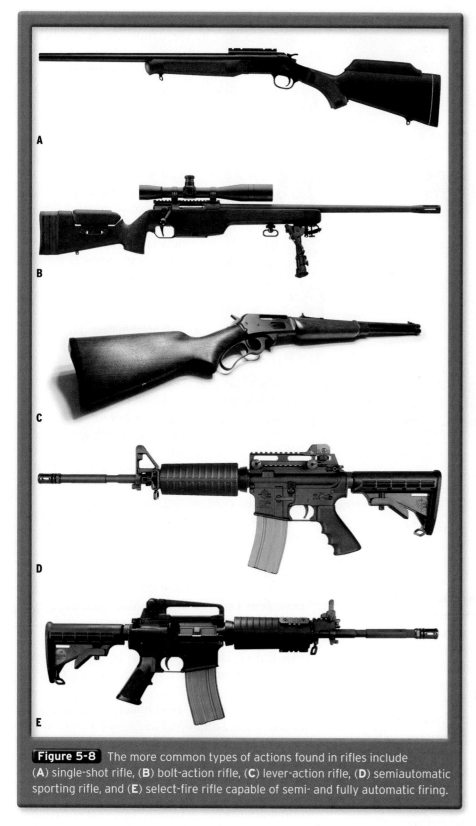

Figure 5-8 The more common types of actions found in rifles include (**A**) single-shot rifle, (**B**) bolt-action rifle, (**C**) lever-action rifle, (**D**) semiautomatic sporting rifle, and (**E**) select-fire rifle capable of semi- and fully automatic firing.

also be referred to in millimeters, as in a bullet diameter of 9 millimeters, or 9-mm pistol.

Metric calibers for small arms are usually expressed with an "×" between the width and the length; for example, 7.62 × 51 NATO. This indicates that a bullet with a diameter of 7.62 mm is loaded in a cartridge case 51 mm long, which is commonly used by the NATO (North Atlantic Treaty Organization) countries. The same firearm can be referred to by its caliber and manufacturer: .308 Winchester.

Common calibers of rifle ammunition used by law enforcement are the .223 Remington (5.56 × 45 mm) in the Colt AR-15 and M-4 style rifles, and the .308 (7.62 × 51 mm NATO) used in marksman rifles. Common pistol calibers used by law enforcement include 9 mm, .357 Sig, .40 Smith and Wesson, and .45 ACP. You should become familiar with your team's weapons by going to a shooting range and using them until you become proficient.

Ammunition

It is important to be knowledgeable about the types of ammunition that may strike a suspect, a bystander, or a SWAT officer. A simplified explanation of the four components of firearm ammunition follows **Figure 5-10** :

- A **round** of ammunition is a functional combination of a cartridge case, propellant, primer, and one or more projectiles (bullets).
- The cartridge case has a primer, which is struck by a firing pin when the trigger

cal (for caliber) is used in place of inches. For example, a rifle with a diameter of 0.22 inch is a .22 cal; however, the decimal point is generally eliminated when spoken, as in a twenty-two caliber rifle. Calibers of weapons can

is pulled, igniting the main charge of smokeless propellant (ie, gunpowder) that pushes the bullet down the barrel and through the muzzle of the firearm. Some weapons use a special type

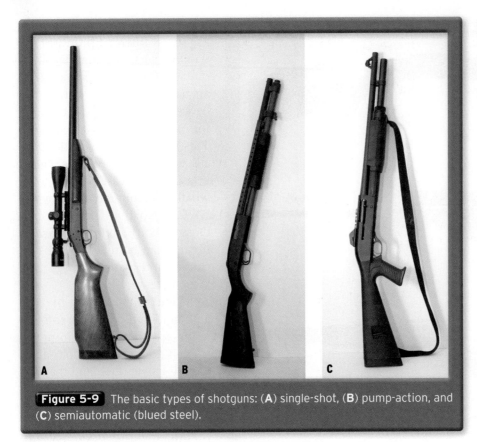

Figure 5-9 The basic types of shotguns: (**A**) single-shot, (**B**) pump-action, and (**C**) semiautomatic (blued steel).

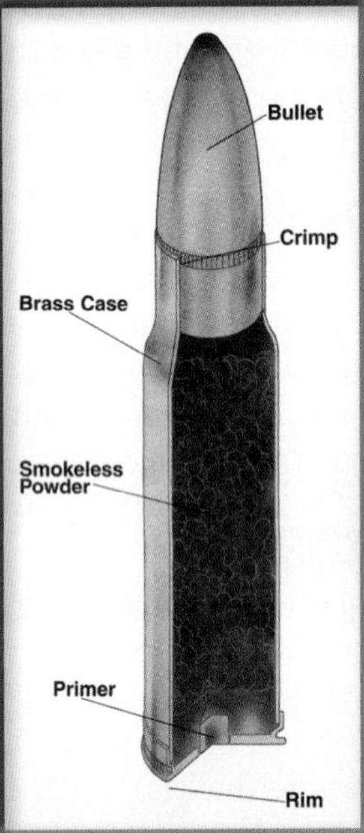

Figure 5-10 There are four parts to a round of ammunition: bullet, propellant, primer, and cartridge case.

that is shot through the muzzle by the ignition of the propellant and resultant expanding gases. Bullets come in many forms. The following are the most common:

- **Full metal case or full metal jacket bullets.** The entire lead core is surrounded by a metal case that does not expand significantly, causing enhanced perforation and deeper penetration. These bullets are often used by the military. Some of these bullets may even have a steel core designed to pierce armor.

- **Soft point bullets.** The front portion of the lead core is exposed, with the copper jacket covering the sides and base of the bullet. These bullets are designed for hunting animals as they have increased expansion with a greater transfer of energy and less penetration into the body.

- **Hollow point or expanding bullets.** The front of the bullet is hollow to facilitate expansion and reduce penetration, thus increasing the transfer of energy, which increases the stopping power of the projectile. The outer copper jacket is often prestressed or thinned so that the bullet will expand in a reliable fashion. When the bullet is fired into a body, it expands, transfers energy, and creates a larger hole. Some bullets have a plastic tip in this hollow space that increases the speed and accuracy of the bullet and helps with expansion.

- **Fragmenting bullets.** These bullets are designed to disintegrate on impact and transfer all their energy into the object struck. These bullets are used when over-penetration or ricochet of a bullet is not desirable. These bullets have the advantage of increased stopping power when shooting criminal suspects, with less likelihood of harming citizens in the background with an exiting or ricocheting bullet.

- **Wadcutter or semiwadcutter bullets.** These have a flat or conical tip with a body that is semirectangular in profile. They are designed to leave a clean, circular

of bullet called a .22-caliber rimfire, which consists of a bullet, powder, and a cartridge case that has a layer of material spun into the rim that contains primer material.

- A shotgun round is also called a shell. It has an additional component called the wadding, which is a plastic or paper divider between the propellant and the lead pellets or other projectile(s).

Bullets are the portion of the round

Safety

Special plastic hollow bullets filled with paint or brightly colored liquid soap that mark the location of the bullet "hit" are manufactured for use by tactical officers when conducting simulated force-on-force training **Figure 5-11**. Products include Simunitions and Force-on-Force.

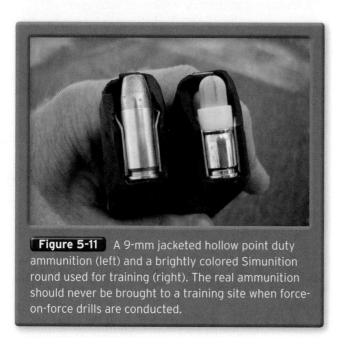

Figure 5-11 A 9-mm jacketed hollow point duty ammunition (left) and a brightly colored Simunition round used for training (right). The real ammunition should never be brought to a training site when force-on-force drills are conducted.

hole in a paper target. They are usually composed of lead and are used as target rounds.

- **Round-nosed lead bullets**. These bullets are solid lead with a rounded, more aerodynamic nose than semiwadcutter bullets. They are also used for target shooting.

Shotgun Ammunition

Shotgun ammunition is commonly called a shotgun shell, and is manufactured in a variety of types and sizes. The most common is lead shot, or birdshot, and varies from very small pellets, to BB-sized turkey-hunting shot, to pea-sized buckshot, or may be a single projectile called a slug or sabot round. More than 100 pellets are held in a small birdshot shell such as No. 8 shot, while there are only 9 or 12 pellets in 12-gauge OO (double-ought) buckshot in 2¾- and 3-inch shells. Shot size is measured in hundredths of an inch, and each size is referred to by a number. Following the archaic and somewhat confusing system of shotgun terminology, the larger the number, the smaller the shot. The smallest lead shot is No. 12, measuring 0.05 inch in diameter.

The next size larger is No. 9, measuring 0.08 inch in diameter. Then come Nos. 8½, 8, 7½, 6, 5, 4, 2, 1, BB, T, and F, which measures 0.22 inch.

A separate category of larger shot is called buckshot, which uses a different numbering system. The smallest buckshot size is No. 4, which measures 0.24 inches in diameter. In order of increasing size, the designations are No. 4, No. 3, No. 2, No. 1, 0, 00 (double-ought), and 000 (triple-ought) buckshot. No. 4 buckshot is slightly larger than .22 caliber. Imagine shooting 21 lead or steel balls in a single shot, each one a little bigger in diameter than a .22 caliber bullet. The four largest sizes of buckshot are comparable to rifle or pistol calibers. The largest size, No. 000, measures .36 caliber, or a 0.36-inch diameter.

There are a variety of **slugs** or single-bullet projectiles that may be fired from shotguns. The simple lead bullet may be a single 1-ounce lead slug; this bullet carries tremendous power and is often used for deer hunting. Also, there are smaller single projectiles that may be sandwiched between two plastic sabot pieces that break free from the sabot bullet, which then travels with greater accuracy and higher speed. The shotgun shell casing is the plastic container that holds the other components, including primer, propellant, shot cup, and shot or slug. Some shot components include tungsten or bismuth metal, which is heavier than steel shot commonly used for duck hunting. Specialty rounds for shotguns include breaching rounds (used for defeating door locks, and for shooting the hinges off doors during entry by SWAT units), **flechettes** (small nail-like projectiles that are used in some military applications), exploding incendiary devices (for signaling or for scaring off birds), **flares** (bright balls of fire that are fired into the air for emergency signaling), and less-lethal rubber bullets or lead-shot bean bags **Figure 5-12**.

Shotgun Gauge

Shotgun gauge is not measured in hundredths of an inch or in millimeters, as are rifle and handgun bore, with one exception. The bore of a shotgun is measured by gauge. Shotgun gauge is calculated by the number of pure lead balls the exact size of that shotgun's bore that it would take to weigh 1 pound. Modern shotguns come in 10-, 12-, 16-, 20-, 28-gauge, and .410. The .410 actually is a caliber designation and is the only exception to the gauge measuring system. The smaller the gauge number, the bigger the bore, since fewer balls are needed to weigh one pound. For example, it would take 12 lead balls the size of the 12-gauge barrel to equal 1 pound of weight. The most common shotgun in the United States is the 12 gauge.

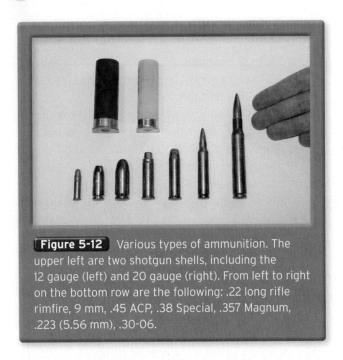

Figure 5-12 Various types of ammunition. The upper left are two shotgun shells, including the 12 gauge (left) and 20 gauge (right). From left to right on the bottom row are the following: .22 long rifle rimfire, 9 mm, .45 ACP, .38 Special, .357 Magnum, .223 (5.56 mm), .30-06.

Bullet Weight

The weight of a bullet is measured by the term **grains**. A common weight of a pistol bullet, such as the 9-mm pistol, is 124 grains. The grain is based on the ancient weight of 1 grain of wheat, where 7,000 grains = 1 pound, and 1 gram = 15.4 grains.

Some handgun cartridges are designed to make a handgun similar to a small shotgun, and shoot a type of ammunition called a **shotshell**. These are designed to function by firing a number of very small bullets in one cartridge, sometimes called snake shot, as they are used for shooting snakes and other pests in some areas of the country.

Accuracy and Range of Bullets

The accuracy and range of different types of ammunition vary greatly and depend on many factors. A .22 rimfire 40-grain bullet can travel over a mile if fired at a 45-degree angle. However, the shotgun pellet that is size 8 (small birdshot) has much less power and range, and will not travel beyond several hundred yards. Rifle bullets from a .308 and .30-06 have accurately struck and killed soldiers at a distance in excess of 1,000 yards.

The accuracy of a shot depends on many factors such as the type of bullet used, the inherent accuracy of the rifle, the velocity of the projectile, the weather conditions, and the skill of the shooter. Rifles have a much greater potential for accuracy over longer distances than handguns. A skilled rifle shooter can accurately and consistently hit a man-sized target at over a mile distance (over 5,280 feet). Common rifle calibers include the 5.56 mm (M-16), the .223 caliber (civilian AR-15), the .270 caliber, the .30-06, the 7.62 mm (M-60 machine gun), and the .308 caliber (sniper round). A common and less expensive round used for hunting small game and for informal target shooting is the .22 long rifle cartridge. It propels a small 40-grain bullet at a fairly high speed (1,300 feet per second) and is capable of penetrating most parts of the human body and potentially causing serious injury and/or death.

Shotshells contain a variety of sizes and numbers of small pieces of "shot." Buckshot can be expected to spread out in a pattern roughly 1 inch per yard traveled. Buckshot retains more of its velocity, and the shot pattern is more concentrated over a longer distance than smaller bird shot. This is a common type of ammunition used by police in shotguns and is also used by deer hunters in the southern United States. Birdshot loses velocity quickly, and the pattern spread tends to be wide. Birdshot may produce serious wounds at close ranges of 10 to 20 feet or less, but loses its energy quickly when shot from over 60 yards away. Heavy clothing may stop birdshot at distances of 50 feet.

You should know the common types of weapons found in your region as well as your tactical team's firearms. Familiarity with types of bullets and other projectiles, energy, the type of round, and the likely path of the bullet while traversing the body may allow you to determine the types of possible injury. The next section discusses the skills and methods to accurately strike a target through the use of a firearm.

Marksmanship

Marksmanship is the acquired ability to shoot a firearm and accurately place a bullet or other projectile into a target **Figure 5-13**. All law enforcement officers are required to complete a basic firearms course as well as maintain a certain level of proficiency tested against department-mandated qualifications. As a TMP, you may or may not be authorized and trained in marksmanship, but in general, you will likely shoot alongside SWAT officers and other TEMS providers during your monthly SWAT training.

Safety

Each police department has training officers who are valuable resources for future training to improve your skills.

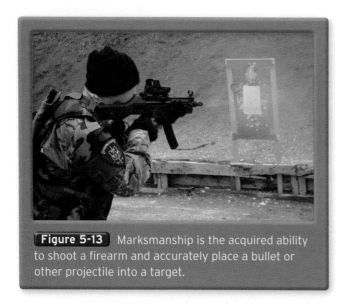

Figure 5-13 Marksmanship is the acquired ability to shoot a firearm and accurately place a bullet or other projectile into a target.

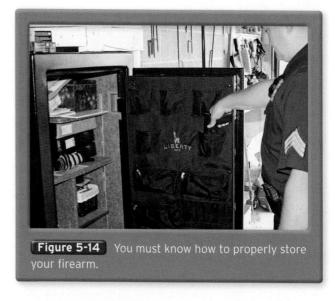

Figure 5-14 You must know how to properly store your firearm.

The ability to hit a target with any type of weapon is often critical to the safe and successful resolution of the mission. Most of us will never be involved in a real gunfight. For the unfortunate few who do end up involved in a life-or-death gunfight, having the skills to use good tactics, shoot accurately and efficiently, retain the ability to think and not panic, move quickly, and seek hard cover may very well make the difference between living and dying.

Handgun Safety

As a TMP, you may or may not be authorized to arm yourself for self-defense. If you are authorized to be armed, it will likely be a semiautomatic pistol; therefore, this section will mainly focus on the essential skill set of safely handling and accurately shooting this type of weapon.

Whether training at the range or engaged in a real-world callout, always practice the five safety rules of firearm handling. Especially when the weapon is drawn and SWAT officers are moving up through the alley to approach a house, or when entering and searching buildings, you must keep the weapon pointed in a safe direction at all times. Muzzle awareness is extremely important. If you flash point other SWAT officers or TEMS providers here and there, either during training or during real events, that will quickly earn you disrespect as an unsafe novice. Even if you happen to be one of the best shots on the team, inappropriate and unsafe weapons handling will lead to revoking your weapons and even dismissal from the TEMS unit.

Safety

Equipment such as the holster, duty belt, and accessories such as handcuff cases, magazine holder, ASP, and other gear should be squared away and coordinated so that use of the pistol is not obstructed or limited. Arrange for appropriate gear, and practice, practice, practice. Find out about the flaws and shortcomings at the firing range, not on the streets. Discover and address your weaknesses during practice, not during actual operations.

Choose the Right Weapon

The choice of handgun is an important decision. The majority of officers choose a quality semiautomatic pistol with several magazines. US law enforcement officers typically carry a 9-mm, .40- or .45-caliber pistol as their primary handgun. Each person has unique hand size and style preference, and there are hundreds of types of handguns to choose from. Some departments may limit or issue the pistol allowed. Regardless of the weapon used, you should become familiar with the weapon, learning how to maintain, clean, and store it properly **Figure 5-14**. Use high-quality ammunition and avoid getting oils, perspiration, water, or other contaminants on the ammunition.

Practice

Most handguns are incredibly accurate. If the handgun is aimed at the target, the trigger is pulled, and the shot is released without moving the pistol, then the bullet will strike the target. The tricky part is getting this to happen in the middle of a combat situation with life-or-death decisions and constantly changing targets.

Proper training and practice will ensure that your skills continually improve. In order to excel in close quarters battle, practice shooting while moving under the trained eye of experienced instructors. Learn to move quickly to cover, shoot on the move, and shoot behind cover. Learn how to scan 360 degrees, all around, and then low and high. Learn how to perform malfunction drills when your gun jams. Learn how to perform speed reloads under all conditions. Learn how to shoot weak-handed, kneeling, lying down, underneath cars, and in the dark with flashlights. Learn how to keep shooting even after you are shot and knocked to the ground. The list of skills and tactics to learn is long. Continue learning and make practice a part of your routine, just like exercise.

Securing a Firearm

Downed SWAT Officer Firearm Security

The threat of firearms is always present during tactical operations, regardless of whether they are discharged by SWAT officers or suspects using them unlawfully. An unintentional discharge could cause a bullet to strike a SWAT officer or TEMS provider. Bullets may unintentionally travel through walls and strike a SWAT officer on the other side. For example, a SWAT callout approximately 10 years ago resulted in a SWAT officer being shot and killed at the back of a house when the tactical team marksman shot a suspect who exited the front door. The bullet struck the suspect and then traveled through several walls; tragically, it struck the SWAT officer who was getting ready to enter the house from the rear.

SWAT officers who are severely injured, cannot breathe properly, are in shock from heavy bleeding, or are confused from a head injury may become involved in an unintentional shooting. Due to confusion, the SWAT officer may be unable to make appropriate decisions. If disoriented and lying on the ground severely injured, the downed SWAT officer may shoot reflexively at an approaching SWAT officer or TMP, mistakenly believing that the looming figure approaching is a threat.

Because of this risk, you must cautiously approach and immediately assess the mental status of all injured or ill tactical officers (Chapter 11, "Tactical Patient Assessment," discusses the patient assessment process

in detail). The existing scene threats should also be taken into account (eg, Are there more suspects in the building who have yet to be apprehended, or are all suspects neutralized and the situation resolved?). If the SWAT officer needs to remain armed and appears alert and oriented, he or she should be allowed to retain weapons. However, any serious injury or altered mental status should precipitate the removal of all weapons from the downed SWAT officer.

What is the best way to remove a SWAT officer's weapons? An established protocol with your SWAT unit may dictate the procedure. Follow your agency's protocols and procedures. Ideally, a fellow SWAT officer should remove the weapons, and you should focus on patient assessment and medical treatment.

With every method of firearm security, the five rules of firearms safety absolutely must be adhered to.

1. Assume every gun is loaded and treat accordingly.
2. Keep your finger off of the trigger unless you are firing the weapon.
3. Never point the gun at anything you do not want to destroy. When handing the weapon off to a SWAT officer, ensure that the muzzle is pointed in a safe direction.
4. If a sudden threat should appear, make sure of your target and your background.
5. Maintain control of the firearm(s).

There are several ways of removing and securing weapons from downed SWAT officers. One method is to simply switch the firearm safety level to "safe" and pass the weapon off to a SWAT officer. Another method is for you or a SWAT officer to:

1. Safely remove the weapon, keeping the barrel pointed in a safe direction and making sure that the safety selector switch is on "safe." The downed SWAT officer's hand and fingers should be away from the weapon and trigger.

Safety

Routine training with the entire SWAT unit teaches SWAT officers that if they are injured, they will be expected to continue to fight and win. If they are critically injured and clearly unable to effectively fight, their weapons will be removed in most instances. If any serious difficulties arise in the tactical environment, the critically injured SWAT officer should allow a well-trusted and known SWAT officer or TMP to remove and secure his or her weapons.

> **Safety**
>
> You must be knowledgeable and skilled in handling and making safe each type of weapon carried by the SWAT unit. These include the SWAT unit's long rifles, shotguns, submachine guns, pistols, backup weapons, knives, grenade launchers, pepperball guns, TASERs, smoke grenades, gas munitions, distraction devices, explosive entry materials, and other weapons.

> **Safety**
>
> A "blue-on-blue" shooting involves a law enforcement officer mistakenly shooting another law enforcement officer, thinking the other is a suspect with a gun. This happens too often, and is always a tragedy.

2. Completely remove the magazine from the firearm.
3. Open the action and eject the round of ammunition out of the chamber.
4. Lock open the action so that the firearm is completely unloaded before handing it off.

The weapon should be pointed in a safe direction while being passed to a SWAT officer who can safely store and secure the weapons. If the downed SWAT officer's gun was discharged in the incident, then the firearm and ammunition and nearby empty shell casings are all evidence and should be treated accordingly. All weapons and ammunition and their location should be noted, tracked, and a chain of custody should be maintained.

Suspect Firearm Security

A suspect who is injured or has been placed in the prone position and handcuffed should still be considered a significant threat until he or she has been thoroughly searched for handcuff keys (or facsimile) and weapons. Suspects often carry multiple weapons, and therefore they should be searched thoroughly for knives, razor blades, guns, hypodermic needles, and other hazards. You cannot be reasonably certain that a suspect is unarmed until after you have conducted a careful search, ideally with a metal detector wand.

It goes without saying that all firearms should be removed during your search. It may be handled in the standard manner if you are familiar with the weapon. If you are uncertain, then simply keep the weapon pointed in a safe direction with your finger off the trigger, and either hand it off to a SWAT officer, or place it on a secure, flat table nearby while pointed away from any others. Designate a SWAT officer to take possession of the weapon for evidence purposes. If the suspect has a gun removed, then the search should continue, including looking for a second or third gun, knife, or other weapon.

Ready for Review

- The five rules of firearms safety absolutely must be adhered to:
  - Assume every gun is loaded and treat accordingly.
  - Keep your finger off the trigger unless you are firing the weapon.
  - Never point the gun at anything you do not want to destroy.
  - Always make certain of your target and your background before firing, especially if a threat should suddenly appear.
  - Maintain control of the firearm(s).

- Handguns are used most often in officer-involved shootings, and are most likely the weapons you will face.

- Pistols are semiautomatic firearms and are the type most commonly used by law enforcement in the United States. Pistols use a magazine and can be rapidly reloaded.

- Rifles are long-barreled firearms that usually require two hands to operate, are shoulder-fired, and have a barrel with rifling. Rifles are more accurate and more powerful than most handguns and frequently can utilize higher capacity magazines.

- The accuracy of a shot depends on many factors such as the type of bullet used, the inherent accuracy of the rifle, the velocity of the projectile, the weather conditions, and the skill of the shooter. Rifles have a much greater potential for accuracy over longer distances than handguns.

- Marksmanship is the acquired ability to shoot a firearm and accurately place a bullet or other projectile into a target.

- The threat of firearms is always present during tactical operations, regardless of whether they are discharged by SWAT officers or suspects using them unlawfully. Therefore, you must be knowledgeable and skilled in handling and making safe each type of weapon carried by the SWAT unit.

Vital Vocabulary

caliber The measurement of the inside diameter of the barrel of a firearm; may be measured in hundredths of an inch or millimeters.

derringers Small, concealable pistols with one or two barrels, usually loaded by a hinge-style, break-open breech; named after a famous nineteenth century pocket pistol maker, Henry Deringer.

flares Bright bursts of light used to communicate or illuminate; used in shotguns and survival pistols to mark a position.

flechettes Pointed steel projectiles with an appearance of a small nail and with small tails for stable flight; used in shotguns and other weapons in the military.

gauge The diameter of a shotgun barrel.

grains Weight unit used for measuring bullets; the heavier the bullet, the larger the grains.

handguns Firearms designed to be held and operated with one hand.

marksmanship Acquired ability to shoot a firearm and accurately place a bullet or other projectile into the target.

pistols Handguns that do not hold ammunition in a revolving cylinder.

revolvers Handguns with a revolving cylinder that rotates and holds rounds of ammunition.

rifles Firearms designed to be fired from the shoulder, with a barrel that has a helical groove or pattern of grooves and lands cut into the barrel that increase the accuracy of the bullet.

round The entire unit that consists of a case that holds the propellant, primer, and the bullet.

shotshell A self-contained cartridge loaded with shot or a slug designed to be fired from a shotgun.

slugs Large bullets typically fired from a shotgun; primarily used for hunting deer or other large animals.

Conventional Threats and Weapons

OBJECTIVES

- Describe the common tactics of criminal suspects.

- Describe edged weapons and the threat posed to tactical medical providers.

- Describe the threat of firearms to tactical medical providers.

- Describe the types of conventional explosives and the threat posed to tactical medical providers.

- Describe the threat of booby traps to tactical medical personnel.

Introduction

There are many dangers faced by SWAT and TEMS units. This chapter describes the essential threats that may be encountered by tactical medical providers (TMPs). These are discussed in hopes that awareness, along with recognition and countermeasures, will prevent harm from occurring to those who respond to critical incidents.

Each year, over 160 law enforcement officers are killed in the line of duty in the United States. Thousands more suffer significant injuries that result in permanent physical and mental disability. To comprehend the seriousness of this problem, multiply these figures by the number of spouses, children, family members, and friends who are negatively affected by these deaths and injuries. Because of the consequences, it is critical to maintain constant vigilance and anticipate the threats posed by suspects and by accidents, such as motor vehicle crashes.

The solution to countering the criminal threat is not simple, but for SWAT officers and TEMS providers, part of the answer is to become highly educated about criminal tactics and techniques. Survival means being constantly vigilant, protecting yourself and your teammates, wearing appropriate protective gear, completing searches, not trusting anyone who appears to be a bystander or hostage, and always keeping a 360-degree situational awareness for threats. Survival means trusting your intuition (gut instinct) and acting on it appropriately. Chapter 8, "Self Defense and Close Quarters Battle," covers survival tactics in detail. Once properly trained, your intuition about others and the immediate surroundings can be quite accurate. If in doubt or if something does not seem right, immediate action should be taken to create distance between yourself and the threat, to seek cover, or to gather more information before proceeding further. Only then can you decide what the next appropriate action should be.

This chapter reviews a multitude of conventional threats and unique situations faced by TMPs. Some threats can be blocked or prevented with appropriate training and protective equipment. Some threats will be difficult to stop no matter what the warning. Some threats cannot be defeated, but these situations are rare. A substantial number of threats can be anticipated and defeated by knowledge, skill, and equipment. It is up to you to not only obtain a solid education about techniques and devices utilized by alleged perpetrators, but also to continually learn about newer threats and criminal tactics. This can be achieved by routine reading, training, Internet updates, continuing education, seminars, conferences, and learning from the mistakes of others. This knowledge saves lives.

The Human Body and Mind

Criminal Tactics

Tactical medical (TEMS) units must be aware of criminal tactics. Unfortunately, the modern criminal justice system is not perfect, and when a criminal is placed in a jail, he or she often learns *more* about crime. During incarceration, criminals network with other criminals, learning additional criminal techniques, street-fighting skills, and ways to disarm and harm law enforcement officers. Many inmates lift weights so that they are better able to protect themselves in prison, and also to be successful when fighting others once they get out of prison. The modern criminal is a potent adversary who should be taken seriously and never underestimated.

When supporting law enforcement units, most situations are resolved with minimal interaction between the TMP and the uninjured suspect. However, this changes when the suspect is injured. As the TMP, you are required to communicate with and be within touching distance of the suspect to perform a physical examination. If the suspect is significantly injured, you will likely accompany the suspect to the hospital in the confined space of the back of an ambulance. Every encounter provides an opportunity for the suspect to lash out and potentially harm you. Although the list of possible threats is too long to be thoroughly covered here, **Table 6-1** discusses some of the most common criminal tactics. The human mind is creative, thus you must always be aware and beware **Figure 6-1**.

Criminal Suspect Weapons Issues

Criminals use multiple concealed carry tricks that allow pistols, knives, and other weapons to be carried in jackets, vests, undershirts, purses, the groin area, on the ankle, inside shoes, under the arm, in fanny packs, and even in baseball hats. Often criminals illegally carry their handgun at the front of their body tucked into their pants, usually without a holster. Note this fact, remain wary of additional hidden carry locations (such as tucked in between the legs, ankle holsters, inside boots, inside bras, under false bottoms of purses, inside large hairdos, in large books that have

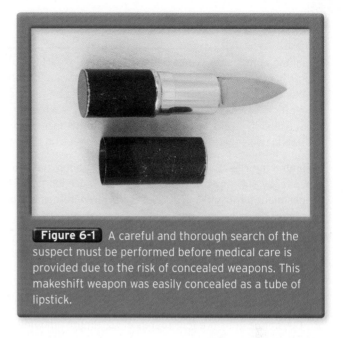

Figure 6-1   A careful and thorough search of the suspect must be performed before medical care is provided due to the risk of concealed weapons. This makeshift weapon was easily concealed as a tube of lipstick.

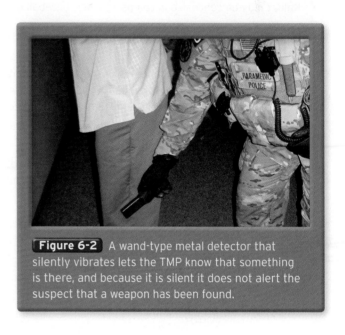

Figure 6-2   A wand-type metal detector that silently vibrates lets the TMP know that something is there, and because it is silent it does not alert the suspect that a weapon has been found.

the pages carved out), and search patients thoroughly before any medical care is provided. SWAT officers should arrest and handcuff suspects and then search them before allowing you to administer medical care. If you do not observe the search directly, you should assume that it was not fully completed and perform the search again. A handheld metal detector can be very helpful in performing a thorough search **Figure 6-2**. Do not completely rely on this device, however, because it cannot detect weapons made of plastic or composite materials **Figure 6-3**.

Table 6-1   Criminal Tactics

Feigning compliance. While being arrested, criminals will often hide their pistols by tucking them into the front of their pants beneath their shirt. Arresting officers, unaware of this hidden gun, may make the criminal turn and put his or her hands against the wall. The suspect may seem to be fully compliant, so the officer may let down his or her guard a bit. The officer places a handcuff around one hand, reaches for the other hand, when the suspect grabs the hidden gun and shoots blindly over the shoulder directly into the face of the officer. In 2007, two Texas deputies were killed in the same month in two separate incidents by ex-convicts using this technique.

Feigning injuries. Suspects pretend to have abdominal pain or injured extremities, knowing that they will be taken to a hospital by only one or two armed guards, which increases their chance of successfully escaping from the emergency department or hospital. In 2009, several law enforcement officers, doctors, and nurses in California were shot by prison escapees doing exactly this.

Hiding weapons. The following hidden weapons have all been used:

- More than 95% of criminals carry their pistol concealed in the front inner belt line, without a holster. Most are right-handed and thus carry it on the left front side of their inner pants. Watch for suspects who touch that area occasionally, especially after running or standing up. They are adjusting their weapon or making sure it did not shift.

- Cell phone guns fire four rounds of .22 rimfire ammunition and look exactly like a real cell phone.

- Knives may be concealed in combs, brushes, baseball hats, belt buckles, boots, and other locations.

- Concealed guns that fire six shots may be located in the handle of a large knife. Beware of the suspect who is pointing a large knife; it could be a gun.

- Hidden handcuff keys sewn into the rear belt line of jeans are easily recovered by a handcuffed suspect who can use them to escape. A simple bobby pin located in the rear pocket of a suspect's pants can be retrieved while being transported and used to unlock handcuffs—even if handcuffs are double-locked. Many Internet sites have handcuff-picking instruction videos.

- Hidden hypodermic needles in pockets and cuffs of pants may puncture the fingers of officers searching the suspect and put the officers at risk for the transmission of bloodborne pathogens. Remember to use metal detectors and the hard plastic edge of these or other devices to screen and/or rub against clothing while searching for hidden weapons, needles, bobby pins, keys, and hidden weapons.

- Razor blades may be tucked into shirt sleeves or the edges of baseball hats.

- Pistols of all types may be tucked inside underwear into the crotch.

- Many gang members will have a girlfriend carry their pistol for them. The location is often the groin area where male police officers are hesitant to search.

- A nickname for a gang member's gun is "wifey." If you hear, "Hey, Pete, get out your wifey," then watch for the gun and beware.

- Hardened plastic "letter opener" knives may be stashed inside sleeves or pants and suddenly retrieved even by properly handcuffed suspects. A metal detector will not detect these.

Painting pistols orange. Sadly, some young criminals paint their guns or the barrel end of their gun orange to simulate a toy pistol. Thus, if the gun is discovered during arrest, the 14- or 15-year-old suspect may say, "It's just a toy gun," and pull it out. The officer may see what he or she interprets as an orange plastic toy pistol and let down his or her guard, while the criminal fires the gun.

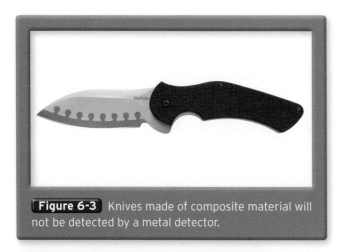

Figure 6-3 Knives made of composite material will not be detected by a metal detector.

At the Scene

Establish a warning system (verbal and sign language) with your SWAT unit to inform the nearby SWAT officers that a hidden weapon has been found.

If a weapon is found, continue the search, looking for additional weapons hidden elsewhere on the suspect. Many criminals carry multiple weapons. For example, in 2009 a deranged patient in Washington was seen in an emergency room and law enforcement was called. Law enforcement searched the patient and removed two handguns; unfortunately, they missed a third gun. Later, when the patient became more agitated, he drew out this third gun and, in the struggle, the involved law enforcement officers were forced to shoot him. Resuscitation efforts were unsuccessful.

Edged Weapons

Edged weapons are deadly threats and should be treated accordingly **Figure 6-4**. If a suspect is armed with a knife or other sharp-edged weapon, he or she can sprint 21 feet and stab an officer in 1.5 seconds, which is the same amount of time it takes the average law enforcement officer to draw a pistol from the holster and fire the first bullet. A substantial number of public safety personnel are injured and killed each year by edged weapons.

Knives are often disguised as combs, pencils, brushes, letter openers, belt buckles, or other common objects **Figure 6-5**. After the suspect is initially handcuffed, you must perform a thorough search to look for these and other weapons before initiating medical

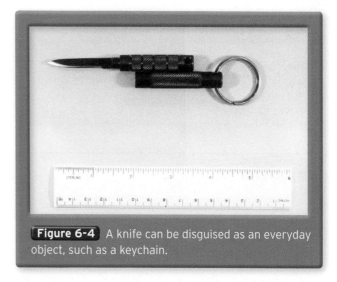

Figure 6-4 A knife can be disguised as an everyday object, such as a keychain.

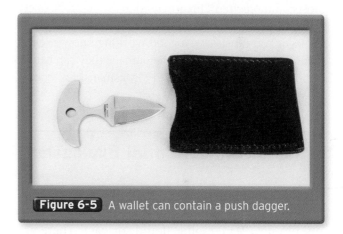

Figure 6-5 A wallet can contain a push dagger.

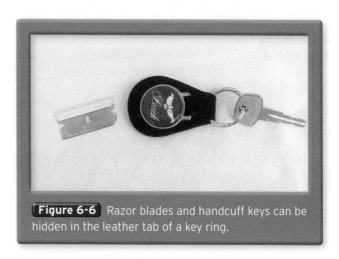

Figure 6-6 Razor blades and handcuff keys can be hidden in the leather tab of a key ring.

care. Any long, thin metal device may be sharpened on the point and used as a **shank** or improvised stabbing tool; such devices can kill even if only 3 inches long. These weapons are easily hidden in sleeves, boots, hats, inside of pants, and other locations **Figure 6-6**.

Firearms

Firearms are the most common lethal threat for public safety personnel. The long-range capability of bullets makes it easy to assault responders from a long distance. A bullet fired from a rifle can penetrate law enforcement vehicles and multiple indoor walls. Handguns are the most common type of firearm used to shoot public safety responders, although any type of firearm can inflict lethal damage. You must have a good working knowledge of firearms, ammunition, and the damage they can cause. Chapter 5, "Firearm Safety and Marksmanship," covers firearms in detail.

Types of Conventional Explosives

Conventional explosives are compounds of nitrogen, oxygen, carbon, and hydrogen. They may exist in any physical state (solid, liquid, or gas). There are two categories of materials used in explosive devices. **Primary high explosive materials** are sensitive to heat, friction, open flame, or pressure and are difficult to handle. Primary explosive materials include substances such as lead azide or mercury fulminate that may be used in blasting caps in mines, rock quarries, and road construction. **Secondary explosive materials** are less sensitive (to prevent unintended explosions) and can be handled relatively safely. Secondary explosive materials include compounds such as trinitrotoluene (TNT), pentaerythritol tetranitrate (PETN), and cyclotrimethylene trinitramine (RDX) explosives. High temperatures and shock usually do not affect these less-sensitive materials.

Most military munitions consist of a **fuse**, a booster, and a main charge. The fuse is a device used for setting an explosion, and there are several types. A fuse may be a narrow tube filled with combustible material, or a wick saturated with such material, or it may be a simple electrical wire that sets off a small flame when current is connected for setting off an explosive charge. The

booster is a small explosive that is designed to detonate the large main charge of explosive material.

Most conventional terrorist weapons are improvised and assembled from common materials. For example, ammonium nitrate is an agricultural fertilizer and it was used in the New York 1993 World Trade Center and Oklahoma City attacks as an explosive material in truck bombs.

The most common type of improvised explosive is the pipe bomb. Pipe bombs are simply built by filling a pipe with gunpowder and are capable of blowing off an arm or leg. In a crowd, they can kill and injure multiple persons. A metal "Maglite" style flashlight, or similar container with black powder, flash powder, or other fast-burning gunpowder is sometimes found as a booby trap in meth labs. A simple cannon-type fuse may be lit or a timer may be used. The flashlight switch itself may serve as the ignition switch. Because flashlights are an increasingly popular pipe bomb booby trap, you should not touch or disturb flashlights you find at a crime or bombing scene; consider them to be bombs until proven otherwise.

The backpack is also a common, convenient method of concealment; it was successfully employed at the Olympic Park bombing in Atlanta in July 1996, as well as in the 2002 bombing in Bali. A medium-sized backpack bomb is capable of killing 20 to 30 people in a location where people are close together. Remain suspicious of anything that seems out of place.

Secondary Explosive Device Threats

Secondary explosions are a very real threat directed at law enforcement and rescue personnel who respond to terrorist incidents. For example, on January 30, 1998, a bomb exploded near the front door of an abortion clinic in Birmingham, Alabama. As the responding personnel gathered, investigators believe the bomber was watching and detonated a remote-controlled secondary bomb, killing a law enforcement officer and seriously injuring a nurse.

In October 2002, an initial explosion from a bomb in a backpack in a hotel on the Indonesian island of Bali killed more than 20 people and was followed soon afterward by a large secondary explosion. This second bomb was detonated near the front of the hotel in a van and killed more than 150 people, with a total casualty count of 202 **Figure 6-7**.

Israel has had multiple incidents where secondary bombs and terrorists firing weapons have threatened and killed rescuers who responded to an initial explosion.

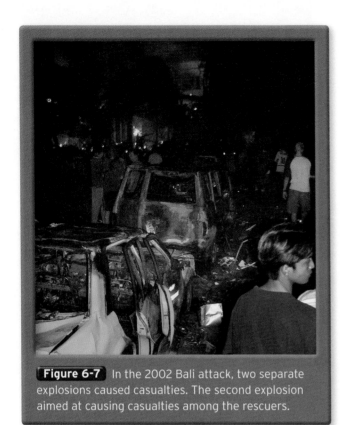

Figure 6-7 In the 2002 Bali attack, two separate explosions caused casualties. The second explosion aimed at causing casualties among the rescuers.

Geiger counters, chemical testing kits, and other newer detector kits as they are developed.

Use extreme caution in approaching the site of any explosion. Unless immediate rescue and lifesaving patient care is required, you should not enter the explosion area. A good indicator of the location of the bomb blast area is broken glass. Stay alert and look for people, vehicles, and packages that appear out of place or any other suspicious activity. Minimize the time spent in the explosion area, stay as far away from the explosion area as possible, and use any solid object (eg, vehicle, building) to shield yourself from a potential secondary explosion. Use care to avoid areas near windows or places where rubble could fall and cause injury.

Booby Traps

Booby traps are devices activated by the victim and intended to inflict harm or death. In the tactical environment, you will need to remain hyper-vigilant for booby traps. These traps include light switches wired to explosive devices; fishing lines with treble hooks hung at eye level; piano wire hooked to hand grenades and strung across the lower part of a doorway at ankle level; mock videotape cassettes that detonate when viewed; pipe bombs; hydrogen cyanide gas generators; attack dogs in closets; buckets of battery acid balanced on the door that spill on tactical officers; power cords with exposed wire ends inside gasoline containers; light bulbs filled with gasoline; mouse traps wired to explosives; and many others. The human imagination knows no bounds when designing devious devices that can injure or kill. Exercise caution when inside buildings. *Nothing* should be picked up or touched unless absolutely necessary, including light switches and objects on tables.

Over time, Israeli first responder teams have adapted their response tactics and now have specific protocols to rapidly establish scene safety. They first remove or inspect suspicious vehicles and packages before providing medical care to those in need.

Explosions and the damage from the blasts present a variety of hazards, including structural collapse; unstable buildings; fires; debris; leaking natural gas, water, and sewers; and partially consumed explosives. Beware of these hazards in addition to secondary devices. It is important that all suspicious blast sites be tested for chemical, biologic, and radiologic contamination using

Ready for Review

- As the TMP, you are required to communicate with and be within touching distance of suspects. The opportunity for the suspect to attack you exists in each encounter.

- SWAT officers should handcuff suspects and search them for weapons prior to you beginning the administration of medical care.

- If you do not observe the search directly, then you should assume that it was not fully completed and perform the search again.

- Firearms are the most common lethal threat for public safety personnel. The long-range capability of bullets makes it easy to assault responders from a long distance. Always be aware of your surroundings—especially above you.

- The most common type of improvised explosive is the pipe bomb, which can be easily concealed in a backpack. Because of the threat of a secondary explosion, you should be suspicious of any object that seems out of place.

- Be alert for booby traps, especially when inside buildings.

Vital Vocabulary

fuse A mechanical or electrical device used for setting off (detonating) an explosive charge or mechanism.

primary high explosive materials Explosives that are extremely sensitive to stimuli such as impact, friction, heat, static electricity, or electromagnetic radiation; often used to help trigger an explosion.

secondary explosive materials Explosive compounds that are less sensitive to handling and require more energy for an explosion to occur.

shank A makeshift knife made out of various materials including wood, metal, plastic, glass shard, and others.

Medical Intelligence and Support

OBJECTIVES

- Describe the role of the tactical emergency medical support (TEMS) unit in ensuring the health and safety of SWAT officers during training.

- Describe the role of the TEMS unit in creating a medical plan for a potential incident site.

- Describe the role of the TEMS unit in creating a medical plan for a special event.

- Describe the role of the TEMS unit in providing medical support and a rehabilitation station during training or a prolonged callout.

- Describe the role of the TEMS unit in creating and maintaining medical records for the SWAT unit personnel.

- Describe the role of the TEMS unit in creating a medical plan for a mission or training event.

- Describe the role of the TEMS unit in collecting medical intelligence and creating a medical threat assessment (MTA).

Introduction

In order to have a successful mission, the TEMS unit must plan before, during, and after the mission. The TEMS unit works with the SWAT unit in pre-event planning to ensure that the proper medical resources, gear, and personnel will be in place when the mission or event occurs. During the callout, the TEMS unit works with the SWAT unit by providing critical medical intelligence and an MTA for the tactical operations leader to consider when the tactical plan is created and revised. After the mission, the TEMS unit may provide feedback on how certain tactics worked in relation to the medical care that was needed, provided, or could be required in the future. Whether you are distributing hot packs in preparation for a prolonged hostage barricade callout in January, replenishing emergency medical supplies in the raid van, or treating a SWAT officer with a minor laceration during the mission, it is only through proper medical planning and proper preparation that optimal outcomes can occur **Figure 7-1**.

Medical Planning for Safe Training

The TEMS unit is responsible for providing tactical emergency medical support during both training and missions. Ensuring that SWAT officers remain healthy is critical on the training ground and in the tactical environment. As a tactical medical provider, you will be responsible for planning how to ensure the health of your SWAT officers on the training ground by assembling the proper medical gear, planning for environmental hazards, setting up a rehabilitation station for especially exhausting training scenarios, and conducting preventive medicine.

When live-fire firearms range training is occurring, you should work with the SWAT unit's safety officer to ensure good compliance with safety. When the SWAT unit uses air-soft, Simunitions, or other simulated scenario-based training, it is extremely important to help maintain a safe environment and keep all real ammunition out of the area. For each training day, you will also ideally perform an MTA. How to perform an MTA is discussed in detail later in the chapter.

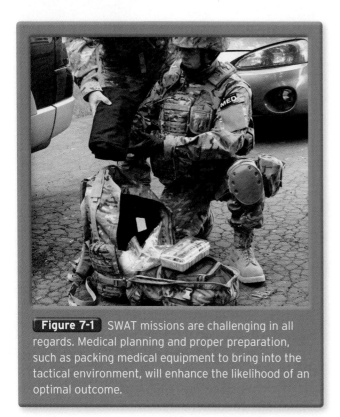

Figure 7-1 SWAT missions are challenging in all regards. Medical planning and proper preparation, such as packing medical equipment to bring into the tactical environment, will enhance the likelihood of an optimal outcome.

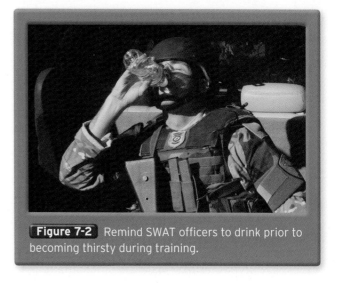

Figure 7-2 Remind SWAT officers to drink prior to becoming thirsty during training.

Law Enforcement Training Injuries and Deaths

SWAT units practice in realistic conditions and often utilize live-fire training drills to keep their skills sharp. Unfortunately, training for SWAT missions is accompanied by the risk of injury and death from accidents. Therefore, the TEMS unit should participate in all unit training sessions and work with the SWAT unit leader to assist in running a safe training day. Considerations for what to bring to these training sessions and what to prepare for are outlined in the following sections. You should consider multiple factors when deciding what additional supplies and equipment to bring or arrange for, including the type of training, expected injuries or illness, distance from a hospital and EMS backup, weather conditions, duration of training, level of physical exertion, and the number of persons undergoing tactical training. Work with the SWAT unit leader and safety officer to help establish a safe training day.

Hot Weather Considerations

Training in hot weather increases hydration needs; therefore, plenty of liquids with electrolytes and nutritional food should be made available. Remind SWAT officers to drink prior to becoming thirsty **Figure 7-2**. In extreme heat with exertion, it is possible for a SWAT officer to drink 1 liter of liquid every hour and still become dehydrated. Adequate water, hydration fluids, shade, and a breeze (electric fan) should be arranged for in advance. Cooling bandanas, several coolers of ice, and additional cooling measures should be considered. TMPs and team leaders should closely observe SWAT officers for early signs of heat illness. In addition, TMPs should help set up hydration stations. The TEMS unit leader will make recommendations to command staff regarding limiting the length of training and how often to schedule breaks. In extremely warm and humid conditions, command staff may decide to limit the risk of heat injury by cancelling or shortening the training session.

Medical Gear

Every year, SWAT officers die during training from sudden death, often associated with cardiac arrest, gunshot wounds, falls, and other traumatic injuries. As a TMP, you need to be as prepared as possible to address any traumatic injuries and medical illnesses according to your level of training. If the training site is remote and without water, shelter, or electricity then additional supplies should be arranged for and brought to the site.

Cold Weather Considerations

During cold weather operations and training sessions, encourage the consumption of hot fluids, utilize air-activated or battery-operated individual hand and foot warmers, wear appropriate clothing, and take steps to help protect SWAT officers from the elements. Dry air associated with cold climates, coupled with significant exertion, can lead to dehydration, so fluid consumption remains important.

Advise SWAT unit leaders to arrange for shelters (tent, building, other) that are warmed and close at hand to decrease exposure to the cold and allow a place for SWAT officers to warm up. Observe SWAT officers for signs of cold injury such as frostbite, altered mental status, and hypothermia. Make recommendations to command staff about rotation of marksmen and other SWAT unit personnel who may be deployed remotely. Remember that SWAT officers take pride in being physically tough and will rarely complain when on a real-world mission or during training. They may easily become lethargic and hypothermic when lying quietly in a cold environment for extended periods of time, especially if it is windy and there is a lot of contact with the cold ground and snow. You will learn the personalities and voices of your SWAT officers, and if you hear radio conversations that suggest the marksman (or other SWAT officer) is becoming lethargic, you should consider the possibility of hypothermia and take appropriate action such as replacing the marksman and getting the officer out of the cold and warmed up.

Additional Environmental Threats and Prevention

The environment is a source of many threats. These threats include weather-related issues such as heat and cold, wind, rain, lightning, and other challenges related to the outdoors such as animals, insects, snakes, and poisonous plants (see Chapter 22, "Environmental Injuries"). The training environment is important to monitor, such as prescreening an old building by doing a walk-through with SWAT unit leaders before the day's training begins. Look for and remove any rusty nails sticking out from floorboards, make sure that the stairs are strong enough for a team of 250-pound SWAT officers, and remove sharp glass and dangerous items from the training site. The MTA should identify these environmental threats and enable SWAT unit leaders to implement policies and procedures to prevent or minimize the likelihood of injuries and illness. You must monitor weather conditions (rain, lightning, severe storms, heat waves) and make suggestions to

the incident commander about limitation of physical activities and perhaps seeking shelter if indicated.

Specific Regional Threats

Tactical missions may be carried out in areas at risk for locally occurring diseases for which SWAT officers may not have adequate immunity or protection. When performing duties in an area with known endemic disease risk, such as mosquito-borne diseases (eg, West Nile fever, eastern equine encephalitis, malaria, dengue), have an effective mosquito repellant available.

Ticks are also a threat in many regions **Figure 7-3**. Insect repellant applied to the legs and arms (skin and external clothing) will help repel ticks. Teach SWAT officers how to perform tick surveillance on themselves and each other when they remove their equipment and uniform. Basic education about Lyme disease and other tick-borne infections during training is a good idea. You should make yourself available for informal medical consultation when questions arise from SWAT officers; if you are uncertain about a particular question, you should research the answer or refer the SWAT officer to the unit's physician or other medical source.

Other threats that may vary depending upon the region of the country and the season of the year include snakebites (venomous), stray dog and other animal bites with possible rabies, brown recluse **Figure 7-4** and black widow spider bites, fire ant bites, and scorpion stings. You should instruct the SWAT unit to identify and avoid dangerous versus harmless snakes, spiders, and scorpions in your area. Identification of potential threats and plans for their mitigation will help lead to a successful mission.

Establish relationships with local hospital emergency medicine experts in your areas and decide in advance

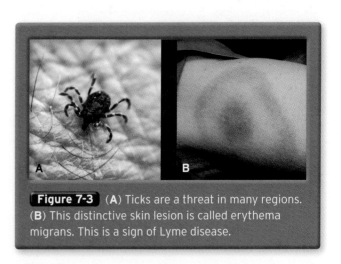

Figure 7-3 **(A)** Ticks are a threat in many regions. **(B)** This distinctive skin lesion is called erythema migrans. This is a sign of Lyme disease.

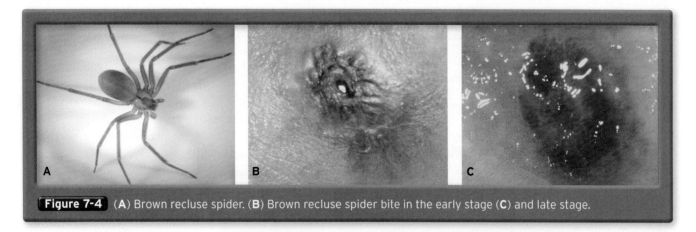

Figure 7-4 (**A**) Brown recluse spider. (**B**) Brown recluse spider bite in the early stage (**C**) and late stage.

the best out-of-hospital treatment and notification system. Poison control centers may be helpful, and knowledge of the nearest antivenom and antidotes should be acquired before a mission.

Prevention of these injuries and bites is important. Remind long-rifle marksmen about examining closely the area where they plan to establish a hide—it may also be hiding vermin and other biting creatures. Permethrin or DEET will decrease mosquito bites and allow the SWAT officer to focus on the mission instead of swatting at insects.

Cross-Agency Training

For SWAT and TEMS units, training with the public safety agencies who may also respond to a callout or a mass-casualty incident is a critical aspect of a successful mission **Figure 7-5**. The National Incident Management System (NIMS) requires public safety agencies to create strategic plans and conduct drills with area partners. When a critical incident strikes a community, the time to plan and prepare is over—it is time to respond.

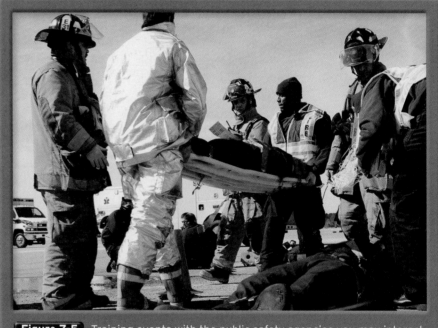

Figure 7-5 Training events with the public safety agencies you may interact with during a mass-casualty incident will ensure that if an emergency occurs, agencies will work together in unison.

Medical Planning for Incident Sites

The TEMS unit must acquire as much information about the types of possible callouts and more likely incident sites prior to a callout. The sites of possible

tactical emergencies include business offices, banks, jails, government buildings, courthouses, hospital emergency departments, stadiums, schools, and other dense-occupancy structures such as shopping malls. Each occupancy structure has its own set of specific concerns. For example, a tactical emergency in a hospital setting may present a substantial number of people who are at risk from a variety of medical conditions and cannot be moved or evacuated quickly.

Special Event Planning

For special events, such as a large controversial demonstration parade with a known travel route or a music festival at a fairground, the TEMS unit can plan

Safety

Many computer programs now allow the SWAT unit to rapidly access architecture building plans and create three-dimensional simulated visual computer programs of the inside and outside of the building. Some computer programs will store actual images taken from inside of the rooms of these important buildings. Work with your SWAT unit to build a reference library of your community's important buildings for rapid reference.

in advance the gear that will be needed, the number of resources that may be needed, and the number of TEMS personnel needed. Some locales and special events may present unique medical threats. For example, a concert in August requires preparation for possible heat emergencies. Many communities have a large civic center or conference facility that routinely holds large gatherings for events such as concerts. SWAT units will often train at these locations once every year or so in order to gain familiarity with the building layout, movement, vulnerable points, roof access, and medical extraction tactics **Figure 7-6**. If the special event is expected to be controversial or there is a risk of a riot, then the SWAT unit may be activated to be available on-site.

Planning for large crowd gatherings is important. For example, large music concerts may have a concentration

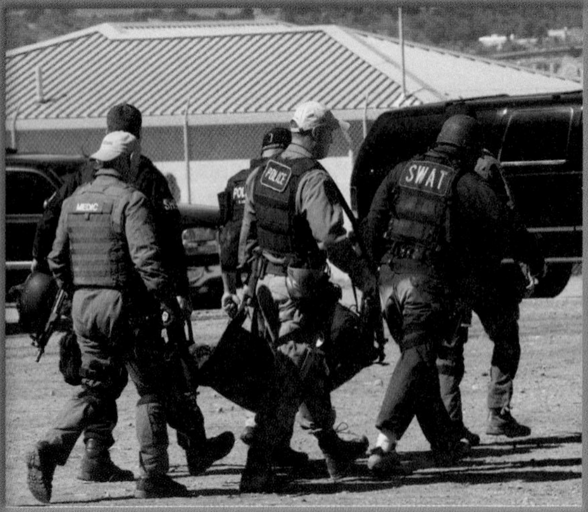

Figure 7-6 SWAT units will often train at locations that host special events in order to gain familiarity with the layout and to perfect medical extraction and transportation tactics.

of younger adults who may be under the influence of alcohol or illegal drugs, which increases the risks for bad behavior. Outdoor summer events could occur during hot humid weather, causing a substantial heat load with subsequent potential for heat injury and dehydration. The same location in a different season could present the threat of cold injuries and hypothermia during wintertime events. During the planning phase, personnel from the TEMS unit will meet with SWAT unit leaders, special event planners, administration of the involved event or building, and other agencies to plan in advance all aspects of the possible SWAT deployment, including the medical response and interaction with regional EMS and fire and rescue agencies.

Planning for Medical Support During a Mission or Training

Nutrition, Hydration, and Sleep Factors

SWAT officers should be educated and trained to be self-sufficient when they arrive at the scene of a callout. Water, nutrition, and sleep are important factors. The prepared SWAT officer takes responsibility and carries healthy snacks and bottles of drinking water in his or her vehicle trunk. In a prolonged callout, these can be eaten, and the water may be carried in bottles and/or emptied into their own Camelbak or canteen hydration systems.

The type of mission will be a factor in planning and preparation. If the SWAT unit is simply going from the police station to a neighborhood at the other end of the city for a high-risk search warrant, they will not need much food for this short 1- to 2-hour event. Perhaps a small energy bar would be appropriate to carry at the most. However, even a short operation in hot weather can cause significant sweating and overheating that can lead to heat exhaustion, decreased performance, and compromised mental sharpness. On all missions, remind SWAT officers to rehydrate often, hand out water bottles, and assist the SWAT officers with keeping their hydration system full of fresh water. Store several cases of water, just in case, as a backup plan. For any prolonged callout or training event, food that is nutritious and well balanced should be available at the command center and rehabilitation station. Make contingency plans in advance with command staff, and choose several acceptable and practical ways to arrange hydration and nutrition. For example, arrange for an American Red Cross vehicle and crew to come to the

At the Scene

The following are easily obtainable liquids and foods that will keep the SWAT unit hydrated and provide them with nutritious food sources.

Hydration

- Water
- Orange juice diluted with water
- Sports drinks/electrolyte solutions
- Minimize use of caffeinated soda; if officers do choose to buy or bring these, then recommend that for each can of soda, the SWAT officer drink an equal amount of water.
- Encourage use of Camelbak-style hydration systems (100- or 70-oz bags).
- In hot weather, keep ice available for cooling drinks.

Nutrition

- Granola bars and protein bars are relatively inexpensive, easy to buy, and can be stored for long periods of time. These should be kept with gear in the SWAT vehicle and the individual officer's vehicle. These foods are heat and cold stable, and create little or no mess.
- Local restaurants may deliver healthy sandwiches and other food for the SWAT unit. If the callout is prolonged more than several hours, then the TEMS unit must provide food surveillance involving routine inspections to make sure the food does not spoil or sit out in the hot sun unrefrigerated for too long. When in doubt about the food quality, throw it away, as food poisoning from spoiled food is not good for mission success.
- Apples, dried fruit, beef sticks, and other portable foods will add variety and allow the SWAT officers to take it with them to their posts.

fresh water and soap and/or hand-cleansing materials.

- **Fatigue.** Rotate the SWAT officers when necessary, and allow them to take 20- to 30-minute power naps. In general, most SWAT officers will not want to sleep if their unit is facing danger. If the TMP insists and command staff orders it, then compliance with a brief period of sleep is beneficial in numerous ways.
- **Low morale.** Provide telephones so that SWAT officers can notify their families of their safe status. Be nice; a friendly TMP who is cheerful and upbeat is always a positive factor at a callout or long training event.
- **Boredom and exhaustion.** Establish a rest area in the rehabilitation station for SWAT officers to safely relax, unwind, and take a break or a power nap.
- **Illness.** Establish proper toilet facilities that are convenient to get to and use without risking safety; establish hand washing and eating areas. Inform the SWAT unit of the location of tactical medical personnel who can assist the SWAT officers if they should feel ill or become injured. Many SWAT officers will tend to not want to admit that they are not feeling good, so try to make an area where discussions and examinations can be performed in private.
- **Dehydration.** Provide plentiful good water and rehydration sources.
- **Other support.** Other agencies and vendors (eg, Red Cross, disaster support agencies, local restaurants, supply stores, portable outhouses) should be contacted and arrangements made in advance and activated when needed. Prepackaged kits and necessary supplies for extended operations may be prepared ahead of time by the TEMS unit, and used when needed.

command post to supply water and snacks in the event of a prolonged callout.

Preventive Care and Support

Advise the incident commander or tactical operations leader on how to provide support for and prevent the following:

- **Heat or cold casualties.** Use proper clothing/gear, rotate staff, provide proper shelter, and drink plenty of fluids.
- **Food poisoning.** Rotate out the food supply; ensure provision of fresh, nutritious food; and provide

Rehabilitation Stations

A necessity on prolonged callouts is establishment of a quiet, protected environment where SWAT officers and TMPs can remove their equipment, warm up or cool down, drink and eat, make telephone calls to loved ones, and rest or sleep. During prolonged callouts, rehabilitation efforts are directed toward keeping the SWAT and TEMS units healthy and rested. The TEMS unit leaders should work with the incident commander to rotate SWAT officers and TMPs through a quiet, safe location called a **rehabilitation station** (or rehab station). There, SWAT officers and TMPs receive a medical evaluation and steps are taken to help personnel rest, hydrate, and regain normal body temperature, blood pressure, and pulse rate.

Vital signs are checked when SWAT officers or TMPs arrive at the rehabilitation area, and the assessment should be repeated prior to departure. Any abnormal vital signs should be double-checked and dealt with appropriately. The goal is for SWAT officers and TMPs to return to duty rehydrated, fed with nutritious food, and rested both mentally and physically. SWAT officers or TMPs should not return to duty if they are experiencing concerning symptoms, have abnormal vital signs, or are experiencing significant psychological stress.

Medical Records

Another component of medical planning is creating, maintaining, and making available medical records. An important precept for TEMS units is to maintain a file of pertinent medical information on any person who may be involved in tactical training and callouts. These include all SWAT officers, medical personnel, negotiators, bomb team members, riot team or mobile field force officers, K-9 officers and their dogs, and command staff (up to and including the chief, sheriff, or other commander). These records should conform to HIPAA regulations and their confidential nature should be maintained. Access should be limited to medical staff and select SWAT unit leaders.

Individual medical histories should note previous surgeries, medical problems, medications, allergies, and adverse drug reactions, which should be documented for later retrieval in a confidential manner. Immunizations, tuberculosis (TB) annual testing, tetanus status, and other pertinent medical records should be tracked and updated appropriately in association with the agency's occupational health providers. The occupational health physician and staff ideally will work with TMPs to help ensure that immunizations and medical records are up to date. If on-the-job injuries or medical issues occur (such as a SWAT officer who injured his or her back during a callout), an employee health follow-up may be organized by the occupational health medical staff.

You will find it worthwhile to have basic medical information immediately available for all SWAT officers and others who may be present at the scene of a callout. One method is to keep a small laminated card for each of these persons, including the SWAT officer's name (which may include an abbreviated last name

for security purposes); religious preference; preferred family physician and surgeon; and name of dentist and location of dental records in case of need for identifying a deceased officer. Allergies and adverse medication reactions should be clarified and specially highlighted if they involve anaphylactic or life-threatening reactions.

Medical Plan

The **medical plan** for training sessions and actual callouts is essentially the MTA coupled with a list of recommendations that impact the medical issues, safety, and health of the SWAT unit. Ideally, the tactical operations leader will use the medical plan and critical information from the MTA when developing the tactical plan for the mission. For each callout, the TEMS unit will work closely with the tactical operations leader to determine the tactics of any rescue team, prepositioning of TMPs (who, where, when, how), the location of relative points of safety, casualty collection points (CCPs), triage areas, and EMS staging areas.

Many aspects of the medical plan are predetermined and will be the same for a wide variety of callouts—for example, the contact number for the local EMS agency. The medical plan coordinates the interaction of all medical assets including those internal to the SWAT unit (TEMS) and those accessible within the surrounding medical community (EMS). The medical plan should list all helicopter and fixed-wing air medical transport agencies within the region, and have the names, phone numbers, and other contact information of key agency leaders who can be contacted in a confidential manner and have been cleared with the SWAT command staff as a part of planning a known tactical operation, or, in callouts without prior notification, may be contacted with urgency if needed.

Medical Intelligence

Medical intelligence involves gathering data on what the SWAT and TEMS units may encounter at the scene of an incident or training site that may impact their health and safety. It also involves gathering medical and psychological information on the involved suspect(s), hostages, and others at the scene. This information may play a role in medical care decisions as well as the tactics and approach used by the SWAT team. Much of the medical intelligence and MTA should be accomplished prior to the mission, and updated continuously once the mission is underway.

Medical Threat Assessment

Medical intelligence is also used to help create the **medical threat assessment (MTA)**. The MTA identifies the threats that may have an impact on the physiological and psychological health and performance of the SWAT and TEMS units. Like the medical plan, the MTA is used when formulating the tactical plan for the mission. The MTA contains both fixed pieces of information (predetermined medical tactics, outside agency contact information, possible staging areas), as well as dynamic information that is constantly evolving and updated, such as the names and medical information of involved suspects, hostages, and others involved. All TMPs in the TEMS unit collect information for the MTA, but it is the single TEMS unit leader who puts all of the information together into the MTA.

The MTA must take into account any potential injury or medical care scenario that could affect the health or performance of the SWAT unit during training or mission operations. It should have a risk assessment of hazards thought to be present at the scene and measures to respond to these risks (for example, a threat of sulfuric acid burns at a battery warehouse, with the response being immediate availability of on-site water hoses in addition to a standby Hazardous Materials Response Team several blocks away). Another consideration is the availability of on-site wound care and suturing capability if the SWAT unit is involved in a prolonged callout located several hours away from a nearby medical center.

The MTA should include an assessment of the on-scene witnesses, family members, and relatives who may have important information regarding suspects' medical issues. This can include type of medications and whether or not they have been compliant with taking their psychiatric medications. Also important are the names of trusted psychiatrists or counselors who can be consulted for advice about the predicted response of emotionally disturbed persons (EDP), and sometimes can be brought to the scene to assist negotiators.

The information to be included in the MTA includes:

- Medical database (also found in the medical plan)
  - List of regional support agencies and contact numbers/radio frequencies
  - Medical resources information: Local medical facilities, nearest Level I trauma facility, nearest burn facility, local air medical helicopter information, local fire and EMS agencies, emergency veterinary services
- On-scene database
  - Environmental threats: Weather threats, plants, hazardous materials, biologic threats, terrain threats, heat, cold, mosquitoes, bathroom facility availability, and local factors
  - Training site evaluation: The name of safety officer, results of the physical site inspection, and other safety measures
  - Callout scene evaluation: The number of occupants/hostages, age and gender of occupants, medical intelligence on occupants including psychiatric history and medications, compliance with medications, animal threats, surrounding people (eg, adjacent schools, medical facilities), and other factors

The MTA should be individualized and mission-specific. The information gathered before SWAT training and callout deployments can and should be used to better prepare for and deal with all predictable medically related threats and issues. This process is dynamic in that additional information can be obtained in real time as the callout progresses. During the actual mission, the MTA should be updated and used to make important decisions. The command staff will be updated with this new information by the TEMS unit leader.

MTA Briefing to Command Staff

The TEMS unit leader should be prepared to present a brief summary of the MTA to commanders and SWAT officers before a mission. The extent and format of the MTA depends on the time available for planning and the nature of the callout. For example, a routine planned search warrant service allows time for a formal MTA that can be presented at the mission briefing. The basic MTA one- or two-page document can then remain in place for the next high-risk search warrant in the same area; it will only take a brief amount of time to update the specifics for the next callout (See Appendix B).

A more urgent scenario, such as a barricaded suspect with a hostage, may require that the TEMS unit deploy and rapidly gather specific medical intelligence on-site as the callout progresses. This medical intelligence must be gathered without jeopardizing operational security. The TEMS unit leader may elect to brief only the tactical operations leader, or may brief the entire SWAT unit about the MTA and pertinent medical intelligence.

If the situation is tense and stress levels are high, then the tactical command staff may not want to be interrupted for more than 30 seconds to receive the information in the MTA. The key issues that require immediate action

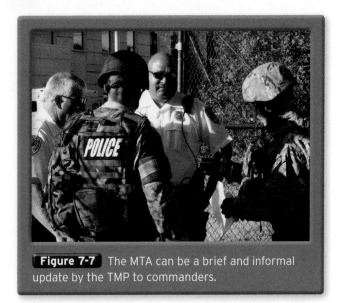

Figure 7-7 The MTA can be a brief and informal update by the TMP to commanders.

by the SWAT unit commander should be identified and stressed. Depending upon the duration of the mission, situation, hostage negotiations, and further intelligence, there may be a need for several MTA briefings. This will keep the SWAT unit commander updated with medical information as the mission unfolds, which will assist in appropriate decision making.

Collecting Medical Intelligence for the MTA

When collecting medical intelligence about suspects, hostages, or others involved in a callout, you should take into account their past medical history, prior surgical procedures, current medical diagnosis, and medications taken. The use of psychoactive drugs, alcohol, or other substances can make suspects more volatile, unpredictable, or medically unstable with regard to their decision making and physical condition. For example, geriatric hostages and bystanders may not tolerate heat

and stress well, especially if they take medications that slow their evaporative heat loss. Another concern is patients who are taking psychotropic medications who may decompensate without their medicine.

The MTA should include medical information on all involved citizens, if you are able to obtain it, including types of medical conditions and required medication. The patient's physician would also be an excellent source of additional medical intelligence, if you are able to make contact. Although HIPAA laws may cause medical staff to hesitate to release information over the phone, proper explanation of the life-threatening situation will usually decrease barriers to obtaining needed information.

If medical intelligence shows that patients with lung disease are on scene, the tactical use of chemical agents should be avoided. This also may be true with younger patients who have severe reactive airway problems such as asthma or a history of anaphylaxis. Patients with diabetes are a particular concern. Many sensitive diabetics require insulin and food to maintain a normal blood sugar. Other concerns may include dehydration, deficiency of food and nutrition, limited restroom facility access, environmental temperature extremes, and other issues.

Post-Mission Medical Planning

After the mission, the TEMS unit will participate in post-incident debriefing and review, assist the command staff with an analysis of the mission or training event, and help to make any necessary improvements to the medical plan, TEMS unit, policies, and procedures. Incorporating the lessons learned into future unit training and preparedness is a critical component of future success for the SWAT and TEMS units.

Ready for Review

- Medical planning occurs before, during, and after every mission or training event.

- You will be responsible for planning how to ensure the health of your SWAT officers on the training ground by assembling the proper medical gear, planning for environmental hazards, setting up a rehabilitation station for especially exhausting training scenarios, and conducting preventive medicine.

- The TEMS unit must acquire as much information about the types of possible callouts and more-likely incident sites prior to a callout.

- For special events, the TEMS unit can plan in advance the gear that will be needed, the number of resources that may be needed, and the number of TEMS personnel needed.

- During prolonged operations, it is important that the TEMS unit provide support and preventive medical care through rehabilitation stations.

- TEMS units must maintain a file of pertinent medical information on any person who may be involved in tactical training and callouts. These include all SWAT officers, medical personnel, negotiators, bomb team members, riot team or mobile field force officers, K-9 officers and their dogs, and command staff.

- The medical plan for each training session or real-world callout is basically the MTA coupled with a list of recommendations that impact the medical issues, safety, and health of the SWAT unit.

- Medical intelligence involves gathering data on what the SWAT and TEMS units may encounter at the scene of an incident or training site that may impact their health and safety.

- The MTA identifies the threats that may have an impact on the physiological and psychological health and performance of the SWAT and TEMS units.

- Like the medical plan, the MTA is considered and used when formulating the tactical plan for the mission.

- The MTA contains both fixed pieces of information as well as dynamic information that is constantly evolving and updated.

- After the mission, it is important to participate in a review and incorporate the lessons learned into future unit training and preparedness as a critical component of future success for the SWAT and TEMS units.

Vital Vocabulary

medical intelligence Gathering of data and medical information about prospective patients and mission conditions that may impact tactical medical care and decision making.

medical plan A medical predeployment plan that coordinates the interaction of all medical assets to include both those internal to the SWAT unit and those accessible within the surrounding medical community.

medical threat assessment (MTA) An assessment that identifies the threats that can have an impact on the physiological and psychological health and performance of the SWAT and TEMS units.

rehabilitation station A protected location in the outer perimeter where SWAT officers and TMPs can rest, recover, and be medically evaluated for a short period of time during a prolonged callout or significantly challenging training session.

Self-Defense and Close Quarters Battle

OBJECTIVES

- Describe the possible techniques a tactical medical provider (TMP) can use to provide self-defense in the tactical environment.

- Describe the body's response to the stress of the tactical environment.

- Describe the restraint devices and techniques that are used to restrain a suspect.

Introduction

In most circumstances, the tactical medical provider (TMP) is able to remain relatively safe and protected by hard cover and the immediate presence of nearby armed law enforcement officers who have encircled and isolated the criminal threats. In a perfect world, there would be zero threat to TMPs.

Unfortunately, this is not a perfect world. All TMPs, even those unarmed TMPs who remain outside the outer perimeter, choose to enter the arena of the uncontrolled, hazardous, and unpredictable tactical environment. In the tactical environment, no place is completely safe. All TMPs must be prepared to simultaneously provide medical care and protect themselves, downed SWAT officers, and patients. This self-defense capability includes the knowledge of combat physiology, criminal tactics, unarmed fighting skills such as defensive blocking moves and strikes, as well as armed close quarters battle (CQB) combat skills. These self-defense techniques are mentioned and discussed in this chapter; however, additional hands-on training is essential.

The authors highly recommend that every TMP attend and complete as much law enforcement training as possible, including self-defense, CQB, firearms, and less-lethal weapons training. An armed TMP must also be thoroughly trained in countering disarming moves by suspects.

Principles of Self-Defense

The topic of self-defense is broad and encompasses many aspects that simply cannot be contained in one chapter or even one book. It is up to individual TEMS units to work with their law enforcement agency to obtain the education, strength training, physical combat skills, and weapons familiarization and competency, as well as continually maintain and improve their self-defense and combat skills.

Depending upon the weapons that are authorized in your agency, you should develop the ability to rapidly and smoothly choose the right tool from your toolbox of unarmed defense techniques, weapons, and tactics. Decisions will need to occur in milliseconds, leaving no time for you to think consciously—only to react. Self-defense blocking techniques

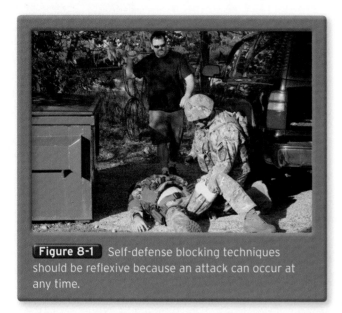

Figure 8-1 Self-defense blocking techniques should be reflexive because an attack can occur at any time.

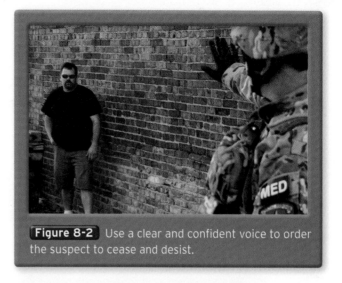

Figure 8-2 Use a clear and confident voice to order the suspect to cease and desist.

and other skills should be reflexive, because often the first sign of an attack is the pain and shock of suddenly being hit, stabbed, or shot **Figure 8-1**. Your mental attitude and physical preparation must be established well before any altercation occurs.

Self-defense usually refers to the use of violence for protection and is justification for this otherwise illegal act of violence. Its legal status varies from state to state, and courts generally find that the degree of violence used in self-defense must be comparable to the threat faced. Therefore, deadly force should only be used in situations of life or death.

Preemptive self-defense is the act of landing the first blow in a situation where there is no hope for de-escalation or escape. Many self-defense instructors and experts believe that if the situation is so clear-cut as to feel that certain violence is unavoidable, the defender has a much better chance of surviving by landing the first blow and gaining the immediate upper hand. That being said, it is important as a TMP to know your agency's use of force policies. In some agencies, preemptive self-defense may not be permitted. Learn and remember the use-of-force policies for your own agency.

As the TMP, you are involved with the SWAT unit on a mission and committed to providing medical support, but if a criminal threat arises, then you may have to support the SWAT unit in other ways, including helping to neutralize threats. Only in extremely rare circumstances should you actually be involved in a life-or-death struggle, but since this may occur, you must learn and maintain the skills necessary to win any confrontation. These skills may range from using a calm and confident voice **Figure 8-2** to physical blows.

Safety

Consult your local law enforcement agency's policies to determine the level of self-defense proficiency that is expected of TMPs. Law enforcement policies should discuss the initial and continuing training procedures that are in place to ensure proper maintenance and improvement of skills. The plan for strength training, physical combat skills, weapon system familiarization, and defense tactics should be included in the policies.

You may have a significant handicap in a fight if there is a SWAT officer downed under your care and a threatening suspect suddenly appears. Your choice will likely be limited to maintaining your position and defending the downed SWAT officer. The goal is to win this confrontation if it does arise.

Winning a Confrontation

In most fights, there is no second place. As stated by US Special Forces Sergeant and self-defense expert instructor John Holschen, "If you're going to fight, fight like a bear. If you're going to be a bear, be a grizzly and fight to win."

You do not have to become a black belt in karate to become competent in self-defense. There are some very basic blocking maneuvers that are fairly easy to learn and remember. These techniques can be used for SWAT callouts, and have additional value for protection in the emergency department, ambulance, and in the streets as a citizen. The key is to work with your TEMS and SWAT units to seek, obtain, and become competent in unarmed and armed combat (per your local protocols).

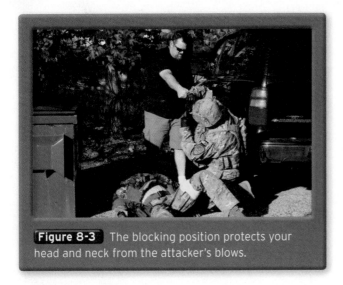

Figure 8-3 The blocking position protects your head and neck from the attacker's blows.

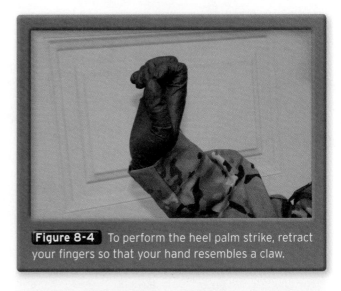

Figure 8-4 To perform the heel palm strike, retract your fingers so that your hand resembles a claw.

Fight or Flee

Remember the goal of self-defense is to prevent harm to yourself and those you are obligated to protect. If there is no reason to "stick around" and if you are under attack, then you may use a defensive block followed by a few strikes to break free and run to safety, especially if there are multiple attackers.

However, if you are a TMP and a sworn law enforcement officer and there is a one-on-one combat situation, then it is inappropriate to simply strike the suspect and then run away, allowing the suspect to remain free and at risk of hurting others, including nearby innocent citizens. Keep a good situational awareness, think, use your best weapon (your brain) effectively through good tactics, and if no other option is available, then use an appropriate level of force to deal with and neutralize the attacker(s).

Self-Defense Moves

Self-defense moves include the simple blocking position. In this position, your fists are both placed behind your neck, with your bent elbows and arms pressed gently against the side of your head. This protects your head and the sides of your neck from the attacker's strikes and blows while you attempt to crouch down and back away **Figure 8-3**. If and when the opportunity and indication arises for you to physically strike the attacker, the elbow strike, the heel palm strike, knee strike, and other blows may be delivered.

Heel Palm Strike

Generally speaking, open hand strikes are preferred over closed fist strikes, due to the fact that a solid strike with a fist will often result in painful hand and finger fractures that render the hand ineffective. When using heel palm strikes, the heel of the palm is used to strike, while the

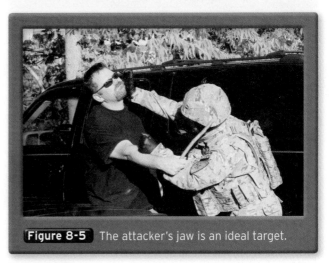

Figure 8-5 The attacker's jaw is an ideal target.

fingers are pulled back out of the way, resembling a claw **Figure 8-4**. The heel of the hand is more resistant to being broken when struck against the hard bony surfaces of the head, face, and jaw of the opponent, allowing you the option of striking multiple times. The energy is more focused in a narrow spot, instead of spread over the wide surface of the fist. In addition, the biceps muscle tends to remain relaxed and does not interfere with the production of speed as your triceps muscle extends your arm and the wrist is extended, allowing the heel palm to strike the target faster and harder. The target on the attacker will be variable and will depend upon many things including the body position and location of the defender and attacker, threat level, and other dynamics.

Your foot position and body stance are critical to throwing an effective heel palm strike. Your feet should be solidly planted shoulder width apart. As you thrust your palm forward to strike the attacker, you should swing forward from the hip to increase the strike force. Your target may be the attacker's jaw, face, skull, neck, abdomen, groin, or other open location **Figure 8-5**.

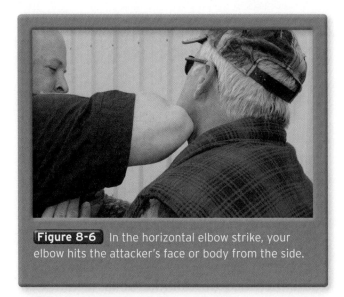

Figure 8-6 In the horizontal elbow strike, your elbow hits the attacker's face or body from the side.

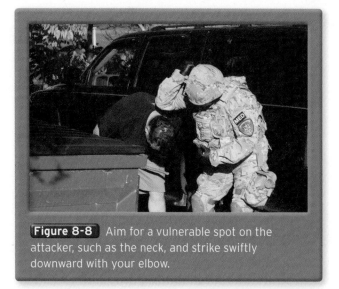

Figure 8-8 Aim for a vulnerable spot on the attacker, such as the neck, and strike swiftly downward with your elbow.

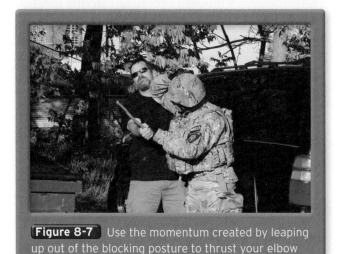

Figure 8-7 Use the momentum created by leaping up out of the blocking posture to thrust your elbow into the attacker's jaw.

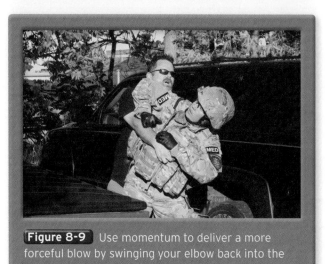

Figure 8-9 Use momentum to deliver a more forceful blow by swinging your elbow back into the attacker.

Elbow Strikes

The elbow joint is made up of a hard bone that is a particularly effective weapon. The point of the elbow is very difficult to break and is a devastating weapon in CQB combat. There are several variations of the elbow strike, based upon how the arm and elbow are swung:

- **Horizontal elbow strike.** The elbow comes at the attacker's face or body from the side, with the forearm tucked against the upper arm **Figure 8-6**.
- **Rising elbow strike.** This strike is very effective in conjunction with the blocking posture. If the attacker closes in and begins hitting you, keep your fists behind your neck, arms folded against the side of your face, and crouch down. When the attacker is close enough, suddenly stand up, thrusting the point of your elbow into the attacker's lower jaw and face **Figure 8-7**. Immediately follow this by issuing heel palm strikes repeatedly until the threat is neutralized.

- **Downward elbow strike.** This strike works effectively in many circumstances, including fighting on the ground. This elbow strike is performed by maintaining a bent elbow and raising it vertically in the air, then striking downward against the attacker's face or other body structure, again, avoiding the hard skull surfaces if possible **Figure 8-8**.
- **Back elbow strike.** This strike works remarkably well when an attacker grabs you from behind, or when fighting on the ground. This elbow strike is performed by moving your bent arm forward then rapidly swinging your elbow back, striking your attacker in a vulnerable soft spot **Figure 8-9**.

Head Butt Strikes

The head butt strike uses the front of your head (the hard bone about 1 inch above your eyebrow), side of

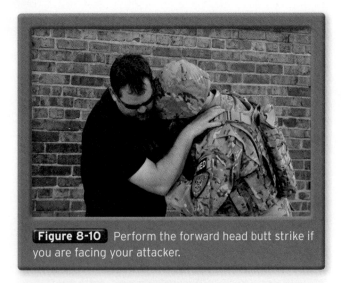

Figure 8-10 Perform the forward head butt strike if you are facing your attacker.

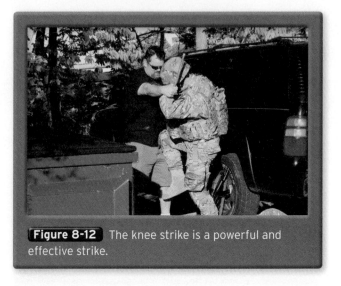

Figure 8-12 The knee strike is a powerful and effective strike.

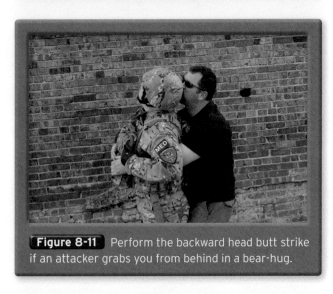

Figure 8-11 Perform the backward head butt strike if an attacker grabs you from behind in a bear-hug.

while dragging a downed officer or carrying medical gear. To perform the knee strike, spring your striking knee forward and up by suddenly pushing off from your toes. The knee is swung directly into a soft target such as the groin, abdomen, or a low-hanging head **Figure 8-12**. Attackers of similar size can be pulled into the knee to make the strike more effective. Some knee pads are manufactured with a hard pointed section making this strike even more painful for the attacker. Follow up by delivering additional strikes until the attacker is neutralized.

Combat Physiology

No discussion of self-defense is complete without discussing combat physiology. The human body has predictable responses to the stress of a fight, especially in a life-threatening confrontation. In recent years, several law enforcement and military researchers have closely investigated what exactly happens in the human mind and body during intense life-or-death confrontations. It is important to know these facts because it may happen to you, and the knowledge of what you will or will not see, hear, feel, and do during the intense few seconds of battle can literally help to save your life.

What happens inside of your body when you are faced with a deadly criminal adversary with the intent to kill? What skills and defense tactics will you be able to use when that moment comes? What will your body actually do? Will you perform exactly as you wanted to? What will you think? Will you have trained your mind and developed the proper combat mindset that will allow you to successfully initiate a reasonable use of force, and then successfully finish that encounter as the winner?

your head, and back of your skull as a weapon. If you are facing your attacker, perform the forward head butt strike. Clench your teeth, tilt your head slightly downward, aim for your attacker's nose, and lunge forward with sudden forceful movement of your head, neck, and upper body, as if you are violently sneezing **Figure 8-10**. Avoid striking the hard bony parts of your attacker's skull.

Perform the backward head butt strike if an attacker grabs you from behind in a bear-hug. Clench your teeth, bend your neck forward, and then suddenly extend your back and neck, throwing your head backward. The goal is to strike your attacker's face or nose **Figure 8-11**. After successfully delivering the blow, twist away, and throw repeated strikes until your attacker is neutralized.

Knee Strikes

The knee strike is a very powerful self-defense technique, especially if you have one hand occupied

The human response to combat is affected by many things. Much of your body's response is based on nerves, hormones, and limitations of function of your entire body, including the heart, lungs, brain, senses, and muscles. You can use your knowledge of how your body works to maximize your performance in the combat environment. You will also know the limitations that your adversary is experiencing. This knowledge can be used to stack the cards in your favor in a deadly force encounter.

Hormones and Nerves

The human body has two nervous systems: the sympathetic and parasympathetic nervous systems. The parasympathetic system takes over during relaxation and allows us to digest our food, sleep, repair, and grow. During stressful times, the parasympathetic system is suppressed and the **fight-or-flight response** is enhanced by the sympathetic system. The sympathetic nervous system deals with fight-or-flight stress. It releases stress hormones that have very specific effects on the body that aid in combat. Epinephrine and norepinephrine are types of adrenaline or catecholamines that are produced and released by the body during times of high stress. These hormones affect the body in many ways, including increasing the heart rate and blood pressure, contracting certain blood vessels and dilating air passages, which all help the body to fight or run away better. They will increase strength also, but will decrease the ability to use fine motor control, so the ability to use medical instruments or perform advanced medical procedures may be adversely affected.

The bottom line is our body is designed to survive, and processes such as digesting food get tossed to the wayside as the body increases blood flow to our muscles, thus rendering the body better able to survive by fighting or fleeing.

Blood Vessels

The heart pumps blood out to the body via the arteries, and returns blood to the heart via the veins. Branching out from the arteries are the capillaries or blood vessels. The average human has about 5 liters of blood circulating within the blood vessels. Blood constantly circulates through the blood vessels and contains essential nutrients that the body tissues need, including oxygen and glucose. Blood vessels can widen (dilate) or shrink (constrict). During the stress of a fight, the skin's blood vessels shrink, the blood flow to the intestines and less-vital organs decreases while the large skeletal muscles that allow us to run and fight receive increased blood flow. The net effect is a positive increase in muscle strength.

The Brain

In combat, a similar shift occurs in the brain, as blood flow to *survival* centers or the more primitive areas of the brain is enhanced. This has several results:

- Thinking is simplified, making it difficult to think through complex problems. For example, if attacked, the brain will normally automatically revert to simple self-preservation mental tasks such as fighting or running, and will less likely be able to remember complex medical tasks. This results in fewer mental distractions, as the brain can focus on simple decisions and trained reflex responses. It is also more difficult to recall the specific details of the fight.
- It is more difficult to interpret and process multiple stimuli.
- Preplanning or immediate action drills become easier to recall and allow a more reflexive response.
- Emotion is prevented from negatively interfering with the potentially repulsive mechanics of battle and allows the focus to solely be on survival.
- Individuals may be less aware of loud noises (auditory exclusion), and thus are less distracted.
- The individual may experience brief temporary visual changes (tunnel vision), which allow greater concentration on the center of attention, the adversary.

The Heart

The cardiac function is also affected during combat. With the need for more energy and oxygen, the strength of heart contractions increases as do the heart rate and blood flow. The heart reacts to the epinephrine and nerve input, which is why an exciting or life-threatening event will cause a pounding heart. A normal resting heart rate (pulse rate) ranges from 60 to 100 beats per minute. The optimal heart rate during stress is faster, within the range of 115 to 145 beats per minute.

The Eyes

Vision is also affected by the stress of combat. Changes include tunnel vision, dilation of pupils, and change in lens shape, which results in difficulty focusing. You can increase your odds by remembering to scan and look in all directions or perform a 360-degree check. This is especially important after being involved in a gun fight where the possibility of an additional criminal suspect always exists.

If you remember that a suspect will also have a narrow field of view, then you can take advantage of this at the beginning of the confrontation by "getting off the X." The "X" represents the physical spot on the ground where you are standing at the initial moment of the attack. The opponent sees you there and will focus his or her energy and weapons toward this location. To get off the X, move laterally away from the spot, ideally toward and behind hard cover, decreasing the chance of getting shot or stabbed. This involves rapid movement at an angle of about 45 degrees to create distance and to get out of the line of attack. Move quickly and use cover. If armed for self-defense, then shoot carefully. While moving, remember that you will have **tunnel vision**; therefore, quick glances in the exact direction you are moving will help decrease the chance of collision with a telephone pole or accidentally tripping over an object. After the first suspect is down and neutralized, immediately scan with your eyes all around, up and down, in a 360-degree circle, realizing that your vision is compromised for a short period of time.

The Ears

Hearing is affected in combat. Quite commonly, law enforcement officers involved in an officer-involved shooting testify that they did not hear any gunshots but only muffled noise; this is referred to as **perceptual narrowing**. They may also report thinking that a partner 50 yards away had shot at the suspect when in fact it was their own gun. Some officers did not know that it was they who shot, until they looked in their own hands and saw a gun with smoke coming out of the barrel. Some noises, even gunshot blasts, are not heard at all, and this is termed **auditory exclusion**. Sometimes officers actually yell "show me your hands" over and over again, yet they do not remember ever saying that in some cases. The human body's adaptation to combat is unique and will vary considerably among different officers. If a TMP is involved in an officer-involved shooting or other near-death self-defense situation, the TMP will likely encounter many of these physiologic changes.

The Gastrointestinal and Genitourinary Tracts

The gastrointestinal tract is negatively affected by combat stress, and a significant stressful event or fight will quite commonly cause loss of bowel and/or bladder control, diarrhea, nausea, and vomiting, most of which may

occur during, but sometimes after, the fight. Soldiers returning from war often feel a sense of relief when they realize that they were not the only ones who had lost control of their bowels or bladder, or had vomiting after their first few firefights. Often, this effect is not seen in the more experienced veterans who are mentally less affected by combat and whose bodies have adapted to these intensely stressful situations. The genitourinary (GU) tract is mainly affected by the loss of bladder control, which is always socially embarrassing but in fact a normal response to a highly stressful event.

The Skin

The skin is an organ. It is the largest organ of the body and has a large number of blood vessels. In times of stress, the body adapts to shrink these blood vessels, which allows the blood to go to more important organs such as the heart and muscles and brain. This explains why the skin can appear pale white in some people as intense blood vessel shrinkage occurs.

Restraint Devices and Techniques

When placing a suspect in a position for questioning or when arresting a suspect, SWAT officers will nearly always use some type of restraint. The most common method is a simple two-point restraint, which uses proper protocol and backup to place the suspect in a position where the suspect can be easily physically controlled and then handcuffed followed by a thorough search ("Control, then Cuff, then Search") **Figure 8-13**.

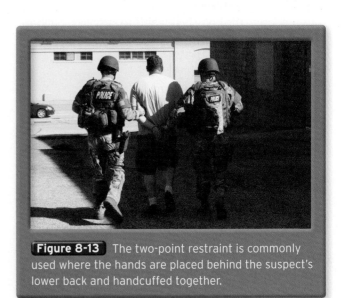

Figure 8-13 The two-point restraint is commonly used where the hands are placed behind the suspect's lower back and handcuffed together.

The two-point restraint is commonly used where the hands are placed behind the suspect's lower back and handcuffed together. This is quite effective and allows the suspect to be controlled and placed into a squad car or transportation van to be taken to the police station or jail for incarceration.

It is extremely dangerous to handcuff a suspect. Each year law enforcement officers are hurt or killed during altercations with suspects who choose to make the handcuffing the exact moment that they begin fighting. A common tactic is to fake compliance and to go along with all instructions while smiling and talking in a friendly manner with the arresting officer. But once the officer places hands on the suspect or immediately after the first handcuff is snapped into place, a violent attack occurs with a life-or-death struggle. Hidden weapons may be produced or the attached handcuff may suddenly be used as a weapon. Do not attempt to handcuff a suspect unless you are thoroughly trained and experienced, and have at least one or more backup officers who are prepared to use deadly force if the circumstances require it.

The use of four-point restraints may be indicated when the suspect is extremely agitated and kicking violently with his or her legs. Four-point restraint is simply the restriction of all four extremities **Figure 8-14**. There are various formations of four-point restraint, so the policies and procedures of the local law enforcement

agency should be consulted and followed. The suspect may be placed on his or her side or back when four-point restraint is utilized. At the scene and during transport, the patient's vital signs should be reassessed frequently to ensure that the suspect is stable. If the patient has abnormal vital signs, pulse oximetry readings, or cardiac activity; has a significantly altered mental status; or if a prolonged struggle was involved, then the suspect should be transported as soon as possible for further medical evaluation and remain under close monitoring en route.

Weapons and the TEMS Unit

The TEMS unit may potentially be armed with batons, TASERs, firearms, OC spray, and other weapons. Your agency will decide which, if any, weapons the TEMS unit may carry into the tactical environment. The agency will also provide the proper training for these weapons.

Firearms

Whether or not your TEMS unit is armed is determined by your law enforcement agency. Whether your TEMS unit is armed or not, you must be able to safely handle, unload, and render safe any and all SWAT weapons including less-lethal weapons. Always follow the local policies and procedures of the local law enforcement agency. It is advantageous to be competent in loading, clearing malfunctions, and accurately firing all of the SWAT unit firearms for the rare circumstance where the TMP is alone with a SWAT officer who is incapacitated and a significant threat continues to exist. Many SWAT units utilize four to six different types of long guns and eight to twelve different types of pistols. Chapter 5, "Firearms Safety and Marksmanship," discusses firearms safety in detail.

Batons

The actual use of a baton, night stick, or other striking weapon by TMPs is extremely rare. If a TEMS unit is authorized to carry these weapons, they must be fully trained and certified according to law enforcement guidelines. In general, the most commonly carried baton is the extendable baton, often named the "ASP" after the company that designed it. The baton can cause death if the suspect is struck on the head, neck, or other critical area. There are target areas you should try to hit, including the actual weapon that is being held (stick, knife, other), nerves (such as the common peroneal

---

Safety

You can learn additional restraint methods by attending formal law enforcement training.

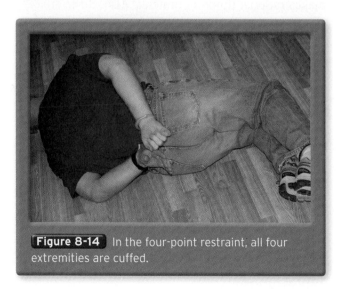

Figure 8-14 In the four-point restraint, all four extremities are cuffed.

nerve in the leg), and large muscle groups of the body. Areas to avoid include the head, neck, spine, sternum, and groin.

OC Spray

Oleoresin capsicum pepper (OC), also referred to as pepper spray or pepper foam, is a tool that is not 100% reliable but often is successful when used for stopping a physical attack. It should be noted that a small percentage of humans and dogs are not affected at all by the OC. Also, some emotionally disturbed persons are essentially immune to it. The range of a handheld small OC dispenser is 4 to 5 feet. The tight stream dispenser has a range of 10 feet. The fogger can reach 10 to 12 feet. It acts almost immediately. Wind is a factor to consider when deploying OC.

Illumination Tools

A powerful light beam can be used as a nonlethal method of temporarily blinding and overwhelming a threatening suspect. The blinding effects of certain extremely powerful illumination tools can impact a suspect up to 300 feet away. The visual disorientation experienced by the suspect will cause the suspect to feel unbalanced, giving the TMP a temporary tactical advantage. Newer flashlight technology has enabled a miniature strobe feature to rapidly flash the bright light on and off, which further disables and confuses the suspect. During the confusion following the use of light to blind a suspect, SWAT officers may have an opportunity to more closely approach the suspect and effect an arrest and capture.

At the Scene

When OC spray is utilized, be prepared to immediately go to a backup plan as it is not 100% reliable in stopping an attacker.

Several companies (Surefire, Streamlight, Blackhawk, and others) have developed compact law enforcement and EMS lighting tools that are very bright and are small enough to be carried at all times. They have switches that allow the flashlight to be turned on and off rapidly, which allows a tactical advantage. These flashlights are very dependable, and many use lithium batteries that have a shelf life of 10 years and function in below-freezing temperatures, which add to reliability.

Knives

Most SWAT officers and TMPs carry the common folding knife, although in most instances it is used as a tool and not a weapon. Few law enforcement agencies teach any knife fighting techniques because keeping a substantial distance away and using other methods of achieving compliance are much better ways of dealing with a suspect with a knife. If it can safely be accomplished, less-lethal weapons should be used to gain compliance. Overall, knives are effective tools, but limited in use as defensive weapons and should not be used or counted on in combat except in extreme situations.

TASER and Other Conducted Electrical Weapons

It is rare for a TMP to be authorized and issued a TASER or similar device at this time, unless they are full-time law enforcement officers. TASERs are discussed in detail in Chapter 3, "SWAT Unit Essentials." The indications for use of a TASER are to enforce compliance with directions and to more safely resolve a confrontation with an adversary, especially if that attacker is under the influence of PCP or other mind-altering substance that makes rational thinking difficult. Also, if the attacker is very large and strong, it has been shown that use of these devices results in less physical harm to both law enforcement officers and the suspects.

Ready for Review

- All TMPs must be prepared to simultaneously provide medical care and protect themselves, downed SWAT officers, and patients.

- Consult your local law enforcement agency's policies to determine the level of self-defense proficiency that is expected of TMPs. Law enforcement policies should discuss the initial and continuing training procedures that are in place to ensure proper maintenance and improvement of skills. The plan for strength training, physical combat skills, weapon system familiarization, and defense tactics should be included in the policies.

- Depending upon the weapons that are authorized in your agency, you should develop the ability to rapidly and smoothly choose the right tool from your toolbox of unarmed defense techniques, weapons, and tactics.

- Do not attempt to handcuff a suspect unless you are thoroughly trained and have the legal authority to do so. At least one or more backup SWAT officers should be present.

Vital Vocabulary

auditory exclusion A temporary loss of hearing that occurs as part of the fight-or-flight stress response during confrontation with danger; serves to remove background noise allowing for a sole focus on survival.

fight-or-flight response The sympathetic nervous system's automatic response to fear: stress hormones are released, which temporarily increase the blood flow to the skeletal muscles, thereby increasing the body's ability to run or fight, and focusing the mind purely on survival.

perceptual narrowing A temporary reduction of higher brain center processing of sensory information that occurs as part of the fight-or-flight stress response during confrontation with danger; serves to simplify decision-making and help a person focus on survival.

tunnel vision A temporary reduction in the field of vision that occurs as part of the fight-or-flight stress response during confrontation with danger.

Operational Tactics

Introduction

As a TMP, you must be familiar with the dangers you may face when supporting special weapons and tactics (SWAT) units. Many of these threats occur suddenly and without notice. You may go from sitting calmly at the dinner table to donning tactical gear and entering a highly dangerous area 20 minutes later. In order for you to assist in safely completing the SWAT unit's mission and return safely home, it is critical that you obtain and interpret important information, develop mission plans, and operate as an integrated unit with your SWAT officer colleagues **Figure 9-1**.

Activation

SWAT Unit Activation

In general, patrol officers attempt to contain and resolve less-hazardous incidents with fellow patrol officers. Truly dangerous situations occur when an experienced criminal with a "nothing-to-lose" mentality has weapons to inflict harm on responding law enforcement officers and citizens. These situations and others call for a specialized unit that can contain, negotiate, neutralize any threats, and resolve the dangerous situation as peacefully as possible **Figure 9-2**.

Recently, there has been an increased use of less-lethal weapons such as the shotgun beanbag round and electronic control devices such as TASERs. Less-lethal weapons have reduced the need for SWAT callouts because patrol officers can often team up and convince the criminal suspect to surrender. If the situation is initially particularly high risk, however, the SWAT unit leadership must determine whether the SWAT unit should be activated. Many police departments have automatic callout criteria, while other departments make the decision on a case-by-case basis after discussion with command staff.

The decision to activate a SWAT unit is not taken lightly due to the risk of injury and death to SWAT officers, and also due to the

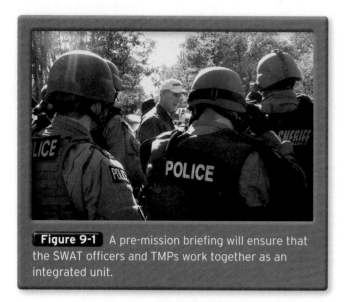

Figure 9-1 A pre-mission briefing will ensure that the SWAT officers and TMPs work together as an integrated unit.

TEMS Unit Activation

Each TEMS unit will have protocols for calling out and activating its personnel. While training with your unit, you will learn the specific protocols and procedures followed by your TEMS unit. An all-unit simultaneous activation via pager, cell phone, or home phone notification is a very efficient system for TEMS unit activation. In this system, each time the law enforcement agency activates its SWAT unit, the TEMS unit is also automatically activated. In fact, some SWAT units will not perform an elective high-risk mission without the presence of their TEMS personnel.

At a minimum, two TMPs should be involved in entry during a SWAT callout. For a routine, high-risk, search-and-arrest warrant SWAT callout, it is ideal for two TMPs to accompany the entry team (to post nearby or enter with the team, depending on local protocols), while a third TMP remains at the tactical operations center (TOC) with the command staff. For larger buildings or more complex and lengthy callouts, more TMPs are desirable.

Not everyone on the TEMS unit is needed for a straightforward, high-risk search warrant. A system should be developed within each TEMS unit that allows for each TMP to participate in a fair and equal number of callouts in order to maintain a balance of field experience among TMPs within the TEMS unit. This system should allow a partial or full callout of TEMS personnel so that the resources can be matched to the callout indications. For example, if a standard high-risk arrest warrant is being served by the SWAT unit and undercover vice agents, then three TMPs should be involved and a selection system should be used to choose which three members out of the ten-person TEMS unit it will be. On average, when accounting for employee vacations and routine work schedules (outside of their tactical service), a TEMS unit composed of ten people will on average have three or four people available to deploy at any given time.

expense of paying 20 to 30 specially trained tactical officers overtime salary for several hours, which can cause budgetary concerns. The use of a SWAT unit is very likely the safest and most reliable way to neutralize a high-risk situation and apprehend or neutralize dangerous suspects.

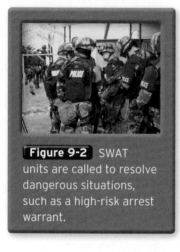

Figure 9-2 SWAT units are called to resolve dangerous situations, such as a high-risk arrest warrant.

Once the decision is made by command staff to activate the SWAT unit, the SWAT officers, who are typically on call 24 hours a day and 7 days a week, are contacted by phone, radio, or pager. The SWAT officers typically call back to the communications center or law agency headquarters where they verify that they are responding and receive specific directions informing them of the mission and assembly point. The SWAT unit will often gather at the law enforcement headquarters, but in some circumstances, such as a hostage barricade scenario, it is best to have SWAT officers assemble several blocks from the actual incident location. The goal is to gather at an appropriate, safe location, become organized, determine the facts of the situation, develop contingency plans, and prepare to resolve the situation in the best way possible.

Callout Formation

When the SWAT and TEMS units are activated, the SWAT officers and TEMS providers report to either agency headquarters or directly to a specified site near the incident. If the SWAT and TEMS units are meeting at the agency headquarters, the SWAT and TEMS units will first receive a rapid but thorough briefing. After the briefing, the SWAT and TEMS units will travel in one or multiple vehicles to the callout site. Often one or several raid vans are used, which may be plain and unmarked. If an armored vehicle such as the BearCat is utilized, eight or more SWAT officers with one or two TMPs will ride in it to the scene and be ready to respond to dangerous threats immediately.

If the SWAT callout involves meeting at or near the scene of the incident, take a few moments before leaving in the car to identify the exact travel route. This will prevent you from accidentally driving into high-crime areas alone, and prevent you from sitting in your car in a bad neighborhood while trying to figure out where you are. When a callout requires SWAT officers and TEMS providers to respond directly to the incident, then the dispatch center must provide accurate and specific directions to SWAT and TEMS personnel regarding the best approach in order to prevent personnel from getting too close to the suspect or driving through a field of gunfire. You should have good communication with knowledgeable dispatchers or fellow officers regarding the situation, threats, travel route to the scene, location to park, and a general idea of what to do upon arrival. Text messaging works well with pagers and cell phones and can provide much information. Do not read or send text messages while driving.

All SWAT and TEMS personnel meet and gear up upon arrival at the designated callout location. A majority of SWAT units have their SWAT officers carry all of their own personal tactical gear and weapons with them in their department vehicles to maximize the speed of response.

SWAT Officer Data Cards

Ideally you will be given up-to-date information on each SWAT officer's medical history, allergies, and medications in the event that illness or injury occurs. This information can be easily summarized on **SWAT officer data cards**, which do not include the entire name of the SWAT officer but instead have the first name and the first initial of the SWAT officer's last name, along with pertinent medical information. This way, if a data card is accidently dropped at the scene then the security of the SWAT officer data cards may be compromised, but the information cannot be used against the SWAT unit officers. If a member of the SWAT support team or bomb squad does not have a data card, take a moment to fill out some basic information.

Medical Threat Assessment

The incident commander and the tactical operations leader will be too occupied to explain the situation to each arriving TMP; therefore, the TEMS unit leader should gather information about the specific suspects, nature of the callout, current plans, and the tasks that need to be completed by the TEMS unit. The TEMS unit leader will update TEMS personnel as they arrive. This TEMS unit leader will also participate in mission planning and use information gathered by all TMPs to develop the mission-specific medical threat assessment (MTA). If any suggestions are made during the assessment and planning, such as setting up a rehabilitation station if the callout is projected to be prolonged, the TEMS unit leader will convey information to the incident commander and the tactical operations leader at a convenient and appropriate time.

Personnel Tracking

A roster of on-site SWAT unit and TEMS unit personnel should be created and updated accurately until the mission is complete. All SWAT and TEMS unit personnel who enter and leave the area must be accounted for.

Safety

Keeping track of individual SWAT officers in the tactical environment is a major task for the tactical operations leader. SWAT officers should have identical or at least similar uniforms and insignia subtly displayed. If some SWAT officers or TMPs leave the scene without notifying anyone, it may present a time-consuming, frustrating, and dangerous experience if someone has to go searching for the missing SWAT officer or TMP. SWAT officers and TMPs need to keep close contact, and when dismissed, inform the tactical operations leader that they are leaving the scene. It is also a good idea for personnel to "buddy up" and remain with their partners during callouts, especially in dangerous areas and at nighttime.

At a complex scene, and especially at nighttime, it is easy to lose track of individual SWAT officers or TEMS providers. The tactical operations leader will post and maintain an updated name board of who is present, as well as the specific team they are assigned to.

Tactical Plan Development

The incident will determine how much time is available to make plans for the mission. The collective wisdom and common sense of the tactical operations leader is needed to determine the best methods of approaching the scene, arranging negotiations if necessary, assigning marksmen their positions, scouting the area, and delegating responsibilities.

The tactical operations leader will arrange for an immediate reaction team in the event that violence breaks out before the SWAT unit is fully organized and operational. While the immediate reaction team is deployed immediately and stands by prepared to respond if gunfire or other violence erupts, the remainder of the SWAT unit and the tactical operations leader will perform other duties, such as reconnaissance, organizing contingency plans, and beginning the negotiation process. Contingency plans, rescue teams, officer-down immediate action drills, points of no-turn-around, and medical extraction plans should be determined before initiating any approach or assault. Marksmen will deploy to hidden positions and report on any activity. The rules of engagement will be reviewed and information disseminated about the physical descriptions of suspects and hostages, as well as known innocent bystanders or undercover agents inside the building.

Safety

Clear labeling of "POLICE," "SHERIFF," "SWAT," or other law enforcement title displayed on the front and back of an exterior uniform or vest will identify exactly who is involved in the mission in the tactical environment. Without proper identification, a law enforcement officer or TMP could be mistaken for a criminal suspect, with tragic results.

If time allows, you may want to consider a brief pratice session where SWAT officers actually load and unload into the SWAT unit vehicles several times, practice their approach, and practice their response roles. It is important for entry team leaders to acknowledge and point out who will be involved in the initial entry (dynamic entry or stealth entry) as well as any narcotics or vice squad officers who will be along on the callout.

There will likely be several patrol officers and detectives who will help in perimeter access control and the later investigation. Occasionally an assistant district attorney may be present to observe and assist in providing legal advice to ensure the successful prosecution of the suspects.

Immediate Action Drills

During the planning phase, the tactical operations leader will decide what to do if a SWAT officer is injured or downed during each key phase of the mission. The tactical operations leader must convey this plan to the SWAT and TEMS personnel so that if the unexpected injury does occur, the SWAT and TEMS units can perform an **immediate action drill (IAD)** to quickly stabilize the scene, provide stabilizing first aid, and extract and transport the SWAT officer or patient to the appropriate location at the most optimal time.

These hasty rescues may be accomplished by an entry team using ballistic shields, and possibly covering fire, to immediately remove a downed SWAT officer to a position of relative safety. You should smoothly integrate with the SWAT officers to assist in the assessment, stabilization, and extraction of the SWAT officer. Depending upon the mission and the objectives, the SWAT unit should then either continue with the entry or immediately recover the downed SWAT officer and withdraw. At least one of the TMPs will be expected to remain with the downed SWAT officer as the SWAT and TEMS units continue with the mission, while several SWAT officers perform an extraction and transportation of the downed SWAT officer.

Each situation will vary and everyone on the entry team should know which point of the mission is the no-turning-back phase. For example, if a high-risk search warrant is served and the entry team is shot at during the approach with a SWAT officer downed by a bullet, then the plan may be to perform an IAD to remove the SWAT officer and then have the entire entry team withdraw. However, if a hostage-barricade scenario occurs and the situation deteriorates to the point where the hostage is thought to be at high risk of being harmed, then an assault will be ordered. The IAD will likely be to continue the dynamic entry with the remaining SWAT officers running past the downed SWAT officer in full dynamic assault, while one TMP and a guard SWAT officer remain with the injured SWAT officer. When the main goal—the safety of the hostage—is ensured, then the entry team can work together to extract the downed SWAT officer.

TEMS Unit Placement

Perimeters and Zones at Callouts

At the site of a SWAT callout, the area surrounding the suspect is divided by circular or square city-block boundaries, known as perimeters **Figure 9-3**. These areas are defined as follows:

- **Inner perimeter**. Inside of the inner perimeter is the most dangerous area at a tactical callout, where the suspect can potentially attack and use weapons to cause casualties. Each agency has local protocols on the use of TMPs in the inner perimeter. TEMS providers may routinely accompany the entry team inside the inner perimeter to perform medical care and assist with the entry. Other SWAT units do not utilize TMPs inside the inner perimeter until all suspects are neutralized and the building has been cleared.
- **Tactical warm zone**. In the area between the inner and outer perimeters, TMPs may find variable degrees of hard cover that represent areas of relative safety from bullets and/or weapons. There is some risk of violence to personnel but less than in the inner perimeter. This is a common area for the TMP to detach from the entry team and remain nearby, within visual range of the exact building entry point, but outside and behind hard cover. From a point of relative safety, the TMPs can wait with a SWAT officer for the mission to be completed. If a SWAT officer is shot or otherwise downed, then that officer can be extracted to the TMPs or the TMPs can go to the injured officer with a SWAT officer or two guiding and protecting them.
- **Outer perimeter**. The outer perimeter is the area at a tactical callout that is considered to be safe from weapons and violence. Its boundary is generally enforced by perimeter patrol officers to keep bystanders out and to watch for and apprehend any potential suspects trying to escape. Some SWAT units will keep their TMPs waiting behind hard cover at this location until the downed SWAT officer is brought out to them, or if circumstances demand it, they may be escorted by armed SWAT officers into the tactical warm zone or inner perimeter to provide emergency care.

Placement of the TEMS Unit in the Tactical Environment

The location of the TEMS unit and the tactics used by SWAT units vary. Some SWAT units use TMPs who are law enforcement officers with medical training on the initial entry team. Other SWAT units place TMPs at a nearby **point of relative safety**—an area located at either the outer perimeter or just inside it in the tactical warm zone where TMPs can more safely provide stabilizing medical care. In this setup, TMPs will remain outside the outer perimeter until they are called to enter the tactical warm zone as needed when injured SWAT officers are brought to them. Some SWAT units keep their TMPs entirely outside of the outer perimeter. Their IAD is to have fellow SWAT officers bring any injured or ill victims to the TEMS unit near the TOC. Other SWAT units use a hybrid of these and other tactics. There is no one correct strategy. Follow the strategy of your agency.

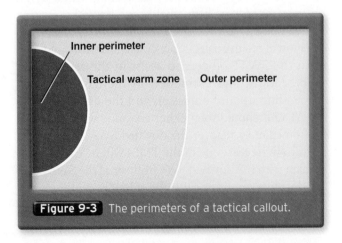

Figure 9-3 The perimeters of a tactical callout.

Many TEMS units use the following strategy. When a critical incident develops to the point where SWAT entry is required, the TEMS unit moves forward with the entry team to a point of hard cover. The TEMS unit remains at a point of relative safety—close enough to the entry site to allow a fast response time, just outside of the inner perimeter. Ideally, a TMP will be able to respond to a downed SWAT officer in less than 30 seconds. If the scene is not secured but a SWAT officer is injured and can be moved, then the downed SWAT officer is extracted and brought to the point of relative safety for first aid. If conditions or manpower limitations dictate it, the TMP may consider entering the inner perimeter to go to the downed officer's side, but always with either a SWAT officer on guard or another TMP who is armed and assumes the role of a guard while medical care is provided. As always, follow your local protocols.

Positioning of EMS Transportation

TEMS units are often nontransport units, so the EMS system is required for transport of injured persons to the hospital **Figure 9-4**. This must be considered during the planning of the mission, especially the location of the ambulance, the safety of EMS personnel, communication with the EMS personnel, and coordination of transportation efforts.

If multiple persons are involved in an incident and may potentially become victims, then the TEMS unit leader will advise the command staff during the MTA briefing on the recommended number of ambulances that should be prestaged in case of a worst-case scenario. These EMS units should be updated appropriately with necessary information about the ongoing event, possible outcomes, possible transportation needs, and

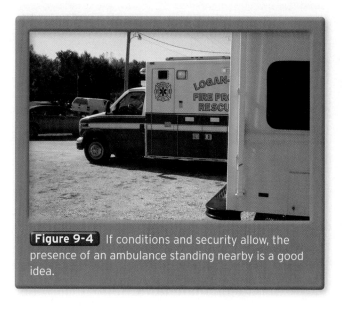

Figure 9-4 If conditions and security allow, the presence of an ambulance standing nearby is a good idea.

coordination of medical care. At the conclusion of the callout, the supporting ambulance agencies and personnel should be appropriately and personally thanked, updated, and dismissed from the callout scene.

Entry

As a TMP, you must be well trained in the specific tactics and strategies utilized by your SWAT unit. The exact methods will vary considerably depending upon the SWAT leadership, training, and past experiences of your unit.

Indications for Dynamic or Stealth Entry

There are two primary methods for entering a structure: dynamic or stealth entry. Depending on the incident, only one type of entry may be used or both types of entry may be used. The type of entry will be determined by the tactical operations leader during the preplanning phase of the callout.

Dynamic Entry

Dynamic entries are usually made with rapid team movement inside of a building with forcible mechanical tools, distraction devices, and/or with explosive breaches utilized. Dynamic or fast entry is done when there is substantial danger to the entry team or to innocent persons or hostages inside, or there is a need to move quickly during drug search warrants to prevent drugs and other evidence from being destroyed. Many SWAT units have abandoned this strategy of entry for simple drug or evidence recovery due to the higher risks to entry team members. Typically, TMPs do not participate in these high-risk entries as part of the entry team unless they are fully trained SWAT officers. The role of the TEMS unit in this mode of operation is to remain at a point of relative safety and come forward when requested, or remain at their fixed point and have SWAT officers bring the injured officer to them.

Safety

Tactical teams must have escape routes planned in advance and known to the entire team. Avoid situations in which there is only one path out.

Stealth Entry

Stealth entries or slow entries are usually made when there is a need to conduct surveillance and locate threats in a manner that is not time sensitive. Stealth entries may be used to search for a hidden felony suspect in a building or house using a slow, methodical search with mirrors and video cameras. The stealth entry is also sometimes used to rescue persons who are in close proximity to hostage takers but not held at gunpoint. The rationale for this type of entry is to conduct reconnaissance carefully to locate the suspects, rescue any persons in danger, and neutralize threats. If the SWAT officers are suddenly discovered, the stealth entry may then become dynamic. In some circumstances, particularly in larger buildings with multiple rooms and floors, TEMS unit personnel will accompany SWAT officers toward the end of the stack formation to initiate stabilizing treatment of any injured persons.

Entry Team Operations

The entry team should approach the target location as silently and discreetly as possible. Depending on the circumstances, the entry team may choose a dynamic entry and enter hard and fast. Such an approach allows less time for suspects to react and retrieve any weapons or get rid of any drugs. In less time-urgent situations, the entry team leader may choose to use chemical agents to force the suspect out, or perform a stealth entry using mirrors and video cameras on a pole to slowly enter the building and search the rooms, identify the suspect(s), and rely on the negotiations team to convince the suspect(s) to surrender.

Depending on the size of the building and many other factors, TMPs providing support to the entry team may remain outside a small building while the search and arrest are accomplished. In a large building, the TMPs may be assigned to stay with the main entry team or rescue team. In such cases, TEMS personnel will enter and search the building to help look for and care for injured victims. Also, the TEMS unit will be immediately available to care for downed SWAT officers.

The Stack Formation

TEMS personnel participating in a SWAT unit movement will usually be placed in the more secure rear third of the **stack formation** [Figure 9-5]. The entry team will want to enter a building or room as efficiently as possible, and one of the best ways to do this is to line up in a single-file formation. When the door is opened or breached, then the SWAT officers can efficiently enter the structure using either a stealth or dynamic method. TMPs who are armed and trained should enter toward the rear of this stack, but should not be the last one in line. A SWAT officer should provide the final rear guard and be prepared to deal with an ambush or unexpected suspects.

Stairs Tactics

Entry teams that encounter stairs must recognize that going up or down a set of stairs is a significant hazard and must be done in a cautious and tactically correct manner in order to minimize the threat of being shot. Although the risks for any TMPs at the end of the stack formation are significantly less than for those SWAT officers in the front, when an entry team negotiates a stairwell or multilevel stairway, any doorways that are encountered must be cleared or covered by an armed SWAT officer.

The Pie Tactic

Doors are referred to as "fatal funnels" because past experience has shown that law enforcement officers who stand in doorways for too long may be shot. If a suspect

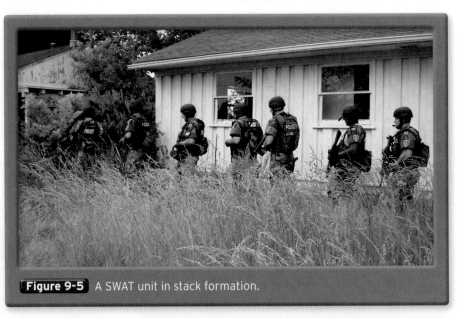

Figure 9-5   A SWAT unit in stack formation.

is waiting inside a room or structure, then the doorway is the funnel entry point. The suspect can simply aim a gun at the door and shoot when a SWAT officer or TEMS personnel enters into the funnel.

Before entering a room in a stealth approach, SWAT officers will use a mirror, perform a quick peek, or "pie" the room. A quick peek is done at a low level, avoiding the eye level of the suspect. A quick peek can provide an idea of what lies in the next room without unnecessary exposure. To "pie" the next room with unknown suspects inside, the SWAT officer will point his or her weapon into the room while remaining to the side of the doorway. The SWAT officer will then slowly take one step sideways, viewing one portion of the room or "one slice of the pie." As the SWAT officer gradually moves sideways, the officer is exposed to larger portions of the room while remaining ready to spring out of the doorway and shoot if appropriate. This tactic can also be used with corners.

When a room or structure is entered, you should continue moving and make observations. Entering the room should be a team effort with the entry team leader scanning left to right and another SWAT officer scanning right to left, or vice versa depending upon the room obstacles and threats. The entry team should scan the entire room for hazards or threats as they enter, and should prepare to take evasive action and eliminate threats. TMPs who arrive later should maintain a situational awareness and not be complacent in thinking that every threat has already been eliminated. Watch for the unexpected—that nice wool blanket hanging on the wall may be hiding a closet with an armed and dangerous suspect inside.

When moving along a hallway, walk near the wall about 1 foot away but not in contact with the wall to avoid skipped bullets. The entry team should move in single file trying to stay out of the middle of the hallway. The last person should scan the rear to look for suspects approaching. Use care when crossing doorways or cross-halls. Threats can come from any direction.

Safety

Note that one or two interior walls of normal drywall or sheetrock construction do not provide ballistic protection. Shooting through interior walls is possible even with pistols.

Clearing Rooms: Entry and Egress

When entering a structure or location, you should ideally identify an egress (exit) route and have a backup route established. Windows normally do not provide a good egress route because most will need to be broken to facilitate an exit, and above-ground locations may preclude this route due to height. Emergency exits from multistory structures with an elevator may be restricted to the stairs. Some doors may lock once closed and thus require movement to the ground or roof level. Newer egress techniques include the use of slings and ropes to lower victims to the ground level, but the situations where this is needed are extremely rare.

SWAT units may need to use simple tools such as a saw or sledgehammer to create an emergency exit location by sawing holes in drywall or knocking apart a block-stone wall to create a way to egress from a building with a casualty. Ingenuity and creativity are valuable assets in these situations.

Victim Restraint

Any person or victim who is not personally known to the SWAT unit or TEMS unit is a threat until proven otherwise. In many circumstances, when the identities of the suspects are not clearly known, all persons at a scene are handcuffed and restrained until the suspects are positively identified. This may require the use of handcuffs or plastic Flexcuffs, or the suspects will need to be held at gunpoint. The TMP is *not* to handcuff or restrain suspects or even seemingly innocent hostages unless the TMP has received appropriate training, is experienced, and has maintained up-to-date skills in restraining suspects properly. Many suspects have been street-trained and know how to escape or assault SWAT officers during the handcuffing process.

When rendering medical assistance, leave restraints in place until the individual is determined not to be a threat. Prior to that, restraints are removed only if they will interfere with life-saving procedures. Do not remove restraints without the permission and standby assistance of a SWAT officer. If a suspect needs to be restrained with handcuffs to a backboard, one method is to place the suspect on his or her back and restrain one hand to the board or stretcher near the lower hip area and secure the other hand above the level of the shoulder, which will prevent the suspect from sitting up and moving about.

TEMS Operational Procedures

Recognition of Danger and Threats

Danger can come from a variety of sources. Suspects are the source of some hazards, while other threats are a result of the tactical environment (booby traps, low-light conditions, abandoned buildings). Watch where you step during low-light situations and carry a flashlight. Many older structures have poor lighting and dilapidated stairs or steps. Listen for sounds of an altercation and persons opening doors or windows. Do not forget to look up to see if you are being observed.

Cover and Concealment

Cover and concealment are important principles. Concealment protects you from the view of suspects, but it does not provide protection from small arms fire or explosions **Figure 9-6**. Concealment usually consists of shrubs, bushes, camouflage netting, interior walls of struc-

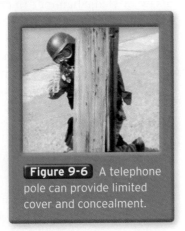

Figure 9-6 A telephone pole can provide limited cover and concealment.

tures, garbage cans, utility poles, or normal vehicles. Although concealment may afford some protection from suspects, cover should be chosen over concealment whenever possible.

Cover provides substantial protection from small arms fire and explosion shrapnel **Figure 9-7**. Examples of cover include a large 3-foot diameter tree trunk, fire hydrant, masonry or concrete structure, and other substantial objects. Remember that high-velocity center fire

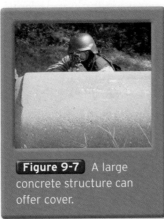

Figure 9-7 A large concrete structure can offer cover.

rifle bullets may even penetrate some of the cover such as trees, large mailboxes, or thin masonry walls. Interior walls of houses or vehicles do not provide substantial cover. Most rifles, shotguns, and pistol rounds will penetrate interior walls of homes and commercial buildings and the sheet metal, glass, and plastic of vehicles.

Safety

Ballistic threats include bullets that, when fired against a solid surface such as pavement or concrete, deform and may ricochet and travel at high speed parallel to the surface. This means that shots that strike pavement or a hard surface in front of an officer will follow that surface. This makes it possible to skip bullets under a vehicle or along a wall. Bullets will follow the wall parallel to its surface making a person walking along the side of a wall susceptible to being struck. When walking down a hallway, walk at least 1 foot away from a wall to avoid skip shots **Figure 9-8**.

You should constantly think about what cover is nearby, plan how to stay hidden, and try to maximize use of cover during the mission. When selecting a potential escape route or patient evacuation route, you should consider the types of cover and concealment available.

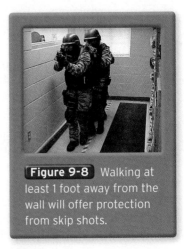

Figure 9-8 Walking at least 1 foot away from the wall will offer protection from skip shots.

Vehicles as Protection

Vehicles do not offer substantial protection from rifle fire, and some pistol bullets will easily penetrate vehicles. If a vehicle must be used for cover or concealment, a wise choice is to stay behind the engine block and front tire. The engine block and tire or wheel may deflect or stop some rounds. Remember that bullets will skip under vehicles and also skip off the surfaces of metal structures, and that quick peeks should not be made over the hood, roof, or trunk as bullets will spall and follow these structures.

Moving from Cover

It typically takes a suspect about 1 second to note and react to movement, and 1 to 2 seconds to aim and fire at the target. If the suspect is prepared, this length of time

Safety

Ordinary glass provides no ballistic protection.

may be shorter. Therefore, when moving from cover to cover, limit your exposure to no more than 2 seconds. Before moving out, know where you are moving to and how long it will take. Avoid leaving good cover simply to gain a better vantage point. If the exposure will last more than 2 seconds, rethink your decision. If you must expose yourself moving from one point of cover to another for more than 3 seconds, then make random movements in a serpentine zigzag weaving pattern to make target acquisition more difficult for the suspect. Although this movement lengthens your exposure time, it will be more difficult for the suspect to obtain target acquisition.

Quick Peeks

Quick peeks are a method for observing a specific setting while minimizing exposure. The 2-second rule applies: Never expose yourself for more than 2 seconds because doing so makes you an easy target. Another rule is never to peek from the same location more than once. If a suspect can target your location, a second look also makes you an easy target. Crouch down before peeking because the suspect will be expecting to see someone at his or her eye level, not beneath it.

Light Tactics

When moving with the SWAT unit through dark areas, you should not turn on a flashlight or light source unless it is acceptable to the entry team commander and nearby fellow teammates. Remember: *If you can see the enemy, the enemy can see you.*

Use the light source to your advantage. Divide the search areas. While searching a dark area by scanning it with a flashlight, it may be tempting to keep the flashlight on and take in everything all at once; however, the light and your vision will only cover so much area. Be systematic in the search and create overlapping zones, and make certain that one area is clear before moving on to the next.

While searching with flashlights, you should turn the light on briefly (fraction of a second), then move a step or two to a new location to flash the light briefly over a new area. When searching for potentially armed suspects, remember that the light beam will tell the suspect exactly where you are. Whenever the light is turned on, it is the adversary's target.

Sound and Light Discipline

Sound and light discipline are essential in the tactical environment. Essentially this means keeping quiet and not being seen or heard. Portable radios, ringing cellular telephones, chiming watches, or beeping pagers all present hazards as the suspect can hear them and learn the location of the entry team. Consider using a nonaudible alerting system on these devices, such as the vibrate function, and use quiet tactical headsets for radio communication. Some rubber-soled shoes and boots can squeak loudly on hard floors, so choose and test your footwear appropriately. Dried leaves and branches will make noise in an outdoor setting, as will a vehicle door. Jingling keys and coins in the pocket are another source of noise. Work to noise-proof your gear, and then test by jumping up and down to see if any gear or items move and make noise.

Night operations may result in a situation where the suspect fires on any light source and the gunshot victims are downed within eyesight of the suspect. These situations require the TMPs to work in the dark with no visible light that may be seen by the suspect. Low-light and no-light medical care requires the tactile use of your hands in assessing the patient, as well as use of instruments and treatment without light.

For many years, the military has successfully used night vision monocular or binocular goggles for patient assessment and medical care. The military has also employed special red lights (low visibility from a distance) and some prefer low-intensity green lights, which facilitate blood identification. Night operations require good light discipline in order to protect both you and the patient. Light use should be very limited when threats exist. However, the use of a low-powered flashlight to negotiate stairs or other hazardous locations may be critical.

Using Other Senses to Maintain Situational Awareness

You may be able to detect air currents from opening doors or windows from some distance away, which can alert you to suspect movement. You may also use your sense of smell to detect a suspect's location. Intense-smelling colognes or other body sprays and body odor may allow detection by smell. Many of the clandestine drug laboratory chemicals have a distinctive smell. Some toxic agents such as natural gas odorant, solvents, hydrogen sulfide, or anhydrous ammonia are easily detected by smell. The sense of touch may also alert you to vibration in floors that indicate suspect movement. Be sensitive to this in the tactical environment.

Covert Communications

A method of covert communication such as hand signals for your SWAT unit will be demonstrated to you during training with your TEMS unit. This system will include methods to communicate danger, intent, or situational information, even while under observation of a suspect. For example, when faced with an uncooperative suspect who is not obeying commands, knowing a hand signal or other communication for a partner to deploy and use his or her TASER may be instrumental in resolving the crisis. It is especially important for you to be able to signal to rescuers in a covert manner to indicate your status if you are wounded and exposed to a suspect's view.

Radio Communications

You will become intimately familiar with the radio language and communication procedures used by the SWAT unit during training. Most SWAT units use discreet signals, codes, and brevity phrases. Many of these are the same as normal police communications such as "10-4" ("Okay"). This allows a standard thought, observation, or finding to be transmitted with brevity and some security **Figure 9-9**.

Each SWAT unit will incorporate a specific terminology to identify various parts of structures,

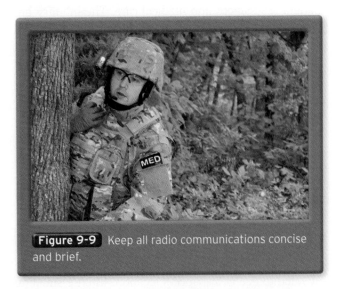

Figure 9-9 Keep all radio communications concise and brief.

directions, movement in formation, and related activities. For example, some SWAT units use directional names to describe structures, while others use numbers for each side of a building and floors, while an additional technique is to color-code each side of a structure (eg, white is the front, red is the right side of house when facing the front of the house). You must be familiar with this language as it may be life-threatening to approach the wrong side of a building if you are called forward for a downed SWAT officer during a crisis.

If a situation involves non-SWAT law enforcement personnel or other agencies, then it is a good idea to use plain common language. If a regional disaster draws government response agencies, then law enforcement and NIMS mandate use of common terminology during agency operations.

Adhere to radio discipline and do not transmit unless emergency conditions warrant or unless you are requested to respond.

Mission Completion

Through effective SWAT unit planning, training, and teamwork, high-risk situations can be resolved without injury more often. Statistically, suspects are unlikely to be hurt or ill. If suspects are injured, provide appropriate on-site evaluation, emergency medical care, and make recommendations to the SWAT/TEMS leaders as to whether or not the suspect should be taken to the hospital for formal evaluation. The suspect(s) may need to be taken to the hospital for a complete evaluation, or they could be referred to the jail facility medical site for minor medical care and observation. Any bystanders or hostages who are apparently injured or seriously ill should be evaluated and stabilized by either the TMPs or the EMS system providers.

Post-Mission Debriefings

The tactical operations leader will usually want the TEMS unit to remain on site until it is certain that there are no further threats or additional suspects. After the mission, most SWAT units will hold a debriefing session at the headquarters so all SWAT unit and TEMS unit personnel can comment and provide feedback. The goal is to improve tactics and future performance. If the callout occurs late at night or lasts for several days, then the debriefing may be arranged within a day or two after SWAT officers and TEMS providers have rested. These sessions ensure that TEMS unit callout protocols are current and high quality.

Mission debriefings should be conducted in a nonjudgmental manner so that the session remains constructive. The discussion should allow each SWAT officer and TMP to discuss what went right and what needs to be improved. If properly organized, this debriefing is very helpful for the SWAT unit and TEMS unit, and leads to improvement of the units, equipment, and tactics.

Consideration should be afforded to improving individual and unit performance, communications, medical equipment and packs, transportation, security (adequate protection of the TMPs), teamwork, and, in cases where medical attention was needed, evaluation of the care provided. HIPAA regulations should be followed

Safety

Only through self-analysis and constructive criticism can SWAT units and TEMS units make worthwhile changes to their operations.

when discussing patient care, especially if it involved medical care of a SWAT officer.

An essential aspect of operating in a dangerous or violent environment is the understanding of the legal and justifiable use of force by law enforcement officers. To truly understand the principles of use of force by law enforcement officers—including the issues of self-defense, defense of others, and making arrests—law, policy, and procedure must be studied. After classroom study, force-on-force training with simulations requires participants to make real-time, life-or-death decisions and provide after-action explanations for their actions based on law and policy. Through study and training, TMPs will gain a true understanding of use of force by law enforcement. If weapons were used to end the incident, then the involved SWAT officer as well as all involved law enforcement officers and any public safety officers should be supported and arrangements made for further support and consideration of critical incident stress debriefing counseling.

Ready for Review

- When the SWAT and TEMS units are activated, the SWAT officers and TEMS providers report to either agency headquarters or directly to a specified site near the incident.

- The TEMS unit will bring SWAT officer data cards to the scene. These data cards have the first name and the first initial of the SWAT officer's last name, along with pertinent medical information.

- During the planning phase, the tactical operations leader will decide what to do if a SWAT officer is injured or downed during each key phase of the mission.

- Local protocols will dictate the placement of your TEMS unit at a callout.

- Many TEMS units use the following strategy at callouts: the TEMS unit moves forward with the entry team to a point of hard cover and remains at a point of relative safety just outside of the inner perimeter. If a SWAT officer is injured, the injured officer is either brought to the TMPs or the TMP is escorted to the injured officer.

- If suspects are injured, provide appropriate on-site evaluation, emergency medical care, and make further recommendations to the TEMS leader as to whether or not the suspect should be taken to the hospital for formal evaluation.

- Post-mission debriefings ensure that TEMS unit callout protocols are current and high quality.

Vital Vocabulary

dynamic entries Rapid entries by an entry team into an incident scene; designed to overwhelm those inside.

immediate action drill (IAD) A tactic or approach to a situation that is planned and practiced in drills by the SWAT unit so it may be performed smoothly and efficiently if needed during a callout.

inner perimeter The most dangerous area at a tactical callout, where the suspect can potentially attack and use weapons to cause casualties.

outer perimeter The area at a tactical callout felt to be safe from weapons and violence; boundary generally enforced by perimeter patrol officers to keep bystanders out and to watch for and apprehend any potential suspects trying to escape.

point of relative safety An area located at either the outer perimeter or just inside it in the tactical warm zone, where TMPs can more safely provide stabilizing medical care.

quick peeks A method for observing a specific setting while minimizing exposure.

stack formation Single-file formation of SWAT officers designed to allow rapid entry and overwhelming response; used during the entry phase.

stealth entries Slow and silent entries by an entry team into an incident scene; often used if there is no time urgency.

SWAT officer data cards Cards carried by TMPs and SWAT unit leaders; contain essential medical and personal data for each SWAT officer in case of injury.

tactical warm zone Located between the inner and outer perimeters, this is an area of increased threat and risk, but does not have direct risk due to the contained suspects within the hot zone.

Types of SWAT Callouts

OBJECTIVES

- Describe the role of the tactical medical provider (TMP) when responding to a hostage situation or high-risk warrant in a single simple structure.

- Describe the role of the TMP when responding to a callout involving an emotionally disturbed person.

- Describe the role of the TMP when responding to an active shooter scenario.

- Describe the role of the TMP when responding to a search for a suspect or fugitive.

- Describe the role of the TMP when responding to a mass gathering event.

- Describe the role of the TMP when responding to a riot.

- Describe the role of the TMP when responding to an injured patient in an exposed position.

- Describe the role of the TMP during an executive protection callout.

- Describe the role of the TMP during a high-risk prisoner transport.

Introduction

An estimated 40,000 SWAT callouts occur in the United States annually. Every one of these callouts is a uniquely different situation with unique challenges. However, many callouts fall into common categories and occur at common settings, thus enabling SWAT units to create standard tactics for common types of callouts. As a TMP, you will learn the specific tactics of your SWAT unit during training. This chapter provides an overview of the common types of SWAT callouts and the general tactics for each callout.

Single Simple Structure

A common callout site that the SWAT unit responds to is a residential house or small building. A common situation involves the presence of suspects who are selling drugs illegally or are involved in other illegal activities and now have an arrest or search warrant issued. If the suspect is armed and thought to have high risk of "fighting it out" or is known to have rifles or machine guns, or if multiple high-risk suspects are involved, the law enforcement agency will typically arrange for a few SWAT officers or the entire SWAT unit to be involved in the high-risk warrant service.

Another type of callout is the barricaded suspect(s) who refuses to surrender and come out of a house or small building. This type of callout is handled through teamwork between the SWAT unit and the negotiations team, and ideally will result in the suspect(s) choosing to peacefully surrender. Hostage situations are also ideally resolved peacefully through negotiations. If the suspect begins to harm or kill hostages, then immediate entry with a goal of saving the hostages will need to occur. There is a high risk for violence and shooting in these situations.

Tactics

In a high-risk warrant callout, the TEMS unit will usually be called in advance and informed about the basics of what is planned and when to meet at the police headquarters. Upon responding to the headquarters, the SWAT unit leader and law enforcement commander will give a briefing about the mission, including the location and

At the Scene

In a high-risk warrant callout, notice may be given several days in advance or may occur within 45 minutes of notification. Therefore it is important for TMPs to carry their essential gear and supplies in their car or close by at all times.

description of the house. The role, location, and expected position of the TEMS unit will be specified. During the briefing, it is important to discuss the plan for an officer-down or subject-down incident per local protocols and tactics.

In a hostage callout, the TEMS unit initially is best located at the TOC or a location nearby where TMPs are relatively safe. Here, TMPs can provide medical support; gather medical intelligence from witnesses, family, or friends; and help generate a medical threat assessment (MTA). As a TMP, you may provide preventive medicine to SWAT officers and arrange for food and water in the rehabilitation station. Later, if negotiations fail or if the SWAT unit decides to make an entry, you may move forward with the SWAT unit to take up a closer position behind hard cover or remain with the entry team on the entry depending on what the tactical operations leader designates.

Emotionally Disturbed Persons

Emotionally disturbed persons (EDPs) are commonly the cause of critical incidents that result in a SWAT callout. EDPs include persons with acute or chronic

Safety

Be aware that another potential weapon exists with EDPs: bloodborne pathogens. An EDP might claim to have an infectious disease, such as HIV, and may threaten to bite or spit on the TMP or SWAT officer. At the moment, it will be unknown if the person is telling the truth or not. This is one reason why appropriate standard precautions must be taken to safeguard SWAT officers and TMPs. All SWAT and TEMS personnel who will be near the suspect should have eye, nose, and mouth protection and several pairs of nitrile gloves on to decrease the chance of incurring a bloodborne pathogen.

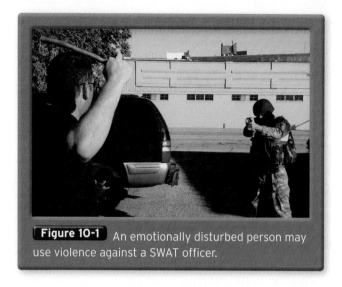

Figure 10-1   An emotionally disturbed person may use violence against a SWAT officer.

mental illness such as paranoid schizophrenia or suicidal behavior. An EDP may not be taking prescribed antipsychotic medications; may be addicted to PCP or methamphetamine; may exhibit abnormal behavior; or may be intoxicated, suicidal, or mentally unstable. If the EDP has a weapon, the likelihood that responding SWAT officers will have to use force to resolve the situation increases greatly **Figure 10-1** .

Sometimes there is an underlying medical illness that causes mental status changes, such as a calm, rational individual with diabetes who develops hypoglycemia (low blood sugar) and becomes angry and irrational. If the situation can be medically resolved, then these patients can return to a rational state within minutes. For example, in 2003 an EDP stopped his car in the middle of a Vancouver, Oregon, interstate highway and yelled at anyone who approached, threatening them with a knife. The SWAT unit was activated. Law enforcement ran the driver's license plate through the system to find his personal information, including his home phone number. The driver's wife was contacted. She revealed that her husband had diabetes and that sometimes he became very angry and upset when his glucose levels dropped. Slowly, SWAT officers coaxed him to surrender by dropping the knife and keeping his arm out of the window. He then gave up his knife and allowed an IV with glucose to be started by a TEMS unit nurse on the SWAT unit. The glucose stabilized his condition, his mental status returned to normal, and the incident was resolved peacefully. He later thanked the SWAT officers.

Tactics

At callouts, it is important to obtain the psychiatric and medical history of EDPs from relatives or counselors, if available. You may assist SWAT negotiators by enlisting additional resources from psychiatric counselors and support from an appropriate relative or friend. The negotiations team will want to take optimal steps toward a peaceful resolution.

You should speak with relatives and witnesses to try to identify the likely cause of the behavior and gather medical information. For example, if a suspect is barricaded and has a history of psychiatric illness, then you may want to talk with relatives at the scene (or by telephone) who may know the location of the medical pharmacy where the EDP purchases medications. The type of medications and frequency of refills may be helpful information. Sometimes the EDP can be coaxed into taking his or her medications immediately, which may lead to more rational behavior and a peaceful resolution of the conflict.

The ultimate goal is to convince the EDP to surrender, lay down any weapons, allow law enforcement to safely take him or her into custody, and eventually be placed in the care of the appropriate psychiatric resources. The SWAT unit, TEMS unit, and support resources such as the negotiations team and mental health professionals can work together to resolve the situation.

Often, less-lethal measures are needed because these individuals do not make rational decisions and their behavior is unpredictable. For example, an EDP with paranoid schizophrenia who has not taken his medication may feel that someone is out to get him and may be fearful of anyone in uniform. If his house is suddenly surrounded by law enforcement vehicles and his family has fled the house due his potentially violent behavior, then it will be very difficult to convince him to simply walk out the front door and surrender to police. Whether the EDP is hearing voices or exhibiting paranoid behavior, often a shotgun beanbag round or TASER will be necessary to resolve the crisis effectively.

Only after the EDP is taken into custody by a SWAT officer and in a safe location should you begin patient care. First, ensure that the scene is safe, that the EDP is handcuffed, and that there are no weapons on the EDP. SWAT officers should maintain a presence to help control any sudden violent behavior. Protect the EDP from harm to self or others. Conduct a thorough patient assessment, and initiate both medical and mental health support. If the EDP is very upset and physically violent, then consider contacting medical control or if your protocols and training permit, consider giving the EDP sedative medications.

Do not touch a patient with a mental illness without telling him or her what your intent is in advance. Verbally attempt to calm and reorient the patient to reality. Do not participate in a patient's delusions or hallucinations.

Determine if the patient is a threat to himself, herself, or others, or if the patient is unable to care or provide for him- or herself. Contact medical control as early as possible if restraints or force are needed.

If restraints are used, document the reason for restraints, time of application, the condition of the patient before and after restraints were applied, method of restraint, and the law enforcement involvement (including law enforcement equipment used). Reassess the patient in restraints every 5 minutes.

Initiate transportation when indicated by communicating with SWAT command staff to let them know what is needed in terms of medical assets and transportation to the hospital. If the patient is felt to be fairly medically stable and does not need a trauma evaluation or major medical workup, then the EDP should be taken to a mental health facility or to jail where authorities can arrange a mental health evaluation. Use law enforcement personnel to help further restrain the patient if necessary and to help guard the EDP.

Document the patient's behavior, statements, actions, or surroundings that substantiate threatening behavior, if witnessed. An example would be a suicidal male who threatens on the phone to negotiators to shoot any SWAT officers who enter his home. Continue to watch for violent outbursts and potential violence such as striking with the fists or hands, kicking, spitting, and headbutting. Self-defensive blocking moves may be used to prevent injury.

Active Shooter Scenarios

Active shooter scenarios range from a violent, disgruntled employee shooting coworkers in an office building to a gunman running loose on a college campus, to a terrorist group shooting commuters in a train station. The suspect(s) actively shooting and killing human targets will continue to shoot and kill until the suspect(s) commits suicide, runs out of ammunition, or is stopped.

Multiple active shooter scenarios have occurred throughout the world, and are not limited to the United States. Active shooter scenarios have occurred in schools, churches, college campuses, shopping malls, business locations, and elementary schools **Figure 10-2**. Many solitary shooters intentionally choose a "gun-free zone" such as a school, church, college campus, or shopping mall because they know that their victims will be unarmed. Sometimes the shooter is stopped quickly, but other times the shooter may use tactics such as using

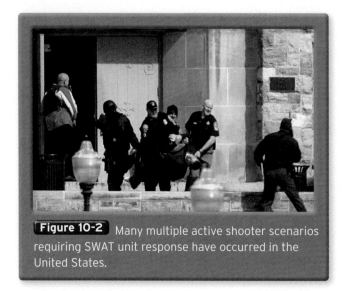

Figure 10-2 Many multiple active shooter scenarios requiring SWAT unit response have occurred in the United States.

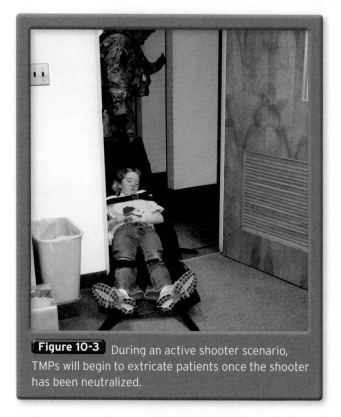

Figure 10-3 During an active shooter scenario, TMPs will begin to extricate patients once the shooter has been neutralized.

chains to lock doors to the building shut to prevent a rapid response by local law enforcement, resulting in more casualties. This was the case during the Virginia Tech shooting on April 16, 2007.

Tactics

Statistically, an active shooter scenario, such as the school shooting in Columbine or at Virginia Tech, is resolved when the shooter commits suicide when confronted by regular patrol officers or security staff before the SWAT unit can arrive at the scene. However, even after the active shooter is neutralized, the building must still be expertly and carefully searched for unknown additional suspects as well as to find and treat any wounded bystanders. In this setting, TMPs may join up with SWAT officers as they arrive and advance with the SWAT unit as part of the rescue team **Figure 10-3**.

Special tactics have been developed and utilized by SWAT and TEMS units across the country for entering and clearing an unsecured building and simultaneously providing emergency medical care. These tactics often involve use of rescue teams with armed SWAT officers providing protection toward the front, sides, and rear of the rescue team, with TMPs protected and relatively secure in the middle of the rescue team. Rescue teams enter the building to systematically search for and neutralize additional shooters, clear rooms, and locate innocent victims who can be stabilized and extracted. All victims in the tactical environment should be screened to verify that they are not actual suspects who are trying to get away by acting like an innocent victim.

As the rescue team moves through the site, TMPs are able to provide the focused rapid medical assessment needed to stabilize and rescue victims, while SWAT officers use ballistic shields, Kevlar blankets, hard cover, and other tactics to protect TMPs and victims from active shooters. This allows TMPs to safely assess and manage patients in the tactical environment and extract victims to a safer casualty collection area. The SWAT officers with shields can provide ingress and egress coverage and protection, allowing the victims the benefits of a protected rapid extraction.

After providing medical care, nondisposable equipment should be gathered up because the entire area is a crime scene. Medical backpacks and gear may be picked up as long as it does not disturb any evidence. Any medical gear not gathered up will be claimed as evidence by investigators and it may be months or longer until it is released. Medical gear is valuable and essential, and may be needed later that same day for unexpected events such as a secondary attack.

At the Scene

If gunfire is exchanged, after all victims are extracted and evacuated, closely examine all SWAT officers and law enforcement personnel for injuries. TEMS unit personnel should also check each other closely if there is any chance of injury from gunfire or explosion.

Safety

In active shooter scenarios, Level IV ballistic vests with ceramic hard plates; rigid, individually carried ballistic shields; clear, wheel-mounted ballistic shields; hand-carried, pole-mounted 9 foot × 4 foot Kevlar ballistic blankets; armored vehicles; remote control robots; and other devices may be of benefit in addition to standard body armor and personal protective equipment.

Occasionally, the SWAT unit is activated and deployed at the incident before any shooting occurs. This may occur in cases where the shooter barricades him- or herself in an office or other location where there may be multiple hostages, with limited windows and doors. In these cases, an immediate reaction team (IRT) will be formed by the SWAT unit to be located nearby the building with the goal of neutralizing any active shooter(s) if and when indicated. The IRT will run to the sound of the shooting and will not stop for treatment of the wounded even if a SWAT officer is downed. Soon afterwards, or possibly simultaneously, a rescue team will be formed and deploy that will ideally include TMPs. TMPs will be expected to move quickly to find victims, perform rapid triage, provide basic expedient lifesaving care, and rapidly extract salvageable patients with security support by SWAT officers as the rescue team moves through the building, systematically clearing rooms, and eliminating any additional threats or booby traps.

If the TEMS unit is armed, then TMPs can work in pairs or with SWAT officers in the rescue team to gather additional patients, stabilize critical injuries, and bring the wounded to a collection point inside the inner perimeter where additional TEMS personnel can perform additional triage, provide expedient treatment, and extract patients to the EMS transport area **Figure 10-4**.

Escaped Fugitive or Suspect

A SWAT unit may be called out to search for an armed and dangerous felon(s) or suspect(s) who ran away from the crime scene or perhaps escaped from prison. This type of situation has occurred in many communities and in many types of challenging settings such as outdoor woodland and urban areas.

Tactics

The proper way to capture the felon(s) or suspect(s) is to set up a perimeter to prevent escape and then organize a group of law enforcement officers to systematically search the terrain for the suspect(s). Several techniques may be used, but in general, a SWAT unit may be joined by other law enforcement officers to form a line of officers to walk through the area carefully searching for the suspect(s) **Figure 10-5**. Leaders and commanders typically will follow along about 30 to 50 yards behind the line. This central rear location is where the TEMS unit may be placed as well. The advantage of this location is its central position, in case the TEMS unit needs to respond quickly to a downed officer, and its relative safety, especially if the TMPs are unarmed.

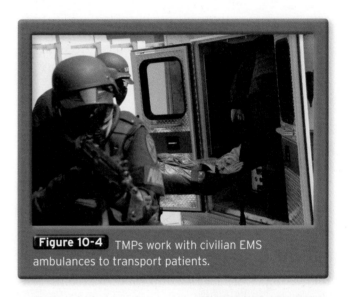

Figure 10-4 TMPs work with civilian EMS ambulances to transport patients.

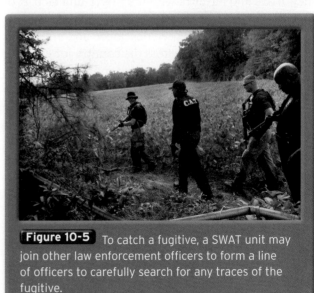

Figure 10-5 To catch a fugitive, a SWAT unit may join other law enforcement officers to form a line of officers to carefully search for any traces of the fugitive.

Mass Gathering Events

SWAT units often respond to potentially violent incidents at mass gathering events **Figure 10-6**. Conditions may rapidly deteriorate during a demonstration or special planned event such as a large music festival. The role of the TEMS unit will usually be to provide medical support for law enforcement personnel. Depending on the situation, medical support for citizens at the scene may be needed as well.

A **mass gathering event** is a gathering of more than 1,000 people at a single site for an event that is planned in advance **Figure 10-7**. Cooperation between the event sponsor or promoter and the public safety agencies involved should be worked out in advance. When working with the tactical operations leader in preplanning for these types of events, temperature, humidity, rain or snow, amount of direct sunshine,

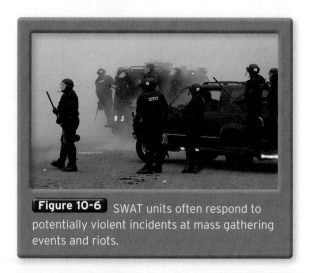

Figure 10-6 SWAT units often respond to potentially violent incidents at mass gathering events and riots.

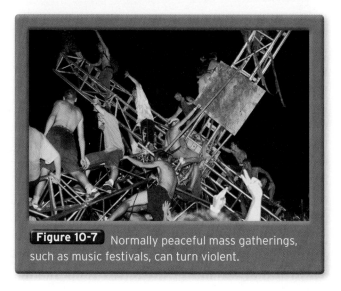

Figure 10-7 Normally peaceful mass gatherings, such as music festivals, can turn violent.

and other environmental factors should be taken into consideration in the MTA.

Tactics

Appropriate planning should be coordinated by the SWAT leadership and the TEMS unit leader for a mass gathering event, including:

- Medical threat identification
- Ensuring adequate security measures
- Ensuring that adequate medical supplies are on-hand
- Clarifying evacuation routes
- Transportation arrangements
- Communications/channel selections along with backup channels

During the mass gathering event, the TEMS unit should ensure that they maintain good communications with the SWAT unit and local law enforcement commanders so that they can respond effectively to the site of any injured or ill patients. The TEMS unit may perform roving patrols at a peaceful event, where they help monitor the large crowd for signs of illegal activities and recognize any developing medical issues, such as mass overheating on a hot, sunny, and humid day. By setting up mass cooling stations, the risk of heat-related emergencies will decrease.

Riots

A **riot** is a public act of violence by an unruly mob or state of disorder involving group violence. The violence may be sudden and intense, and may be directed against people or property. The actions are typically chaotic and exhibit herd behavior, where the individuals may not usually be violent but in the presence of others will participate in violent acts in reaction to a perceived grievance or out of dissent. Law enforcement agencies are usually the primary group tasked with keeping the peace in these situations and may call on SWAT units for assistance. SWAT units may act as part of a Mobile Field Force. This is an organized group of law enforcement officers that train and respond together to help maintain the peace in crowd mass disturbances (riots).

Tactics

When creating the medical plan in response to a riot, the level of protective equipment that you should don or bring with you into the tactical environment should be determined. Hard body armor, ballistic helmets with clear face shields, and air-purifying respirators (APRs) may be needed along with flame resistant Nomex clothing. Remember that the normal bullet-resistant Kevlar ballistic vest in use by patrol officers and SWAT units may not stop an edged or pointed weapon such as a knife or shank. If knives or similar weapons are expected to be carried by rioters, then a special type of knife-resistant vest may be chosen. Some riot crowds have thrown urine and other noxious fluids on police, and therefore splash protection and water-resistant clothing may be needed. At a minimum, you should wear the same level of protection as the SWAT officers that you are supporting.

You should work with police detectives and other intelligence departments to obtain medical intelligence regarding any weapons or substances that might be used against SWAT officers and include this information in the MTA. Because of the unpredictable nature of a riot, bring medical supplies for treating large numbers of patients, both law enforcement and civilian. Medical gear backpacks with multiple compression dressings and other medical supplies are essential if you need to treat large numbers of injured patients.

Possible injuries include chemical agent exposure, heat illness, blunt and penetrating trauma from thrown bricks, rocks, sticks, and other objects. Thermal burns from **Molotov cocktails** are rare, but can occur. Molotov cocktails are improvised weapons that are lit and thrown at police or other targets. The injuries incurred by demonstrators may be of a similar nature but may include impact injuries from less-lethal projectiles, baton strikes, pepper balls, chemical munitions, common abrasions, and other injuries. Although rare, penetrating trauma from firearms and knives is a possibility during riots and should be prepared for. Patient assessment and the management of these injuries are covered in detail in Section 2, "Assessment and Management of Injuries."

At the Scene

If a crowd disturbance breaks out during a mass gathering event or you respond to a riot, avoid being separated from your TEMS unit and the SWAT officers protecting you. Remain aware of and be prepared for the use of chemicals or other agents by police and/or rioters.

Downed SWAT Officer or Bystander in an Exposed Position

SWAT and TEMS units may face the rare instance where a SWAT officer or bystander is injured and in an exposed position with the suspect still at large **Figure 10-8**. The downed SWAT officer or bystander may be unable to move out of a location that is under direct gunfire threat. The challenge is determining how to safely gain access to the injured person(s) to allow SWAT officers and TEMS providers to stabilize and evacuate the patient from a hostile fire zone.

Tactics

If sufficient cover is available and the benefits of rescuing a downed officer outweigh the risk of death or injury, then you will render expedient care and extract the patient. However, the ability to evacuate a patient may not be immediately possible in this setting; therefore, it may be necessary to provide care for an extended time until the threats are neutralized. Whatever the technique used, you must be vigilant of your personal safety during the event or when entering an area subject to hostile fire.

If cover is not available, it may be advisable to utilize observation of the patient from a distance, and perform a remote patient assessment (see Chapter 11, "Tactical Patient Assessment"). The risks of rescue must be weighed against the benefits of reaching the downed patient(s) to provide medical care. If observing from a distance reveals that there is no movement or evidence of breathing, the possibility of death should be strongly considered. If death is likely, then rescue attempts are

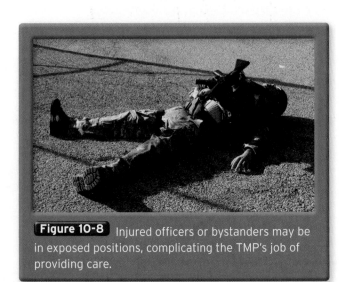

Figure 10-8 Injured officers or bystanders may be in exposed positions, complicating the TMP's job of providing care.

nothing more than body recoveries, and are simply unnecessary. These should be postponed until the threats are neutralized.

Executive Protection

With political power, wealth, and fame comes the risk of harm from terrorists, criminals, or mentally unstable persons. In response to these threats, a field of protective services called **executive protection** (also known as dignitary protection) has grown and expanded during the modern era. From Secret Service agents protecting the president of the United States to a retired law enforcement officer protecting a pop star from the paparazzi, the level of protection, experience, and training in this field varies. As a TMP, you may receive a request to become involved in executive protection if a foreign or domestic dignitary such as the president of the United States visits your city or town.

The person who is being protected is known as the protectee, principal, or dignitary. The key priority for each executive protection mission is to keep the protectee(s) safe and healthy. This goal is accomplished by performing a thorough threat assessment while working with law enforcement dignitary protection staff, and planning, preparing gear, incorporating the planned activities of the person(s) being protected, training, and equipping personnel. There are two components to the executive protection mission: basic physical protection and mission support, including medical support. The role of the TEMS unit during an executive protection mission is primarily supportive.

The Role of the TMP

TMPs may be requested to work with executive protection specialists to provide medical support for the protectee, as well as for the security specialists, law enforcement officers, and others who form the **executive protection detail team**. In many cases, the TMP becomes involved because his or her SWAT unit is asked to provide security as part of the executive protection detail team or act as protective detail. During a visit by the president of the United States, the entire SWAT unit may be involved. In other situations (such as an important governor or executive from overseas), the executive protection detail team may only comprise three or four SWAT officers, in addition to several security personnel from a federal or state agency, such as Secret Service and state police, plus one or two TMPs.

The TEMS unit leader should communicate in writing with the appropriate dignitary staff and executive protective detail team leadership to document exactly what is expected from medical support and how they should perform their mission. Some protectees do not want any medical personnel within sight of the media, because they do not want to appear frail and old. Other protectees want to have TMPs remain close by in case they are needed.

Ideally, TMPs should obtain in advance the essential medical information on the protectee and accompanying security personnel, family, and staff who will be traveling with the protectee. This information can be incorporated into the MTA. Any special needs and medical conditions must be prepared for, such as a child with disabilities, food restrictions, or an unusual medical illness that will require specialized gear.

It should be decided beforehand by command staff whether or not the medical personnel will provide support for anyone other than the SWAT unit or the protectee at the scene. TMPs may be paired with specific security detail personnel and should follow their advice and guidance provided it is reasonable, such as a location to stand or sit down during the event. Searches of TEMS personnel and their equipment for weapons by the executive protection detail team may occur depending upon their protocols. An example would be a visit by a Saudi Arabian prince whose security staff may inspect all bags and medical equipment.

Tactics

The mission requirements must be reviewed beforehand and an MTA should be developed and implemented to help determine the number of medical personnel and medical supplies that should be utilized, as well as the appropriate medical facilities to respond to during all travel routes. The type of mission, location, weather, time of the day, and the activities of the protectee will dictate what the TEMS unit should prepare for.

The TEMS unit should work alongside the executive protection specialists to perform an advance survey, route survey, and site survey with the goal of identifying undesirable elements and physical hazards, taking necessary action to reduce risk or harm to the protectee. The TEMS unit will then want to assemble a comprehensive MTA for all aspects of the mission.

Hopefully the protection mission runs smoothly and nothing happens but the expected. However, if there is an attack, sudden illness, car accident, or other unexpected incident, then the TEMS unit will engage in operational emergency medicine, which is essentially tactical emergency medicine in one of many potential environments, from a highway tunnel to a government building. Each location will present unique challenges and hazards that should be considered in advance by the involved TMPs.

Explosive Ordnance Disposal Search

The **Explosive Ordnance Disposal (EOD) search** involves searching for explosive devices along the route the protectee will take or at the event site prior to the arrival of the protectee. Although TMPs are not directly involved in an EOD search and response, the TEMS unit should be aware when this activity takes place because of the risk to the team in the event an explosive is discovered or detonates. The personnel who perform the search are specially trained and equipped. Once the routes and area close to the event have been searched for bombs and other threats, these areas are typically "sealed," and no unauthorized persons are allowed to enter the area until the event is over.

Presidential Executive Protection

The United States Secret Service is an exceptional group of highly trained professionals. One of their top missions is to protect the president and the vice president of the United States. They travel with the president, vice president, and other dignitaries, along with their families, with the goal of keeping them safe and healthy. The Secret Service is responsible for the security of the president at all times, whether the president is in the White House, at a campaign rally in Iowa, or attending an overseas conference. For presidential visits within the United States and elsewhere throughout the world, Secret Service agents work with local law enforcement and military units in such tasks as assisting in blocking off roads and controlling large groups of people. Often the local SWAT unit is asked to maintain a nearby presence to provide additional assistance if required.

The SWAT unit commander will contact the TEMS unit leader with information on when and where a mission briefing on the SWAT unit's role in assisting the Secret Service will take place. The president's visit may be a surprise or it may be public knowledge. Until it has been announced publicly in the local newspapers or on television, information about the president's arrival, visit, and departure should be treated confidentially. Any detailed security information exchanged is limited to personnel on the SWAT unit on a need-to-know basis.

The exact times of arrival and departure, the route of travel, stops along the route, the length of speech, or

the location of an overnight stay are all highly classified and should not be communicated to anyone who is not authorized to receive that information. If the Secret Service wants you to know the information, they will tell you. Most of the information is given at a series of meetings about 1 week to several days before the visit. It is not unusual for the Secret Service to choose not to divulge the president's travel itinerary and exact travel route to local law enforcement. The hectic schedule of the president is often determined mere days or hours in advance, and it is simply impossible for the Secret Service to perform a security background check of all the leaders of law enforcement agencies and their officers as they travel throughout the world. Therefore, they keep the detailed information limited in distribution to enhance the true mission, which is to keep the president and other dignitaries safe and healthy.

Depending on the type of mission and the president's activities, the SWAT and TEMS unit may or may not be subject to a search and background clearance. When determining who will be present on a protective services detail, it is important for all personnel to be accurately listed and accounted for. If there are any last-minute personnel changes or substitutions, the SWAT unit commander and the Secret Service need to know immediately.

The medical care for the president and his close family is provided for by the president's personal physician and medical staff members. Therefore, if an attack does occur, then this special medical team and ambulance that travels with the Secret Service motorcade will be used to transport the president and provide medical care using their advanced medical equipment and skills. The primary responsibility of the TEMS unit will be to provide tactical medical support to their SWAT unit only; however you should be prepared to treat any member of the motorcade.

The Formal Motorcade

The motorcade will vary depending on the perceived risks, location, and size of the city. Anywhere from 10 to 40 vehicles may be involved, including one or two scout

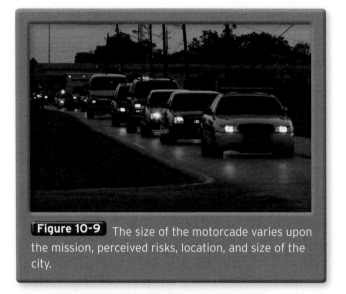

Figure 10-9 The size of the motorcade varies upon the mission, perceived risks, location, and size of the city.

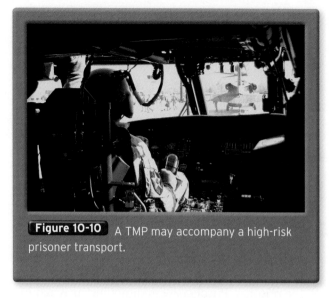

Figure 10-10 A TMP may accompany a high-risk prisoner transport.

At the Scene

The involvement in a presidential motorcade is exciting, challenging, and requires excellent teamwork. Fortunately, the day's work tends to result in a successful mission.

patrol cars, the lead motorcade car, lead car, limousines, follow car, staff cars, tactical car, presidential ambulance vehicle with medical staff, intelligence car, major crimes car, press buses, civilian ambulance, local police squad cars, SWAT unit vehicles, and tail cars to prevent anyone from joining or passing the motorcade **Figure 10-9**. The TEMS unit is often limited to two TMPs who travel with the SWAT unit.

High-Risk Prisoner Transport Medicine

This type of tactical medical support is unique in that the protectee is a federal criminal, military detainee, or terrorist who has committed or is accused of a major crime and has been captured or arrested. When a TMP is tasked with accompanying a protective detail transporting these high-risk federal prisoners, it is called **high-risk prisoner transport medicine** **Figure 10-10**. During this type of mission, the TMP is asked by law enforcement personnel to perform medical support during the high-risk tactical operation of transporting a federal felon or terrorist. Local, state, or federal SWAT

officers and possibly special operations soldiers from the military will be involved during these high-risk transportation missions. This may include travel between the site of capture and prison, between two prisons, or perhaps back and forth to a courtroom at a trial location that may need to be repeated daily for several weeks. Many of these high-risk missions are performed by the Special Operations Group (SOG) with the United States Marshals, as well as the Immigration and Naturalization Service (INS), and sometimes local SWAT officers.

In the United States, the Justice Prisoner and Alien Transportation System (JPATS) is a federal government agency charged with the transportation of persons in legal custody between prisons, detaining centers, courthouses, and other places in the United States where they must be transported. This agency is also known as "Con Air" (convict air transportation). It was formed in 1995 when the INS and the United States Marshals merged their air fleets. They use airplanes to transfer more than 300,000 prisoners each year, along with other vehicles in a network that involves cars, vans, and buses.

Tactics

The threats involved with high-risk prisoner protective detail include assassination attempts by enemies of the prisoner (ie, mob hit), a direct attack on the motorcade or transportation vehicle in order to aid in the escape of the prisoner, and escape attempts by the prisoner. Prior to transport, the federal corrections facility officers will search the prisoner thoroughly and ensure that the prisoner is disarmed, handcuffed, and often blindfolded or made to wear blackened soft goggles that prevent identification of personnel, and to hide the location and travel routes. The interior of the vehicle is carefully searched by federal corrections officers prior to transport for hidden handcuff keys, weapons, drugs, and other items. When possible, female prisoners are transported by at least two female guards or law enforcement officers for multiple reasons, including escort during bathroom visits. If transporting more than one prisoner, members of rival gangs are transported separately. When terrorists or organized crime figures are transported they are usually kept isolated and not allowed to communicate with other prisoners.

The physical well-being of prisoners should be monitored during transit. Potentially violent prisoners should be fully restrained and watched at all times. Any wheelchairs, crutches, prosthetic devices, or medication should be transported with, but not in the possession of, the prisoner. Prisoners with disabilities may require special equipment during transportation. High-risk prisoners should never be left unattended.

The usual transportation risks are always present, such as motor vehicle collisions, extreme weather conditions (slippery roads), mechanical problems (tire blow-out), or aircraft mechanical problems (which may cause an emergency landing). Therefore, the preparation and MTA should focus on the transportation method, type of vehicle, route, medical facilities, EMS agencies along the way, backup vehicles, environmental conditions, anticipated threats, as well as the medical history and known active medical conditions of the prisoner as well as the involved law enforcement officers and other protective escort personnel. Emergency medical gear should be accessible by protective escort personnel as well as TMPs.

It is possible for the TMP to become a casualty. Therefore, before the mission begins, take a moment to talk with the protective escort personnel and review all of the emergency medicine plans, possible EMS ambulance intercepts, contact information for the air medicine helicopter, and other key information. Emergency contact information and preplanning should involve learning about all local assets of the EMS system including air medicine assets, helicopter support, and advanced life support intercept agencies. The use of GPS (global positioning system) coordinates is beneficial if the transportation will involve air transfer or long-distance ground transfer. Share this information (with rapid reference paperwork to hand out) with all members of the protective escort team. Do not share any potentially embarrassing information that HIPAA patient privacy rules would not allow, unless it truly affects operational security. For example, if the prisoner has been diagnosed with a rare cancer and is likely to die soon, the prisoner may be more likely to take extreme risks to gain freedom. Print key phone numbers and important information from the MTA on a small sheet, copy it, and hand it out to all of the protective escort personnel. The protective escort personnel may need to call for medical help if you are seriously injured.

Scene Safety First

Prior to providing any required medical care, search the prisoner. Even though the prisoner has been incarcerated and likely has been searched, blindfolded, and double-cuffed on the wrist and ankles, the prisoner must be searched again prior to providing any medical care. If there is a vehicle accident during transport, then there will be multiple distractions for all protective escort personnel, the prisoner may obtain a handcuff key, screwdriver, or handgun, and may hide that weapon until an escape opportunity presents itself. Trust no one.

Remain cognizant of the fact that the incarcerated prisoner represents a deadly threat. Get at least two armed guards to assist you with security before approaching the prisoner. At least one officer should cover and point a weapon at the prisoner; another officer (or more) should ensure the prisoner is properly handcuffed and has no weapons, and can help maintain a 360-degree threat awareness.

Ready for Review

- A common callout site that the SWAT unit responds to is a residential house or small building for either a high-risk arrest warrant or a hostage situation.

- Emotionally disturbed persons (EDPs) are commonly the cause of critical incidents that result in a SWAT callout. Try to contact family, friends, and medical professionals to obtain more information about the individual.

- Even after an active shooter is neutralized, the building must still be carefully searched for additional suspects. The search also allows you to locate and treat any wounded bystanders.

- During a search for a fugitive in the woods or open terrain, the TEMS unit may be positioned 30 to 50 yards behind the search line of officers. At this position, the TEMS unit will be relatively safe while still able to respond immediately to a downed officer.

- At a mass gathering event, the role of the TEMS unit will usually be to provide medical support for law enforcement personnel. Depending on the situation, there may be a need to provide medical support for citizens at the scene as well.

- During a callout for a riot, you should work with police detectives and other intelligence departments to obtain medical intelligence regarding any weapons or substances that might be used against SWAT officers and include this information in the medical threat assessment.

- The role of the TEMS unit during an executive protection mission is primarily supportive.

- The risks during a high-risk prisoner protective detail include assassination attempts by enemies of the prisoner (ie, mob hit), a direct attack on the motorcade or transportation vehicle in order to aid in the escape of the prisoner, escape attempts by the prisoner, and usual transportation hazards.

Vital Vocabulary

emotionally disturbed persons (EDPs) People who are functionally impaired due to a mental, behavioral, physical, or emotional disorder.

executive protection Techniques and tactics used to mitigate the threat of violence or kidnapping of a very important person or family member with a large amount of money, power, or fame.

executive protection detail team Group of professionals tasked with the job of protecting a very important person or family member from harm or kidnapping.

Explosive Ordnance Disposal (EOD) search Methods and techniques used by specially trained experts to search for, neutralize, and prevent bombs from detonating.

high-risk prisoner transport medicine When a TMP is tasked with accompanying a protective detail transporting a high-risk prisoner.

mass gathering event A gathering of more than 1,000 people at a single site for an event that is planned in advance.

Molotov cocktails Improvised weapons made of glass bottles filled with gasoline with a cloth rag acting as a wick.

riot A public act of violence by an unruly mob, or state of disorder involving group violence.

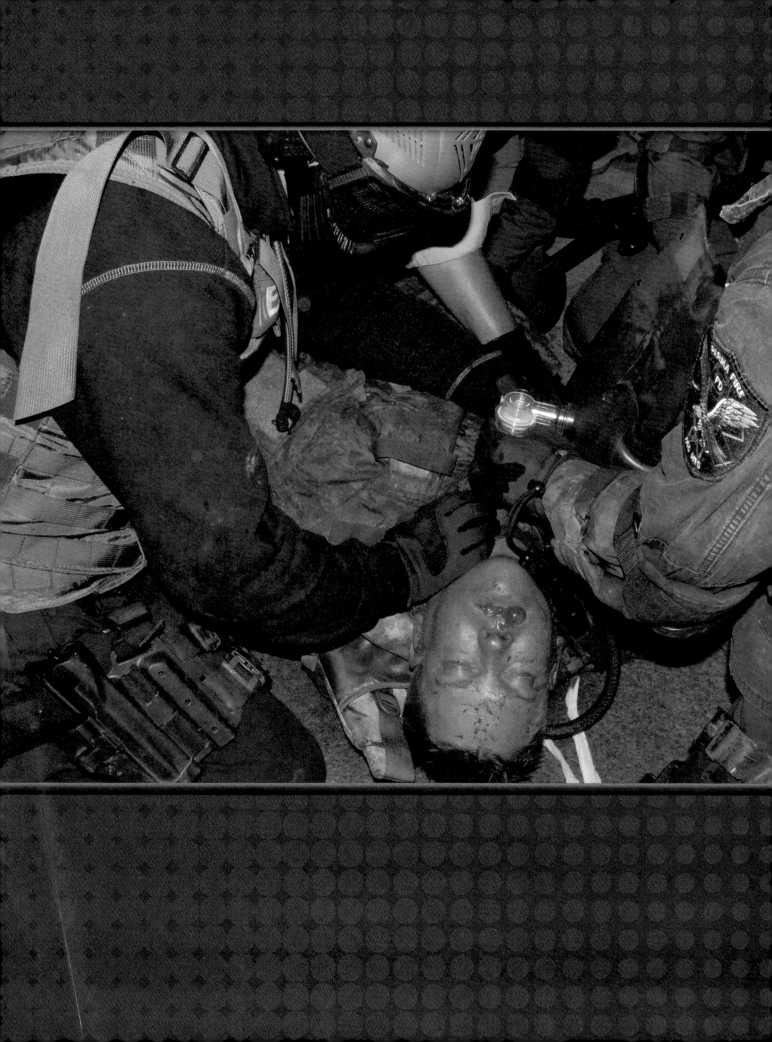

SECTION

. . . .

2

Assessment and Management of Injuries

CHAPTERS

Tactical Patient Assessment

Introduction

In the tactical environment, rapid systematic assessment of a patient increases the likelihood that life-threatening injuries are identified and priortized **Figure 11-1**. If life-threatening injuries are identified during the assessment, lifesaving treatment and interventions can be initiated immediately. This chapter provides a clear and comprehensive approach to tactical patient assessment.

Scene Safety

As a tactical medical provider (TMP), what is your first priority at a callout? In the tactical environment, the patient is not usually the highest priority. Your highest priority is your personal safety. If the SWAT and TEMS units are going to be able to continue to neutralize threats and help others in need of medical care, then your priorities must be kept in the proper order at all times.

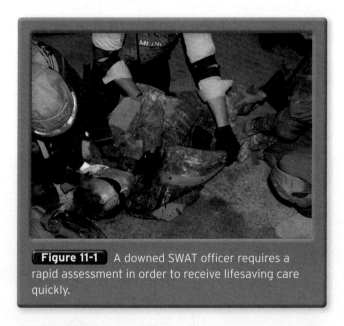

Figure 11-1 A downed SWAT officer requires a rapid assessment in order to receive lifesaving care quickly.

The goal of the SWAT unit is to resolve the callout with as few injuries and deaths as possible. As a TMP, your role is to medically support the SWAT officers and help the SWAT unit achieve its goals by providing medical care to patients in the tactical environment. Specifically, your priorities are:

- Your personal safety is your first and highest priority.
- The safety, health, and medical care of SWAT officers and TEMS providers are your second priority.
- Care for other patients, such as hostages, bystanders, and suspects is your third priority.

Although the order of these priorities may sound self-serving, this order is based on the principle of ensuring the full availability of the SWAT and TEMS units who can then provide the maximum resources during the entire callout. Simply put, if you are injured, you will not be able to help others. Additionally, you will have made the situation worse by becoming a patient, adding one more person to the list of patients who need to be assessed, stabilized, and evacuated.

360-Degree Situational Awareness

You can maximize your safety and maintain a high level of alertness by utilizing 360-degree situational awareness. A complete circle contains 360 degrees; thus this concept describes the need to maintain a functional awareness of the situation around you at all times. This includes being able to rapidly recognize friends versus foes and deal with threats. Maintaining proper 360-degree situational awareness requires keeping track of multiple issues simultaneously as they occur or develop around you. To maintain 360-degree situational awareness during the mission, you should:

- Stay within a 30-second response time of the SWAT unit.
- Know where your unit is, where they are going, and the mission plan.

At the Scene

The SWAT officer's priorities differ from the TMP. The SWAT officer's priorities begin with first helping hostages or other innocent citizens, then fellow SWAT officers, and finally any suspects.

- Know the danger zones versus known safe areas, and maintain a high suspicion for danger in all areas at all times.
- Remember that unexpected threats can appear any time and from any direction.
- Memorize and recall the mission plan, building layout, and description of the wanted suspect(s).
- Make and adjust immediate reaction drills and backup plans for all officer-down contingencies.
- Remain able to respond with the rescue team to rapidly intervene at a crisis location (such as a downed officer) at all times.
- Update the medical threat assessment continually with mission-specific and accurate medical intelligence, including optimizing medical evacuation methods and routes, and maintain the ability to communicate with and link to regional EMS assets.
- Know the exact location of and maintain the ability to communicate with the tactical operations center (TOC) and incident command (IC) center.
- Maintain a constant awareness of the likely locations of suspects, hostages, injured victims, nearby neighbors, and other persons who may be impacted by the SWAT deployment.
- Watch for curious citizens, differentiate between threatening versus innocent bystanders, and know how to deal with each decisively.
- Always pay attention to your intuition (gut instinct) and act on it without hesitation. When in doubt, move to a new location or a safer position.

Partners-in-Safety

To remain safe and provide tactical emergency care to a patient, a minimum of two TMPs are required. This model allows one TMP to focus on maintaining a defensive, protective position and neutralize any threats that may arise, while the other TMP provides tactical emergency medical care for the patient.

In the partners-in-safety system, prior to initiating tactical emergency medical care to a patient, you should ideally have someone designated to watch your back. This may be your TEMS partner, a SWAT officer designated by command to protect the TEMS element, or perhaps a patrol officer who is accompanying the mission. The in-depth procedures of assessing patients and providing medical care will absorb your attention. If you can trust your partner to provide cover, then your attention can be more fully devoted to patient assessment and providing

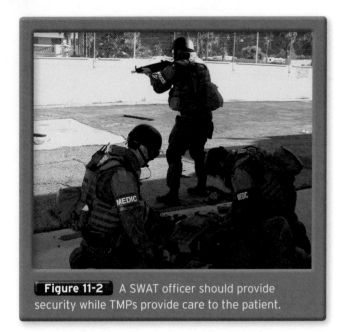

Figure 11-2 A SWAT officer should provide security while TMPs provide care to the patient.

Table 11-1	Call-A-CAB 'N Go
Call	Call out for help and communicate.
A	Abolish all threats.
CAB	Circulation, followed by Airway, and Breathing
'N	Neurologic status check
Go	Go to the appropriate advanced medical facility.

Modified from Wipfler III, J. Combat medicine: new things a tactical officer should know. *The ITAO News.* Reproduced with permission of the Illinois Tactical Officers Association.

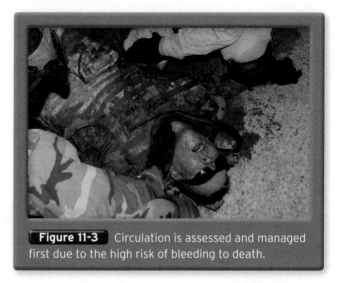

Figure 11-3 Circulation is assessed and managed first due to the high risk of bleeding to death.

high-quality medical care. An ideal situation is for one or more SWAT officers to provide security while two TMPs work together to assess, manage, and extract the patient **Figure 11-2**.

Safety When Treating Suspects

If a suspect is shot or injured by the SWAT unit, the suspect should be handcuffed and fully searched before any medical care takes place. In addition, you must assume that every one of your patients in the tactical environment is going to try to kill you. This is true for anyone with an unknown or uncertain identity, from hostages to the seemingly innocent bystander. Use caution and proper protective tactics at all times.

Safety

Any medical care provided to the suspect must be balanced and properly prioritized with the need for personal and unit safety.

Tactical Patient Assessment: Call-A-CAB 'N Go

In the tactical environment, a useful mnemonic is the "Call-A-CAB 'N Go" tactical patient assessment process **Table 11-1**. The standard EMS approach consists of assessing and maintaining the ABCs (airway, breathing, and circulation) during the primary assessment. Due to the demands and dangers of the tactical environment,

the tactical patient assessment must differ. The rationale behind the reversal of ABC to CAB is the following: a SWAT officer who is entering a building to pursue a suspect is healthy and well oxygenated, and has no serious medical problems—a SWAT officer is a fit athlete. When a SWAT officer suffers penetrating trauma from a bullet, knife, or explosion, the most common cause of death is bleeding (hemorrhage) **Figure 11-3**.

Although the airway and breathing may be at risk, the SWAT officer is generally oxygenated sufficiently for the first few minutes after traumatic injury; stopping major hemorrhage is the top priority, and C therefore comes before A and B. Once the bleeding is under control, the airway and breathing can be assessed and managed. Penetrating trauma can cause death in a matter of minutes, so immediate control of bleeding is essential.

Call-A-CAB 'N Go stands for:

- **Call:** Call out for help and communicate with your unit in order to tell them what is happening. Use appropriate communication such as hand signals, voice, and/or a portable radio to ensure that your unit and the tactical operations leader know what is happening and where the threats are, to obtain help with neutralizing threats, and to help with medical care, extraction, and evacuation. This may need to occur simultaneously with the next step—A.

- **A:** Abolish threats; identify and abolish all threats appropriately. When the threats are abolished, the patient is extracted to hard cover where the tactical patient assessment process can begin. Medical care is not provided by the TMP until the patient has reached hard cover or hard cover is brought to the patient.
- **CAB:** Circulation, followed by Airway and Breathing.
- **'N:** Neurologic status check; a rapid neurologic assessment to determine the patient's mental status and identify any significant spinal cord injury.
- **Go:** Go to the appropriate advanced medical facility. The patient is evacuated and transported in an appropriate vehicle at an appropriate speed according to the seriousness of the patient's condition.

Call

When an entry team is making the approach to a building or after they have entered a building, they are at risk of being attacked by suspects. Immediately upon witnessing an attack upon the entry team, the nearby SWAT officers or TMPs should utilize their voice, radio, hand signals, or other communication devices to call out to let the tactical operations leader and the entire unit know what is happening and where the threat is. By calling out what happened, the tactical operations leader and the rest of the unit will gain a sense of what just happened, where the threat is, who is injured, and where you are. Without this information, additional injuries may occur.

As a TMP, you should work with the entry team to respond to the injured SWAT officer as you have trained and the appropriate immediate action drills (IADs) should be implemented. The downed SWAT officer may be extracted by nearby SWAT officers to you or you may move forward to the downed officer, depending on your agency's tactics. If you and others from the TEMS unit are called to come forward to treat downed SWAT officers or other victims, a SWAT officer who is familiar with the geography and safe travel paths should lead you to the patient(s).

As you approach, it is important to call out to the SWAT unit that you are moving toward them, such

as, "medic coming through," and also call out prior to entering and exiting each room. Calling out to the SWAT unit helps to ensure your safety—you do not want to surprise a SWAT officer with your sudden presence. Call out to the downed SWAT officer when approaching and tell the downed officer what you and the rest of the SWAT unit are doing, such as "rescue." This will reassure the downed officer that you are a friend and not a foe.

A: Abolish Threats

Abolish all threats appropriately. Note that all of the following should be done by the SWAT unit *before* you initiate any medical care in the tactical environment. SWAT officers will nearly always be the ones neutralizing threats. However, you are responsible for your own safety. This step includes:

- **Abolish risks from the shooter or other threat(s).** The injured SWAT officer, if properly trained and in possession of the proper combat mindset, will continue the fight even after being shot once or multiple times, and will continue shooting and pressing forward with the attack in order to neutralize the threat(s). If the suspect runs behind cover or runs away from the firefight, then the injured SWAT officer can break away from the assault to seek hard cover and begin self-care **Figure 11-4** . This attitude of "you are never

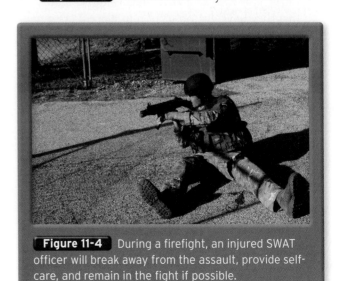

Figure 11-4 During a firefight, an injured SWAT officer will break away from the assault, provide self-care, and remain in the fight if possible.

down" is the winning mindset, even after being shot or otherwise injured. Nearby SWAT officers will neutralize or contain the criminal threat(s) and then render buddy-aid behind hard cover. When the immediate threats are abolished, the TMP will become involved.

- **Abolish needless rescue.** Use remote assessment techniques if there is any question about the viability and/or possible death of patients who are at a distance and under direct active threat. Do not risk personnel to approach and recover a dead body. If a SWAT officer is struck in the head by a large caliber rifle bullet and has obvious signs of massive brain injury, then consider that unfortunate person as effectively dead.

- **Abolish the risk of further gunfire; abolish further casualties.** Move behind hard cover or bring it to protect the patient(s), and do not approach the injured patient(s) unless the benefits outweigh the risks. For example, rather than run out into an open parking lot to extract an injured officer, an armored vehicle should be deployed to cover the injured officer, decreasing risk of gunfire, so that the officer can be extracted safely.

- **Abolish the risks of secondary explosions in active shooter and/or terrorist scenarios.** A designated experienced SWAT officer should scan for nearby boxes, briefcases, cars, or other items that may be a secondary device targeted at responding rescue personnel. If you see something that appears suspicious, notify command and pull back.

- **Abolish the risks of bloodborne pathogens.** Wear PPE to protect yourself and make certain that any nearby SWAT officers who provide hands-on assistance with medical care also wear PPE. Issue nitrile gloves to all SWAT officers and ensure that they have eye protection in place. Personnel who are close to the patient should also wear face masks.

- **Abolish any risk of injury from HazMat agents.** Watch for chemical, biologic, and radiologic contamination, especially after a suspicious explosion. Monitor for symptoms, use a personal dosimeter to screen for radiation, and protect yourself and your unit.

- **Abolish risks from seemingly innocent individuals.** At the scene, remember that all hostages and any involved citizens at the scene who are not personally known and trusted should be handcuffed and searched prior to medical assessment and management. All hostages and bystanders, regardless of how innocent or injured they seem, should be treated as highly dangerous individuals.

- **Abolish weapons dangers.** If a gun is discovered during the search, use proper firearm safety and management, safely hand off weapons to SWAT officers or secure them nearby, and continue to search and find all hidden or disguised weapons and other threats. Many criminals carry two or more guns; if you find a gun, then search carefully for the second or third gun and a knife or two.

- **Abolish all threats from incomplete searches.** Unless you personally witnessed the complete and thorough search of a suspect or patient, then assume it was not performed correctly. The best way to ensure that the job is done right is to do it yourself. Search the patient again if there is any doubt as to whether the initial search was done correctly.

- **Abolish threats using a metal detector.** Criminals of both genders carry weapons in their chest or groin area, which can be a difficult and awkward area to search. A metal detector that can detect metal from an inch away can assist when searching this area of the body, as well as other private areas such as the chest area of women.

- **Abolish all threats from SWAT officers' less-lethal weapons.** For a downed officer, ensure that all distraction devices, less-lethal devices, pepper spray, and smoke and chemical gas grenades are secured. These have a canister or grenade-like appearance and are typically found in a pouch on the SWAT officer's vest. The best tactic is to leave these devices inside the vest pouch or holster when the vest is removed. If they fall out or are found outside a holster, do not handle them unless you have been trained in their use and safety. If the pin is solidly in place, there is little risk of injury.

- **Abolish threats from curious bystanders.** A common tactic used by criminals and terrorists is to try to escape a crime scene by acting like an innocent bystander. They may slip into a building and remove or change clothing to modify their appearance, and then walk out as if nothing happened. If anyone attempts to stop them, they may use violence and lethal force to escape arrest. The criminal may be brazen and simply walk up to law enforcement officers asking questions, provide false information, and walk away. Use caution, ask questions, and report anyone who is acting strangely.

- **Abolish the continued threat of weapons that are removed.** Any weapons that are found should be secured per your SWAT unit's protocols. Pistols and rifles that are removed from injured SWAT officers or from suspects may be safely handed off to nearby SWAT officers or TEMS providers. Some SWAT units may require that the weapon be unloaded and secured by placing the unloaded weapon or knife into a secure location such as a utility bag or pouch attached to the TMP.
- **Abolish personal bombs, booby-traps, and hidden devices.** Although extremely rare, all suspects and even hostages should be checked for bombs and booby-traps in appropriate situations. For example, if a suspect is known to make and use homemade bombs, then a careful search for explosives and other devices should always be performed by appropriately trained personnel. Only begin medical care after a patient is restrained and is found to possess no weapons, IV needles, hidden razor blades, cuff keys, cell phones, contact wires, switches, or bombs, and

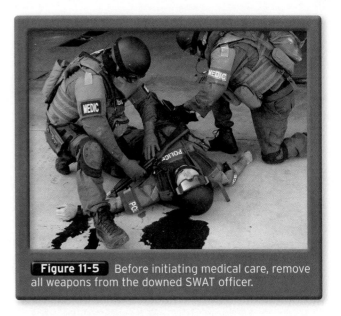

Figure 11-5   Before initiating medical care, remove all weapons from the downed SWAT officer.

the patient is located in a relatively safe place away from direct threat of gunfire or other serious harm.

CAB: Circulation, Airway, and Breathing

Once any threats have been abolished and the patient is behind hard cover, then assessment and management can begin.

Circulation

First, immediately stop any significant external extremity bleeding by rapidly applying a compression dressing or tourniquet (Chapter 12, "Controlling Bleeding," covers

At the Scene

If an injured SWAT officer is in shock or is at risk for developing shock, fellow SWAT officers will need to remove all weapons from the injured officer before you initiate care **Figure 11-5**. The reason is simple. The seriously injured SWAT officer may be (or soon will be) unable to think clearly or make rational decisions. Thus, the confused SWAT officer may actually think that the approaching fellow SWAT officer or you are a criminal suspect and take defensive action such as shooting at you. The injured SWAT officer may have been engaged in shooting or apprehending a suspect when the injury occurred. Most SWAT officers have excellent reflex defense mechanisms, and if they interpret your actions as threatening, the confused SWAT officer may try to injure you. However, if the injured SWAT officer is only lightly wounded and is alert and stable and likely to remain that way, then this SWAT officer likely should keep his weapons, stay in the fight, and remain able to protect himself and the unit. In fact, the SWAT officer should remain ready to fight and return fire, even during the extraction and evacuation phase.

Safety

Many SWAT callouts occur at night or in low-light situations such as a dark garage or basement. You should be trained to search and assess patients in a no-light or low-light environment **Figure 11-6**. The use of palpation to find and assess for injuries may be required, and restricted use of light may be mandated due to the presence of persistent threats nearby. You should learn to feel for slick or wet skin and clothing that may indicate blood, holes in uniforms and skin, deformed or painful tender extremities, and crepitus (air under skin); you should also know how to conduct a brief neurologic examination in darkness.

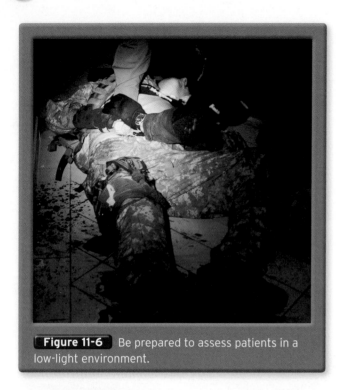

Figure 11-6 Be prepared to assess patients in a low-light environment.

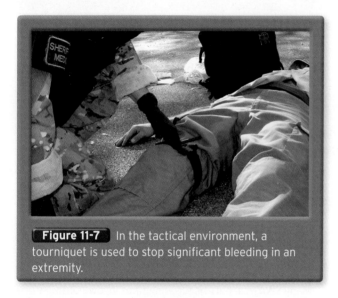

Figure 11-7 In the tactical environment, a tourniquet is used to stop significant bleeding in an extremity.

these skills in detail) **Figure 11-7** . Then rapidly assess the patient's pulse rate, pulse quality, pulse rhythm, and skin.

External Bleeding The average adult body contains approximately 5 to 6 liters (L) of blood and can normally lose 1 to 2 pints of blood (the usual amount given by donors, about one-fourth of an IV bag) without any harmful effects. The severity of hemorrhage depends on the amount of blood lost in relation to the physical size of the patient. The amount of visible blood is often not a good way to

judge the severity of an injury; for example, serious injuries, such as open femur fractures from a gunshot wound, do not bleed heavily externally but may bleed significantly internally. Relatively minor injuries, such as a scalp laceration, will bleed profusely externally.

Arterial bleeding is rapid, profuse, and pulsating, with the blood escaping in spurts synchronized with the pulse. It is usually bright red because it is rich in oxygen. Venous bleeding is a steady flow. It is usually dark red or maroon in color because it is oxygen-poor. Capillary bleeding is slow and oozing. It often clots spontaneously.

To perform a rapid scan of major external bleeding, look for signs of blood loss including active bleeding from wounds and/or evidence of bleeding such as blood on the clothes or near the patient. When you evaluate an unconscious patient, do a sweep for blood quickly and lightly by running your gloved hands from head to toe, on both the front and back of the patient's body, pausing periodically to see if your gloves are bloody.

If you find external bleeding, control it through direct pressure, a compression bandage, or a tourniquet in severe cases. Chapter 12, "Controlling Bleeding," reviews these skills in detail.

Pulse The patient's pulse is most easily felt at a pulse point where a major artery lies near the surface and can be palpated gently against a bone or solid organ. The locations for assessing a patient's pulse are **Figure 11-8** :

- Radial pulse
- Brachial pulse
- Posterior tibial pulse
- Dorsalis pedis (pedal) pulse
- Carotid pulse
- Femoral pulse

After you have determined that a pulse is present, next determine its adequacy. This is done by assessing the pulse rate, pulse quality, and pulse rhythm. For an adult, the normal resting pulse rate should be between 60 and 100 beats/min. The dramatic situations encountered in a SWAT callout will likely cause tachycardia (more than 100 beats/min) in healthy, uninjured personnel. Therefore, a SWAT officer in the early stages of shock will likely have a pulse rate of 110 to 130 beats/min or higher. The pulse rate, along with the pulse quality and pulse rhythm, are indicators that can call out if the patient's condition is serious.

Skin Assessing the patient's skin helps you to determine the adequacy of the patient's blood perfusion. Adequate perfusion meets the current needs of the cells; inadequate perfusion causes cells and tissues to die. Examine the patient's skin, nail beds, and eyes. Pale or cyanotic

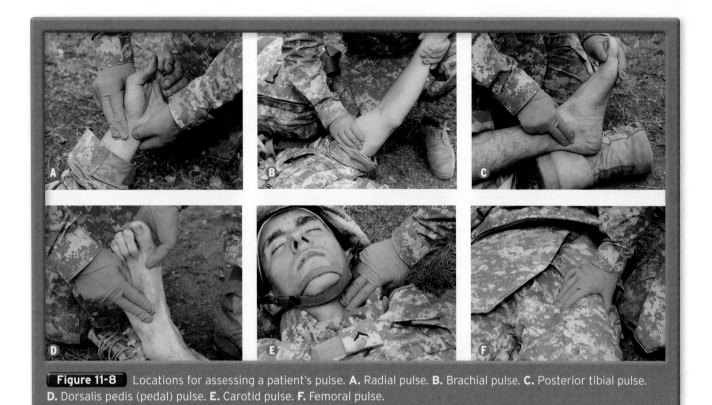

Figure 11-8 Locations for assessing a patient's pulse. **A.** Radial pulse. **B.** Brachial pulse. **C.** Posterior tibial pulse. **D.** Dorsalis pedis (pedal) pulse. **E.** Carotid pulse. **F.** Femoral pulse.

At the Scene

If the patient is witnessed to have collapsed due to medical (nontrauma) full cardiac arrest, then it is critical to administer an AED during the circulation phase. If there is a delay in getting the AED from a squad car or ambulance, then begin CPR immediately.

(bluish) skin indicates low oxygen levels in the blood. Flushed and red skin may indicate high blood pressure, fever, or severe overheating.

Normal skin temperature is warm to the touch (98.6°F). Abnormal skin temperatures are hot, cool, cold, and clammy (moist). In the tactical environment, feeling the patient's forehead or neck with the back of your hand is usually adequate to determine whether the patient's temperature is elevated or decreased. Keep in mind that during training or callouts many SWAT officers may be overheated from wearing heavy gear and thick vests and will likely be hot and sweating when assessed.

Airway

The next step is the assessment of the patient's airway, checking to make sure he or she is moving air while breathing. This is done while considering the mechanism of injury (how the patient was injured) and your ability to maintain cervical spine motion restriction. If a significant mechanism of injury is involved (fall from roof, collision with a motor vehicle), then apply a cervical collar and maintain spinal precautions (see Chapter 19, "Head, Neck, and Spine Injuries").

During the airway assessment, always be alert for signs of airway obstruction. Regardless of the cause, a mild or severe airway obstruction will result in inadequate or absent air flow into and out of the lungs.

Listen to the patient. Patients who are talking have an open airway. A conscious patient who cannot speak or cry most likely has a severe airway obstruction. Signs of airway obstruction in an unconscious patient include

Safety

Unconscious patients should be considered to have possibly experienced a traumatic event such as a fall, and cervical spine precautions may be indicated. With these patients, consider the mechanism of injury; a patient who has fallen from a second story window is more likely to have spinal injuries than a patient who fell to the floor after being shot.

noisy breathing (gurgling, snoring, or bubbling) or extremely shallow or absent breathing. If you identify an airway problem, stop the assessment process and obtain a patent airway (see Chapter 13, "Basic Airway Management," and Chapter 14, "Advanced Airway Management").

Breathing

Assess the patient's breathing by *watching* the patient's chest rise and fall, *feeling* for air through the mouth and nose during exhalation, and *listening* to breath sounds when possible. In the tactical environment, a stethoscope is often not used during this phase; however, it should be kept available. Assess the patient's respiratory rate and depth of breathing. Watch for bilateral chest rise and the use of accessory muscles, indicators of breathing issues that require management.

A normal respiratory rate varies widely in adults, ranging from 12 to 20 breaths/min. Due to the stress and physical requirements of the callout, a SWAT officer's respiratory rate may be normally elevated prior to injury. Due to the noise issues of the tactical environment, when determining the patient's respiratory rate it may be easier to watch the chest rise or to place your hand on the patient's chest and feel it rise and fall **Figure 11-9** . While counting the patient's respirations, also note the rhythm (regular or irregular).

Observe how much effort is required for the patient to breathe. Normal respirations are not usually shallow or excessively deep. Shallow respirations can be identified by little movement of the chest wall or poor chest excursion. Deep respirations cause a significant rise and fall of the chest.

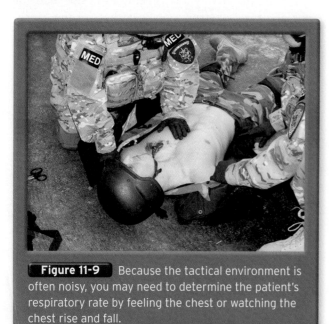

Figure 11-9 Because the tactical environment is often noisy, you may need to determine the patient's respiratory rate by feeling the chest or watching the chest rise and fall.

Observe the patient for signs of respiratory issues. The presence of retractions (indentation of skin pulled inward with deep breathing, located above the clavicles, below the ribs, and in the spaces between the ribs) or the use of accessory muscles of respiration (neck, chest, and abdominal muscles) are signs of inadequate breathing and require ventilation assistance (see Chapter 13, "Basic Airway Management," and Chapter 14, "Advanced Airway Management"). A patient who can speak only two or three words before pausing to take a breath, a condition known as two- to three-word dyspnea, has a serious breathing problem (see Chapter 18, "Torso Injuries").

'N: Neurologic Status Check

Check for any major neurologic disability by performing a rapid neurologic exam. Check the patient's level of consciousness, check for possible spinal cord injury by rapidly examining the sensation and strength in the patient's extremities, and examine the pupils if the patient is unresponsive.

In the tactical environment, you need to ascertain only the gross level of consciousness (LOC) by determining which of the following categories best fits your patient:

- Conscious with an unaltered LOC (normal mental status)
- Conscious with an altered LOC
- Unconscious

Mental status and level of consciousness can be evaluated in just a few seconds by testing for responsiveness and orientation. The **AVPU scale** is a rapid method of assessing the patient's level of consciousness using one of the following four terms:

A   Alert
V   Responsive to Verbal stimuli
P   Responsive to Pain
U   Unresponsive

The AVPU scale is based on the following criteria:

- **Alert**. The patient's eyes open spontaneously as you approach, and the patient appears to be aware of you and responsive to the environment. The patient appears to follow commands, and the eyes visually track people and objects.
- **Responsive to Verbal stimuli**. The patient's eyes do not open spontaneously. However, the patient's eyes do open to verbal stimuli, and the patient is able to respond in some meaningful way and follow commands when spoken to.
- **Responsive to Pain**. The patient does not respond to your questions but moves or cries out in

response to painful stimuli, such as gently but firmly pinching the patient's earlobe, pressing down on the bone above the eye, or pinching the muscles of the neck. Be aware that some methods may not give an accurate result if a spinal cord injury is present.

- **Unresponsive**. The patient does not respond spontaneously or to verbal or painful stimuli.

For a patient who is alert and responsive to verbal stimuli, evaluate orientation by testing the patient's ability to remember four things:

- **Person**. The patient is able to remember his or her name.
- **Place**. The patient is able to identify his or her current location.
- **Time**. The patient is able to tell you the current year, month, and approximate date.
- **Event**. The patient is able to describe what happened.

If the patient is conscious with an unaltered LOC, perform a quick strength and sensation assessment of the arms and legs. Ask the patient to squeeze your fingers as you place two fingers into each of the patient's hands, which tests grip strength. Next, test the patient's legs by lightly rubbing the patient's lower leg then ask the patient to raise that leg. After the patient raises the leg, switch, and test the other leg **Figure 11-10**. This tests sensation as well as gross strength of the legs. If the patient has a suspected spinal or extremity injury, then you can modify the test by asking the patient to wiggle and raise his or her toes. If you note a definite weakness or absence of muscle strength and sensation of the arm(s) and/or leg(s), there may be a spinal cord injury so apply full spinal immobilization with a backboard and the cervical collar (see Chapter 19, "Head, Neck, and Spine Injuries").

If the patient is unconscious or conscious with an altered LOC, then valuable information may be obtained by assessing the pupils' response to light with a flashlight (if tactically appropriate). A patient with significant head trauma and one pupil dilated will likely need immediate evacuation and transport to the hospital for emergency brain surgery in order to survive. A patient with fixed and dilated pupils and no pulse is essentially dead and further medical efforts are likely futile.

Go

After assessing and managing the CAB 'N, it is time to determine if you have a load-and-go situation. The term *load and go* (also known as scoop and run) means that a patient has been diagnosed with a life-threatening or limb-threatening condition and should be rapidly assessed, stabilized, evacuated, and then loaded into the ambulance (or other emergency transport vehicle) to be transported to the hospital **Figure 11-11**. Only the minimal essential assessment and stabilizing treatment

Special Populations
....

Immediately evacuate and transport every pediatric trauma patient with any abnormal findings, severe pain, or a serious mechanism of injury. These are load-and-go patients.

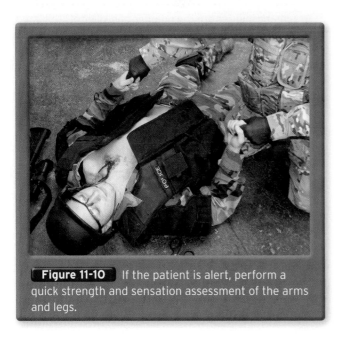

Figure 11-10 If the patient is alert, perform a quick strength and sensation assessment of the arms and legs.

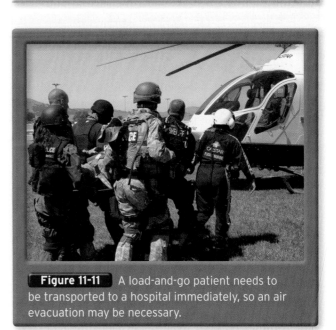

Figure 11-11 A load-and-go patient needs to be transported to a hospital immediately, so an air evacuation may be necessary.

Table 11-2   Load-and-Go Indications

- Penetrating or blunt trauma to extremities with major uncontrolled hemorrhage

- Hypovolemic shock

- Signs of traumatic conditions that may rapidly lead to hypovolemic shock:
  - Tender, distended abdomen
  - Pelvic instability
  - Bilateral femur fractures
  - Amputation
  - Penetrating trauma (knife, bullet, shrapnel) to the head, neck, or torso

- Head injury with unconsciousness, unequal pupils, or decreasing level of consciousness

- Airway obstruction that cannot be quickly relieved by mechanical methods such as suction, forceps removal of foreign body, intubation, or surgical airway

- Conditions resulting in possible inadequate breathing or shock:
  - Large open chest wound (sucking chest wound)
  - Large flail chest
  - Tension pneumothorax
  - Major blunt chest injury
  - Blunt trauma to the larynx or trachea
  - Anaphylactic shock
  - Acute chest pain
  - Burns or severe smoke inhalation injury
  - Abdominal pain after trauma
  - Pregnancy
  - Significant penetrating or blunt trauma

- Cardiopulmonary arrest (if potentially survivable and/or recently wounded)

At the Scene

The leader of a well-prepared TEMS unit will meet with the local ALS and BLS agencies on a recurring basis to discuss the TEMS unit's capabilities, training, and any unique procedures (expanded protocols) that they are authorized to perform in the field. Any questions or issues revolving around the transition of medical care or transfer of care from the tactical environment to the emergency medical transport vehicle (ambulance or helicopter) should be discussed during these meetings. From BLS-level TMP to a civilian ambulance paramedic to a physician TMP, the goal is to follow local protocols and to provide the highest continuum of care for the patient.

delayed until the patient is en route to the hospital. However, since these patients are not experiencing life- or limb-threatening injuries, you may spend more time on managing the patient's injury (splinting, bandaging, controlling pain) in the field, if appropriate.

Patient Assessment During Evacuation

Once the patient evacuation is underway or while waiting for the vehicle or aircraft that will evacuate the patient, you should continue to further assess the patient.

Special Populations

Traumatic injuries are the number one killer of children in the United States. More children die of injuries annually than of all other causes combined. Common causes of traumatic injury and death in the tactical environment include falls, fires, gunshot wounds, chemical inhalation and exposure from clandestine drug laboratories in the home, and child abuse. If children are found during a callout, child and family protective service agencies should be notified to help ensure the best welfare for the children.

Because of a child's small size, high-energy blunt impacts, such as a motor vehicle crash, fall from a height, and assault can lead to multisystem trauma, including the head, chest, abdomen, and the long bones in the extremities. In addition, high-energy and penetrating wounds that cause severe hemorrhaging can quickly lead to hypovolemic shock. In pediatric patients, shock can quickly lead to cardiac failure, with bradycardia and respiratory failure, and then to cardiac arrest.

should be done at the scene. What critically injured patients need is either an operation or the intensive care that can only be provided at a hospital. Table 11-2 lists the indications for load and go.

Load-and-go patients are evacuated (see Chapter 16, "Extraction and Evacuation") as bleeding is controlled and the patient's airway and breathing are stabilized. Less critical procedures such as starting an IV, splinting, or bandaging must not delay transport in a load-and-go patient. Secondary assessment and management will be given as needed in the ambulance en route to the hospital. If appropriate, a TMP may accompany this patient to the hospital.

In patients without load-and-go indications, the secondary assessment may be performed on scene or

SAMPLE History

Ideally, if your patient is a SWAT officer, a detailed medical history for your patient will be known and available. However, if your patient is a suspect, victim, or bystander, then you will not have a known medical history for the patient, so you should conduct a **SAMPLE history**. Find out:

S Signs and symptoms of the chief complaint.

A Allergies that the patient has to medications. If the patient is unable to communicate, then checking a purse, wallet, or medical alert bracelet may provide additional information.

M Medications that the patient takes daily.

P Past medical and surgical history.

L Last meal or drink.

E Events leading to the illness or injury.

Use whatever data are available. Ask fellow officers or witnesses exactly what happened, prior to leaving the scene if possible.

Secondary Assessment

If time allows, a secondary assessment should be performed while the patient is being transported to the hospital. The purpose of the secondary assessment is to perform a systematic head-to-toe physical examination of the patient. Once transportation is under way or while waiting for transportation, you can begin the secondary assessment by taking the patient's vital signs.

Vital Signs

Assess the patient's vital signs and place the patient on a cardiac monitor, pulse oximeter, and an electronic blood pressure device.

Head-to-Toe Assessment

Remove any ballistic gear, loosen any tight clothing, and reassure the patient. If a patient has a suspected spinal cord injury, then consider leaving the ballistic vest in place until arrival at the hospital to avoid further movement of the spine. Then perform a systematic head-to-toe assessment:

1. Look at the face for obvious lacerations, bruises, or deformities.

2. Inspect the area around the eyes and eyelids **Figure 11-12**.

3. Examine the eyes for redness and for contact lenses. Assess the pupils using a penlight **Figure 11-13**.

4. Look behind the patient's ears to assess for bruising (Battle's sign).

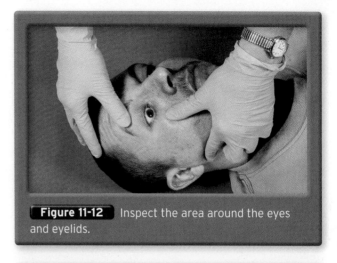

Figure 11-12 Inspect the area around the eyes and eyelids.

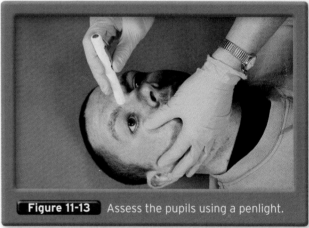

Figure 11-13 Assess the pupils using a penlight.

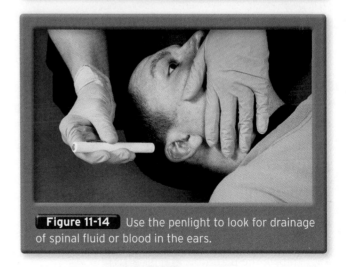

Figure 11-14 Use the penlight to look for drainage of spinal fluid or blood in the ears.

5. Use the penlight to look for drainage of spinal fluid or blood in the ears **Figure 11-14**.

6. Look for bruising and lacerations about the head. Palpate for tenderness, depressions of the skull, and deformities.

7. Palpate the zygomas for tenderness or instability **Figure 11-15**.

8. Palpate the maxillae **Figure 11-16**.

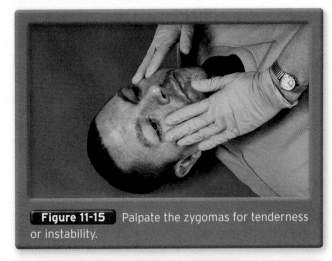

Figure 11-15 Palpate the zygomas for tenderness or instability.

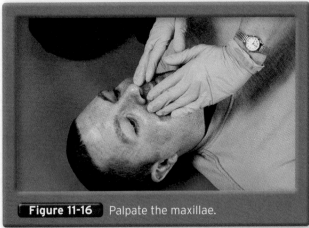

Figure 11-16 Palpate the maxillae.

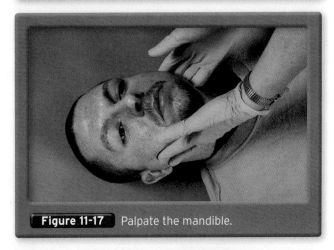

Figure 11-17 Palpate the mandible.

9. Palpate the mandible **Figure 11-17**.

10. Assess the mouth and nose for cyanosis, foreign bodies (including loose teeth or dentures), bleeding, lacerations, or deformities.

11. Check for unusual odors on the patient's breath.

12. Look at the neck for obvious lacerations, bruises, and deformities.

13. Palpate the front and the back of the neck and spine for tenderness and deformity.

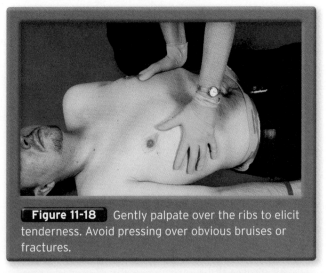

Figure 11-18 Gently palpate over the ribs to elicit tenderness. Avoid pressing over obvious bruises or fractures.

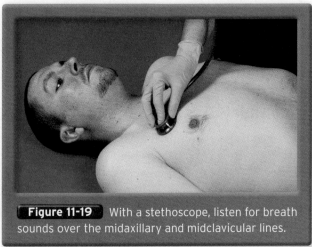

Figure 11-19 With a stethoscope, listen for breath sounds over the midaxillary and midclavicular lines.

14. Look for distended jugular veins. Note that distended neck veins are not necessarily significant in a patient who is lying down.

15. Look at the chest for obvious signs of injury before you begin palpation. Be sure to watch for movement of the chest with respirations.

16. Gently palpate over the ribs to elicit tenderness. Avoid pressing over obvious bruises or fractures **Figure 11-18**.

17. With a stethoscope, listen for breath sounds over the left and right midaxillary (sides of the chest) and midclavicular lines (top of the chest) **Figure 11-19**. With a stethoscope, listen also at the bases and apices of the lungs.

18. With a stethoscope, listen briefly to the heart. Listen for a muffled heartbeat, abnormal rhythm, abnormal sounds, or murmurs.

19. Look at the abdomen and pelvis for obvious lacerations, bruises, and deformities.

20. Gently palpate the abdomen for tenderness **Figure 11-20**. If the abdomen is unusually tense, you should describe the abdomen as rigid.

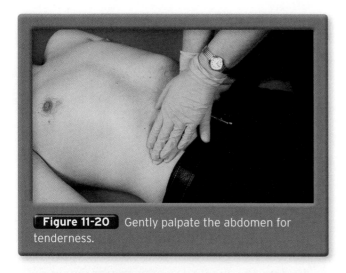

Figure 11-20 Gently palpate the abdomen for tenderness.

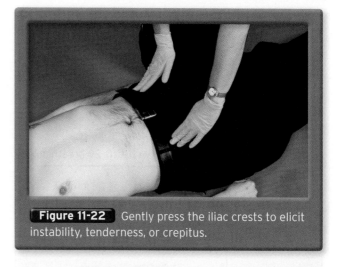

Figure 11-22 Gently press the iliac crests to elicit instability, tenderness, or crepitus.

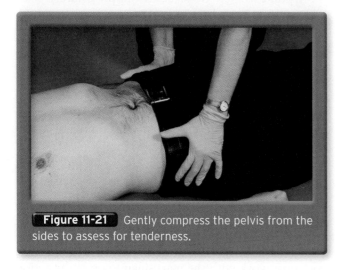

Figure 11-21 Gently compress the pelvis from the sides to assess for tenderness.

21. Gently compress the pelvis from the sides to assess for tenderness **Figure 11-21**.
22. Gently press the iliac crests to elicit instability, tenderness, or crepitus **Figure 11-22**.
23. Inspect all four extremities for lacerations, bruises, swelling, deformities, and medical alert anklets or bracelets. Also assess distal pulses and motor and sensory function in all extremities.
24. Assess the back for tenderness or deformities. Remember, if you suspect a spinal cord injury, use spinal precautions as you log roll the patient.

Trauma Scoring Systems

When applicable, calculate the patient's **Glasgow Coma Scale (GCS) score** and possibly the patient's revised trauma score. The GCS scoring system is used to determine a patient's level of consciousness by measuring and assigning point values, or scores, for eye opening, verbal response, and motor response. The highest score is 15; the lowest score is 3. The GCS chart shown in **Figure 11-23** shows how the numerical values are determined.

GLASGOW COMA SCALE

Eye Opening

Spontaneous	4
To voice	3
To pain	2
None	1

Verbal Response

Oriented	5
Confused	4
Inappropriate words	3
Incomprehensible sounds	2
None	1

Motor Response

Obeys command	6
Localizes pain	5
Withdraws (pain)	4
Flexion (pain)	3
Extension (pain)	2
None	1

Glasgow Coma Scale Maximum Score	Total	15
Glasgow Coma Scale Minimum Score	Total	3

Figure 11-23 Glasgow Coma Scale scores are used to assess a patient's level of consciousness—for example, in patients with head injuries. The lower the score, the more severe the extent of brain injury.

Table 11-3	Components of the Revised Trauma Score

Revised Trauma Score	Components
4	• GCS: 13-15 • Systolic blood pressure: > 89 mm Hg • Respiratory rate: 10-29 breaths/min
3	• GCS: 9-12 • Systolic blood pressure: 76-89 mm Hg • Respiratory rate: > 29 breaths/min
2	• GCS: 6-8 • Systolic blood pressure: 50-75 mm Hg • Respiratory rate: 6-9 breaths/min
1	• GCS: 4-5 • Systolic blood pressure: 1-49 mm Hg • Respiratory rate: 1-5 breaths/min
0	• GCS: 3 • Systolic blood pressure: 0 mm Hg • Respiratory rate: 0 breaths/min

Abbreviation: GCS, Glasgow Coma Scale.
Source: Reproduced from Revised Trauma Score.
© Trauma.org

The **revised trauma score** is a system that measures the following three physiologic parameters: respiratory rate, systolic blood pressure, and GCS score Table 11-3 . The total score will range from 0 to 13, with the more debilitated patient receiving a lower score. Often there is not time during the rapid transport to calculate this score. However, if there is a delay in transport or if a longer transportation time allows for this score to be determined, then this information will be used at the trauma center.

Reassess Vital Signs

Recheck and record the patient's vital signs and responses. Do this at least every 15 minutes for stable patients, every 5 minutes for critical patients, and also after each intervention, noting the times and vital signs obtained.

Reassess Airway, Breathing, and Circulation

Reassess the patient's airway, breathing, and circulation to identify and treat changes in the patient's condition.

Recheck Interventions

If time allows, expose the patient's injuries and adjust bandages, stabilize fractures, improve spine stabilization measures if indicated, administer medications per local protocols, and monitor for signs of worsening status.

Update the medical center appropriately with estimated time of arrival (ETA) and status every 10 minutes. Reassure the patient and provide support.

Remote Assessment Medicine

Remote assessment medicine (RAM) is a unique aspect of tactical medicine in which a TMP, without direct physical contact, can visually assess injured patients from a safe distance with a goal of determining whether the patient is dead or alive. Usually an optical magnifying device is used, such as a good quality pair of binoculars; however, a spotting scope or rifle scope may be used as well. When using weapon systems to inspect a scene, you must work with the marksman to open the action (lock bolt back) and keep your finger off the trigger. Night vision devices should be considered in low-light scenarios.

Situations that require RAM may include a SWAT officer or other patient who is injured and lying out in the open within range from a suspect's gunfire, which prevents initial rescue efforts. These patients may be observed by the TMP or marksman for signs of life or signs of injury such as movement of the chest, arms, legs, or head; respirations; nature of the injury; and other factors (exposed brain matter, massive trauma). A large blood pool, white pale skin, and lack of movement also suggest death.

The incident commander is then apprised of the likely medical condition of the patient lying in the open. Rescue decisions can be made more strategically based on this information. If the patient is moving or breathing, then signs of life exist, and rescue may be pursued more aggressively. Conversely, a patient without movement or respirations is likely dead and therefore does not merit a rapid rescue mission and the unnecessary risk of further

Tactical Combat Casualty Care

Three Phases of Care

Tactical Combat Casualty Care (TC-3) is the military's protocol for battlefield medicine.

Some principles of TC-3, including the continuum of care, have been adapted by TEMS medical directors for the tactical environment when creating protocols and tactics. Unlike the battlefield, where combat medics are sent out into the heat of battle to treat wounded soldiers, *very rarely* does a TMP engage in patient care in the inner perimeter during an active gunfight in which the shooter(s) has not been neutralized. *Very few SWAT commanders willingly send forward TMPs unless their safety can reasonably be ensured.* The rules of engagement and acceptable casualty rates differ between citizen law enforcement and the military.

In TC-3, there are three phases of care on the battlefield:

1. Care Under Fire
2. Tactical Field Care
3. Tactical Evacuation Care

Care Under Fire is the care rendered by the combat medic at the scene of the injury while the combat medic and the casualty are still under effective hostile fire. During this phase, the available medical equipment is limited, and the key priority is to get to a safer area where a more thorough medical exam and treatment can be given. Tactical Field Care is the care rendered by the combat medic once the combat medic and the casualty are no longer under effective hostile fire. Tactical Evacuation Care is the care rendered once the casualty has been picked up by an aircraft, vehicle, or boat.

Care Under Fire

When under enemy fire, there is very little time to provide comprehensive medical care to a casualty. Suppression of enemy fire and movement of the casualty to cover are paramount **Figure 11-24**. The risk of injury to other personnel and additional injury to casualties will be reduced if immediate attention is directed to the suppression of hostile fire.

The combat medic may initially need to assist in returning fire instead of stopping to care for the casualty. The best medicine on any battlefield is fire superiority. The combat medic may be able to direct the casualty to hard cover and direct the casualty to provide self-aid for life-threatening hemorrhage, if the casualty is able. If the casualty needs to be moved, a tourniquet that can be applied rapidly by the casualty or a buddy may help to stop major extremity bleeding.

Tactical Field Care

During the Tactical Field Care phase, the combat medic has more time to provide care and there is a reduced level of hazard from hostile fire. The time available to render care varies. In some cases, tactical field care may consist of rapid treatment of wounds with the expectation of a reengagement of hostile fire at any moment.

At other times, care may be rendered once the mission has reached an anticipated evacuation point, without further pursuit, and while the combat medic is awaiting casualty evacuation. In this circumstance, there may be ample time to render whatever care is feasible in the field. The time prior to extraction may range from half an hour to many hours.

Although the combat medic and the casualty are now in a somewhat less hazardous setting, lengthy and detailed assessments and management procedures are not performed during this phase. Patient assessment and management are directed to airway, breathing, and circulation. The combat medic may insert an airway or perform a surgical cricothyrotomy to ensure a patent airway. If the casualty has a major chest-penetrating trauma or deformity, the combat medic may perform a needle thoracostomy to ensure breathing. If the casualty has lost a great deal of blood, the combat medic may apply a hemostatic dressing and begin an IV to prevent shock. After ensuring that the casualty's airway, breathing, and circulation are stable, all wounds are dressed to prevent further contamination. The combat medic monitors the casualty's condition, provides pain control, and documents all casualty findings and care until the casualty is evacuated.

Tactical Evacuation Care

At some point in the battle or military operation, the casualty during wartime will be scheduled for evacuation; however, evacuation time may vary greatly, from minutes to hours to days. For civilian law enforcement tactical operations, the transportation and evacuation care typically is measured in minutes and seconds, with a majority of the cases going immediately to a hospital. A multitude of factors affect the ability to evacuate a casualty, including availability of evacuation assets (aircraft or vehicles), weather, tactical situation, and mission.

(continues)

Tactical Combat Casualty Care (continued)

Only minor differences exist between the care provided in the Care Under Fire and the Tactical Field Care phase. Once en route, stabilizing treatment can be continued. Additional medical personnel may accompany the casualty and assist the combat team on the ground. Additional medical equipment, such as oxygen and monitors, can be brought with the evacuation asset to augment the combat medic's equipment.

Continuum of Care

The continuum of care concept may be adapted from the battlefield to the tactical environment. Continuum of care is the spectrum of tactical emergency medicine: self-aid, buddy-aid, and care provided by TMPs. If the downed SWAT officer is under fire and conscious, then the SWAT officer may perform self-aid by stopping any heavy bleeding by applying a tourniquet. When it is safe to approach and extract the downed SWAT officer to hard cover, buddy-aid occurs. When the injured SWAT officer is moved to hard cover, care is provided by the TMP.

The continuum of care extends from the tactical environment into training. The TEMS unit assists in developing the mindset of self-aid in the SWAT officers through self-aid emergency medical training. After the immediate threats are neutralized, the wounded SWAT officer cannot simply lie there and wait for the TMP. Instead, self-aid is initiated if possible, and then later buddy-aid through evacuation, and when the downed SWAT officer is behind hard cover, the TMP will provide care safely. The hospital is the conclusion of the continuum of care.

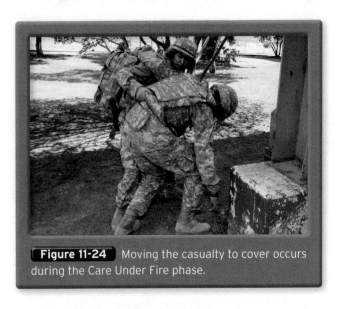

Figure 11-24 Moving the casualty to cover occurs during the Care Under Fire phase.

loss of life. The remote assessment can provide essential information that may change the whole dynamic of the response and save lives.

Barricade Medicine

SWAT units and negotiation teams may be called for an armed, barricaded suspect who may or may not have hostages. Many barricade situations are of the type that the TEMS unit can provide helpful information, advice, and support. The negotiation team may request assistance from the TEMS unit in an over-the-phone medical evaluation of an injured or ill barricaded suspect, as well as any hostages. Because very few TMPs are trained as negotiators, it is unlikely that the need will arise for an actual telephone conversation with the suspect or hostages. However, there may be important medical questions that need to be answered in certain circumstances. If possible, you should work alongside the negotiation team to assess the suspect and hostages and obtain their medical history, medications, current impairment, mental health issues, alcohol or illicit substance use, and stress tolerance. You may obtain valuable information by talking with the hostages' and suspect's family members, the suspect's psychiatrist, or other sources in order to gain medical intelligence and help with the medical threat assessment.

Fortunately, these callouts are resolved peacefully most of the time; however, hostages may have medical problems that are exacerbated by the stressful situation or they may be injured and in need of immediate stabilizing medical care. If the suspect can be convinced to release the injured or ill hostage, that is of course a positive step. However, if the injured or ill hostage is forced to remain inside the barricaded building, then the TEMS unit may work with the negotiation team to assist in providing emergency medical care directions to the suspect or other hostages who can then help the injured or ill patient. This situation is barricade medicine.

Medical Complaints

During the course of a callout or training, a SWAT officer might come to you with a medical complaint. There are certain complaints that may be associated with a serious underlying medical condition or be the result of environmental stressors. Seemingly minor complaints may be early signs or symptoms of a life-threatening condition. Many SWAT officers may ignore the warning signs of a serious medical condition and may want to remain on-site with the SWAT unit. The SWAT officer may not want to be seen as weak, and may try to minimize or even hide certain symptoms.

The following symptoms or complaints indicate the need for an immediate referral to an on-scene TEMS unit physician or transport to the emergency department:

- Chest pain (heart attack, pneumothorax, pulmonary embolus)
- Sudden unexplained shortness of breath (pulmonary embolus, congestive heart failure [CHF], pulmonary edema, collapsed lung)
- Severe back pain between the shoulder blades (aortic dissection)
- Severe abdominal pain (infection, obstruction, appendicitis, perforated ulcer, aortic rupture, ectopic pregnancy if female)
- Sudden onset of "the worst headache of my life" (brain aneurysm, spontaneous brain hemorrhage, meningitis)
- Fever with collapse (sepsis/life-threatening infection)
- Sudden fainting with no prior warning, or dizziness (lethal heart arrhythmia, heat stroke, dehydration)
- Neurologic symptoms such as loss of vision, abnormal visual acuity, weakness of one arm/leg/muscles of face, difficulty speaking, dizziness (seizure, stroke)

Barricade medicine includes providing directions on how to stop bleeding from a gunshot wound, how to provide CPR, or how to administer glucose to a patient with a diabetic emergency.

Triage

Mass-Casualty Incident

If the callout results in multiple civilian patients or you respond to a mass-casualty incident, then the TEMS unit will need to perform triage on the multiple patients to determine which patient should be treated

At the Scene

In the rare event that you speak with a suspect during a hostage callout, work with a partner. Your partner can help remind you what to say, how to describe a procedure, and offer you support. Speak in simple terms and avoid medical terminology. Work closely with the negotiation team in order to maximize your attempt to de-escalate and defuse the situation, allowing for a peaceful resolution.

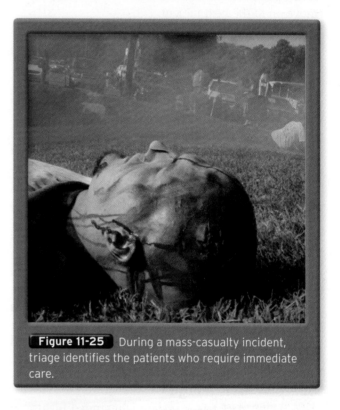

Figure 11-25 During a mass-casualty incident, triage identifies the patients who require immediate care.

first **Figure 11-25**. **Triage** simply means "to sort" your patients based on the severity of their injuries. The goal of doing the greatest good for the greatest number means that the triage assessment is brief and the patient condition categories are basic. Triage starts with ensuring that the scene is relatively safe, followed by quickly screening all patients with an abbreviated evaluation system such as START.

START Triage

START triage is one of the easiest methods of triage. The first step of the START triage system is performed on arrival at the scene by calling out to patients, "If you can hear my voice and are able to walk . . ." and then directing patients to an easily identifiable landmark. The injured persons in this group are the "walking wounded" and are considered minimal (green) priority or third-priority patients.

The second step in the START process is directed toward nonwalking patients. You move to the first nonambulatory patient and assess the breathing status. If the patient is not breathing, you should open the airway by using a simple manual maneuver (see Chapter 13, "Basic Airway Management"). A patient who still does not begin to breathe is triaged as expectant (black). If the patient begins to breathe, tag him or her as immediate (red), place the patient in the recovery position, and move on to the next patient.

If the patient is breathing, a quick estimation of the respiratory rate should be made. A patient who is breathing faster than 30 breaths/min or slower than 10 breaths/min is triaged as an immediate priority (red). If the patient is breathing between 10 to 29 breaths/min, move to the next step of the assessment.

The next step is to assess the circulation status of the patient by checking for bilateral radial pulses. An absent radial pulse implies the patient is in shock, is potentially dying, and should be triaged as an immediate priority. If the radial pulse is present, go to the next assessment.

The final assessment in START triage is to assess the patient's mental status, which simply means to assess the patient's ability to follow simple commands, such as "show me three fingers." This assessment establishes that the patient can understand and follow commands. A patient who is unconscious or cannot follow simple commands is an immediate priority patient. A patient who complies with a simple command should be triaged in the delayed category.

JumpSTART Triage

The **JumpSTART triage** system is intended for use in children younger than 8 years or who appear to weigh less than 100 lb. As in START, the JumpSTART system begins by identifying the walking wounded. Infants or children not developed enough to walk or follow

At the Scene

Hazardous materials and weapons of mass destruction incidents force the fire department's hazardous materials response team to identify patients as contaminated or decontaminated before the regular triage process can begin. Contamination by chemicals or biologic weapons in a treatment area, a hospital, or trauma center could obstruct all systems and organizations coping with the mass-casualty incident.

commands (including children with special needs) should be taken as soon as possible to the treatment sector in the outer perimeter for immediate secondary triage. This action assists in getting children who cannot take care of their own basic needs into a caregiver's hands. The JumpSTART system has several differences in the breathing status assessment compared with that in START. First, if you find that a pediatric patient is not breathing, immediately check the pulse. If there is no pulse, label the patient as expectant. If the patient is not breathing but has a pulse, open the airway with a manual maneuver. If the patient does not begin to breathe, give five rescue breaths and check respirations again. A child who does not begin to breathe should be labeled expectant. The primary reason for this difference is that the most common cause of cardiac arrest in children is respiratory arrest.

The next step of the JumpSTART process is to assess the approximate rate of respirations. A patient who is breathing less than 15 breaths/min or more than 45 breaths/min is tagged as immediate priority, and you should place the patient in the recovery position before moving on to the next patient. If the respirations are within the range of 15 to 45 breaths/min, the patient is assessed further.

The next assessment in JumpSTART triage is also the circulation status of the patient. Just like in START, you are simply checking for a distal pulse. This does not need to be the brachial pulse; assess the pulse that you feel the most competent and comfortable checking. If there is an absence of a distal pulse, label the child as an immediate priority and move to the next patient. If the child has a distal pulse, move on to the next assessment.

The final assessment is for mental status. Because of the developmental differences in children, their responses will vary. For JumpSTART, a modified AVPU score is used. A child who is unresponsive or responds to pain by posturing or with incomprehensible sounds or is unable to localize pain is considered an immediate priority and tagged as such. A child who responds to pain by localizing it or withdrawing from it or who is alert is considered a delayed priority patient.

Triage Categories

There are four common triage categories. Use the mnemonic IDME to help you remember each category: Immediate (red), Delayed (yellow), Minimal (green; hold), and Expectant (black; likely to die or dead) **Table 11-4** . This is the order of priority for the treatment and transport of patients.

Immediate (red-tag) patients are your first priority. They will need immediate care and transport. They

Table 11-4   Triage Priorities

Triage Category	Typical Injuries
Red tag: first priority (immediate) Patients who need immediate care and transport; treat these patients first, and transport as soon as possible.	• Airway and breathing difficulties • Uncontrolled or severe bleeding • Severe medical problems • Signs of shock (hypoperfusion) • Severe burns • Open chest or abdominal injuries
Yellow tag: second priority (delayed) Patients whose treatment and transport can be temporarily delayed.	• Burns without airway problems • Major or multiple bone or joint injuries • Back injuries with or without spinal cord damage
Green tag: third priority (walking wounded) Patients who require minimal or no treatment and transport can be delayed until last.	• Minor fractures • Minor soft-tissue injuries
Black tag: fourth priority (expectant) Patients who are already dead or have little chance for survival. Treat salvageable patients before treating these patients. Law enforcement investigators and coroners will want the bodies disturbed as little as possible in order to determine what happened and to maximize evidence collection.	• Obvious death • Obviously nonsurvivable injury, such as major open brain trauma • Respiratory arrest (if limited resources) • Cardiac arrest

usually have problems with ABCs, head trauma, or signs and symptoms of shock.

Delayed (yellow-tag) patients are the second priority and will need treatment and transport, but it can be delayed. Patients usually have multiple injuries to bones or joints, including back injuries with or without spinal cord injury.

Minimal (green-tag) patients are the third priority. Patients may require no field or only "minimal" treatment. These patients are the "walking wounded" at the scene. If they have any apparent injuries, they are usually soft-tissue injuries such as contusions, abrasions, and lacerations.

The last priority is the expectant (black-tag) patients who are dead or whose injuries are so severe that they have, at best, a minimal chance of survival. This category may include patients who are in cardiac arrest or who have an open head injury, for example. If you have limited resources, this category may also include patients in respiratory arrest. Patients in this category receive treatment and transport only after patients in the other three categories have received care.

Triage Tags

It is vital that a patient has a tag or some type of label. Tagging patients early assists in tracking them and can help keep an accurate record of their condition. Triage tags should be weatherproof and easily read

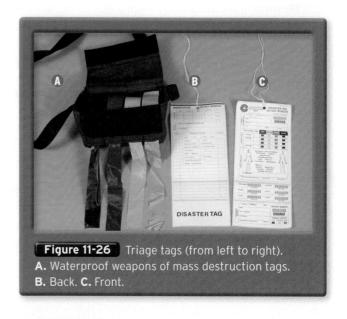

Figure 11-26 Triage tags (from left to right). **A.** Waterproof weapons of mass destruction tags. **B.** Back. **C.** Front.

Figure 11-26. The patient tags or tape should be color-coded and should clearly show the category of the patients. The use of symbols and colors to indicate the triage categories is important in case some rescuers are color blind.

The tags will become part of the patient's medical record. Most have a tear-off receipt with a number correlating with the number on the tag. If the patient is unconscious and cannot be identified at the scene, the tag will be an identifier for tracking purposes.

At the Scene

A TMP who becomes sick or injured during a callout should be handled as an immediate priority and be stabilized and transported off the site efficiently in order to optimize the morale of remaining TMPs.

Triage Area

In the triage area or casualty collection point, patients should be reassessed and physically grouped according to triage category. All patients triaged as immediate (red) should be staged closest to the ambulance arrival point outside the outer perimeter. This site should ideally be uphill and upwind from the incident site in a relatively safe location. These patients should be treated, closely monitored, frequently reassessed, and transported as soon as possible.

SWAT Assessment Triage

In the event of gunfire, explosions, or weapons of mass destruction that cause mass casualties in the warm tactical zone, the TMP should evaluate and provide stabilizing care to all patients at the scene who urgently need emergency medical care. However, the role of a TMP is to provide medical support and care for the SWAT unit. If there are multiple casualties needing treatment simultaneously, the first patients to be evaluated should be SWAT unit casualties. This is often referred to as SWAT Assessment triage, and it has a practical and legally defendable basis. In SWAT Assessment triage, the second priority is to triage, evaluate, and provide lifesaving emergency medical care *to other patients at the scene*. There are three reasons why SWAT officers receive first priority:

1. In nearly all circumstances, SWAT officers are willing to accept help and will not fight or attempt to hurt rescuers. In the rare circumstance where a suspect and a SWAT officer are both injured, you can assess and treat both patients faster if you treat the SWAT officer first. The SWAT officer is likely to cooperate and assist you, rather than possibly fight you and resist treatment.

2. SWAT officers are mission-focused. A rapid patient assessment can determine whether the SWAT officer has potentially lethal injuries.

3. The downed SWAT officer is an individual with *known weapons*. These weapons need to be secured so they cannot be stolen or used by suspects, nor mistakenly used by the injured SWAT officer. The suspect may or may not have a weapon, so the suspect should be monitored, handcuffed, and watched at gunpoint, but not assessed and treated until the injured SWAT officer has been stabilized.

Ready for Review

- In the tactical environment your highest priority is your own personal safety. You can help to maintain your safety by practicing 360-degree situational awareness, having a partner-in-safety, and searching all suspects prior to assessment.

- Call-A-CAB 'N Go is the tactical patient assessment mnemonic that stands for:

  - Call out for help and communicate with your unit in order to tell them what is happening.

  - Abolish all threats.

  - Assess and manage all threats to the patient's Circulation.

  - Assess and manage all threats to the patient's Airway.

  - Assess and manage all threats to the patient's Breathing.

  - Assess the patient's Neurologic status.

  - Go to the appropriate advanced medical facility.

- Remote assessment medicine is a unique aspect of tactical medicine in which a TMP without direct physical contact can visually assess injured patients from a safe distance with the goal of determining if the patient is dead or alive.

- In barricade medicine you may assist the negotiation team by gathering medical intelligence on the hostage taker and any hostages.

- In a mass-casualty incident, adults may be screened with the START triage process and pediatric patients may be screened with the JumpSTART process.

Vital Vocabulary

AVPU scale A method of assessing level of consciousness by determining whether the patient is alert, responsive to verbal stimuli or pain, or unresponsive; used principally early in the assessment.

Glasgow Coma Scale (GCS) score An evaluation tool used to determine level of consciousness, which evaluates and assigns point values (scores) for eye opening, verbal response, and motor response, which are then totaled; effective in helping predict patient outcomes.

JumpSTART triage A sorting system for pediatric patients younger than 8 years or weighing less than 100 lb. There is a minor adaptation for infants since they cannot walk on their own.

remote assessment medicine (RAM) Visually assessing injured patients from a safe distance with a goal of determining if the patient is dead or alive.

revised trauma score A trauma scoring system that rates injury severity by comparing the Glasgow Coma Scale score, the systolic blood pressure, and the respiratory rate and assigning a score between 1 and 13 based on those factors.

SAMPLE history A brief history of a patient's condition to determine signs and symptoms, allergies, medications, pertinent past history, last oral intake, and events leading to the injury or illness.

START triage A patient sorting process that stands for Simple Triage and Rapid Treatment and uses a limited assessment of the patient's ability to walk, breathing status, circulation status, and mental status.

triage The process of establishing treatment and transportation priorities according to severity of injury and medical need.

Controlling Bleeding

OBJECTIVES

- Describe how to identify external and internal hemorrhage in a patient.
- Describe the differences between controlled hemorrhage versus uncontrolled hemorrhage.
- Describe the principles of tourniquet use.
- Describe how to apply a commercial tourniquet.
- Describe how to apply an improvised tourniquet.
- Describe the types and use of hemostatic agents.

Introduction

Bleeding can be external and obvious or internal and hidden **Figure 12-1**. Either way, it is potentially dangerous, first causing weakness and, if left uncontrolled, eventually shock and death. The most common cause of shock following trauma is bleeding. Generally the shock from trauma is caused at least in part from bleeding. This chapter discusses how to manage bleeding in the tactical environment.

Identify Hemorrhage

Hemorrhage (bleeding) is the escape of blood cells and plasma from capillaries, veins, and arteries. The average adult body contains approximately 5 to 6 liters (L) of blood. The average adult can normally lose 1 to 2 pints of blood without any major harmful effects (1 liter equals 2.11 pints). The severity of hemorrhage depends on the amount of blood lost in relation to the physical size of the patient. The amount of visible blood is often not a good way to judge the severity of an injury. For

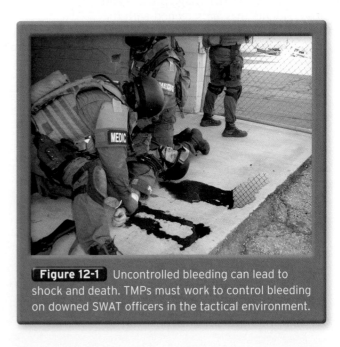

Figure 12-1 Uncontrolled bleeding can lead to shock and death. TMPs must work to control bleeding on downed SWAT officers in the tactical environment.

example, serious injuries, such as open femur fractures, may not bleed heavily externally whereas relatively minor injuries, such as a scalp laceration, will bleed profusely.

Suspicion and severity of internal bleeding should be based on the **mechanism of injury (MOI)** or how the injury occurred (fall, gunshot, knife, motor vehicle crash). Although not usually visible, internal bleeding can result in serious blood loss from the vascular system. This blood can collect inside the chest, abdomen, or extremities, resulting in low blood pressure, shock (hypoperfusion), and subsequent death. A patient with serious internal bleeding will often develop shock before you realize the extent of the patient's injuries.

Traumatized, painful, swollen, and deformed extremities will often contain long bone fractures and should be recognized and properly managed due to the significant hemorrhage that may occur. Chapter 20, "Extremity Injuries," covers the management of these injuries in detail. A fractured humerus or tibia may be associated with the loss of up to 750 mL of blood. A femur fracture is commonly associated with a loss of 1,500 mL, and several liters of blood may accumulate in the pelvis from a pelvic fracture.

Sources of Bleeding and Characteristics

Typically, bleeding from an open artery (arterial bleeding) is brighter red (high in oxygen) and spurts in time with the pulse. The pressure that causes the blood to spurt also makes this type of bleeding difficult to control. As the amount of blood circulating in the body drops, so does the patient's blood pressure and, eventually, the spurting will decrease.

Blood from an open vein (venous bleeding) is darker (low in oxygen) and flows slowly or severely, depending on the size of the vein. Because it is under less pressure, most venous blood does not spurt and is easier to manage; however, it can be profuse and life-threatening. Major trauma to the proximal extremities will often cause both venous and arterial hemorrhaging as these blood vessels are located next to each other. Capillary blood (bleeding from damaged capillary vessels) is dark red and oozes from a wound steadily but slowly. Venous and capillary blood is more likely to clot spontaneously than arterial blood **Figure 12-2**.

Hemorrhage

External bleeding can usually be easily controlled by using direct pressure or a compression bandage. Internal bleeding is usually not controlled until a surgeon locates

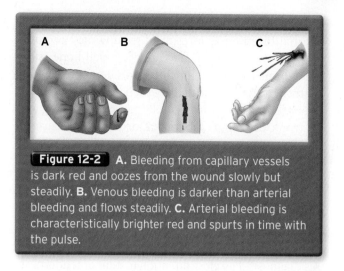

Figure 12-2   **A.** Bleeding from capillary vessels is dark red and oozes from the wound slowly but steadily. **B.** Venous bleeding is darker than arterial bleeding and flows steadily. **C.** Arterial bleeding is characteristically brighter red and spurts in time with the pulse.

the source in an operating room and sutures it closed. Because internal bleeding is not as obvious, you must rely on signs and symptoms to determine the extent and severity of the hemorrhage.

External Hemorrhage

External bleeding results from a break in the skin and injury to the underlying blood vessel. External bleeding includes lacerations, puncture wounds (gunshot wounds), amputation, abrasions, and incisions. These injuries are discussed in detail in Chapter 21, "Soft-Tissue Injuries." Its extent or severity is often a function of the type of wound and the types of blood vessels that have been injured.

Arteries may spurt initially, but as the patient's blood pressure decreases, often the blood simply flows. In addition, an artery that is cut directly across will often recoil and contract due to small muscle cells in the arterial wall and result in slowing and potentially stopping the bleeding. By contrast, if the artery is cut in an elderly patient with arteriosclerosis (hardening of the arteries) then the calcium and other deposits will prevent the artery from contracting and shrinking, thus leading to a great deal of bleeding and death if not properly treated.

Some injuries that you might expect to be accompanied by considerable external bleeding do not always have serious hemorrhaging. For example, a SWAT officer who is near an explosion may have amputations of one or more extremities due to a building collapse and heavy concrete smashing the limbs, yet experience little bleeding because the wound and blood vessels were pinched and smashed, resulting in significant blood vessel damage and fast clotting of the veins and arteries. Conversely, a police officer who is cut with a knife or shot with a high-velocity bullet striking the upper thigh and femoral artery will very likely have severe bleeding, with the only effective means of bleeding control being use of a tourniquet.

Internal Hemorrhage

Internal bleeding as a result of trauma may occur in any part of the body. A fracture of a small bone (such as the humerus, ankle, or tibia) produces a somewhat controlled environment in which a relatively small amount of bleeding can occur. By contrast, bleeding into the trunk (ie, thorax, abdomen, or pelvis), because of its much larger space, may be severe, uncontrolled, and difficult to diagnose in the tactical environment.

Any internal bleeding must be treated promptly. The signs of internal hemorrhage (such as discoloration or bruising) do not always develop quickly, so you must rely on other signs and symptoms and clinical suspicion, including an evaluation of the MOI to make this diagnosis. Pay close attention to pain or tenderness, tachycardia (rapid pulse), dizziness, altered mental status, and other signs of shock such as pale skin. Management of a patient with internal hemorrhaging focuses on the treatment of shock (see Chapter 15, "Shock Management"). Research has shown that many cases of blunt trauma and internal bleeding can be managed without surgery, but for the TMP, any patient with suspicion for major internal bleeding should be rapidly evacuated and transported to a hospital for further diagnosis and management based on the injury and the patient's condition.

Controlled Versus Uncontrolled Hemorrhage

External bleeding that can be controlled by direct pressure or a tourniquet can be managed by the wounded SWAT officer, a nearby SWAT officer, or a TMP **Figure 12-3**. If there is moderate or minor bleeding and no other injuries, then simple stabilization, evacuation, and transport to a hospital within an hour or two will usually result in a good outcome.

Most external bleeding can be managed with direct pressure, although arterial bleeding may take 5 or more minutes of direct pressure to form a clot. For this reason, a tourniquet may need to be used to control external bleeding to an extremity that cannot be controlled with direct pressure and a compression bandage.

Any major bleeding that you cannot control is a serious emergency. As a consequence, the assessment of the patient includes a search for life-threatening bleeding. If found, the hemorrhage must be controlled; if the hemorrhage cannot be controlled in the tactical environment, all of your efforts should concentrate on attempting to stabilize the patient as you work rapidly to extract and transport the patient to a hospital where further diagnosis and treatment can hopefully stop the bleeding.

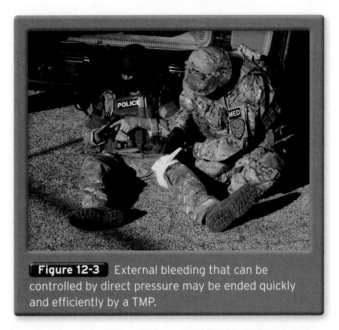

Figure 12-3 External bleeding that can be controlled by direct pressure may be ended quickly and efficiently by a TMP.

Physiologic Response to Hemorrhage

Typically, bleeding from an open artery is bright red (because of the high oxygen content) and spurts in time with the pulse. The higher arterial pressure that causes the blood to spurt also makes this type of bleeding difficult to control. As the amount of blood circulating in the body decreases, the blood pressure will eventually decrease, and the bleeding will decrease. However, the healthy person who is bleeding to death will have a significant increase in the heart rate as the body tries to compensate for the lower blood pressure, which will cause the amount of blood flowing out to increase. It is essential to compress killer bleeds as soon as possible.

On its own, bleeding tends to stop rather quickly, within about 10 minutes, in response to internal clotting mechanisms and exposure to air. In most healthy persons under the age of 65, when blood vessels are lacerated, blood flows rapidly from the open vessel. The open ends of the vessel then begin to narrow, which reduces the amount of bleeding. Platelets collect at the site, plugging the hole and sealing the injured portions of the vessel. Bleeding will not stop if a clot does not form unless the injured vessel is externally compressed or a tourniquet squeezes the blood vessels closed and shuts it off from the main blood supply. Direct contact with damaged body tissues and fluids or the external environment commonly triggers the blood's clotting factors.

Hemorrhage Treatment

First, ensure that you are wearing standard bloodborne personal protective equipment, including gloves, face

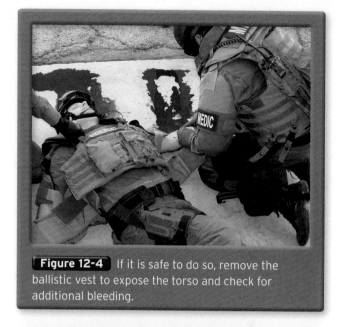

Figure 12-4 If it is safe to do so, remove the ballistic vest to expose the torso and check for additional bleeding.

mask, and eye protection, before you perform the CAB portion of the "Call-A-Cab-'N-Go" tactical patient assessment process. Rapidly scan for any bleeding and injuries. The uniform or clothing will appear dark or red. There may be only a slight oozing of blood from the SWAT officer's ballistic vest where it meets the neck. A major hemorrhage may have occurred and by the time you are able to respond or the wounded SWAT officer is brought to you, the patient may be in shock with minimal bleeding. Ask witnesses how much blood was seen at the site of injury. Use your eyes and ask questions to determine the approximate amount of bleeding that may have occurred.

Your gloved hands should sweep hidden body regions, such as under the head, neck, back, buttocks, and legs, with a quick visual scan of the gloves in between these sites so you know where the blood came from. If possible, ask fellow SWAT officers to help you remove gear and expose the bleeding torso or extremity **Figure 12-4**. Use scissors or a knife to cut clothing and expose any sites of bleeding **Figure 12-5**. Occasionally, you will need to loosen a ballistic vest to assess the chest and abdomen while ballistic threats still exist; in these cases, consider keeping the ballistic vest on the patient

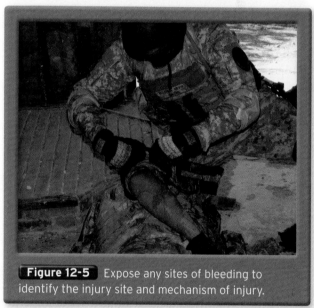

Figure 12-5 Expose any sites of bleeding to identify the injury site and mechanism of injury.

during extraction for protection from additional injury. These guidelines also apply to a ballistic helmet.

The goal of treating hemorrhage is to stop the bleeding. There is no single correct way to control bleeding, and the method selected will depend on many variables. Remember: extremity hemorrhage that is severe should be treated with a tourniquet immediately and any penetrating trauma to the torso is an immediate load-and-go situation.

Treatment for a downed patient who is bleeding during an under-fire situation is extremely limited. The main priority is to abolish threats and get the patient behind hard cover. Only in the rarest circumstance with severe bleeding will a tourniquet be applied by TMPs when there is a direct threat of deadly hazards. A rapid extraction to hard cover (either self-extraction or buddy

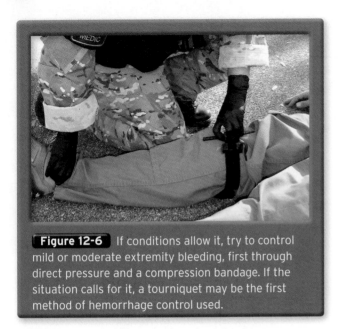

Figure 12-6 If conditions allow it, try to control mild or moderate extremity bleeding, first through direct pressure and a compression bandage. If the situation calls for it, a tourniquet may be the first method of hemorrhage control used.

extraction) will then enable the safe application of a tourniquet or compression dressing.

If you are in a fairly safe area behind hard cover when treating a downed SWAT officer or other patient, then mild or moderate bleeding may initially be controlled by direct pressure. Direct pressure is the quickest method to control bleeding. To accurately control bleeding through direct pressure, first completely expose the wound.

Place a sterile dressing or trauma bandage on the wound, apply firm pressure with your gloved hand, and then use the elastic wrapping to tightly hold continued pressure over the wound. If only a gauze dressing is used, use separate cravat or elastic wrap to hold continued pressure. Ensure that the bandage is only tight enough to control the bleeding. If the bleeding is not controlled, either apply a tourniquet or consider applying additional compression dressings and/or firm pressure directly over the wound for several minutes. This increased pressure may help to control the bleeding. Secure the compression dressing in place so it will not slip. The emergency (Israeli) bandage and Olaes bandages are very effective compression dressings that can control mild or moderate hemorrhage.

If the patient is conscious, has no other serious injuries, and will be under your or other TMPs' direct observation, then you can try to stop the bleeding by applying firm pressure and a compression bandage. However, if there are multiple injuries including torso trauma with load-and-go indications, or if there are multiple casualties at the scene and the TMP cannot remain at the patient's side, then a tourniquet is the best solution for any major extremity hemorrhage **Figure 12-6**.

In the past, medical personnel were taught to elevate an injured arm or leg above the level of the heart in conjunction with direct pressure. This may not be a wise idea if threats exist or if there is no time for this extra step. Do not elevate an extremity if you suspect a long-bone fracture until it has been properly splinted and you are certain that elevation or other movement will not cause further injury. The patient may be alert and stable enough to raise his or her own extremity, or it may be necessary to use a nearby object to maintain elevation, such as a medical gear backpack.

Splinting or immobilization is an effective means of controlling bleeding from a fractured long bone or other large bone (see Chapter 20, "Extremity Injuries"). Broken bone fragments may continue to move and may cut and damage nearby major blood vessels and increase bleeding if they are not immobilized; muscular activity can also increase the rate of blood flow. Pneumatic (air) splints may be used to apply direct circumferential pressure over an

Medical Gear

The Olaes modular bandage is a combat compression bandage. This bandage was developed by special operations soldiers who learned important lessons in direct combat. The bandage includes a gauze pad area that uses as its absorbent pad a total of 3 meters of gauze that can be removed to pack into a large gunshot wound or other devastating injury to help stop bleeding. It also has an occlusive small clear plastic sheet tucked in behind the dressing pad, which can be pulled out, unfolded, and used to create a one-way-valve-type dressing to cover sucking chest wounds. Additionally, it has an attached clear plastic pressure cup that allows focal pressure over the wound, and this can also be used when reversed as a rigid cup for covering an eye injury. Another Olaes feature is the roll of elastic wrap that has small Velcro control strips attached every several inches that prevent it from accidentally unrolling entirely if it is dropped during the wrapping and application process **Figure 12-7**.

The emergency bandage (also know as the Israeli combat dressing) is another excellent compression bandage that is widely used. It consists of an absorbent gauze pad (some versions have two pads) that is applied to the wound with an elastic bandage that holds the dressing in place **Figure 12-8**. In addition, a flattened D-shaped plastic bar (pressure bar) is attached near the gauze dressing that allows it to be tightened with focal pressure over the wound. Both the Olaes and emergency bandage have a plastic clip on the tail of the dressing that is designed to be used as a windlass and thus used to twist the bandage to cause further compression. It is possible to twist these bandages tight enough to form a tourniquet, but the stretch and friction of the ACE-type bandage makes it more difficult to occlude arterial blood flow. Both the Olaes and emergency bandage are made in 4- and 6-inch versions, and are double-wrapped and vacuum-sealed to help maintain a compact sterile package.

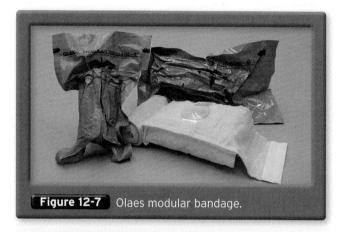

Figure 12-7 Olaes modular bandage.

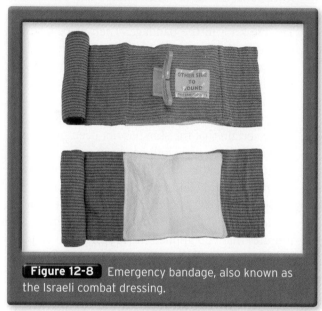

Figure 12-8 Emergency bandage, also known as the Israeli combat dressing.

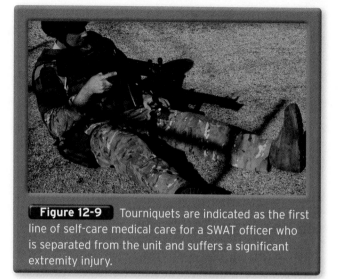

Figure 12-9 Tourniquets are indicated as the first line of self-care medical care for a SWAT officer who is separated from the unit and suffers a significant extremity injury.

Safety

Never use wire or rope to improvise a tourniquet! The narrow width of wire or rope does not provide proper compression.

extremity, compressing the extremity, its soft tissues, and the bleeding vessels. Splinting using a pneumatic splint gives a double benefit: splinting and direct pressure.

Principles of Tourniquet Use

In a tactical environment when compression dressings and other techniques do not stop bleeding or if there is severe arterial bleeding, a tourniquet is a very reliable means of stopping major extremity hemorrhage. Direct pressure is almost impossible to maintain during evacuation. Tourniquets are indicated as the first line of self-care medical care for a severely wounded SWAT officer who is alone or separated from the unit **Figure 12-9**.

Tissue and nerve damage are rare if the tourniquet is left in place for less than 2 to 3 hours. In fact, surgeons routinely apply tourniquets to reduce bleeding in the operating room and leave them in place for that length of time without any adverse effects to the limb. Longer tourniquet times are possible without injury, but the longer a tourniquet is left in place, the more likely ischemia or nerve damage will occur. With massive

hemorrhage and amputations, it is better to accept the small risk of tissue and nerve damage than lose a casualty to blood loss and hypovolemic shock.

Direct pressure, elevation, or compression dressings will not control some bleeding; prompt application of a tourniquet may be lifesaving. If the nature of the wound is such that direct pressure will not be effective, go directly to a tourniquet. Traumatic amputation of an extremity is one of those situations. Forceful, severe arterial bleeding from an extremity wound will often benefit from early use of a tourniquet. In this case, do not waste time attempting a compression dressing.

A tourniquet is ideally 1 to 2 inches in width; this width decreases the amount of nerve and tissue damage occurring under the tourniquet. If a commercial device such as a CAT or SOFTT is not available, use any equipment that will create an effective tourniquet.

Tourniquet Procedures

Every SWAT officer should carry a tourniquet in the exact same location where it can be accessed easily in any emergency situation. When providing treatment for a patient, use the patient's own tourniquet.

To apply a Combat Application Tourniquet (CAT) or a Special Operations Forces Tactical Tourniquet (SOFTT), follow these steps:

1. Apply the tourniquet several inches above the bleeding wound.
2. Adjust the friction adaptor buckle until the tourniquet is tightened and securely in place **Figure 12-10**.

3. Twist the windlass rod to slowly increase direct pressure to the extremity; twist and tighten the tourniquet until the arterial bleeding stops. Note that some oozing from the wound may continue for a minute or two.

4. Lock the windlass rod in place with the locking device **Figure 12-11**.

5. Ensure the bleeding has stopped. If it has not, then check to see if the bleeding is above or below the level of the tourniquet, look for a second injury and bleeding site; consider tightening the tourniquet further, or consider placing a second tourniquet just above (proximal) the first tourniquet.

6. Mark the time of tourniquet application, using a triage tag or patient care note, or writing a "T" or "TK" on the patient's forehead along with the time it was applied. Complete the tactical patient assessment and determine the best way to evacuate and transport the patient to the hospital. The tourniquet must be left in place until the patient is evaluated at the hospital.

If a commercial tourniquet is not available, or if a mass-casualty situation requires more tourniquets than

you have, follow these steps to apply a tourniquet using a triangular bandage and a stick or rod:

1. Cut fabric from the patient's pants or other nearby appropriate material that is long enough to improvise a tourniquet. If available, a cravat or triangular bandage may be folded until it is about 3 or 4 inches wide and several layers thick.

2. Wrap the bandage around the extremity twice if possible. Choose an area only slightly proximal to the bleeding (about 1 or 2 inches) to reduce the amount of tissue damage to the extremity. If conditions do not allow you to cut away clothing to visualize the injury, then apply the tourniquet at the proximal arm or leg.

3. Tie one knot in the bandage. Then place a sturdy stick or rod on top of the knot, and tie the ends of the bandage over the stick in a square knot.

4. Use the stick or rod as a handle (windlass) and twist it to tighten the tourniquet until the bleeding has stopped; then stop twisting **Figure 12-12**.

5. Make certain that the skin has not been pinched or damaged where the cloth has been twisted.

6. Secure the stick in place so it will not become loose during extraction and transportation, and make the wrapping neat and smooth to minimize tissue damage.

7. Write "T" or "TK" and the exact time (hour and minute) that you applied the tourniquet on a piece of adhesive tape, triage tag, or the patient's forehead. If possible, use the phrase "time applied." Securely fasten the tape to the patient's forehead. Hospital personnel should also be notified that the patient has a tourniquet in place. Record this information on the patient care report.

8. As an alternative, you can use a blood pressure cuff as an effective tourniquet. Position the cuff proximal to the bleeding point, and inflate it just

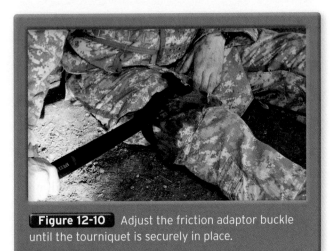

Figure 12-10   Adjust the friction adaptor buckle until the tourniquet is securely in place.

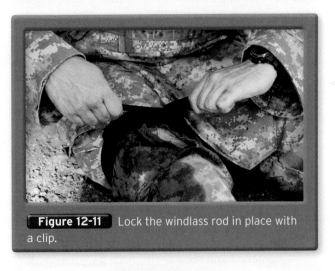

Figure 12-11   Lock the windlass rod in place with a clip.

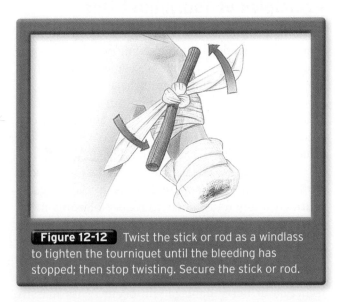

Figure 12-12   Twist the stick or rod as a windlass to tighten the tourniquet until the bleeding has stopped; then stop twisting. Secure the stick or rod.

enough to stop the bleeding. Leave the cuff inflated. If you use a blood pressure cuff, monitor the gauge continuously to make sure that the pressure is not gradually dropping. You may have to clamp the tube with a padded hemostat leading from the cuff to the inflating bulb to prevent loss of pressure.

Avoid loosening or removing a tourniquet once it has been applied. The loosening of a tourniquet may dislodge clots and/or cause continued bleeding resulting in enough blood loss to cause shock and possibly death. Tourniquet removal should not be attempted if the anticipated evacuation time is less than 2 hours. Direct pressure, compression dressings, or hemostatic agents can be used in conjunction with a tourniquet to control hemorrhage.

Hemostatic Agents and Dressings

Hemostatic agents and dressings are used to control life-threatening external hemorrhage that is not amenable to tourniquet use. It may be used as an adjunct to tourniquet removal (if evacuation time is anticipated to be longer than 2 hours). Work with your medical director to determine which, if any, hemostatic agent or dressing will be used in the tactical environment. The hemostatic dressings may be used on any significant bleeding wound in accordance with each manufacturer's specific recommendations. Always consult the manufacturer's recommendations carefully prior to use of any hemostatic agent.

The QuikClot combat gauze is a 3-inch-wide roll of thin gauze that is 12-feet long and comes rolled up in a waterproof plastic package **Figure 12-13**. It has zeolite (kaolin clay), a natural blood-clotter, added to the gauze, which reportedly decreases bleeding according to several research studies. It was approved for use by the US Armed Forces and other military units and is currently a first-line hemostatic product recommended by the Committee on Tactical Combat Casualty Care since 2008. This long gauze roll is stuffable and can be placed or packed into a large wound cavity, or can be unrolled and packed down into the wound to stop bleeding. It later needs to be removed in the controlled setting of the emergency department or operating room.

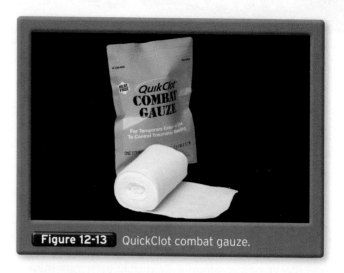

Figure 12-13 QuickClot combat gauze.

Special Populations

Commercial tourniquets will not fit infants. If an infant has significant extremity bleeding, use a cloth or other soft material to make an improvised 1.5- to 2-inch-wide field expedient tourniquet.

The HemCon bandages are varying-sized (1.5-, 2-, and 4-inch squares) foam-backed dressings that contain chitosan, made from the sterilized exoskeleton of shrimp, which has clotting and antibacterial properties. Although the manufacturer reports there have been no known allergic reactions, they recommend exercising caution using this product on individuals with severe shellfish allergies.

The new HemCon ChitoFlex dressing is available in several sizes (1 × 3-, 3 × 9-, and 3 × 28-inch length) as well as GuardaCare 2 × 2-inch and 4 × 4-inch 8-ply gauze squares. A new product is ChitoGauze, which has a z-folded dressing that is 4 inches wide and 4 yards long intended for combat environments. The longer strips are stuffable. The ChitoGauze is packaged prefolded in an accordion-like z fashion, which allows it to be removed from the packaging without having to unroll it or worry about it falling out onto the ground.

Celox is a chitosan-based product marketed by Medtrade Products LTD (England). A variety of products are made including Celox granules, Celox Pro (for hospitals), Celox A (deep applicator), Celox First Aid (for home use, several granule and gauze products), and Celox gauze in a 3-inch × 10-foot roll that has chitosan embedded in the stuffable gauze roll to stop bleeding faster.

There are a number of other products that are being marketed for hemorrhage control, including TraumaDex, D-Stat Dry, ActCel gauze, and others. Medical directors, with input from TMPs, should review and evaluate available data on all new products before approving them for field use.

Medical Gear

In addition to commercial tourniquets, carry an assortment of rip-proof cloth strips that could adequately serve as tourniquets in an emergency. Several windlasses should also be carried.

Ready for Review

- Bleeding is the most common cause of trauma-associated shock.

- External bleeding may be controlled by using direct pressure, a tourniquet, or a hemostatic agent.

- Internal bleeding requires evacuation and transport to a hospital.

- Tourniquets are indicated as the first line of medical self-care for a wounded SWAT officer who is alone or separated from the unit if that SWAT officer suffers a significant extremity injury.

- Tissue and nerve damage are rare if the tourniquet is left in place for less than 2 or 3 hours.

- To be effective in saving a life, the decision to apply a tourniquet needs to be made very quickly (seconds, not minutes), and the application needs to be equally fast (seconds, not minutes).

- Hemostatic agents and dressings are intended to be used to control life-threatening external hemorrhage that is not amenable to tourniquet use. It may be used as an adjunct to tourniquet removal (if evacuation time is anticipated to be longer than 2 hours).

Vital Vocabulary

hemorrhage The escape of blood cells and plasma from capillaries, veins, and arteries; bleeding.

hemostatic agent Powder, packet, gauze, or other dressing that is specially mixed with or coated with an agent or material that increases the speed and efficiency of the body to form clots and stop bleeding.

mechanism of injury (MOI) The way in which traumatic injuries occur; the forces that act on the body to cause damage.

Basic Airway Management

- Describe the conditions that can cause an airway obstruction in the tactical environment.

- Describe indications and contraindications for performing the head tilt–chin lift in the tactical environment.

- Describe indications and contraindications for performing the jaw-thrust maneuver in the tactical environment.

- Describe indications and contraindications for using a nasopharyngeal airway in the tactical environment.

- Describe indications and contraindications for using an oropharyngeal airway in the tactical environment.

- Describe the special equipment considerations for the tactical medical provider when providing ventilation in the tactical environment.

- Demonstrate the bag-mask device technique in the tactical environment.

- Describe the special equipment considerations for the tactical medical provider when suctioning a patient's airway in the tactical environment.

Introduction

After any circulation issues are resolved, it is time to assess and secure the patient's airway **Figure 13-1**. After the immediate dangers are abolished, a point of relative safety is reached or created, and circulation is stabilized, then the patient's airway should be addressed **Figure 13-2**. Ensure that you are wearing proper PPE when assessing and stabilizing the airway.

The objective is to rapidly establish and maintain a **patent** (open) airway. First determine whether the patient is breathing or attempting to breathe. Remember that awake, alert, and talking patients rarely require airway intervention. However, if the airway is not open, then it is up to you to fix it. An obstructed airway is extremely serious, and if a patient cannot breathe, then irreversible brain damage begins after 4 to 6 minutes.

Causes of Airway Obstruction

A multitude of conditions can cause an airway obstruction, including the tongue, trauma, and aspiration. In the unconscious patient, the jaw relaxes and the tongue tends to fall back against the posterior wall of the pharynx, closing off the airway. A patient with mild obstruction from the tongue will have snoring respirations; a patient whose airway is severely obstructed will have no respirations. Fortunately, obstruction of the airway by the tongue is simple to correct using a manual maneuver (eg, head tilt–chin lift, jaw-thrust).

With trauma, the airway may be obstructed by loose teeth, facial bone fractures, tissue, clotted blood, or a neck wound. In addition, penetrating or blunt trauma may obstruct the airway by fracturing or displacing the larynx, allowing the vocal cords to collapse. If an obstruction, such as teeth or vomitus, is allowed to enter the lungs (aspiration), the result can be life threatening. In addition to obstructing the airway, aspiration destroys delicate lung tissue, introduces pathogens into the lungs, and decreases the patient's ability to ventilate (or be ventilated). Suction should be readily available for any patient who is unable to maintain his or her own airway. Always assume that the patient has a full stomach. Suctioning should be used to clear the airway of secretions as needed. Suctioning is covered in detail later in this chapter.

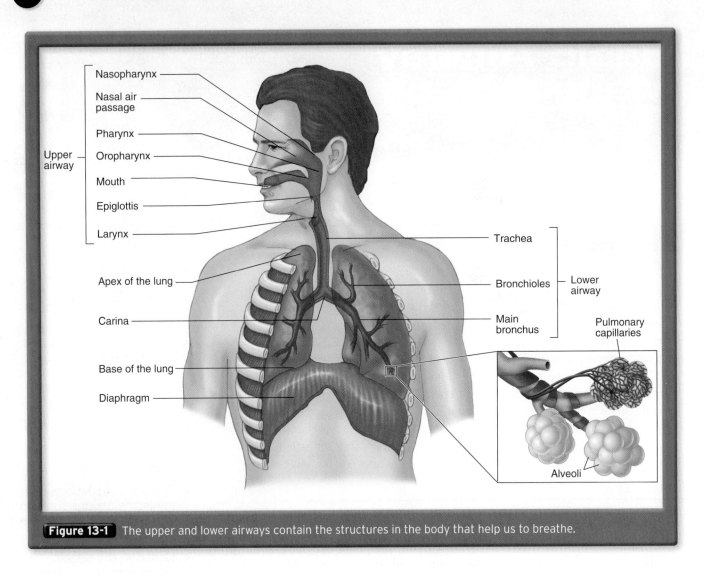

Nasopharynx

Nasal air passage

Pharynx

Upper airway

Oropharynx

Mouth

Epiglottis

Larynx

Apex of the lung

Carina

Base of the lung

Diaphragm

Trachea

Bronchioles — Lower airway

Main bronchus

Pulmonary capillaries

Alveoli

Figure 13-1   The upper and lower airways contain the structures in the body that help us to breathe.

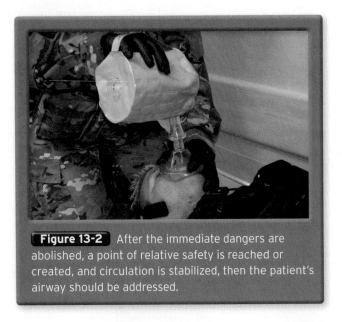

Figure 13-2   After the immediate dangers are abolished, a point of relative safety is reached or created, and circulation is stabilized, then the patient's airway should be addressed.

Manual Maneuvers

Sometimes the simplest, most low-tech techniques are the fastest and most effective ways to open a patient's airway. In the unresponsive patient, the most common cause of airway obstruction is the patient's tongue **Figure 13-3**. To correct this problem, manually maneuver the patient's head and jaw to move the tongue forward and open the airway. Simple techniques used to accomplish this include the head tilt–chin lift maneuver and the jaw-thrust maneuver.

Head Tilt-Chin Lift Maneuver

Opening the airway to relieve an obstruction can often be accomplished by simply tilting the patient's head back and lifting the chin. The **head tilt-chin lift maneuver** is

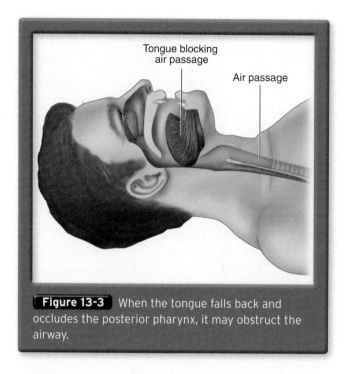

Figure 13-3 When the tongue falls back and occludes the posterior pharynx, it may obstruct the airway.

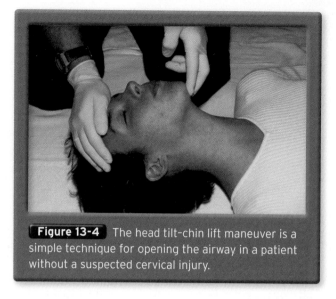

Figure 13-4 The head tilt–chin lift maneuver is a simple technique for opening the airway in a patient without a suspected cervical injury.

the preferred technique for opening the airway of a patient who has not sustained significant neck or facial trauma. Occasionally, this simple maneuver is all that is required for the patient to resume breathing. Following are some considerations when using the head tilt–chin lift maneuver:

- **Indications.** An unresponsive patient who has no significant mechanism for cervical spine injury, who is unable to maintain or protect his or her own airway.
- **Contraindications.** A responsive patient or a possible cervical spine injury.
- **Advantages.** No equipment is required, and the technique is simple, safe, and noninvasive.
- **Disadvantages.** It is hazardous to patients with spinal injury and does not protect from aspiration. It requires one TMP to maintain the open airway. It is difficult to maintain this maneuver when extracting or transporting patients.

Perform the head tilt–chin lift maneuver in the following manner:

1. With the patient in a supine position, position yourself beside the patient's head.
2. Place one hand on the patient's forehead, and apply firm backward pressure with your palm to tilt the patient's head back. This extension of the neck will move the tongue away from the back of the throat and palate and help to open the airway.

3. Place the fingertips of your other hand under the lower jaw near the bony part of the chin. Do not compress the soft tissue under the chin, because this may block the airway.
4. Lift the chin upward, bringing the entire lower jaw with it, helping to tilt the head back. Do not use your thumb to lift the chin. Lift so that the teeth are nearly brought together, but avoid closing the mouth completely. Continue to hold the forehead to maintain backward tilt of the head **Figure 13-4**.

Jaw-Thrust Maneuver

If you suspect that the patient has experienced a cervical spine injury, open the airway using the **jaw-thrust maneuver**. In this technique, you open the airway by placing your fingers behind both sides of the angle of the jaw and lifting the jaw forward. The jaw is displaced forward at an angle. You can seal a mask around the patient's nose and mouth while performing this maneuver. Following are some considerations when using the jaw-thrust maneuver:

- **Indications.** Unconscious patient, possible cervical spine injury, or unable to protect his or her own airway.
- **Contraindications.** Conscious patient or resistance to opening the mouth.
- **Advantages.** May be used in a patient with a cervical spine injury, may use with cervical collar in place, and does not require special equipment.
- **Disadvantages.** Cannot maintain if the patient becomes conscious or combative, difficult to maintain for an extended period of time and while moving patient, very difficult to use in conjunction

with bag-mask ventilation, fingers must remain in place to maintain jaw displacement, requires a second TMP for proper bag-mask ventilation, and does not protect against aspiration.

Perform the jaw-thrust maneuver in the following manner:

1. Kneel above the patient's head. Place your fingers behind the angles of the lower jaw, and move the jaw upward. Use your thumbs to help open the mouth by adjusting the position of the lower jaw to allow breathing through the mouth and nose.
2. The completed maneuver should open the airway with the mouth slightly open and the jaw jutting forward.

Once the airway has been opened, the patient may start to breathe on his or her own. Assess whether breathing has returned, and support as needed **Figure 13-5** .

Basic Airway Adjuncts

If the patient is semiconscious or unconscious, an artificial airway may be needed to help maintain an open air passage. *An artificial airway is not a substitute for proper head positioning.* Even after an airway adjunct has been inserted, the appropriate manual position of the head must be maintained.

Nasopharyngeal Airway

The **nasopharyngeal airway (NPA)** is a soft rubber tube that comes in various sizes that is inserted through the nose into the pharyngeal area of the airway, preventing the tongue from blocking air movement, thereby allowing passage of air from the nose to the lower airway. The purpose of the NPA is to maintain an artificial patent airway or to provide airway management when suctioning is necessary. The NPA is much better tolerated than an oral airway in conscious or semiconscious patients who have an intact **gag reflex** **Figure 13-6** . Do not use this device when the patient has experienced trauma to the nose, or if you have reason to suspect a skull fracture (eg, **cerebrospinal fluid [CSF]** leaking from the nose), the roof of the mouth is fractured, or brain matter is exposed. Inserting the NPA in such cases may cause it to enter the brain through the hole caused by the fracture.

The following are considerations when using an NPA:

- **Indications.** Conscious or semiconscious patient, casualty with an intact gag reflex, mouth injuries (broken teeth, massive oral tissue damage).

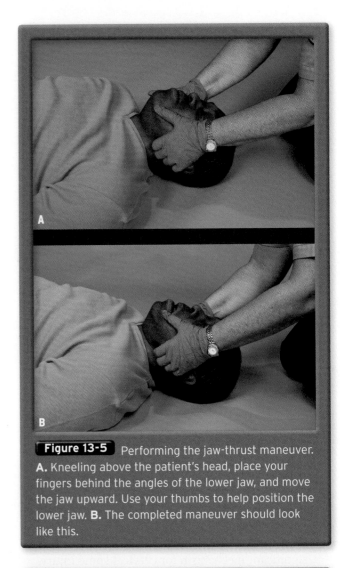

Figure 13-5 Performing the jaw-thrust maneuver. **A.** Kneeling above the patient's head, place your fingers behind the angles of the lower jaw, and move the jaw upward. Use your thumbs to help position the lower jaw. **B.** The completed maneuver should look like this.

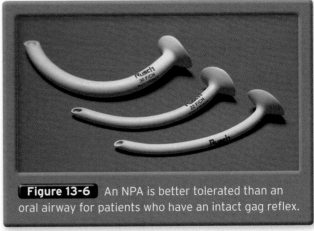

Figure 13-6 An NPA is better tolerated than an oral airway for patients who have an intact gag reflex.

- **Contraindications.** Any evidence of head injury, traumatic injury to the roof of the mouth, exposed brain matter; CSF draining from nose, mouth, or ears.
- **Complications.** Minor tissue trauma (nosebleeds). This is not an indication to remove the airway. In some patients, a nasal airway will trigger the gag reflex.

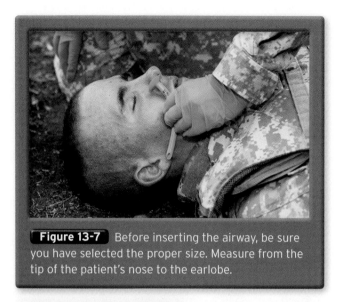

Figure 13-7 Before inserting the airway, be sure you have selected the proper size. Measure from the tip of the patient's nose to the earlobe.

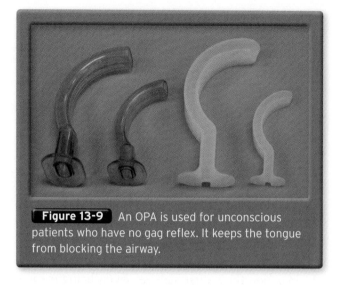

Figure 13-9 An OPA is used for unconscious patients who have no gag reflex. It keeps the tongue from blocking the airway.

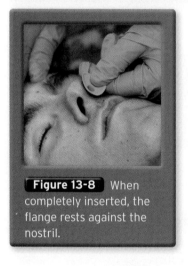

Figure 13-8 When completely inserted, the flange rests against the nostril.

To insert an NPA, follow these steps:

1. Before inserting the airway, be sure you have selected the proper size. Measure from the tip of the patient's nose to the earlobe **Figure 13-7**. In almost all individuals one nostril is larger than the other, so inspect the nostrils closely.
2. Lubricate the NPA prior to insertion.
3. The NPA should then be placed in the larger nostril, with the curvature of the device following the curve of the floor of the nose. For either nostril, the bevel should face the **septum**. Should difficultly arise with initial insertion, orient the bevel more superiorly as it first enters the nostril. Once resistance is met, rotate the bevel toward the septum.
4. Advance the airway gently.
5. When completely inserted, the flange rests against the nostril **Figure 13-8**. The other end of the airway opens into the posterior pharynx.
6. If the patient becomes intolerant of the nasal airway (vomiting, coughing, gagging), adjust the length of the NPA by withdrawing the NPA only until the gag reflex is relieved.

As an alternative, the proper size of the NPA can be determined by measuring from the tip of the nostril to the angle of the jaw rather than the earlobe. If the NPA is too long, it may obstruct the patient's airway. If the patient becomes intolerant of the NPA, gently remove

it from the nasal passage. Although the NPA is not as likely to cause vomiting as the oropharyngeal airway, you should have suction readily available if possible.

Oropharyngeal Airway

The **oropharyngeal airway (OPA)** (or J tube) is a curved, hard plastic device that fits over the back of the tongue with the tip in the posterior **pharynx** **Figure 13-9**. It is designed to hold the tongue away from the back of the throat, thereby preventing an airway obstruction in a casualty without a gag reflex. It also allows for drainage and/or suction of secretions, thereby preventing **aspiration**.

An OPA should be inserted promptly in an unresponsive patient—breathing or not—who has no gag reflex. Because its distal end sits in the back of the throat, this device will stimulate gagging and retching in a conscious or semiconscious patient. For that reason, the OPA should be used only in a deeply unconscious, unresponsive patient without a gag reflex. To assess a patient's gag reflex, use the eyelash reflex. If the patient's lower eyelid contracts when you gently stroke the upper eyelashes, the patient probably has an intact gag reflex. If the patient gags during insertion of the OPA, remove the device immediately and be prepared to suction the oropharynx. Following are some considerations when using an OPA:

- **Indications**. Unconscious patient without a gag reflex.
- **Contraindications**. Conscious patients, patients with a gag reflex present, facial trauma.

The OPA can induce vomiting and aspiration when the gag reflex is present. If the OPA is improperly sized or is inserted incorrectly, it could actually push the tongue back into the pharynx, creating an airway obstruction. Rough insertion of the OPA can injure the hard palate, resulting in oral bleeding and creating a risk of vomiting or aspiration. Prior to inserting an OPA, suction the oropharynx as needed to ensure that the mouth is clear of blood or other fluids.

The steps for inserting an OPA (J tube) are listed here:

1. Place the patient on a flat surface in a supine position.
2. Select the proper size airway by measuring from the patient's earlobe to the corner of his or her mouth or from the center of the patient's mouth to the angle of the lower jawbone **Figure 13-10** .
3. Open the airway using the appropriate maneuver. Use the head tilt–chin lift method for a patient with no risk of spinal injury. Use the jaw-thrust maneuver for a patient with a possible spinal injury.
4. Maintain the patient's airway by utilizing manual techniques and/or mechanical devices.
5. With your nondominant hand, use the cross-finger technique to open the patient's mouth. To perform the cross-finger technique, place your thumb at the corner of the patient's lower lip and your index finger at the corner of the patient's upper lip.
6. Visualize inside the mouth, and suction if necessary. Do *not* use the OPA if you see that the roof of the mouth is fractured or brain matter is exposed. The airway may enter the cranial cavity.
7. Holding the OPA in your dominant hand, position the correct size airway so that the tip is pointing toward the roof of the patient's mouth.
8. Insert the OPA into the patient's mouth by sliding the tip along the roof past the uvula or until resistance is met by the soft palate **Figure 13-11** .
9. Gently rotate the airway 180 degrees, so the tip is positioned behind the back of the tongue. The

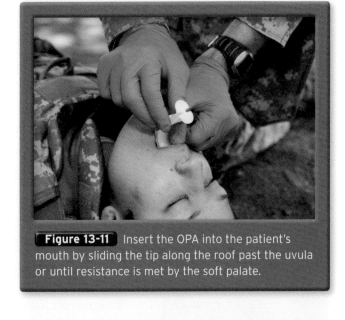

Figure 13-11   Insert the OPA into the patient's mouth by sliding the tip along the roof past the uvula or until resistance is met by the soft palate.

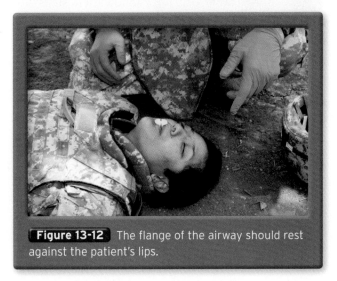

Figure 13-12   The flange of the airway should rest against the patient's lips.

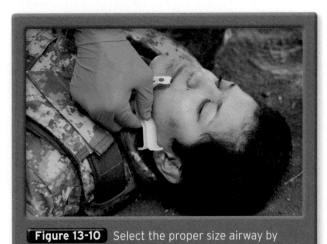

Figure 13-10   Select the proper size airway by measuring from the patient's earlobe to the corner of his or her mouth, or from the center of the patient's mouth to the angle of the lower jawbone.

flange of the airway should rest against the patient's lips **Figure 13-12** .

10. If the OPA is too large for the patient (more than a quarter of its length protruding from the patient's lips), remove it and choose the proper size to prevent occlusion of the airway.
11. Ventilate as necessary, in accordance with local protocols.
12. Monitor the patient closely. If the patient gags or regains consciousness, remove the airway immediately.
13. Remove the airway by pulling it out in line with the natural curvature of the mouth. *Do not* rotate.
14. Vomiting may occur once the airway is removed. Have a suction device ready when removing the airway adjunct.

Ventilations

If a patient is found with inadequate breathing or is **apneic** (not breathing), you must provide adequate ventilation. Two basic techniques are ventilation through mouth-to-mask ventilation or with a bag-mask device. If the TMP is properly trained and the indications exist, then a more advanced airway may be required (see Chapter 14, "Advanced Airway Management").

Mouth-to-Mouth Ventilation

Mouth-to-mouth ventilations are now routinely performed with a barrier device, such as a mask or face shield. A **barrier device** is a protective item that features a plastic barrier placed on a patient's face with a one-way valve to prevent the backflow of secretions, vomitus, and gases. Barrier devices provide adequate standard precautions **Figure 13-13**. Mouth-to-mouth ventilations without a barrier device should be provided only in extreme situations.

Most TMPs do not carry oxygen into the inner perimeter due to the weight and risks of a highly pressurized tank. In addition, the average patient will not necessarily need the extra oxygen, but instead will benefit from simple airway and ventilation techniques prior to evacuation and transportation to a hospital.

Mouth-to-Mask Ventilation

Performing mouth-to-mask ventilations with a pocket mask containing a one-way valve helps to prevent possible disease transmission. The mask may be shaped

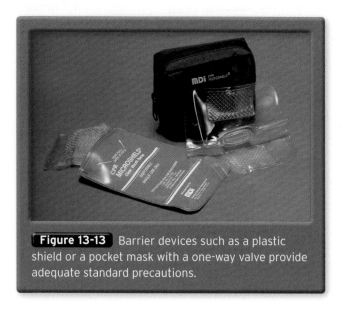

Figure 13-13 Barrier devices such as a plastic shield or a pocket mask with a one-way valve provide adequate standard precautions.

like a triangle, with the apex (top) placed across the bridge of the nose. The wider base (bottom) of the properly sized mask is placed in the groove between the lower lip and the chin. If the mask is round, then the center of the mask should be placed over the patient's mouth, and the air in the rim of the mask should be adjusted for a leak-proof seal. In the center of the mask is a chimney with a 15/22-mm connector that you can attach a one-way valve and either blow into this for mouth-to-mask ventilation, or use a medical airway bag to provide ventilations.

Follow these steps to use mouth-to-mask ventilation:

1. Kneel at the patient's head. Open the airway using the head tilt–chin lift maneuver or the jaw-thrust maneuver if indicated. Insert an oral or nasal airway to help maintain airway patency. Connect the one-way valve to the face mask and place the mask on the patient's face. Make sure the top is over the bridge of the nose and the bottom is in the groove between the lower lip and the chin. If the mask has a large, round cuff around the ventilation port, center the port over the patient's mouth. Inflate the collar to obtain a better fit and seal to the face if necessary. Hold the mask in position by placing your thumbs over the top part of the mask and your index fingers over the bottom half. Grasp and lift up the hard surface of the lower jaw with the remaining three fingers on each hand, making an airtight seal by pulling the lower jaw into the mask. Maintain an upward and forward pull on the lower jaw with your fingers to keep the airway open. This method of tightly securing the mask to the patient's face is known as the EC-clamp method **Figure 13-14**.

2. Take a deep breath and exhale into the open port of the one-way valve. Breathe slowly into the patient's mask until you observe adequate chest rise.

3. Remove your mouth and watch for the patient's chest to fall during passive exhalation.

You will know that you are providing adequate ventilations when you see the patient's chest rise adequately and do not meet resistance when ventilating. You should also hear and feel air escape as the patient exhales.

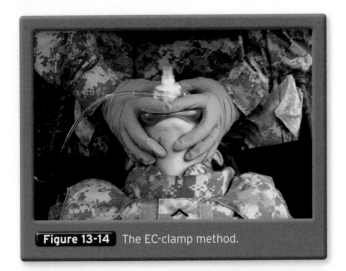

Figure 13-14 The EC-clamp method.

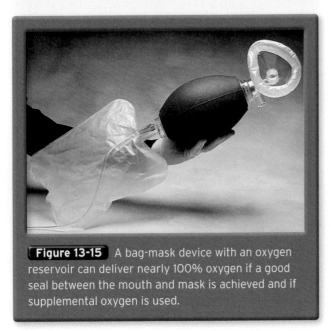

Figure 13-15 A bag-mask device with an oxygen reservoir can deliver nearly 100% oxygen if a good seal between the mouth and mask is achieved and if supplemental oxygen is used.

The Bag-Mask Device

A **bag-mask device** should be used when you need to deliver air to ventilate patients, and it may also be used to provide high concentrations of oxygen to patients who are not ventilating adequately **Figure 13-15**. The bag-mask device may be used with or without oxygen. You should use an oral or nasal airway adjunct in conjunction with the bag-mask device.

Bag-Mask Device Technique

Whenever possible, you should work with a partner to provide two-person bag-mask device ventilation. One TMP can maintain a good mask seal by securing the mask to the patient's face with two hands while the other TMP squeezes the bag. Ventilation using a bag-mask device is a challenging skill: it may be very difficult for one TMP to maintain a proper seal between

the mask and the face with one hand while squeezing the bag well enough to deliver an adequate volume to the patient. This skill can be difficult to maintain if you do not have opportunities to practice. Effective one-person bag-mask device ventilation requires considerable experience. Also, performance of this skill depends on having enough personnel to carry out other actions that need to be done at the same time, such as chest compressions, putting the stretcher in place, or helping to lift the patient onto the stretcher.

Follow these steps to use the two-person bag-mask device technique:

1. Kneel above the patient's head. If possible, your partner should be at the side of the head to squeeze the bag while you use both hands to establish a good effective connection between the mask and the patient's face.

2. Maintain the patient's neck in an extended position unless you suspect a cervical spine injury. In that case, you should immobilize the patient's head and neck with a cervical collar when possible or provide manual in-line stabilization with your forearms and use the jaw-thrust maneuver. If you are alone, use your knees to immobilize the head.

3. Open the patient's mouth and suction as needed. Insert an oral or nasal airway to maintain airway patency.

4. Select the proper mask size. Place the mask on the patient's face. Make sure the top reaches the bridge of the nose and the bottom is in the groove between the lower lip and the chin. If the mask has a large, round cuff around the ventilation port, center the port over the patient's mouth. Inflate or deflate the collar to obtain a better fit and seal to the face if necessary.

5. Hold the mask in position by placing the thumbs over the top part of the mask and the index finger over the bottom half.

6. Bring the lower jaw up to the mask with the last three fingers of each hand. This will help to maintain an open airway. Make sure you do not grab the fleshy part of the neck, as you may compress the tongue and other structures and create an airway obstruction.

7. Connect the bag to the mask if you have not already done so.

8. Hold the mask in place while your partner squeezes the bag with two hands until the patient's chest rises **Figure 13-16**. If a spinal injury is suspected, help maintain manual in-line stabilization of the patient's head and neck with your forearms while maintaining an adequate mask-to-face seal with

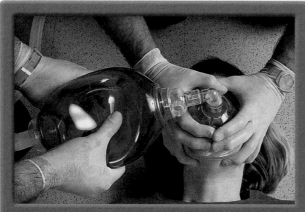

Figure 13-16 With two-person bag-mask device ventilation, you should hold the mask in place with a two-handed EC-clamp method to maintain an open airway while your partner squeezes the bag with two hands.

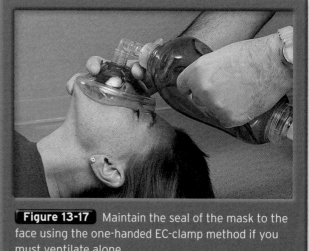

Figure 13-17 Maintain the seal of the mask to the face using the one-handed EC-clamp method if you must ventilate alone.

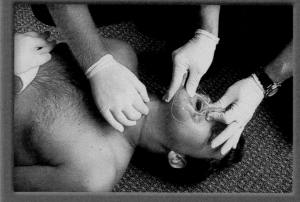

Figure 13-18 The Sellick maneuver, also called cricoid pressure, will help prevent or alleviate gastric distention when artificial ventilations are being performed.

your hands. Continue squeezing the bag once every 5 seconds in an adult, and once every 3 seconds for infants and children.

9. If you are alone, use the one-handed EC-clamp method to maintain an effective face-to-mask seal **Figure 13-17**. Use the head tilt–chin lift maneuver to make sure the neck is extended. If a spinal injury is suspected, maintain the patient's head in a neutral in-line position with your knees as you pull the patient's lower jaw into the mask. Squeeze the bag in a rhythmic manner once every 5 seconds with your other hand. Continue squeezing the bag once every 5 seconds for an adult and once every 3 seconds for infants and children.

As you are assisting ventilations with a bag-mask device, you should evaluate the effectiveness of your delivered ventilations. If there is an abnormal resistance to the inflow and outflow of air, this will affect the rise and fall of the patient's chest, the rate of ventilation, and the patient's heart rate. If the patient's chest does not rise and fall, you may need to reposition the head, use an airway adjunct, or use the **Sellick maneuver**, also called **cricoid pressure** **Figure 13-18**. Note that the Sellick maneuver, however, is contraindicated in a patient who is actively vomiting, as it may cause esophageal rupture.

When using a bag-mask device or any other ventilation device, be alert for **gastric distention**, inflation of the stomach with air. To prevent or alleviate distention, you should do the following: (1) ensure that the patient's airway is appropriately positioned, (2) ventilate the patient at the appropriate rate, and (3) ventilate the patient with the appropriate volume.

At the Scene

Supplemental oxygen should be delivered to any patient in the outer perimeter and during transportation who exhibits signs of difficulty breathing. These signs include shortness of breath, a respiratory rate greater than 20 breaths/min, use of accessory muscles, an altered level of consciousness, cyanosis, head injury, or any indications of shock.

Be mindful of your entire technique and the ultimate goal of the procedure: to deliver oxygen to the patient's lungs, to allow exhalation, and to minimize the amount of air that enters the patient's stomach. If an additional rescuer is available, use the Sellick maneuver, which is covered in detail in Chapter 14, "Advanced Airway

Management." When TMPs are performing a two-person bag-mask device technique, the TMP who is providing ventilations may also be able to perform the Sellick maneuver. Some large or difficult airway patients may require both hands to ventilate, and in this case, a third person should perform the Sellick maneuver if possible.

If the patient's stomach appears to be distending, you should reposition the head and use cricoid pressure. In a patient with a possible spinal injury, you should reposition the jaw rather than the head (that is, use the jaw-thrust). If too much air is escaping from under the mask, reposition the mask for a better seal. If the patient's chest still does not rise and fall after you have made these corrections, check for an airway obstruction. If an obstruction is not present, you should attempt ventilations using an alternate method, such as the mouth-to-mask technique. If you have advanced training and certification, consider advanced airway techniques or request ALS assistance.

Suctioning the Airway

The purpose of suctioning is to keep the patient's airway clear of all foreign matter (eg, blood, saliva, vomitus, and debris), which could be aspirated into the trachea or the lungs. When the patient's mouth or throat becomes filled with vomitus, blood, or secretions, a suction device enables you to remove the liquid material quickly and efficiently, thereby allowing you to ventilate the patient. Ventilating a patient with secretions in his or her mouth will force material into the lungs, resulting in an upper airway obstruction or aspiration. If you hear gurgling, the patient needs suctioning.

The indications for suctioning include:

- Patients who have a decreased level of consciousness and are unable to clear their own airway.
- Patients who cannot clear their airway because of excessive amounts of foreign matter.

You can use a flexible suction catheter, which is a sterile tube used for oral or nasal suctioning of fluids or small foreign particles. The Yankauer (rigid) suction tip (tonsil tip) is used for oral suction only. It is not necessary to measure the distance it is inserted into the mouth, just keep sight of the tip when inserting it. The large-bore opening of the Yankauer suction tip or similar clear tube is the preferred method of removing large particles of foreign material.

To perform suctioning on a patient:

1. Ensure that all nearby personnel have donned proper PPE: eye goggles, face mask, and gloves.
2. Suctioning may cause the patient to sneeze, cough, and vomit, and the heart rate to slow.
3. Position the patient properly. For a nontrauma and conscious patient, position yourself at the patient's head and turn his or her head to the side. For a trauma and unconscious patient, position yourself at the patient's head and maintain spinal alignment while log rolling the patient toward you.
4. Select and measure the suction catheter **Figure 13-19**.
5. Consider the route: mouth or nose.
6. Check the suctioning unit and equipment. Ensure all the pieces are present and functioning. If using an electric unit, ensure that a power source is available and the unit is functioning before beginning the procedure.
7. Cover the proximal port of the suctioning device with your thumb and set the maximum suction vacuum at 100 to 120 mm Hg for an adult or a child and 60 to 100 mm Hg for an infant.
8. Release your thumb from the port before inserting it; do not suction on the way in.

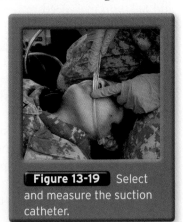

Figure 13-19 Select and measure the suction catheter.

At the Scene

If basic airway techniques do not create or maintain a patent airway in the patient, advanced airway techniques may be required. If you are trained at the BLS level, do not hesitate to call for ALS providers.

9. To perform oral suctioning, open the patient's mouth using the cross-finger technique **Figure 13-20**.
10. If you are using a Yankauer (rigid) tip, insert it with the convex (bulging out) side against the roof of the mouth and stop at the beginning of the pharynx.
11. If you are using a flexible suction catheter, insert the catheter up to the base of the tongue.
12. To perform nasal suctioning, insert the catheter gently into one nostril and then the other.
13. Cover the proximal port to begin suctioning.
14. Suction as you slowly withdraw, moving the tip from side to side **Figure 13-21**.

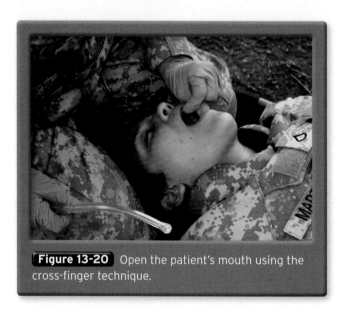

Figure 13-20 Open the patient's mouth using the cross-finger technique.

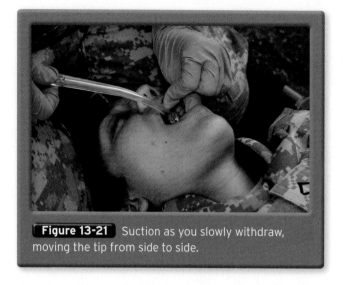

Figure 13-21 Suction as you slowly withdraw, moving the tip from side to side.

15. Suction for 15 seconds or less.
16. Observe the patient for hypoxemia, color change, increased or decreased pulse rate, or a change in breath. Be prepared to provide ventilation support as indicated.

Because of the differences in a pediatric patient's anatomy, medical equipment that is not needed to stabilize an adult patient in the tactical environment may be needed to stabilize the pediatric patient. For example, supplemental oxygen is required in a pediatric patient with difficultly breathing because children have more rapid respiratory rates and a higher oxygen demand that is twice that of an adult. If you have a pediatric patient in the tactical environment, either call out to have an oxygen tank brought to you or evacuate the pediatric patient to an oxygen source.

In order to properly manage the airway of a pediatric patient, you will need immediate access to properly sized equipment in the tactical environment. While gathering medical intelligence, especially at a high-risk warrant or hostage situation, it is critical to determine if any infants or children are involved. If infants or children are present, the proper pediatric-sized equipment needs to be packed and carried with you.

Special Populations

Compared to an adult, the pediatric airway is smaller in diameter and shorter in length, the lungs are smaller, and the heart is higher in a child's chest. The glottic opening (vocal cords) is higher and positioned more anteriorly (toward the front), and the neck appears to be nonexistent. As the child develops, the neck gets proportionally longer as the vocal cords and epiglottis achieve their anatomically correct adult position.

The anatomy of a pediatric airway and other important structures differs from that of an adult's in the following ways **Figure 13-22** :

- A larger, rounder occiput, or back of the head, which requires more careful positioning of the airway. Ensure neutral positioning (sniffing postion) by placing a small towel under the pediatric patient's shoulders to achieve the sniffing position.
- A proportionately larger tongue relative to the size of the mouth and a more anterior location in the mouth. The child's tongue is also larger relative to the small mandible and can easily block the airway, so consider inserting an oropharyngeal airway.
- A long, floppy, U-shaped epiglottis in infants and toddlers is larger than an adult's, relative to the size of the airway that extends at a 45° angle into the airway. Use of a Macintosh blade in a pediatric patient is not appropriate; instead a straight Miller laryngoscope blade should be used when performing endotracheal intubation (see Chapter 14, "Advanced Airway Management").
- Less well-developed rings of cartilage in the trachea that may easily collapse if the neck is flexed or hyperextended.
- Because of the smaller diameter of the trachea in infants, which is about the same diameter as a drinking straw, their airway is easily obstructed by secretions, blood, or swelling. Infants are obligate nose breathers, which may require diligent suctioning of the nasal passages using a bulb suction device to maintain a clear airway.

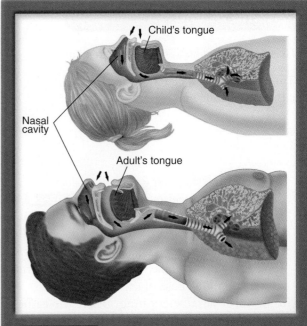

Figure 13-22   The anatomy of a child's airway differs from that of an adult's in several ways. The back of the head is larger in a child, so head positioning requires special care. The tongue is proportionately larger and more anterior in the mouth. The trachea is smaller in diameter and more flexible. The airway itself is lower and narrower (funnel shaped).

Ready for Review

- In the tactical environment, an airway obstruction can be caused by the tongue blocking the airway, a traumatic neck wound, or the aspiration of a foreign object.

- Simple manual techniques, like the head tilt–chin lift maneuver and the jaw-thrust maneuver, are sometimes the most effective way to open a patient's airway.

- Use the head tilt–chin lift maneuver to open the airway of a patient who has not sustained significant neck or facial trauma. If a cervical spine injury is suspected, use the jaw-thrust maneuver to open the airway.

- Use an airway adjunct, such as a nasopharyngeal airway or an oropharyngeal airway, to help maintain an open air passage in a semiconscious or unconscious patient.

- Provide adequate ventilation for any patient found with inadequate breathing or a patient who is apneic. Mouth-to-mask ventilation and bag-mask ventilation are two techniques that may be used in the tactical environment. Due to the dangers of the tactical environment, oxygen may not be available.

- In the tactical environment, suctioning may be performed with a mechanical device or it may be electric-pump generated. Practice suctioning with the device that is used in your agency during training so that you will be able to utilize it under any type of condition.

Vital Vocabulary

apneic Not breathing.

aspiration In the context of airway, the introduction of vomitus or other foreign material into the lungs.

bag-mask device A device with a one-way valve and a face mask attached to a ventilation bag.

barrier device A protective item, such as a pocket mask with a valve, that limits exposure to a patient's body fluids.

cerebrospinal fluid (CSF) Fluid produced in the ventricles of the brain that flows in the subarachnoid space and bathes the meninges.

cricoid pressure Pressure on the cricoid cartilage; applied to occlude the esophagus in order to inhibit gastric distention and regurgitation of vomitus in the unconscious patient.

gag reflex A normal reflex mechanism that causes retching; activated by touching the soft palate or the back of the throat.

gastric distention A condition in which air fills the stomach, often as a result of high volume and pressure during artificial ventilation.

head tilt–chin lift maneuver A combination of two movements to open the airway by tilting the forehead back and lifting the chin; not used for trauma patients.

jaw-thrust maneuver Technique to open the airway by placing the fingers behind the angle of the jaw and bringing the jaw forward; used for patients who may have a cervical spine injury.

nasopharyngeal airway (NPA) Airway adjunct inserted into the nostril of a conscious patient who is unable to maintain airway patency independently.

oropharyngeal airway (OPA) Airway adjunct inserted into the mouth to keep the tongue from blocking the upper airway and to facilitate suctioning the airway.

patent Open, clear of obstruction.

pharynx Chamber that connects the oral cavity with the esophagus.

Sellick maneuver A technique that is used to prevent gastric distention in which pressure is applied to the cricoid cartilage; also referred to as cricoid pressure.

septum The central divider in the nose.

Advanced Airway Management

Introduction

If basic airway techniques do not create or maintain a patent airway in the patient, advanced airway techniques may be required. You may only perform these advanced techniques if you are properly trained, certified, and authorized to do so by off-line or online medical direction, according to your local protocols.

One of the most common mistakes is to proceed with advanced airway management too early, forsaking the basic techniques of establishing and maintaining a patent airway in a patient. *Never abandon the basics of airway management and immediately proceed with advanced techniques simply because you can!* It is equally important to remember that when indicated (ie, a gunshot wound to the neck), you should arrange for a rapid intercept with ALS providers or proceed to performing a more advanced airway technique to establish a protected airway for the patient **Figure 14-1**.

Airway Obstruction

If the basic airway maneuver of suctioning does not dislodge the obstruction and severe airway obstruction remains, advanced airway procedures may be required. If the obstruction is more proximal, direct

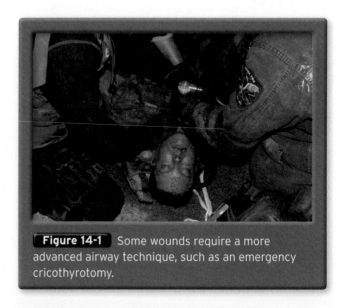

Figure 14-1 Some wounds require a more advanced airway technique, such as an emergency cricothyrotomy.

laryngoscopy with removal of the foreign body with Magill forceps may be successful.

1. Hold the laryngoscope handle with your left hand.
2. Open the mouth by exerting thumb pressure on the chin.
3. Insert a laryngoscope blade into the right side of the mouth, sweeping the tongue to the left.
4. Exert gentle traction upward along the axis of the laryngoscope handle at a 45-degree angle and advance the blade. Do not use the teeth or gums for leverage.
5. Watch the tip until the foreign body is visible. Do not go past the vocal cords.
6. Use suction to improve visibility if secretions are present.
7. Insert the Magill forceps into the mouth with the tips closed.
8. Grasp the foreign object and remove while looking directly at it.
9. Look at the airway to ensure that it is clear of debris. Remove the laryngoscope blade.

If you manage to remove the object, recheck the patient's breathing and circulation and manage as appropriate. If direct laryngoscopy does not reveal the foreign body, use bag-mask ventilation. If bag-mask ventilation does not provide adequate ventilatory support, attempt to insert an advanced airway (such as an endotracheal tube, laryngeal mask airway, or other supraglottic airway). Evacuation and transportation to an appropriate facility is required as soon as it is safe to do so.

Orotracheal Intubation

Orotracheal intubation is the placement of an **endotracheal (ET) tube** orally, through the vocal cords and into the **trachea** **Figure 14-2**. Orotracheal intubation allows direct ventilation of the lungs through the ET tube. **Endotracheal intubation** with a cuffed ET tube is the gold standard of airway care in a patient who cannot protect the airway or who needs assistance with breathing. However, endotracheal intubation requires additional advanced training and practice. It should only be attempted by medical personnel qualified and proficient in the procedure.

Oxygen, medication, and suctioning can be directed into the trachea through an ET tube. The indications for orotracheal intubation include the inability to properly ventilate the patient, severe facial injuries,

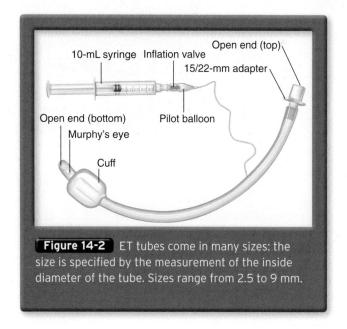

Figure 14-2 ET tubes come in many sizes: the size is specified by the measurement of the inside diameter of the tube. Sizes range from 2.5 to 9 mm.

airway obstruction, anticipated impending airway obstruction (fire/smoke inhalation injury), and the need for a definitive airway in a patient. The advantages of orotracheal intubation include complete control of the airway. The ET tube goes directly into the trachea; when the cuff is inflated, it prevents the tongue, blood, or debris that may be in the upper airway from interfering with the passage of air. It also minimizes risk of aspiration and allows for better oxygen delivery and deeper suctioning of the airway. ET tubes are available in multiple sizes, including pediatric and infant.

The complications of orotracheal intubation include slowing of the heart rate as a result of laryngoscopy and manipulation of the airway. Laryngoscopy also can lead to trauma to the teeth, lips, tongue, gums, and airway structures, although these complications are rare with proper technique. If the procedure takes too long or the patient is critically ill, then hypoxia (lack of oxygen) can occur. In these cases, preoxygenation is a good idea when available, as well as close monitoring of the patient's oxygenation status (by watching skin color and pulse oximetry if available). Other complications include vomiting, aspiration, and esophageal intubation, which prevent any effective ventilation to the lungs and will result in death if undetected. In addition, some medications used to facilitate orotracheal intubation may eliminate any remaining protective airway reflexes or diminish the patient's respiratory effort. This can lead to deadly results if the patient cannot be intubated or ventilated. These medications should only be used if they are absolutely necessary and if the TMP is properly trained.

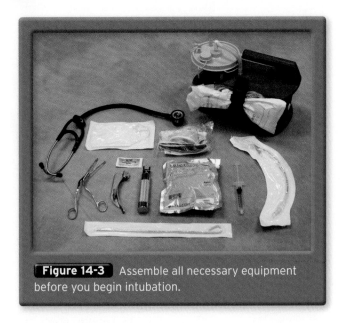

Figure 14-3 Assemble all necessary equipment before you begin intubation.

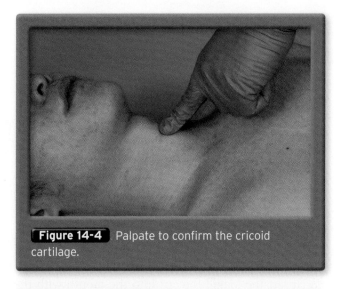

Figure 14-4 Palpate to confirm the cricoid cartilage.

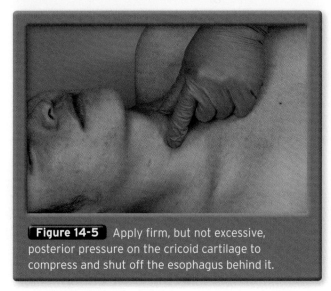

Figure 14-5 Apply firm, but not excessive, posterior pressure on the cricoid cartilage to compress and shut off the esophagus behind it.

Before attempting orotracheal intubation, it is vitally important to assemble all the equipment that you will need **Figure 14-3**. The prepared TMP will have all airway equipment immediately available for use at any time:

- Laryngoscope handle and blade
- Properly sized ET tubes
- Stylet
- 10-mL syringe
- Lubricant for the ET tube
- A suction unit with rigid and soft-tip catheters
- Magill forceps
- Stethoscope
- Commercial securing device
- Secondary confirmation device such as an end-tidal CO_2 detector

Follow local protocols and individual concerns about equipment space.

The Sellick Maneuver

Intubating an unresponsive patient who has no cough and/or gag reflex may cause stomach acid and food to flow up the esophagus into the upper airway and be forced into the lungs, called "aspiration," which can ultimately damage airway tissues and block the lower airway passages. The Sellick maneuver, or cricoid pressure, can be used to help avoid these complications. This procedure is helpful in reducing the chance of regurgitation and aspiration of stomach contents by applying pressure on the esophagus and thereby preventing the stomach contents from flowing into the upper airway. In addition, this also helps to move

the vocal cords into better view during the intubation procedure and increase the speed and ease of placing the ET tube through the vocal cords into the trachea. To perform this maneuver, follow these steps:

1. With the patient's neck slightly extended (only if there is no suspicion of spinal injury), visualize the cricoid cartilage, just below the thyroid cartilage (Adam's apple).
2. Confirm the location of the cricoid cartilage by palpating with the tip of your index finger **Figure 14-4**.
3. Place a thumb and index finger on either side of the midline of the cricoid cartilage. Apply firm, but not excessive, posterior pressure on the cricoid cartilage to compress and squeeze shut the esophagus behind it. Too much pressure could collapse the larynx. Maintain this pressure until the patient is intubated **Figure 14-5**.

The Sellick maneuver should be performed, ideally, by a third TMP and might not be possible if you and your partner are alone. When performing this maneuver, be sure to correctly identify anatomic landmarks to avoid damaging other structures or inadvertently obstructing the airway. Use caution to avoid pressing on the carotid arteries of the neck, as this can cause bradycardia in some people, resulting in hypotension and shock.

The Intubation Procedure: Visualized (Oral) Intubation

Once you are safely behind hard cover or in a point of relative safety and the equipment is assembled, then use standard PPE precautions, including the use of gloves, eye protection, and a mask. Use basic airway methods such as bag-mask ventilation and oxygen, if available, to ensure that the patient is as oxygenated as possible before starting the intubation attempt. Ideally, one or two TMPs should support the airway and ventilate using basic techniques while a third TMP assembles the advanced airway equipment.

An intubation attempt should not take more than 30 seconds. The 30-second time limit begins when ventilation stops and the laryngoscope blade is inserted into the patient's mouth; it ends when ventilation has begun again. If the attempt is not successful, stop, withdraw the tube, oxygenate the patient, and try again according to your local protocols. Follow these steps to perform visualized orotracheal intubation:

1. Open the patient's airway with the head tilt–chin lift maneuver (or the jaw-thrust maneuver if there is risk of spinal injury) and clear the airway of any foreign material.
2. Insert an oral airway and ventilate the patient with a bag-mask device at the appropriate rate, once every 5 seconds in an adult and once every 3 seconds for infants and children. If possible, oxygenate the patient at a rate of 20 to 24 breaths/min for 1 to 2 minutes before attempting intubation. If oxygen is not available, the 30-second intubation attempt should not harm most patients.

Safety

If the casualty is an elderly person, check to make sure any dentures or false teeth or bridges are removed before attempting to intubate the patient.

3. As your partner ventilates the patient, you should quickly assemble and test your equipment. Verify that the bulb on the laryngoscope or lighted stylet is working, select the proper-sized tube, and make sure the ET tube cuff has no leaks. If you are using a nonlighted stylet, insert it in the ET tube and adjust the angle to your liking. You may want to bend the ET tube at a slight angle to make it easier to place properly. Lubricate the tube and stylet as needed.
4. Because you will not likely have a cardiac monitor or pulse oximeter in the field, you should remove the oral airway after 1 to 2 minutes of ventilating.
5. A third TMP, if available, should perform the Sellick maneuver to improve visualization of the vocal cords or positioning of the lighted stylet. This maneuver will also help prevent vomiting and aspiration. If there are only two TMPs, your partner should perform this maneuver with one hand while continuing to ventilate the patient with the bag-mask device.
6. Maintain pressure on the cricoid cartilage until the ET tube cuff is inflated, unless the patient gags or vomits. If this occurs, relax the pressure on the esophagus to prevent potential esophageal rupture. After the retching or vomiting has ended, use suctioning to clear the airway and then resume the Sellick maneuver.
7. Position the patient's head and neck to allow for the best visualization of the vocal cords. In a patient with no spinal cord injury, use the head tilt–chin lift maneuver to align the structures. When you are using the lighted stylet, grasping the tongue and jaw and pulling upward will aid in insertion.
8. To intubate a patient with a suspected spinal cord injury, you should make sure that your partner maintains manual in-line stabilization of the head and neck in the neutral position with a cervical collar in place. You may need to lie on your stomach or straddle the patient's head while leaning back to visualize the vocal cords adequately **Figure 14-6**.
9. Grasp the laryngoscope handle in your left hand. Make sure the blade is locked into place and the bulb is illuminated. Open the patient's mouth with the gloved fingers of your right hand. Gently place the blade in the right side of the patient's mouth and then move it toward the center of the mouth, gently pushing the tongue to the left. The tongue must be displaced for you to visualize the vocal cords **Figure 14-7**.

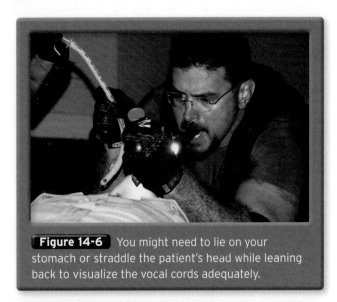

Figure 14-6 You might need to lie on your stomach or straddle the patient's head while leaning back to visualize the vocal cords adequately.

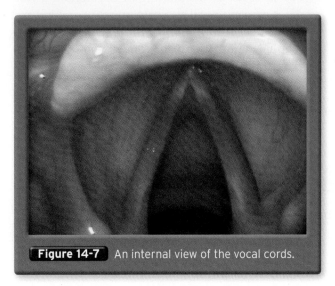

Figure 14-7 An internal view of the vocal cords.

10. Visualize the epiglottis. For those using a Macintosh curved blade, advance it along the base of the tongue until its tip rests at the vallecula, then lift it up sufficiently to allow visualization of the vocal cords. For those using a Miller straight blade, advance it gently but deeply into the pharynx, far enough to gently lift up on the tongue and epiglottis, to visualize the vocal cords. The lifting force is directed straight up, parallel to the long axis of the laryngoscope handle, not rocking back toward the patient's head. Avoid rotation of the wrist. It should feel as if you are picking up the patient's head by the jaw. To avoid breaking the patient's teeth or lacerating the lips, never use the blade as a lever or fulcrum against the upper teeth. Do not lose sight of the vocal cords at any time after you have visualized them. Proper placement of the ET tube depends on

your visualization of the tube as it is placed between the vocal cords.

11. Insert the ET tube with your right hand, keeping the vocal cords and the tip of the tube in sight at all times. Do not advance the ET tube down the center of the laryngoscope blade, or your view of the vocal cords will be obstructed. Advance the tube from the right side of the patient's mouth. Watch the uninflated cuff on the tube as it passes through the vocal cords, then advance the ET tube until the cuff is just past the vocal cords. Document the centimeter markings on the outside of the ET tube at the level of the teeth or lips. It should be approximately 3 times the internal diameter (ET size) at the teeth or gums. Once the tube has been inserted through the vocal cords into the trachea, gently remove the laryngoscope, then remove the stylet if a stylet was used. Do not let go of the ET tube until it is secured.

12. Inflate the soft balloon cuff on the end of the tube with enough air so that the balloon feels appropriately full. It will take anywhere from 3 mL to 10 mL of air **Figure 14-8**. This will seal the trachea so that air can be blown directly into the lungs and little or no air will leak back out. This will also protect against aspiration. Gently squeeze the pilot balloon cuff to verify the amount of air you should use. The pilot balloon should be full but easily compressed between your fingers. Immediately detach the syringe so that the air in the cuff will not empty back into it.

13. The TMP who is not holding the ET tube in place should begin ventilating the patient with a bag-mask device attached to the ET tube. Confirm placement

Safety

The use of light in the tactical environment may be prohibited due to continuing threats such as an active shooter. Any medical assessment or procedure that uses light must be limited or modified so that an external bright light is avoided. Intubating a patient can be performed using a nonlighted technique such as a surgical airway, digital intubation, or nasal intubation. If a lighted laryngoscope is used, it should be inserted into the patient's mouth first and the light turned on (lock blade into position) after it is inserted into the airway. Always protect yourself first and use caution. Modify medical procedures to match the mission requirements.

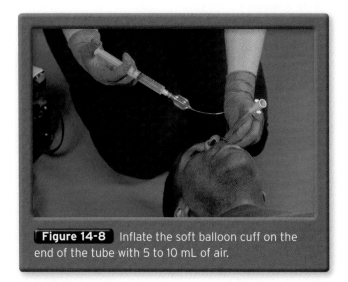

Figure 14-8 Inflate the soft balloon cuff on the end of the tube with 5 to 10 mL of air.

Special Populations

In most pediatric patients, assisting ventilations with a bag-mask device should be sufficient and is the first choice of stabilizing care. Endotracheal intubation should be considered if adequate oxygenation and ventilation cannot be achieved with good bag-mask technique or if transport times are long. Intubation has the advantage of providing a definitive airway and carrying a decreased risk of aspiration, but studies have shown significant failure and complication rates when using this technique in the prehospital setting. Potential complications include damage to teeth and oral structures, aspiration of gastric contents, bradycardia due to a vagal response, bradycardia due to hypoxemia from prolonged attempts, increased pressure within the skull, and incorrect placement. Incorrect placement of the ET tube into the right mainstem bronchus may result in hypoxia and inadequate ventilation. A potentially catastrophic complication is an unrecognized esophageal intubation.

When preparing to intubate an infant or a young child, remember the differences between the adult and pediatric airways. Children have a relatively large tongue, an airway that is positioned more anteriorly, and a flexible trachea that can be easily compressed. Young infants also have a large occiput, and therefore a towel or shirt should be placed underneath the infant's shoulders in order to achieve a neutral position and enable better visualization of the airway.

Access to pediatric-specific equipment is mandatory, including a range of straight Miller laryngoscope blades in sizes 0 to 3 and cuffed ET tubes in sizes 2.5 (for field deliveries of premature infants) to 6.0. Cuffed ET tubes protect the pediatric airway against aspiration of blood and stomach contents.

Any size of laryngoscope handle can be used, although many ALS providers prefer the thinner pediatric handles. Straight (Miller or Wis-Hipple) blades make it easy to lift the floppy epiglottis. A curved (Macintosh) blade should not be used for pediatric patients unless no other alternative exists.

of the ET tube. Listen with a stethoscope over the stomach and both lungs as you ventilate the patient through the tube. You should be able to hear equal breath sounds over the right and left lung fields and no sounds over the stomach. You should also listen at the sternal notch in children. You should see both sides of the chest rise and fall with each ventilation. This is especially important in children because breath sounds in children may be misleading; you may hear them even if the tube is in the esophagus. You should not be able to hear breath sounds in the stomach. If you hear sounds over the epigastrium, remove the tube, ventilate the patient with a bag-mask device, and reattempt intubation.

14. Proper confirmation of ET tube placement is essential. The actual visualization of the ET tube as it passes through the vocal cords followed by chest rise with ventilation and good bilateral breath sounds is the primary method to confirm proper placement. Use of an end-tidal CO_2 detector is an excellent way to confirm proper tube placement in the tactical environment. The detector should turn yellow if the patient is properly intubated. Portable pulse oximetry monitors are becoming more common and digital fingertip pulse oximeters are carried by many TEMS elements; if available, use this device to help confirm improvement of pulse oximetry.

15. Secure the ET tube in position to prevent it from accidently becoming dislodged.

16. Closely monitor the patient for complications of intubation, such as right-mainstem intubation (ET tube is advanced too far and the tip is in the right mainstem bronchus) causing decreased breath sounds on the left side. If there is evidence of right-mainstem

intubation, double-check the ET tube depth and adjust accordingly. Monitor for possible development of tension pneumothorax. During transport, monitor the patient's pulse and blood pressure.

Patient Intolerant of the Endotracheal Tube

Because of the reversal of hypoxia from direct oxygenation, a patient may regain a gag reflex or regain consciousness and try to remove the ET tube. You will

Medical Gear

Light Wands

Several commercially available devices similar to an endotracheal tube stylet are available. These "light wands" are flexible and have a small bright light at the end. These devices are used to place an ET tube into a patient with a difficult airway, such as one that several TMPs cannot intubate. They are designed to light up the larynx and trachea whenever the tip of the ET tube is inside or near the glottis to enable increased accuracy of blind intubation. Light wands do offer some advantages as long as you are not concerned with nighttime light discipline.

Table 14-1	Benefits and Disadvantages of Multilumen Airways	
Benefits	**Disadvantages**
Ease of proper placement	May lose effectiveness (cuff malfunction)
No mask seal necessary	Requires deeply comatose patient
Requires minimal skill and practice to maintain	Requires constant balloon observation
Easily used in spinal injury patients	Cannot be used on patients shorter than 5 feet tall
May be inserted blindly	Requires great care in listening for breath sounds to determine which of the two tubes should be used

need to evaluate the risks and benefits of continued intubation versus removal of the ET tube (**extubation**). If the patient starts to wake up, seems to be aware, has full respiratory effort, and is capable of pulling out the tube, then the ET tube should be removed as long as the airway will likely stay open. If possible and if time allows, try to suction any secretions and blood in the throat first. Then deflate the cuff and carefully withdraw the ET tube as the patient exhales. Provide immediate suctioning if the patient vomits, reassess the airway, and administer supplemental oxygen if it can be provided safely. Be aware that conscious patients are at high risk for laryngospasm (spasm of the larynx) immediately following extubation, and the patient may have a raspy, hoarse voice for a short time. Local protocol may allow sedation for patients who are intolerant of an ET tube if it needs to remain in place.

Multilumen Airways

In addition to endotracheal intubation, other advanced airway devices are available that do not require visualization of the vocal cords for placement **Table 14-1**. **Multilumen airways** such as the **Combitube**, which are inserted without direct visualization of the vocal cords, have been designed to provide lung ventilation when placed in either the trachea or the esophagus, thus making them much easier to insert **Figure 14-9**. If the tube happens to go into the trachea, ventilation is provided directly into the lungs as with an ET tube. If the tube goes into the esophagus, as occurs most often, ventilation can still be provided to the patient. You do not need to maintain a constant face mask seal with these airways because they have a balloon

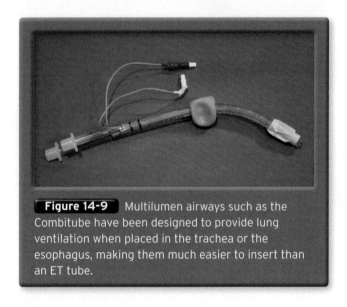

Figure 14-9 Multilumen airways such as the Combitube have been designed to provide lung ventilation when placed in the trachea or the esophagus, making them much easier to insert than an ET tube.

that inflates in the oropharynx; the lungs can be inflated via a tube rather than a mask. Insertion of these devices requires additional training. Your medical director will determine when and how these devices may be used.

Contraindications

Multilumen airways should not be used in the following individuals:

- Conscious or semiconscious patients with a gag reflex
- Children younger than 14 years
- Adults shorter than 5 feet tall
- Patients who have ingested a caustic substance
- Patients who have a known esophageal disease

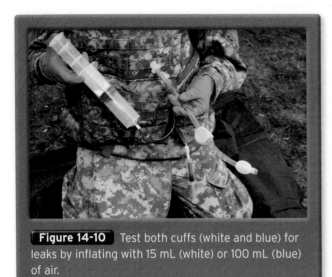

Figure 14-10 Test both cuffs (white and blue) for leaks by inflating with 15 mL (white) or 100 mL (blue) of air.

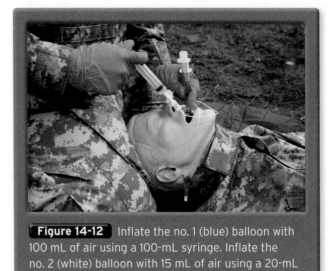

Figure 14-12 Inflate the no. 1 (blue) balloon with 100 mL of air using a 100-mL syringe. Inflate the no. 2 (white) balloon with 15 mL of air using a 20-mL syringe.

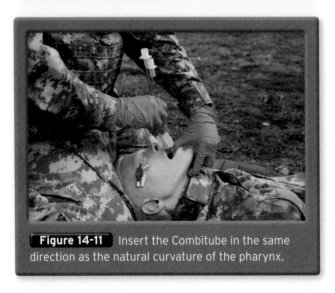

Figure 14-11 Insert the Combitube in the same direction as the natural curvature of the pharynx.

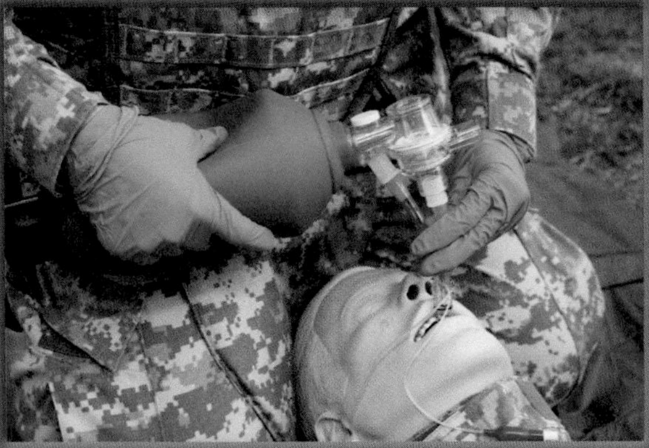

Figure 14-13 Ventilate through the no. 1 (blue) tube.

Combitube

First, always take appropriate standard precautions, including facial protection, because vomiting can occur through the no. 2 tube if the initial placement is in the patient's esophagus. To insert a Combitube, follow these steps:

1. Inspect the patient's upper airway for visible airway obstructions.
2. Use a bag-mask device to provide deep respirations for the patient for 1 to 2 minutes to help maximize the oxygenation of the blood prior to starting the procedure. If possible and safe, provide oxygen.
3. Position the patient's head in a neutral position.
4. Test both cuffs (white and blue) for leaks by inflating the white cuff with 15 mL of air and the blue cuff with 100 mL of air **Figure 14-10**.
5. Insert the Combitube in the same direction as the natural curvature of the pharynx **Figure 14-11**.

6. Grasp the tongue and lower jaw between your thumb and index fingers and lift upward (jaw-lift maneuver).
7. Insert the Combitube gently but firmly until the black rings on the tube are positioned between the patient's teeth.
8. Do not use force with the Combitube. If the tube does not insert easily, withdraw it and retry insertion. Oxygenate the patient between each attempt.
9. Once it is in the proper position, inflate the no. 1 (blue) balloon with 100 mL of air using a 100-mL syringe. Inflate the no. 2 (white) balloon with 15 mL of air using a 20-mL syringe **Figure 14-12**.
10. Ventilate through the no. 1 (blue) tube. If auscultation of breath sounds is positive and auscultation of gastric sounds is negative, continue ventilations **Figure 14-13**.

11. If auscultation of breath sounds is negative or gastric insufflation is heard when bagging air into the no. 1 blue tube, then immediately switch the bag ventilations to the shorter (white) connecting tube no. 2. Confirm tracheal ventilation of breath sounds and absence of gastric insufflation.

12. If you are unable to ventilate the lungs through either tube, the Combitube may have been advanced too far into the pharynx. Deflate the no. 1 balloon/cuff and move the Combitube approximately 2 to 3 cm out of the patient's mouth.

13. Reinflate the no. 1 balloon with 100 mL of air and ventilate through the longer no. 1 connecting tube. If auscultation of breath sounds is positive and auscultation of gastric insufflation is negative, continue ventilations.

14. If breath sounds are still absent, immediately deflate both cuffs and extubate the patient. Insert an oropharyngeal or a nasopharyngeal airway and hyperventilate the patients with a bag-mask device.

The Combitube should not be removed unless the tube placement cannot be determined, the patient can no longer tolerate the tube (begins to gag), or the patient vomits past either the distal or pharyngeal tube. Have suction equipment ready if removal is necessary. Log roll the patient to the side and deflate the pharyngeal cuff using the no. 1 pilot balloon. Deflate the distal cuff using the no. 2 pilot balloon and gently remove the Combitube while suctioning the airway.

Single Lumen Airway

King LT Airway

The **King LT** is a single lumen airway that is blindly inserted into the esophagus **Figure 14-14**. It consists of a curved tube with ventilation ports located between two inflatable cuffs. Both cuffs are inflated using a single valve/pilot balloon. When the airway is properly placed in the esophagus, one cuff is designed to seal the esophagus, while the other is intended to seal the oropharynx. Openings located between these two cuffs provide ventilation of the lungs.

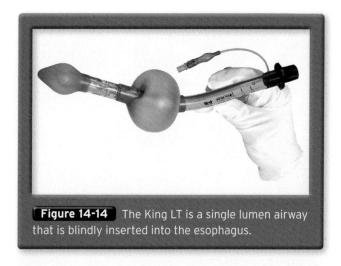

Figure 14-14 The King LT is a single lumen airway that is blindly inserted into the esophagus.

The King LT is intended for airway management in patients who are taller than 4 feet. It does not protect the airway from the effects of vomiting and aspiration. High airway pressures may cause air to leak either into the stomach or out of the mouth. If the trachea is intubated, the airway must be removed and another attempt made to place it in the esophagus.

To insert a King LT, follow these steps:

1. Select the proper device based on the patient's height and local protocols. If possible, prepare a back-up King LT.

2. Position the patient's airway using the appropriate maneuver.

3. Test the cuffs of the King LT. If the cuffs inflate properly, apply a water-based lubricant to the tip and posterior aspect of the tube. Avoid applying lubricant in or near the ventilator openings. Remove all air from the cuffs prior to insertion.

4. Lift the patient's chin with your nondominant hand, hold the mouth open, and apply chin lift unless contraindicated. Insert the tip of the King LT into the corner of the patient's mouth **Figure 14-15** with the tube pointing to the side of the patient's face.

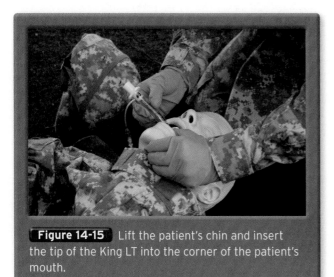

Figure 14-15 Lift the patient's chin and insert the tip of the King LT into the corner of the patient's mouth.

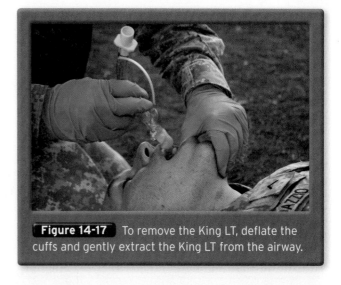

Figure 14-17 To remove the King LT, deflate the cuffs and gently extract the King LT from the airway.

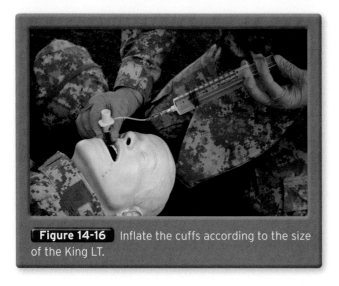

Figure 14-16 Inflate the cuffs according to the size of the King LT.

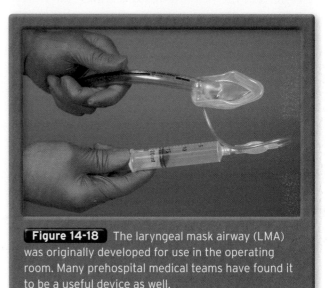

Figure 14-18 The laryngeal mask airway (LMA) was originally developed for use in the operating room. Many prehospital medical teams have found it to be a useful device as well.

5. Advance the tube and ensure that the tube is behind the base of the tongue and then rotate the tube.
6. Advance the tube until the base of the connector is aligned with teeth or gums.
7. Inflate the cuffs according to the size of the King LT **Figure 14-16**.
8. Attach the bag-mask device to the King LT and ventilate the patient per local protocols.
9. To remove the King LT, deflate the cuffs and gently extract the King LT from the airway **Figure 14-17**.

Laryngeal Mask Airway

The **laryngeal mask airway (LMA)** was originally developed for use in the operating room **Figure 14-18**. However, since its inception, its use has been expanded to the field.

The LMA consists of two parts: the tube and the mask or cuff. The device is made of silicone and is available in reusable (after proper sterilization) and disposable types. After blind insertion, the device molds and seals itself around the laryngeal opening by inflation of the mask. The epiglottis is contained within the mask or cuff. The LMA does not protect against gastric regurgitation. The device comes in seven sizes and can be used in children as well as adults.

To insert a laryngeal mask airway, follow these steps:

1. Check the cuff of the LMA by inflating it with 50% more air than is required for that sized airway. Then deflate the cuff completely **Figure 14-19**.
2. Lubricate the base of the device where it will rub against the roof/palate of the mouth during insertion.

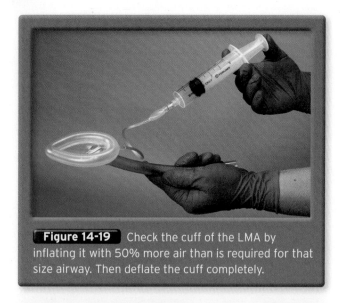

Figure 14-19 Check the cuff of the LMA by inflating it with 50% more air than is required for that size airway. Then deflate the cuff completely.

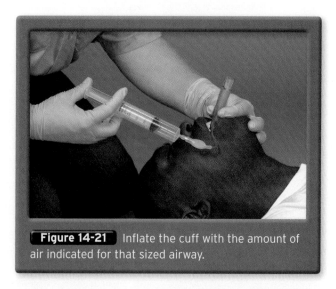

Figure 14-21 Inflate the cuff with the amount of air indicated for that sized airway.

for about a centimeter or two. There should be no detectable air leak when ventilating.

9. Attach the bag-mask device and begin to ventilate the patient. Confirm chest rise and the presence of breath sounds. Monitor the patient closely.

Digital Intubation

Digital intubation is a procedure where the TMP's gloved fingers are used to guide an ET tube blindly into the trachea. This technique should only be performed on a deeply unconscious patient who will not bite. This skill requires substantial training.

Digital intubation may be used in the following exceptional circumstances:

- A laryngoscope is not available or has malfunctioned.
- Other techniques to intubate the patient have failed.
- The patient is in a confined space or is difficult to reach for other airway maneuvers.
- The patient is extremely obese or has a short neck.
- Copious secretions obscure your view of the airway.
- The head cannot be moved due to trauma, or immobilization equipment interferes with direct laryngoscopy.
- Massive airway trauma has made visualization of the intubation landmarks impossible.

Digital intubation is absolutely contraindicated if your patient is breathing, is not deeply unconscious, or has an intact gag reflex.

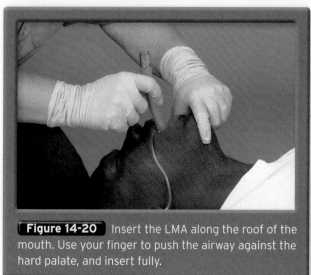

Figure 14-20 Insert the LMA along the roof of the mouth. Use your finger to push the airway against the hard palate, and insert fully.

3. Use a bag-mask device to provide deep respirations for the patient for 1 to 2 minutes to help maximize the oxygenation of the blood prior to starting the procedure. You should provide oxygen if it is available and if it is safe.

4. Ventilation should not be interrupted for more than 30 seconds to accomplish LMA placement.

5. Place the patient's head in the sniffing position.

6. Insert your finger between the cuff and the tube. Place the index finger of your dominant hand in the notch between the tube and the cuff. Open the patient's mouth.

7. Insert the LMA along the roof of the mouth. Use your finger to push the airway against the hard palate, and insert fully **Figure 14-20**.

8. Inflate the cuff with the amount of air indicated for that sized airway **Figure 14-21**. When this is done, the actual LMA will rise up out of the mouth

Because digital intubation does not require a laryngoscope, this technique is advantageous in the event of equipment failure. It is also ideal in situations in which your view of the vocal cords is obscured by copious, uncontrollable oral secretion. Because digital intubation does not require the patient's head to be in a sniffing position, it can be performed on trauma patients and patients whose heads cannot be placed in a sniffing position (eg, obese or short-necked patients).

The major disadvantage of digital intubation is that it requires you to place your fingers in the patient's mouth, thus posing a risk of being bitten. Digital intubation should therefore be performed only in patients who are deeply unresponsive and apneic (not breathing), *and* who have a bite block in their mouth to prevent closure or in patients who have been administered paralytics. There is also potential risk of exposure to an infectious disease. The patient's teeth could easily tear through your gloves and cut your fingers, especially if the teeth are sharp or broken.

Successful placement of the ET tube via digital intubation depends on frequency of practice, experience, manual dexterity, and the size and length of your fingers. Advanced TEMS providers with short fingers or fingers that are large in diameter will have greater difficulty performing digital intubation.

Misplacement of the ET tube is the major complication of digital intubation. Although the intubation is guided by touch, it is easy to misdirect the tip of the tube during insertion. Therefore, diligent attention to tube confirmation is absolutely essential with this technique.

Because it does not require the use of a laryngoscope, digital intubation is associated with a much lower incidence of dental trauma; however, the insertion of a bite block can cause lip trauma, tooth damage, or both. Additionally, vigorous attempts at insertion or improper technique can cause airway trauma or swelling.

Any intubation attempt, regardless of the technique, can result in hypoxia. Therefore, you must carefully monitor the patient's condition (eg, pulse rate, skin color, heart rate) during the procedure. Limit your intubation attempts to 30 seconds, and ventilate the patient appropriately in between attempts.

To perform digital intubation, follow these steps:

1. Take standard precautions (gloves and face shield).
2. Preoxygenate the patient for 1 to 2 minutes with a bag-mask device. If it is available and it is safe, administer oxygen.
3. Check, prepare, and assemble your equipment.
4. Place an appropriate stylet into the ET tube. Bend the ET tube by placing a slight curve at its distal end (like a hockey stick).
5. Place the patient's head in a neutral position.
6. Place a bite block in between the patient's molars to prevent the patient from biting your fingers 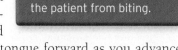.
7. Insert your left middle and index fingers into the patient's mouth and shift the patient's tongue forward as you advance your fingers toward the patient's larynx.
8. Palpate and lift the epiglottis with your left middle finger **Figure 14-23**. The epiglottis should feel like an earlobe.
9. Advance the tube with your right hand and guide it in between the vocal cords with your index finger **Figure 14-24**.
10. Resistance may be felt as the tube enters the larynx. As the resistance increases, the tube should be held firmly in place. Advance the ET tube until it reaches the proper depth.
11. Remove the stylet from the ET tube.
12. Inflate the distal cuff of the ET tube with 5 to 10 mL of air and detach the syringe.
13. Attach the bag-mask device, ventilate, and confirm placement of the ET tube per local protocols.
14. Secure the ET tube.

Figure 14-22 Place a bite block in between the patient's molars to prevent the patient from biting.

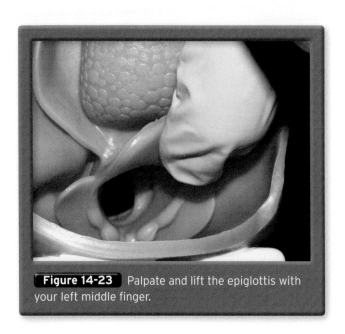

Figure 14-23 Palpate and lift the epiglottis with your left middle finger.

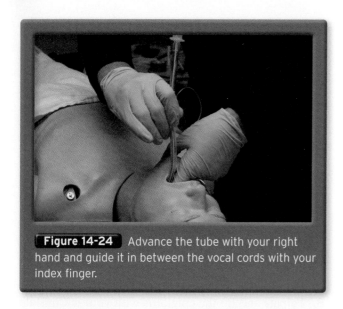

Figure 14-24 Advance the tube with your right hand and guide it in between the vocal cords with your index finger.

Nasotracheal Intubation

Nasotracheal intubation is the insertion of a tube into the trachea through the nose. The introduction of rapid sequence intubation (RSI) has made this procedure less common. In the out-of-hospital setting, it is usually performed without directly visualizing the vocal cords—hence the term "blind" nasotracheal intubation.

Blind nasotracheal intubation is an excellent technique for controlling the airway in situations in which it is either difficult or hazardous to intubate with a laryngoscope. Because the procedure must be performed on patients with spontaneous breathing, it is less likely to result in hypoxia.

Nasotracheal intubation is indicated for patients who are breathing spontaneously but require definitive airway management to prevent further deterioration of their condition. Conscious patients or patients with an altered mental status and an intact gag reflex are excellent candidates for nasotracheal intubation.

Nasotracheal intubation is contraindicated in apneic patients (eg, in respiratory or cardiac arrest); such patients should receive orotracheal intubation. This procedure is also contraindicated in patients with head trauma and possible midface fractures, as evidenced by CSF drainage from the nose following a head injury. In these patients, a nasally inserted ET tube may enter the cranial vault and penetrate the brain. Other contraindications to nasotracheal intubation include anatomic abnormalities, such as in patients with a deviated septum, patients with nasal polyps, or patients who frequently use cocaine. Nasal insertion of an ET tube in these patients may result in severe nosebleeds.

Likewise, you should avoid nasotracheal intubation, if possible, in patients with blood-clotting abnormalities or in those who take anticoagulation medications. These conditions also increase the likelihood and severity of epistaxis following insertion of anything in the nose.

The primary advantage of blind nasotracheal intubation is that it can be performed on patients who are awake and breathing. This procedure does not require that you place anything in the mouth (eg, laryngoscope); the nasotracheal route is associated with much less retching and a lower risk of vomiting in patients with an intact gag reflex.

Another major advantage of nasotracheal intubation is that there is no need for a laryngoscope, which eliminates the risk of trauma to the teeth or soft tissues of the mouth. Because the patient's mouth does not need to be opened, this technique is better suited to patients with limited jaw mobility, such as those with jaw fractures, seizures, or clenched teeth.

Nasotracheal intubation does not require the patient to be placed in a sniffing position, which makes it an ideal technique for intubating patients with a possible spinal injury, unless a midface fracture is suspected. Finally, because the tube is inserted through the nose, the patient cannot bite the tube. Furthermore, it can be secured more easily than a tube that is inserted orally because the nose generally has fewer secretions than the mouth.

Bleeding is the most common complication associated with nasotracheal intubation. If intubation is successful, the airway is protected and the risk of aspiration is eliminated. However, severe bleeding can occur, especially with rough technique, posing an additional threat to an already compromised airway as the swallowing of blood greatly increases the likelihood of vomiting and subsequent aspiration.

The incidence of bleeding associated with nasotracheal intubation can be reduced by gently inserting the tube into the nostril and by lubricating the tip with a water-soluble gel.

The same equipment used for orotracheal intubation—minus the laryngoscope and stylet—is used for blind nasotracheal intubation. Standard ET tubes can be used, although they should be 1.0 to 1.5 mm smaller when inserted nasally. When choosing the size of tube, select one that is slightly smaller than the nostril in which it will be inserted.

Some ET tubes have been designed specifically for blind nasotracheal intubation. For example, the Endotrol tube is slightly more flexible than a standard ET tube and is equipped with a "trigger"—a circular

Special Populations

Do not attempt blind nasotracheal intubation in children younger than 8 years of age!

ring-like plastic piece that is attached to a piece of line, which is itself attached to the tip of the tube. Pulling the trigger moves the tip of the tube anteriorly and increases the tube's overall curvature. This feature replaces the function of the stylet.

The movement of air through the ET tube helps determine proper tube placement following nasotracheal intubation. A number of devices have been developed to allow you to confirm successful nasotracheal intubation without the need to place your face next to the tube and thus risk contact with contaminants in the patient's exhaled breath.

Use these steps to perform blind nasotracheal intubation:

1. Use standard precautions (gloves and face shield).
2. Preoxygenate the patient with a bag-mask device. If it is available and safe, provide 100% oxygen.
3. Check, prepare, and assemble your equipment.
4. Place the patient's head in a neutral position.
5. Pre-form the ET tube by bending it in a circle **Figure 14-25**.
6. Lubricate the tip of the tube with a water-soluble gel.
7. Gently insert the ET tube into the most compliant nostril with the bevel facing toward the nasal septum and advance the tube along the nasal floor **Figure 14-26**.
8. Advance the ET tube through the vocal cords as the patient inhales **Figure 14-27**. If the patient is able to speak, then the ET tube is not in the proper position. When the ET tube is placed properly, the patient may attempt to cough but will not be able to speak.
9. Inflate the distal cuff with 5 to 10 mL of air and detach the syringe **Figure 14-28**.
10. Attach an end-tidal CO_2 detector to the ET tube.
11. Attach the bag-mask device, ventilate, and listen for breath sounds with a stethoscope.
12. Secure the ET tube.

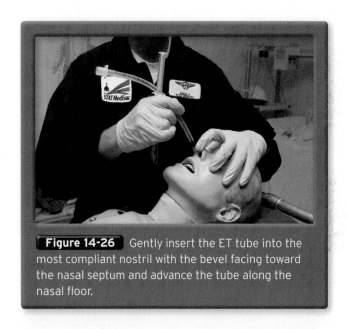

Figure 14-26 Gently insert the ET tube into the most compliant nostril with the bevel facing toward the nasal septum and advance the tube along the nasal floor.

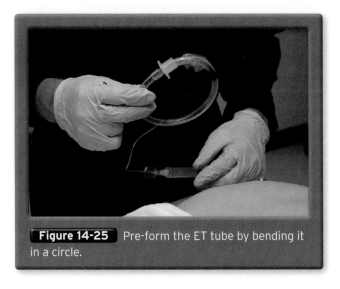

Figure 14-25 Pre-form the ET tube by bending it in a circle.

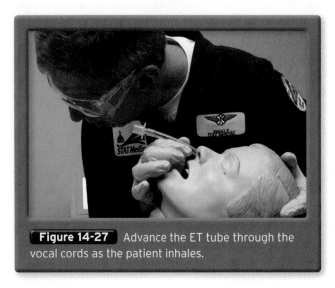

Figure 14-27 Advance the ET tube through the vocal cords as the patient inhales.

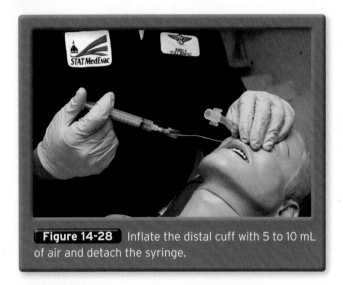

Figure 14-28 Inflate the distal cuff with 5 to 10 mL of air and detach the syringe.

Surgical and Nonsurgical Airways

In some situations, the patient's condition or other factors preclude the use of conventional airway techniques and a more aggressive and invasive approach must be taken to secure the airway and maximize survival. Two methods of securing a patent airway can be used when conventional techniques and methods fail: the open (surgical) cricothyrotomy and translaryngeal catheter ventilation (nonsurgical, or needle cricothyrotomy). To perform these procedures, you must be familiar with the key anatomic landmarks that lie in the anterior aspect of the neck **Figure 14-29**.

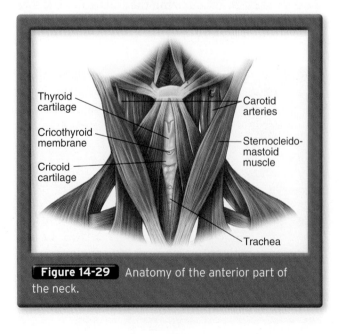

Figure 14-29 Anatomy of the anterior part of the neck.

When performing cricothyrotomy, you should expect to encounter some minor bleeding from the subcutaneous and small skin vessels as you incise the cricothyroid membrane. This bleeding should be easily controlled with light pressure after the tube has been inserted into the trachea, but this should not delay the remainder of the procedure.

Open Cricothyrotomy

Open cricothyrotomy (surgical cricothyrotomy) involves incising the **cricothyroid membrane** with a scalpel and inserting an ET or tracheostomy tube directly into the **subglottic area** (below the vocal cords) of the trachea. The cricothyroid membrane is the ideal site for making a surgical opening into the trachea because no important structures lie between the skin and the airway. The airway at this level lies relatively close to the skin and is easy to enter through the thin cricothyroid membrane. The posterior wall of the airway at this level is formed by the tough cricoid cartilage, which helps prevent accidental perforation through the back of the airway into the esophagus.

Open cricothyrotomy is indicated when you are unable to secure a patent airway with more conventional means. *It is not the preferred means of initially securing a patient's airway.* For example, if you are unable to intubate a patient but can provide effective bag-mask ventilations, cricothyrotomy would not be appropriate.

Situations that may preclude conventional airway management include severe foreign body upper airway obstructions that cannot be extracted with Magill forceps and direct laryngoscopy, airway obstructions from swelling (eg, upper airway burns), massive facial trauma, and the inability to open the patient's mouth. Patients with head injuries and clenched teeth may require cricothyrotomy, especially if you do not have the resources or protocols to perform RSI.

The main contraindication for open cricothyrotomy is the ability to secure a patent airway by less invasive means. Other contraindications include inability to identify the correct anatomic landmarks (cricothyroid membrane), crushing injuries to the larynx and tracheal transection, underlying anatomic abnormalities (eg, trauma or tumors), and age younger than 8 years. In situations where cricothyrotomy is contraindicated, you must rapidly transport the patient to the closest appropriate facility, where an emergency tracheostomy can be performed.

An open cricothyrotomy must be performed quickly. Taking too long to complete a cricothyrotomy will result in unnecessary hypoxia to the patient,

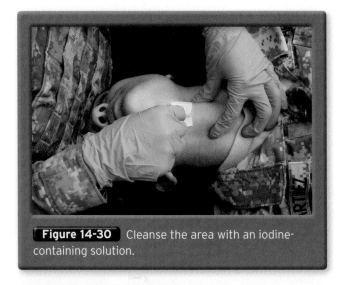

Figure 14-30 Cleanse the area with an iodine-containing solution.

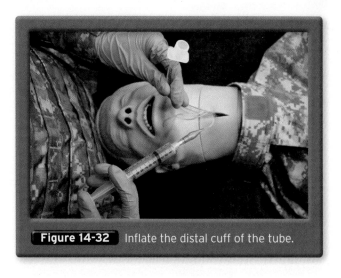

Figure 14-32 Inflate the distal cuff of the tube.

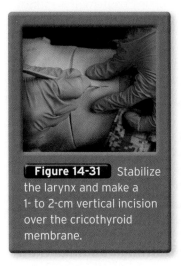

Figure 14-31 Stabilize the larynx and make a 1- to 2-cm vertical incision over the cricothyroid membrane.

which may result in cardiac arrhythmias, permanent brain injury, or cardiac arrest.

Any invasive procedure performed in the tactical environment carries the risk of infection to the patient. Therefore, you should make all attempts to maintain aseptic technique when performing an open cricothyrotomy.

Technique for Performing Open Cricothyrotomy

Follow these steps to perform an open cricothyrotomy:

1. Take standard precautions (gloves and face shield).
2. Check, assemble, and prepare the equipment, which often includes a 6.0-mm ET tube for the average adult.
3. With the patient's head in a neutral position, palpate for and locate the cricothyroid membrane.
4. Cleanse the area with an iodine-containing solution **Figure 14-30**.
5. Stabilize the larynx and make a 1- to 2-cm vertical incision over the cricothyroid membrane **Figure 14-31**. If the anatomy is distorted or an obese patient is being treated, then this incision may need to be 4- to 5-cm to allow increased chance of finding the cricothyroid membrane.

6. Puncture the cricothyroid membrane and make a horizontal cut 1 cm in each direction from the midline.
7. Spread the incision apart with curved hemostats or use the tip of your small finger. If the anatomy is distorted from excessive subcutaneous air or from a nearby expanding hematoma, then consider use of the cricothyrotomy hook to grasp the superior edge of the cricoid ring and stabilize it in place while the ET tube is placed.
8. Insert the tube into the trachea.
9. Inflate the distal cuff of the tube **Figure 14-32**.
10. Attach an end-tidal CO_2 detector in between the tube and the bag-mask device.
11. Ventilate the patient and confirm correct tube placement by auscultating the apices and bases of both lungs and over the epigastrium. The end-tidal CO_2 detector should react appropriately, confirming intubation.
12. Keep the incision site as clean as possible. Apply a dressing to protect the incision and the tube. If bleeding is severe, apply local pressure. Secure the tube with a commercial device or tape. Reconfirm correct tube placement and resume ventilations at the appropriate rate **Figure 14-33**.

Needle Cricothyrotomy

Needle cricothyrotomy also uses the cricothyroid membrane as an entry point into the airway. In this procedure, a 14- to 16-gauge over-the-needle IV catheter (angiocath) is inserted through the cricothyroid membrane and into the trachea. This is used to provide oxygenation and temporary ventilation by injecting

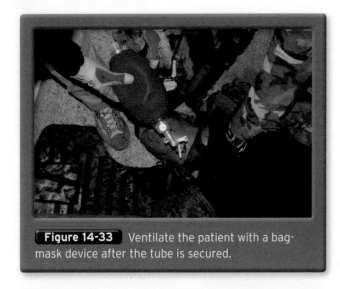

Figure 14-33 Ventilate the patient with a bag-mask device after the tube is secured.

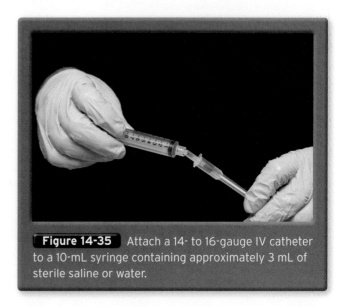

Figure 14-35 Attach a 14- to 16-gauge IV catheter to a 10-mL syringe containing approximately 3 mL of sterile saline or water.

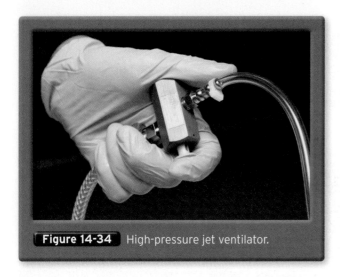

Figure 14-34 High-pressure jet ventilator.

air using a high-pressure jet ventilator to the hub of the catheter **Figure 14-34**. Known as **translaryngeal catheter ventilation**, this procedure is commonly used as a temporary measure until a more definitive airway can be obtained (eg, via open cricothyrotomy).

The indications are essentially the same as for the open cricothyrotomy—the inability to ventilate the patient by other, less invasive techniques; massive facial trauma; inability to open the patient's mouth; and uncontrolled oropharyngeal bleeding. Needle cricothyrotomy is contraindicated in patients who have a severe airway obstruction above the site of catheter insertion. If the equipment necessary to perform translaryngeal catheter ventilation is not immediately available, you should opt to perform an open cricothyrotomy.

Extreme care must be exercised when ventilating the patient with a jet ventilator. The release valve

should be opened just long enough for adequate chest rise to occur. Overinflation of the lungs can result in **barotrauma**, which carries the risk of pneumothorax, which is discussed in detail in Chapter 18, "Torso Injuries." Conversely, opening the release valve for too short a period of time could cause hypoventilation, resulting in inadequate oxygenation and ventilation. This technique can provide a good supply of oxygen, but in some cases does not provide adequate ventilation for long-term use, which results in the buildup of carbon dioxide and acidosis. Therefore, these patients should be taken to an established trauma center where surgeons can establish an improved airway.

Technique for Performing Needle Cricothyrotomy

Follow these steps to perform a needle cricothyrotomy with translaryngeal catheter ventilation:

1. Take standard precautions (gloves and face shield).
2. Attach a 14- to 16-gauge IV catheter to a 10-mL syringe containing approximately 3 mL of sterile saline or water **Figure 14-35**.
3. With the patient's head in a neutral position, palpate the cricothyroid membrane.
4. Cleanse the area with an iodine-containing solution.
5. Stabilize the larynx and insert the needle into the cricothyroid membrane at a 45-degree angle toward the feet **Figure 14-36**.
6. Aspirate with the syringe to determine correct catheter placement. Air should be easily withdrawn if the placement is correct.
7. Slide the catheter off of the needle until the hub of the catheter is flush with the patient's skin **Figure 14-37**.

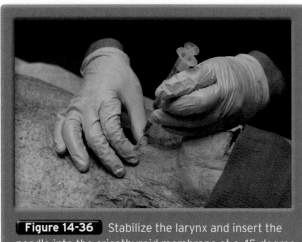

Figure 14-36 Stabilize the larynx and insert the needle into the cricothyroid membrane at a 45-degree angle toward the feet.

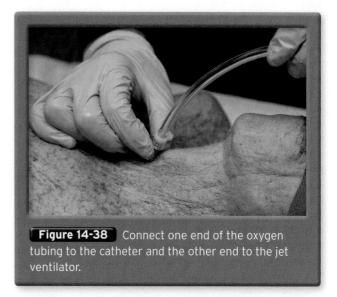

Figure 14-38 Connect one end of the oxygen tubing to the catheter and the other end to the jet ventilator.

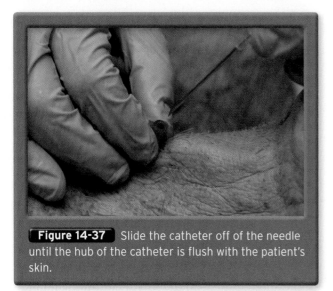

Figure 14-37 Slide the catheter off of the needle until the hub of the catheter is flush with the patient's skin.

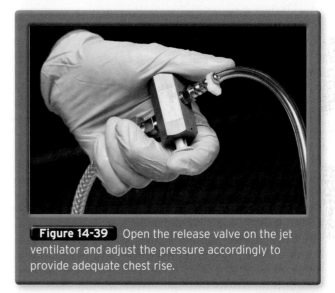

Figure 14-39 Open the release valve on the jet ventilator and adjust the pressure accordingly to provide adequate chest rise.

8. Place the syringe and needle in a puncture-proof container.
9. Connect one end of the oxygen tubing to the catheter and the other end to the jet ventilator **Figure 14-38**.
10. Open the release valve on the jet ventilator and adjust the pressure accordingly to provide adequate chest rise **Figure 14-39**. Ventilate the patient per local protocols.
11. Auscultate the apices and bases of both lungs and over the epigastrium to confirm correct catheter placement.
12. Secure the catheter with a 4″ × 4″ gauze pad and tape. Continue ventilations while frequently reassessing for adequate ventilations and any potential complications **Figure 14-40**.

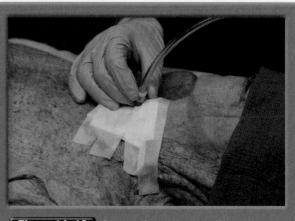

Figure 14-40 Secure the catheter with a 4″ × 4″ gauze pad and tape. Continue ventilations while frequently reassessing for adequate ventilations and any potential complications.

Rapid-Sequence Intubation

The typical patient who undergoes **rapid sequence intubation (RSI)** is critically injured and in need of a patent and protected airway. RSI is generally used for conscious or combative patients who need to be intubated but who are unable or unwilling to cooperate due to clenched jaws or a gag reflex that prevents intubation. The goal is to induce rapid anesthesia using medications that sedate the patient and chemically paralyze the muscles, allowing the advanced-level TMP to open the patient's mouth and intubate.

The TMP who performs this is likely a physician, nurse, or very experienced paramedic. Always follow local protocols.

When performing RSI, remember the eight Ps:

1. **Prepare** and assemble the equipment.
2. **Preoxygenate** the patient. If possible, provide high-flow oxygen by a nonrebreathing mask for 2 to 5 minutes. This may not be possible in the tactical environment.
3. Administer medications to **premedicate**, sedate, and paralyze the patient.
   a. For patients with a head injury or with possible increased intracranial pressure, consider administering a defasciculating dose (typically 10% of a normal dose of a depolarizing neuro-muscular blocking agent) to blunt any further increase in intracranial pressure.
   b. For patients with possible intracranial trauma or increased intracranial pressure, also consider administering 1 mg/kg of lidocaine IV to decrease the increased intracranial pressure associated with upper airway stimulation.
   c. For patients at risk of bradycardia during laryngoscopy (especially children less than 44 pounds or 5 years old), consider administering atropine to decrease any vagal nerve effects from the laryngoscopy.

Safety

Before performing RSI, an airway back-up plan must be in place in case the patient is unable to be intubated due to anatomic damage after receiving the sedation and paralytic medications. A patient who receives these medications will stop breathing and needs oxygen quickly. A TMP must be able to quickly provide an airway through other means, such as an open cricothyrotomy. That equipment should be immediately available before RSI is performed.

Safety

If intubation in children less than 5 years of age is initially unsuccessful and additional paralytics are needed, succinylcholine should *not* be repeated. A nondepolarizing agent should be considered for long-term paralysis in these patients.

   d. For patients with a large amount of anxiety prior to the procedure, consider administering a sedation agent. However, often this is not necessary in the tactical environment. When sedating the patient, use an agent that induces sedation and amnesia, such as benzodiazepine.
4. **Paralyze** the patient using an appropriate medication. Apnea, jaw relaxation, decreased blink response, reduced withdrawal from pain, and decreased resistance to bag-mask ventilations indicate that the patient is sufficiently relaxed to proceed with intubation.
5. Apply posterior cricoid **pressure**.
6. Intubate the patient (**pass** the tube).
7. Confirm ET tube placement (**proof** of placement) and release cricoid pressure.
8. Perform **postintubation** care: ventilate the patient, secure the ET tube, maintain paralysis and sedation.

Table 14-2 lists sedative/induction agents that may be used in RSI, and their doses, onsets, and durations.

Neuromuscular blocking agents are summarized in **Table 14-3**.

At the Scene

When premedicating a patient during RSI, remember the mnemonic "PALS."

P Preparalytic
A Atropine
L Lidocaine
S Sedation

Safety

The contraindications to succinylcholine include patients with large extremity fractures that have not been splinted, as the muscle contractions can cause internal damage. The sharp ends of the fractures may injure nerves and blood vessels.

Table 14-2 — Sedative/Induction Agents

Drug Name	Dose	Onset	Duration
Sodium thiopental (Pentothal)	3-6 mg/kg	< 30 sec	5-10 min
Methohexital (Brevital)	1-3 mg/kg	< 30 sec	5-10 min
Midazolam (Versed)	2-5 mg on induction, 5 mg PRN for sedation	30-60 sec	15-30 min
Lorazepam (Ativan)	0.03-0.06 mg/kg	1-2 min	1-2 hr
Diazepam (Valium)	0.3-0.6 mg/kg	45-60 sec	15-30 min
Etomidate (Amidate)	0.2-0.6 mg/kg	15-45 sec	3-12 min
Ketamine (Ketalar)	1-2 mg/kg	45-60 sec	10-20 min
Propofol (Diprivan)	1-2 mg/kg	15-45 sec	5-10 min
Fentanyl (Sublimaze)	2-3 µg/kg	3-5 min	30-60 min

Table 14-3 — Neuromuscular Blocking Agents

Drug Category	Drug Name	Dose	Onset	Duration
Depolarizing neuromuscular blocking agents	Succinylcholine (Anectine, Quelicin)	1-2 mg/kg	< 1 min	5-10 min
Nondepolarizing neuromuscular blocking agents	Vecuronium (Norcuron)	For intubation: 0.15 mg/kg Postintubation paralysis: 0.01-0.1 mg/kg	90-120 sec	60-75 min
	Rocuronium (Zemuron)	For intubation: 0.6-1.2 mg/kg Postintubation paralysis: 0.1-0.2 mg/kg	< 2 min	30-60 min
	Pancuronium (Pavulon)	For intubation: 0.1 mg/kg Postintubation paralysis: 0.015-0.1 mg/kg	1-2 min	2-2.5 h
	Cisatracurium (Nimbex)	For intubation: 0.15-0.2 mg/kg Postintubation paralysis: 0.03 mg/kg	2-3 min	30-40 min

Ready for Review

- Direct laryngoscopy with Magill forceps may be used to remove a proximal airway obstruction.

- Orotracheal intubation allows direct ventilation of the lungs through the ET tube and is the gold standard of airway care. The prepared TMP will have all airway equipment immediately available for use at all times.

- Intubation should only be performed in a safe environment.

- If an intubated patient regains consciousness, you will need to evaluate the risks and benefits of continued intubation versus extubation.

- Multilumen airways, such as the Combitube, are designed to provide lung ventilation when placed in either the trachea or the esophagus.

- The King LT and the laryngeal mask airway are examples of single lumen airways that are blindly inserted.

- The patient must be unconscious with a bite block or have received RSI medications before digital intubation can be attempted.

- Blind nasotracheal intubation can be performed on patients who are awake and breathing.

- Open cricothyrotomy and needle cricothyrotomy are two methods of securing an airway when conventional methods fail.

- The TMP who performs RSI is likely a physician, nurse, or very experienced paramedic. If the TMP is trained and approved to perform RSI according to local protocols, then those exact medications, medication doses, and timing should be performed.

Vital Vocabulary

barotrauma Injury resulting from pressure disequilibrium across body surfaces; for example, from too much pressure in the lungs.

Combitube A multilumen airway device that consists of a single tube with two lumens, two balloons, and two ventilation ports; an alternative airway device if endotracheal intubation is not possible or has failed.

cricothyroid membrane A thin sheet of fascia that connects the thyroid and the cricoid cartilages that make up the larynx.

endotracheal intubation Insertion of an endotracheal tube directly through the larynx between the vocal cords and into the trachea to maintain and protect an airway.

endotracheal (ET) tube Tube that is inserted into the trachea; equipped with a distal cuff, proximal inflation port, a 15/22-mm adapter, and cm markings on the side.

extubation Removal of a tube after it has been placed.

King LT A supraglottic airway used as an alternative to tracheal or mask ventilation.

laryngeal mask airway (LMA) An advanced airway device that is blindly inserted into the mouth to isolate the larynx for direct ventilation; consists of a tube and a mask or cuff that inflates to seal around the laryngeal opening.

multilumen airway Advanced airway devices, such as the esophageal tracheal Combitube and the pharyngeotracheal lumen airway, that have multiple tubes to aid in ventilation and will work whether placed in the trachea or esophagus.

needle cricothyrotomy Insertion of a 14- to 16-gauge over-the-needle IV catheter through the cricothyroid membrane and into the trachea.

open cricothyrotomy Also referred to as a surgical cricothyrotomy; an emergent procedure that involves incising the cricothyroid membrane with a scalpel and inserting an endotracheal or tracheostomy tube directly into the subglottic area of the trachea.

orotracheal intubation Endotracheal intubation through the mouth.

rapid sequence intubation (RSI) A specific set of procedures, combined in rapid succession, to induce sedation and paralysis and intubate a patient quickly.

subglottic area The area of the trachea below the vocal cords.

trachea The windpipe; the main trunk for air passing to and from the lungs.

translaryngeal catheter ventilation A procedure that provides oxygenation and temporary ventilation to patients with a needle cricothyrotomy by injecting air using a high-pressure jet ventilator to the hub of the catheter.

Shock Management

OBJECTIVES

- Describe the common causes of hypovolemic shock in the tactical environment.

- Describe how to treat hypovolemic shock in the tactical environment.

- Describe how and when to initiate IV infusion in the tactical environment.

- Describe the treatment principles of permissive hypotension.

- Define intraosseous infusion and its benefits in the tactical environment.

- Describe how to perform intraosseous infusion in the tactical environment.

Introduction

As a tactical medical provider (TMP) you must be able to recognize the presence of shock and be able to initiate treatment for shock. The patient who goes into shock is fighting for his or her life, so you must be an expert in recognizing and providing appropriate treatment in the tactical environment **Figure 15-1**. As always, only perform the management techniques that you are trained for and follow your local protocols. This chapter focuses on the most common type of shock you will see in the tactical environment: hypovolemic shock.

Hypovolemic Shock

Hypovolemic shock is a state of inadequate tissue perfusion, with markedly decreased blood flow, oxygen delivery, and glucose supply to vital tissues and organs. In hypovolemic shock, the body's compensatory mechanisms redistribute blood flow to the three vital organs: the kidneys,

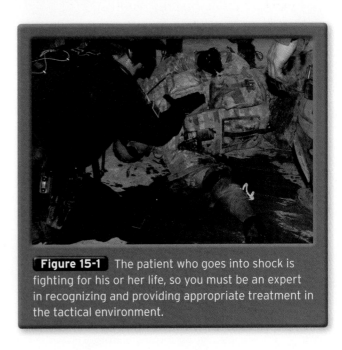

Figure 15-1 The patient who goes into shock is fighting for his or her life, so you must be an expert in recognizing and providing appropriate treatment in the tactical environment.

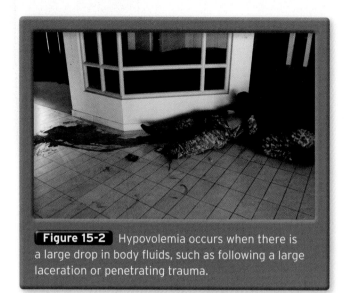

Figure 15-2 Hypovolemia occurs when there is a large drop in body fluids, such as following a large laceration or penetrating trauma.

Signs and Symptoms of Hypovolemic Shock

The patient who goes into shock is fighting for his or her life, so you must be an expert in recognizing the signs and symptoms of hypovolemic shock:

- Rapid, weak pulse
- Changes in mental status (sluggish response, confusion, decreased level of consciousness)
- Cool, clammy skin
- Cyanosis (lips, oral membranes, nail beds)
- Low blood pressure (late sign that may be discovered during the secondary assessment)

heart, and brain. Hypovolemic shock can have many causes; although the two most common in the tactical environment are blood loss (hemorrhage) or fluid loss (dehydration). For many patients in hypovolemic shock, the cause will be immediately apparent (eg, obvious bleeding). Internal hemorrhage may not be so obvious. Any trauma patient who has cool, clammy skin with weak thready pulses and is tachycardic (pulse > 100 beats/min) is in hypovolemic shock until proven otherwise. Almost all patients with multiple injuries will have a degree of hypovolemia. **Hypovolemia** occurs when there is either an absolute decrease in body fluid volume or a shift in body fluids, such as following a large laceration, penetrating trauma, severe burn, severe vomiting, and/or diarrhea **Figure 15-2**. Severe internal bleeding occurs in injuries caused by a violent force (blunt force injury), penetrating trauma (gunshot wounds and knife puncture wounds), and major fractures.

A common sign of hypovolemic shock is cool, clammy, and pale skin. Cyanosis is another sign; it is a bluish tinge of the nail beds, lips, and earlobes. A rapid, weak, and thready pulse is another sign. In later stages of hypovolemic shock, the pulses may be imperceptible. Shallow, rapid breathing and grunting may be heard. Body temperature may be subnormal due to a depressed heat-regulating mechanism. Diminished to absent urine production are additional signs of hypovolemic shock. This occurs due to the body's effort to salvage the two primary organs—the brain and the heart—by shunting blood away from the renal arteries. As shock worsens,

listlessness, stupor, and loss of consciousness occur. Other symptoms include excessive thirst.

Internal signs of hemorrhage with hypovolemic shock may include the above findings, plus:

- Bruising, which indicates bleeding into the skin (soft tissues)
- Tenderness or rigidity of the abdomen or pelvis
- Coughing up blood
- Vomiting blood the color of coffee grounds or bright red (**hematemesis**); the blood may be mixed with food
- Lower intestinal bleeding will result in blood mixed with stool, and it may be red, maroon-colored, or black. This is rarely encountered in a tactical environment.

Pay attention to the patient's pulse (rate and strength), skin, and respirations (rate and quality). Patients in shock will usually have a fast, weak pulse; rapid, shallow breathing; and a pale appearance.

The following points should be remembered when assessing a patient for shock:

- The abdomen should be examined for tenderness or distension, which may indicate internal bleeding.
- The thighs should be checked for deformities or enlargement that indicate a femoral fracture that is causing internal bleeding.
- Check the patient's entire body from head to toe for sources of external and internal bleeding as well as for clues to why the shock is occurring.

Treatment for Hypovolemic Shock

Treatment Goals

The goal of treating hypovolemic shock is to increase tissue perfusion and oxygenation status as soon as possible. In the tactical environment, treatment is directed at stopping the bleeding, maintaining circulation, and providing adequate oxygenation and ventilation.

Treatment Steps

To treat hypovolemic shock in the tactical environment, follow these steps:

1. Control external bleeding through direct pressure, elevation, splinting (see Chapter 20, "Extremity Injuries"), hemostatic agents, or a tourniquet (see Chapter 12, "Controlling Bleeding").
2. Position the patient. If it is safe to do so, expose the hemorrhage sites and use proper techniques to stop any additional bleeding. If the patient is vomiting or bleeding around the mouth, place the patient on his or her side or back with the head turned to the side (except in the case of head injuries or suspected spinal injuries). When exposing the patient, look for associated injuries (eg, gunshot wounds with an entrance injury usually have an exit injury).
3. Ensure an open airway using the head tilt–chin lift or jaw-thrust maneuver.
4. Provide ventilatory support. Use a mouth-to-mask device or bag-mask device with or without oxygen **Figure 15-3** .
5. Perform a neurologic examination to determine the patient's level of consciousness.
6. Attempt to maintain normal body temperature. Remove any wet clothing, and wrap the patient in lightweight Mylar blankets or other insulating materials to prevent hypothermia and minimize the effects of shock **Figure 15-4** .
7. Shock is a load-and-go indication. Evacuate and transport the patient to an emergency department as soon as possible.
8. If appropriate, ALS-level TMPs may provide IV fluid administration during transportation. Do not delay evacuation or transportation to attempt to start an IV in the field.

IV Therapy and Hypovolemic Shock

Insert at least one large-bore peripheral IV line (14 to 16 gauge), using an over-the-needle catheter. If the patient is seriously injured, then two IV lines should

Special Populations

Pediatric patients are difficult to measure blood pressures on, and their blood pressure will remain in normal range while compensating for shock, then suddenly drop. The brachial, femoral, and carotid artery pulses should be monitored. There is a narrower boundary between normal vital signs and shock, and if hemorrhage continues, then their tachycardia of early shock may change to bradycardia, an ominous sign.

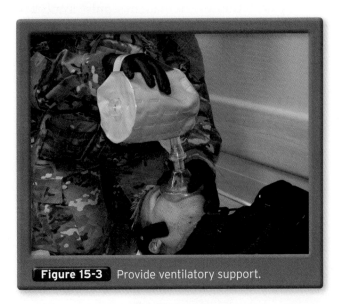

Figure 15-3 Provide ventilatory support.

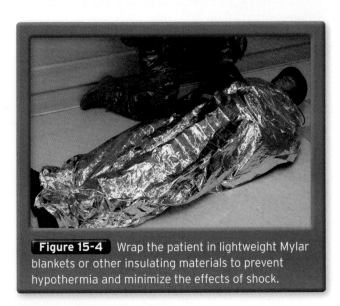

Figure 15-4 Wrap the patient in lightweight Mylar blankets or other insulating materials to prevent hypothermia and minimize the effects of shock.

Special Populations–Pediatrics

Infants and children have less blood circulating in their bodies than adults do, so the loss of even a small volume of fluid or blood may lead to shock. Pediatric patients also respond differently than adults to fluid loss. They may initially respond by increasing their heart rate, increasing respirations, and showing signs of pale or blue skin. Signs of shock in children include tachycardia, poor capillary refill (> 2 seconds), and mental status changes, and in later stages they may develop bradycardia and hypothermia.

Begin treating shock by assessing the CABs, intervening with stabilizing care immediately as required. In assessing circulation, look carefully for bleeding sites and assume that there may be internal bleeding as well. You should pay particular attention to the following:

- **Pulse.** Assess both the rate and the quality of the pulse. A fast or slow but weak, "thready" pulse is a sign that there is a problem. The appropriate rate depends on age; anything over 160 beats/min suggests shock.
- **Skin signs.** Assess the temperature and moisture of the hands and feet. How does this compare with the temperature of the skin on the trunk of the body? Is the skin dry and warm, or cold and clammy?
- **Capillary refill time.** Squeeze a finger or toe for several seconds until the skin blanches, and then release it. Does the fingertip return to its normal color within 2 seconds, or is it delayed?
- **Color.** Assess the patient's skin color. Is it pink, pale, ashen, or blue?

Changes in pulse, skin signs, capillary refill time, and color are all important clues suggesting shock.

Limit your management to simple lifesaving interventions. Time should not be wasted performing field procedures. Stop any bleeding, ensure that the airway is open, and rapidly evacuate the patient to ALS transport. Pediatric patients need high-flow oxygen as soon as possible. If you are permitted to accompany the patient during transport, start IV access. Consider an intraosseous (IO) needle insertion, if vascular access cannot be obtained quickly and the patient is unconscious. Give IV crystalloid fluid at 20 mL/kg boluses to stabilize the patient. Keep giving fluid boluses up to 60 mL/kg as needed to stabilize perfusion based on ongoing reassessment of vital signs. Monitor and treat for low blood glucose levels. Provide immediate transport to the nearest appropriate facility and continue monitoring vital signs en route.

be inserted. Unless local medical policy favors a different resuscitation fluid, give normal saline (0.9% NaCl) solution. For guidance, refer to the IV fluid flow rates in your local protocols.

If the patient is hemodynamically unstable (absence of radial pulse, has a rapid heart rate above 110 to 120 beats/min), has an altered level of consciousness without head injury, or has chest pain, then rapidly infuse an IV bolus of 500 mL to 1000 mL of normal saline, colloid, or other appropriate fluid. The goal is the return of a normal level of consciousness and/or a palpable radial pulse.

A new term called **permissive hypotension** is important in trauma patients with uncontrolled bleeding sites and hypovolemic shock. Treatment using these principles includes limited use of IV fluids to maintain a radial pulse or normal level of consciousness without excessively raising the blood pressure past 90 mm Hg systolic. If the blood pressure is raised higher than this, increased bleeding will occur. The exceptions are patients with traumatic brain injury or with advanced age, as a normal blood pressure may be necessary to improve the patient's outcome.

IV Administration

IV administration is only permitted if you are appropriately trained and certified. Follow your local protocols and the guidance of your medical director. In general, do not delay transportation while attempting to start an IV, especially when the patient has load-and-go indications, such as hypovolemic shock. The IV may be started when possible in the ambulance during transportation. Advanced-level TMPs may start an IV on scene, if circumstances do not allow for immediate extraction and transportation.

One way to ensure proper technique is to develop a routine to follow as you assemble and use the

Safety

The most important point to remember about IV techniques and fluid administration is to keep the IV equipment sterile. Forethought will help prevent mental and procedural errors while starting the IV.

appropriate equipment. The IV supplies should be stored together, which will make the IV insertion faster and more efficient. Experienced TMPs find that a routine will help you keep track of your equipment and the steps necessary to complete a successful IV.

To initiate an intravenous infusion (in an upper extremity), follow these steps:

1. Wash your hands and use antiseptic/germ-free technique.
2. Gather your equipment, clarify the site, identify yourself to the patient, and get permission to start the IV.
3. Only if time allows, clearly identify the patient and explain the procedure. Ask about any allergies.
4. Inspect and assemble the equipment. Check the selected IV bag for proper fluid, clarity, and expiration date. Look for discoloration and for particles floating in the fluid. If found, discard the bag and choose another bag of fluid.
5. Hang the container at least 2 feet above the level of the patient's heart and squeeze the drip chamber until it is half full of solution.
6. Remove the air from the IV tubing.
7. Cut several tape strips and hang them in an accessible location.
8. Select the infusion site.
9. Prepare the infusion site. Apply a constricting band 2 inches above the venipuncture site—tight enough to stop venous flow, but not so tight that the radial pulse cannot be felt. Instruct the patient to open and close his or her fist several times to increase circulation. Select and palpate a prominent vein. Clean the skin with an antiseptic sponge in a circular motion from the center outward **Figure 15-5**.

10. Put on additional sterile gloves if possible.
11. Hold the catheter with your dominant hand and remove the protective cover without contaminating the needle.
12. Hold the flash chamber with your thumb and forefinger directly above the vein or slightly to the side of the vein **Figure 15-6**.
13. Draw the skin below the cleansed area downward to hold the skin taut over the site of the venipuncture.
14. Position the needle point, bevel up, parallel to the vein and about ½ inch below the venipuncture site.
15. Hold the needle at approximately a 20- to 30-degree angle and pierce the skin.
16. Decrease the angle until the needle is almost parallel to the skin surface and direct it toward the vein.
17. Continue advancing the needle until the vein is pierced.
18. Check for blood in the flash chamber.
19. Advance the needle approximately ⅛ inch farther to ensure the proper catheter placement in the vein **Figure 15-7**.
20. Stabilize the flash chamber with your dominant hand, grasp the catheter hub with your nondominant hand, and thread the catheter into the vein to the catheter hub.
21. Remove the flash chamber or needle and lay it aside.
22. With your dominant hand, remove the protective cover from the needle adapter on the IV tubing and quickly connect the adapter into the catheter hub, while maintaining stabilization of the hub with your nondominant hand **Figure 15-8**.
23. Tell the patient to unclench his or her fist and then you can release the constricting band.

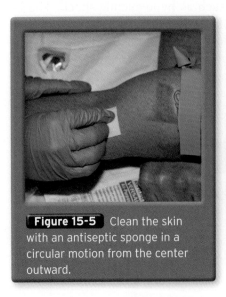

Figure 15-5 Clean the skin with an antiseptic sponge in a circular motion from the center outward.

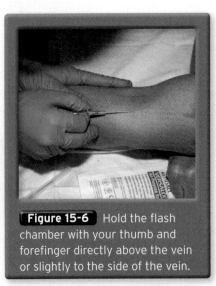

Figure 15-6 Hold the flash chamber with your thumb and forefinger directly above the vein or slightly to the side of the vein.

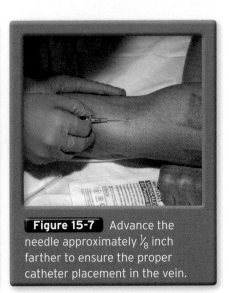

Figure 15-7 Advance the needle approximately ⅛ inch farther to ensure the proper catheter placement in the vein.

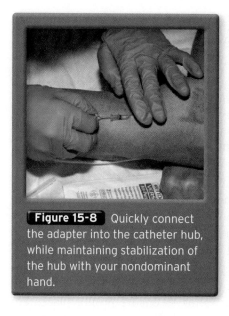

Figure 15-8 Quickly connect the adapter into the catheter hub, while maintaining stabilization of the hub with your nondominant hand.

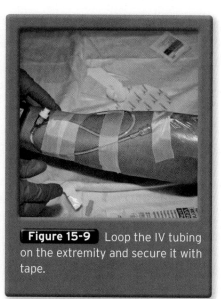

Figure 15-9 Loop the IV tubing on the extremity and secure it with tape.

24. Unclamp the IV tubing and adjust the flow rate to the appropriate drip rate.
25. Examine the infusion site for infiltration such as significant swelling, redness, or edema of the IV site, and discontinue if infiltration is present.
26. Clean the area of blood, if necessary, and secure the hub of the catheter with tape, leaving the hub and tubing connection visible.
27. Apply an antibacterial ointment and a sterile dressing over the puncture site.
28. Loop the IV tubing on the extremity and secure it with tape **Figure 15-9**.
29. Splint the arm loosely on a padded splint, if necessary, to reduce movement.
30. Print the date, gauge of the catheter, time the IV was started, and initials of the person starting the IV on a piece of tape. Secure the tape to the dressing.
31. Print the patient's name, drip rate, date and time the IV infusion was initiated, and the person initiating the IV on another piece of tape. Secure the tape to the IV container.
32. Print the date and time the tubing was put in place and the initials of the person initiating the IV on a third piece of tape and wrap the tape around the tubing, leaving a tab.
33. Re-examine the IV site for infiltration.

IV Troubleshooting

Several factors can influence the flow rate of an IV. For example, if the IV bag is not hung high enough, the flow rate will not be sufficient. Use of a simple IV pressure infuser device will help maintain IV fluid flow regardless of the height or position. It is always helpful to perform the following checks after completing IV administration. Also, if there is a flow problem, rechecking these items will help determine the problem.

- **Check your IV fluid.** Thick, viscous fluids such as blood products and colloid solutions infuse slowly and may be diluted to help speed delivery. Cold fluids run slower than warm fluids. If you can, warm IV fluids before administering them in cold weather as this will decrease hypothermia.
- **Check your administration set.** Macrodrips are used for rapid fluid delivery, whereas microdrips are designed to deliver a more controlled flow.
- **Check the height of your IV bag.** The IV bag must be hung high enough to overcome the patient's own blood pressure. Hang the bag as high as possible or use an IV pressure infuser.
- **Check the type of catheter used.** The wider the catheter (the smaller the gauge), the more fluid can be delivered; 14 gauge is the widest, 27 gauge the narrowest.
- **Check your constricting band.** Make certain that the constricting band is not still on the patient's arm after completing the IV.
- **Use a red or blue low-level flashlight** when starting an IV in dark conditions. Maintain light discipline and avoid giving away your position.

Intraosseous Infusion Administration

Intraosseous (IO) infusion is a technique of administering fluids and medications into the intraosseous space of a long bone. When a patient is in shock, the peripheral veins may collapse, making IV access extremely difficult, if not impossible. However, the spongy interior IO space remains patent, unless the patient has suffered trauma to its bony structure (eg, a fracture). For this reason, the IO space is commonly referred to as a "noncollapsible vein." It quickly absorbs IV fluids and medications and rapidly gets them to the central circulation—as rapidly as is possible with the IV route. Anything that can be given via the IV route—crystalloids, medications, and blood and blood products—can be given via the IO route. IO infusion may be indicated when you are unable to obtain IV access in a critically injured patient in profound shock.

Follow these steps to perform IO infusion (in the lower extremity) using a manually inserted IO needle:

1. Check the selected IV fluid for proper fluid, clarity, and expiration date. Look for discoloration and for particles floating in the fluid. If found, discard the bag and choose another bag of fluid.

2. Select the appropriate equipment, including an IO needle, syringe, saline, and extension set. A three-way stopcock may also be used to facilitate easier fluid administration.

3. Select the proper administration set. Connect the administration set to the bag.

4. Prepare the administration set. Fill the drip chamber and flush the tubing. Make sure all air bubbles are removed from the tubing.

5. Prepare the syringe and extension tubing.

6. Cut several tape strips and hang them in an accessible location. This can be done at any time before IO puncture.

7. Take standard precautions. *This must be done before IO puncture.*

8. Identify the proper anatomic site for IO puncture. There are multiple sites that have been approved for IO use, and the TMP should follow regional EMS protocols. When using the BIG in an adult, go 2 cm from the tibial tuberosity toward the inner leg, and then 1 cm up toward the knee **Figure 15-10**. When using the EZ-IO, go down 2 cm from the patella to the tibial tuberosity, then 1 cm toward the inner leg.

9. Cleanse the site appropriately. Follow aseptic technique by cleansing in a circular manner from the inside out.

10. Perform the IO puncture by first stabilizing the tibia by placing a folded towel under the knee, and holding in a manner to keep your fingers away from both the site of puncture and the path of the needle.

Medical Gear

There are several types of IO needles that may be used in the tactical environment, including the adult Bone Injection Gun (BIG), the EZ-IO, the Jamshidi IO needle, the Sur-Fast IO needle, and the FAST 1 IO needle.

11. Insert the IO needle according to local protocols and the manufacturer's instructions. Unscrew the cap and remove the stylet from the needle.

12. Attach the syringe and extension set to the IO needle. Pull back on the syringe to aspirate air, blood, and particles of bone marrow to ensure proper placement.

13. Slowly inject saline to ensure proper placement of the needle. Watch for fluid leaking into the surrounding tissue (extravasation) and stop the infusion immediately if it is noted. It is possible to fracture the bone during insertion of the IO. If this happens, you should remove the IO and switch to the other leg.

14. Connect the administration set and adjust the flow rate as appropriate. In adults, fluid does not flow as rapidly through an IO catheter as through an IV line; therefore, crystalloid boluses should be given with a pressure infuser device.

15. Secure the IO needle **Figure 15-11**. Be generous when using tape and support it with a bulky dressing. Stabilize in place in the same manner that an impaled object is stabilized. Be careful not to tape around the entire circumference of the leg, as this could impair circulation and potentially result in compartment syndrome.

16. Dispose of all sharps in the proper container.

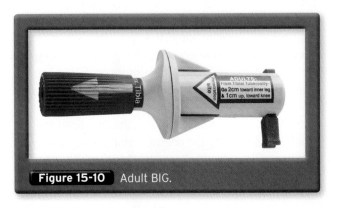

Figure 15-10   Adult BIG.

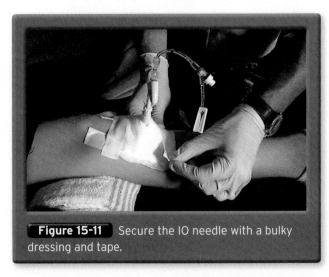

Figure 15-11   Secure the IO needle with a bulky dressing and tape.

Ready for Review

- As a TMP you must be an expert in recognizing and providing the appropriate treatment for a patient in hypovolemic shock.

- The most common causes of hypovolemic shock in the tactical environment are blood loss and fluid loss. Hypovolemia occurs when there is a large decrease in body fluids or a shift of fluid out of the intravascular space into other areas of the body.

- The signs and symptoms of hypovolemic shock in the tactical environment are:

  - Rapid, weak pulse
  - Changes in mental status
  - Cool, clammy skin
  - Cyanosis
  - Low systolic blood pressure

- In the tactical environment, the goal of treating hypovolemic shock is to increase perfusion and oxygenation of the body's tissues. This is done by stopping the bleeding, maintaining circulation, and providing adequate oxygenation and ventilation.

- Never delay transport of the patient to begin IV therapy. IV therapy can be performed during transport.

- Intraosseous infusion may be indicated if the advanced TMP is unable to obtain IV access.

Vital Vocabulary

hematemesis Vomited blood.

hypovolemia An abnormal decrease in blood volume.

hypovolemic shock A condition in which low blood volume, due to massive internal or external bleeding or extensive loss of body water, results in inadequate tissue perfusion.

intraosseous (IO) infusion Administration of fluids and medication into the bone.

permissive hypotension The limited use of IV fluids to maintain a radial pulse or normal level of consciousness without excessively raising the patient's blood pressure past 90 mm Hg systolic in order to prevent further hemorrhaging.

Extraction and Evacuation

OBJECTIVES

- Describe the role of the tactical medical provider (TMP) in patient extraction and evacuation.

- Describe how self-extraction by the injured SWAT officer benefits both the injured SWAT officer and the entire SWAT unit.

- Describe the role of immediate action drills in patient extraction and evacuation.

- Describe the manual extraction techniques used in the tactical environment.

- Discuss how the TEMS unit and civilian EMS interface during the evacuation of a patient.

- Discuss how the TEMS unit safely interacts with air medical evacuation assets and crew.

Introduction

Extraction is the process of moving the patient from the point of injury to a point of relative safety (ie, hard cover) where medical care can be provided **Figure 16-1**. Some situations may allow a downed SWAT officer to perform immediate self-care and self-extraction, while other situations will require one or more SWAT officers and/or TMPs to complete the extraction.

Evacuation is the timely, efficient movement of patients from hard cover to transportation **Figure 16-2**. This is ideally performed by TMPs who can initiate or continue to provide the appropriate level of medical care needed to maintain patient stabilization. This may include dragging or carrying the patient from the initial hard cover to a **casualty collection point (CCP)** where the civilian EMS support crew can meet the patient and the TMPs and initiate transportation to an appropriate hospital. The civilian EMS support crew will have a well-equipped ambulance or aircraft that will allow advanced life support (ALS) measures to be provided en route to the hospital. Chapter 7, "Medical Intelligence and Support," discusses the role of medical planning in achieving a rapid patient evacuation.

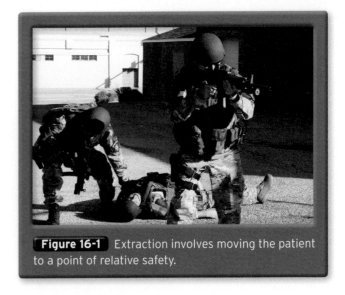

Figure 16-1 Extraction involves moving the patient to a point of relative safety.

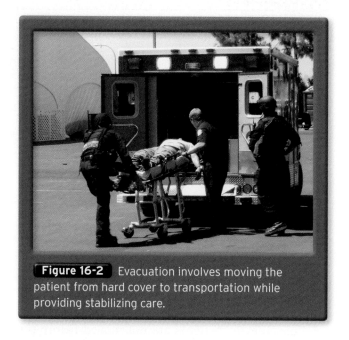

Figure 16-2 Evacuation involves moving the patient from hard cover to transportation while providing stabilizing care.

Extraction

The concept of extraction is simple but can become complex when you consider the many different types of techniques and equipment such as ropes, harnesses, and stretchers that can be used to safely extract the patient. Ballistic blankets, shields, or armored SWAT vehicles may be used to protect the TMP and patient. There are many potential options and combinations of equipment and tactics that may be used to perform extraction. As a TMP you will study the possible tactics and equipment used by your agency and then participate in immediate action drills (IADs) with your SWAT and TEMS units to perfect the various tactics with your agency's equipment. Training drills are critical because if a SWAT officer is injured, training instinctively needs to kick in so the right decisions can be made automatically.

The potential IADs for a downed SWAT officer are discussed before the mission during the premission briefing. Included in the briefing is whether the SWAT officers should press forward with the entry or hold in place and bring the TMPs forward, or abandon the entry attempt and extract the downed SWAT officer as an entire team. These considerations must be communicated to the entire entry team so they will perform with the proper mindset and tactics. For example, suppose an entry team is actively engaged in assaulting a building to rescue

hostages, if a SWAT officer is shot, then the response by the remaining entry team may be to step over the injured SWAT officer and continue the mission. The entry team's primary objective is to rescue the hostages, requiring maximum personnel and speed. The downed SWAT officer may be left behind to be dealt with by TMPs on the tail end of the stack.

Self-Extraction

Ideally, the wounded SWAT officer should attempt self-extraction. The injured SWAT officer may finish the fight by securing the scene immediately around himself or herself by neutralizing threats, and then moving to a point of hard cover. Once behind hard cover, the wounded SWAT officer can assess and self-treat any injuries.

If the injured SWAT officer only has an extremity injury and has effectively tightened a tourniquet on the injured limb, he or she can remain in place behind hard cover for several hours while the remainder of the SWAT unit resolves the callout and clears a safe path for nearby TMPs to respond. Because the injured SWAT officer is behind hard cover administering self-care, additional lives are not placed at risk to perform an urgent assault in a high-threat environment in order to rescue the injured SWAT officer. However, if the SWAT officer has a penetrating torso injury, self-extraction and self-care are not often practical due to the seriousness of the injury; therefore, extraction and treatment likely will be required.

When IADs are practiced during SWAT training, SWAT commanders and TMPs should encourage a "continue to fight for your life" philosophy. SWAT officers should understand that it is a mistake to abandon the

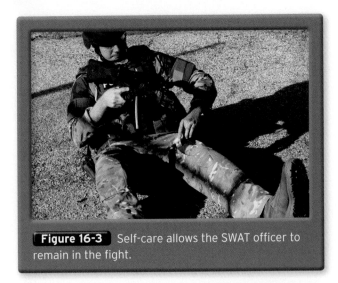

Figure 16-3 Self-care allows the SWAT officer to remain in the fight.

fight and give up when wounded **Figure 16-3**. Do not teach or encourage SWAT officers to simply lie there and expect to be rescued immediately. SWAT commanders should create IADs that train SWAT officers to return fire while moving to hard cover and then performing self-aid. SWAT officers should remain in the fight, even as they are patching themselves up or being dragged down hallways.

Another point to reinforce during training is that individual first aid kits (IFAKs) save lives. The modern IFAK is very small and compact and takes up about the same space as two magazines for an AR-15/M-4 rifle. In fact, a tactical compression bandage, tourniquet, several pairs of nitrile gloves, CPR mask, Band-Aids, and ibuprofen and acetaminophen tablets fit into a double magazine pouch. Remind SWAT officers that these kits will allow lifesaving self-aid and buddy-aid to stop massive external bleeding and to assist in stabilizing a downed SWAT officer. Carrying an IFAK and being ready to provide self-aid and buddy-aid shows the ultimate respect for the lives of fellow SWAT officers. A fellow SWAT officer will not have to risk leaving his or her own hard cover to assist a conscious, injured SWAT officer with a wound that could have been self-treated.

At the Scene

SWAT officers should maintain the attitude that they will continue to fight and function when shot, instead of instantly becoming a victim. This is one of the best lessons you can encourage during training.

Overview of Manual Extraction Techniques

Manual extraction is the process of transporting patients by manual carries and drags. It is accomplished without the aid of a wheeled stretcher or other advanced forms of transport. It is intended to end when a stretcher or ambulance is available.

Patient Handling

Patients evacuated by manual means must be handled carefully when possible. Rough or improper handling may cause further injury to the patient. The extraction effort should be organized and performed methodically. Each movement made in lifting or moving patients should be performed as deliberately and gently as possible. Ideally, patients are not moved before the nature and extent of their injuries are fully evaluated and the required care is administered. Injured SWAT officers need to be extracted rapidly, before any assessment or stabilizing care can be given. This includes patients with suspected spinal injury. The risk of being shot outweighs the risk of worsening the potential spinal injury. When immediate movement of a patient is required, he or she should be moved only far enough to be out of danger and behind hard cover. Only then can tactical patient assessment and stabilizing care be provided.

General Rules for Rescuers

In manual extraction, individuals performing the extraction are referred to as rescuers. Improper handling of a patient may result in injury to the rescuers as well as to the patient. To minimize disabling injuries such as muscle strain or sprains that could hamper the extraction effort, the following rules should be followed:

- Use the body's natural system of levers when lifting and moving a patient.
- Know your physical capabilities and limitations.
- Maintain solid footing when lifting and transporting a patient.
- Avoid walking backwards, as this leads to falls and inefficient movement.
- Use your leg muscles—not your back muscles—when lifting or lowering a patient.
- Use your shoulder and leg muscles—not your back muscles—when carrying or standing with a patient.
- Keep your back straight and use your arms and shoulders when pulling a patient.

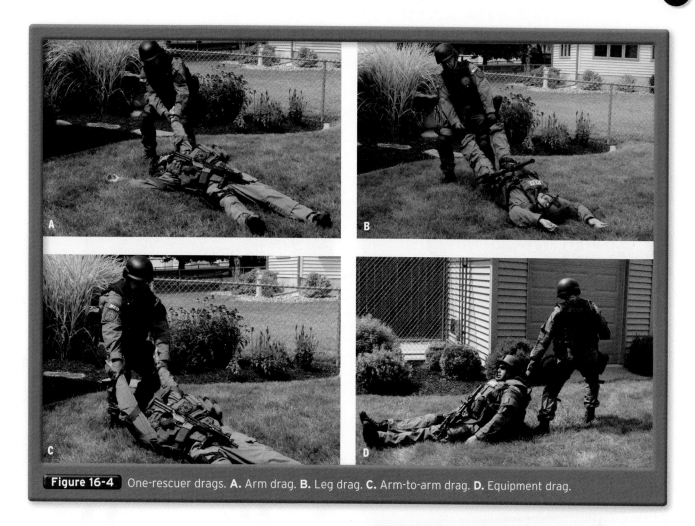

Figure 16-4 One-rescuer drags. **A.** Arm drag. **B.** Leg drag. **C.** Arm-to-arm drag. **D.** Equipment drag.

- Work in unison with other rescuers using deliberate, gradual movements. Slide or roll, rather than lift, heavy persons or objects that must be moved.
- Have a plan for moving patients. If a 250-lb downed SWAT officer requires rapid extraction, either drag the individual or call for help. Do not attempt to carry a 250-lb person yourself.

Dragging

Due to the risks of the high-threat tactical environment, dragging a patient to a point of relative safety may be the simplest and safest extraction technique. When dragging a patient you should pull the patient along the long axis of the body. This will help to keep the spinal column in line as much as possible. By grasping the inside collar of the downed SWAT officer's vest with both hands, you can support the SWAT officer's neck with your forearms and limit the motion of the head and neck. If you follow these guidelines during the move, you can usually move a patient from a life-threatening situation without causing further injury to the patient.

At the Scene

Dragging may result in minor abrasions to the patient, but these are easily treated and nonlife-threatening injuries. If the patient has serious life-threatening injuries, then a few scrapes are offset by the rapid extraction.

One-Rescuer Simple Drag

In the simplest form, the patient is rapidly approached and the rescuer simply does a grab and drag:

- Rotate the patient's arms so that they are extended straight on the ground beyond his or her head, grasp the wrists, and, with the arms elevated above the ground, drag the patient **Figure 16-4A** . You can also apply this concept to the patient's legs **Figure 16-4B** . Also grasp the inside of the patient's boot to use as a handle when dragging the patient by the feet.
- Grasp each of the patient's wrists and drag the patient backward **Figure 16-4C** .

- Grab the straps on the patient's backpack or vest and drag the patient to nearby cover **Figure 16-4D**.

Stretcher Drags

Soft stretchers are designed to roll up or fold up into compact spaces and be carried in backpacks. These soft stretchers have four to eight carry handles, enabling them to be used to both drag and carry patients **Figure 16-8**. These stretchers are primarily used for dragging the patient behind hard cover or outside of a building to the patient collection point **Figure 16-9**. Using one of these stretchers, one rescuer can drag a SWAT officer with one hand to a point of relative safety on the smooth hallway of an office building or school. Two rescuers will be required to drag a patient to safety on concrete or grass for extended distances due to the increased friction. Soft stretchers provide the patient some protection against abrasions and lacerations due to friction.

Medical Gear

A webbing sling loop can be used to help rapidly extract patients. Rescuers can quickly wrap the webbing around both of the ankles and then run the webbing out through the loop, creating a cinch that tightens rapidly and securely, allowing one or two rescuers to drag the patient.

Commercial drag harnesses include the Dragon and the Sling-Link webbing drag systems. The Dragon Handle System is designed for one or two rescuers and is a simple double-loop harness with cushioned drag handles **Figure 16-5**. The Sling-Link can be used to rapidly drag a patient or for vertical extraction (lowering a patient out of a window) **Figure 16-6**. Always follow your agency's tactics and local protocols. Do not attempt maneuvers that you are not trained or authorized to perform.

Other extraction devices include the RAT strap, nylon webbing drag systems, girth hitches, and throw bags containing 8-mm nylon rope **Figure 16-7**. Your TEMS unit leader will investigate and determine which equipment should be used by your agency. Be sure to train extensively with this equipment to ensure that you can use it under any condition.

Safety

One-rescuer drags can be modified into two-rescuer drags. Two-rescuers can drag a 250-lb person more quickly and with less fatigue.

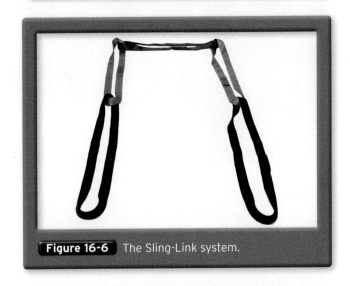

Figure 16-6   The Sling-Link system.

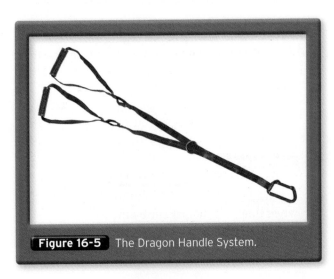

Figure 16-5   The Dragon Handle System.

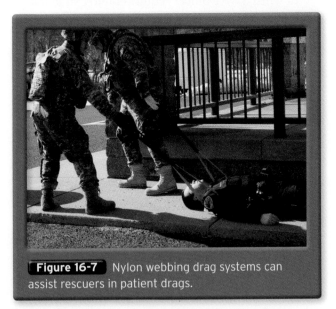

Figure 16-7   Nylon webbing drag systems can assist rescuers in patient drags.

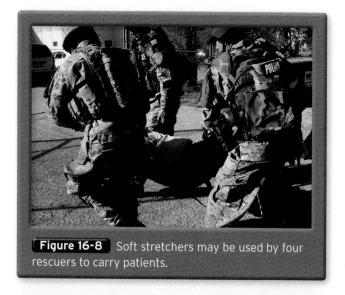

Figure 16-8 Soft stretchers may be used by four rescuers to carry patients.

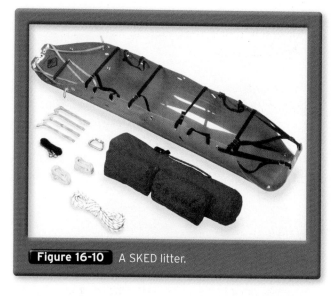

Figure 16-10 A SKED litter.

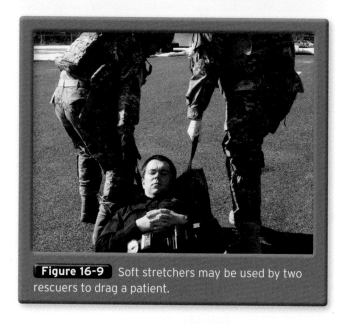

Figure 16-9 Soft stretchers may be used by two rescuers to drag a patient.

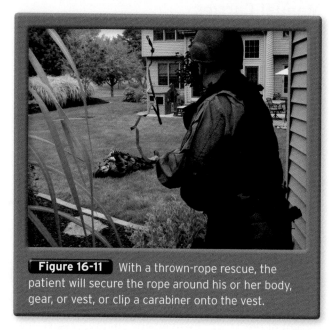

Figure 16-11 With a thrown-rope rescue, the patient will secure the rope around his or her body, gear, or vest, or clip a carabiner onto the vest.

Use caution when using the one-rescuer drag to go down a stairway, as gravity will cause the patient to slide rapidly down the stairway. In order to prevent this, a second rescuer should hold onto the end of the stretcher with the patient's feet to help control the descent. When extracting a patient down or up stairways, it is important to avoid causing further injury to the patient's head or spine. Keep the SWAT officer's helmet and vest in place to protect the body when being dragged over steps.

A rigid or semi-rigid stretcher, such as a SKED, may be used when more protection of the patient is needed **Figure 16-10**. When unrolled and when the patient is properly secured in place, the SKED stretcher provides spinal movement restriction. It is smooth on the outside, making it easier to perform one- to two-rescuer drags.

Thrown-Rope Drag

A technique that rescuers can use to drag a patient to safety is the thrown-rope drag. If a patient is conscious but unable to move and under the threat of direct gunfire, then nearby rescuers may remain behind hard cover and throw a strong nylon rope to the patient. The patient can secure the rope around his or her body or clip a carabiner to the ballistic vest **Figure 16-11**. Once the rope is secure, the rescuers behind hard cover pull the patient toward them and behind hard cover **Figure 16-12**. During training, the drag handle that is attached to the top of a SWAT officer's ballistic vest should be tested to see if it can be used for this purpose or not, as it may break prematurely.

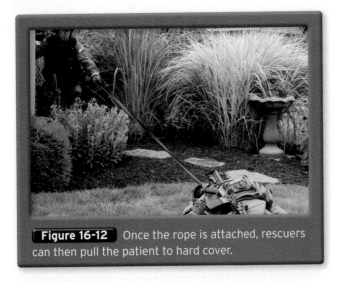

Figure 16-12 Once the rope is attached, rescuers can then pull the patient to hard cover.

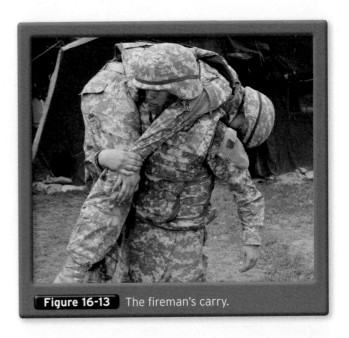

Figure 16-13 The fireman's carry.

Manual Carries

Manual carries are tiring for rescuers and may increase the severity of the patient's injuries. However, in some instances manual carries are essential to save the patient's life. When a stretcher is not available or when the tactical situation makes other forms of patient transportation impractical, a manual carry may be the only means to transport a patient to a relative point of safety. The one-rescuer carry is difficult, considering the weapons, ballistic gear, and typical large frame of the average SWAT officer. If a single rescuer needs to move an injured patient, a simple drag over a short distance to hard cover may be accomplished with greater safety and with less risk of injury to either the patient or rescuer and is preferable.

Minimize Weight and Position the Patient

The first step in any manual carry is to lighten the weight of the patient by removing all unnecessary gear. If there is a ballistic threat, then leave the helmet and ballistic protective vest in place. If the scene is safe from all threats, remove the helmet and vest. Position the patient to be lifted. If conscious, the patient should be told how he or she is to be positioned and transported.

Medical Gear

Appropriate ballistic protection should be used if there is any chance of a suspect shooting at or otherwise attacking rescuers or the patient. Use of multiple ballistic shields, ballistic blankets, hardened armored vehicles, and other precautions should be considered.

This helps to lessen the patient's fear of movement and gains his or her cooperation. It may be necessary to roll patients onto their abdomen or back, depending on their position and the particular carry to be used.

Categories of Manual Carries

One-Rescuer Carries The fireman's carry can be difficult, requires considerable strength, involves the risk of back injury, and makes both the rescuer and the patient larger targets **Figure 16-13**. The advantage of this carry is that one rescuer who is physically fit can move the patient for short distances quickly, including over uneven ground, water, or thick grass. Do not attempt this carry unless you have received training and approval from your agency. This type of carry is rarely used by TEMS units today.

With the supporting carry, the patient must be able to walk or at least hop on one leg using the rescuer as a crutch. This carry may be used to transport a patient as far as he or she is able to walk or hop **Figure 16-14**. Only a conscious patient can be transported by the saddleback carry because he or she must be able to hold onto the rescuer's neck while the rescuer carries the patient on his or her back **Figure 16-15**.

Two-Rescuer Carries Two-rescuer carries are preferable to one-rescuer carries. Two-rescuer carries provide more comfort for the patient, are less likely to aggravate injuries, and are less tiring for the rescuers. The two-person extremity carry is a useful carry for transporting the patient over a long distance **Figure 16-16**. The extremity lift may be especially helpful when the patient is in a very narrow space, such as being carried out

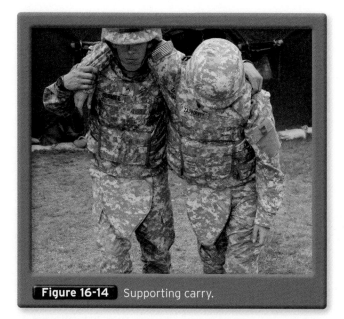

Figure 16-14 Supporting carry.

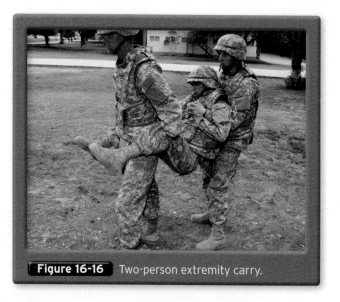

Figure 16-16 Two-person extremity carry.

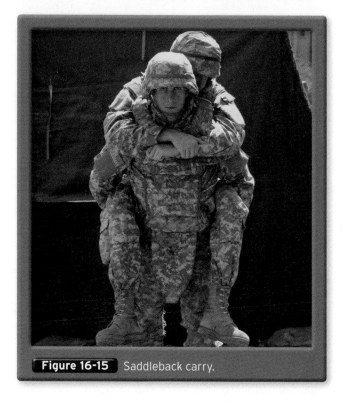

Figure 16-15 Saddleback carry.

At the Scene

In a controlled, safe environment, if a patient has significant potential for or has an actual spinal injury with neurologic deficits, utilize standard spinal immobilization equipment such as a backboard, scoop stretchers, and cervical collars, and consider calling in civilian EMS to assist in extracting and transporting the patient. Less ideal conditions may require ingenuity and makeshift methods, such as using a door as a backboard and the patient's boots taped along the head to limit cervical motion. Always follow your local protocols and tactics.

in a sitting position. The second rescuer moves to a position between the patient's legs, facing in the same direction as the patient, and slips his or her hands under the patient's knees or ankles. As the rescuer at the head gives the command, both stand fully upright and move the patient.

Evacuation

TEMS and EMS Interface

Ideally there will be well-equipped and well-staffed EMS transport at the patient collection point that will allow for ALS measures to be provided en route to the hospital. Many TEMS units rely on an ALS-level ambulance to transport the patient along with one or two ALS-level TMPs to the hospital. In the best of circumstances, there will be seamless interface between the TEMS unit and

through a narrow door in a residence. Communication is the key to success with this lift. Coordinate movements through direct verbal commands.

The first rescuer kneels behind the patient's head as the second rescuer kneels at the patient's feet. The two rescuers should be facing each other. The patient's hands should be crossed over his or her chest. The first rescuer places one hand under each of the patient's armpits. The first rescuer grasps the patient's wrists or forearms and pulls the upper torso until the patient is

At the Scene

In the event that a vehicle is needed to extract a downed SWAT officer from the inner perimeter, the ideal choice would be an armored vehicle that has thick enough glass and outside armor to reliably stop all pistol and rifle gunfire. This armored vehicle should be equipped with emergency medical kits and support gear to allow patients to be cared for by other SWAT officers and possibly any accompanying TMPs. Follow the local protocols and tactics of your agency.

Controversy

Sometimes there may be a significant delay in the arrival of a civilian EMS ambulance. This can be due to poor communication, lack of preparation, or the inability of the community to provide standby ambulance support due to limited resources. In situations where the civilian EMS ambulance is delayed, the severity of injuries must be considered and a decision made on the disadvantages of waiting an unknown length of time for an ambulance versus using other more readily available transportation methods.

If a load-and-go situation exists and there is no ambulance on scene, the command personnel and TEMS leader may decide to have the patient urgently transported in an on-site vehicle. A law enforcement patrol vehicle or a truck belonging to SWAT personnel could be selected to rapidly transport the patient to the hospital.

Each state has strict EMS guidelines and rules regarding inspection, authorization, and certification of ambulances. If an injured SWAT officer is transported to the hospital by a noncertified ambulance, then there will be an investigation. Careful preplanning will limit the variables that could cause such a scenario.

the community EMS agencies, resulting in optimal patient care.

A civilian EMS ambulance is not bulletproof, and any pistol or rifle bullet will likely easily penetrate these vehicles. If a patient is in need of extraction, the ambulance should not be involved. An ambulance does not provide any effective degree of protection from bullets or shrapnel. Ambulances should be staged outside of the outer perimeter where extricated patients are brought to the patient collection point for evacuation.

Communicating with Civilian EMS and Hospitals

It is critical that the TEMS unit have a good system of communication with civilian EMS. While gathering medical intelligence for the medical threat assessment, you should write down the cell phone number and radio frequency used by the civilian EMS ambulance(s) standby crews. If radios are being used for communication, the patient's name should be omitted. If possible, cell phone communication should be used.

The EMS ambulance standby crew should be updated as the situation unfolds, acknowledging the need not to reveal any sensitive information. As a TMP, you should never direct the ambulance to enter the callout scene. Only the incident commander (IC) is permitted to call for the ambulance to approach and enter the scene, and this is done only if it is safe for the civilian EMS ambulance crew. The IC has the entire "big picture" view and knows if there are any threats still at large—the TMP does not.

As a TMP, you should communicate with the hospital or trauma center, especially if you are riding with the patient in the ambulance. Communicate the mechanism of injury, injuries, and the estimated time of arrival which

allows the emergency department and trauma team time to prepare their equipment, personnel, and operating rooms. Ideally you will have a medical card with key information about each SWAT officer that may inform the hospital staff about allergies, known medical history, medications, and other information that will enhance patient care. If you are able to obtain a SAMPLE history from a non-SWAT officer patient, then this information should be reported to the hospital staff.

During the transport of suspects, sometimes the suspect will make statements to the civilian EMS crew or TMPs that could be useful in the prosecution of a crime. This is particularly true in the case of dying suspects. If the suspect is still conscious in his or her last moments, a suspect may confess to crimes or identify others who committed crimes. These statements are afforded special consideration in court. Although it is not your job to probe for such information, you should listen and note all such statements. Record these statements at the earliest possible moment and inform the appropriate investigating officers.

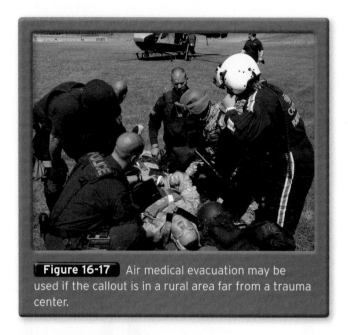

Figure 16-17 Air medical evacuation may be used if the callout is in a rural area far from a trauma center.

Air Medical Evacuation

Air medical evacuation is a viable option for many TEMS units **Figure 16-17**. The use of air transport may play a role in a congested city with highways at a standstill as well as in providing support for a SWAT unit in a rural or distant location far away from ground ambulance crews and hospitals. In most areas, only the air medical evacuation staff may accompany the patient during transport. If a patient is a suspect who is awake and is considered a threat, then the patient should be handcuffed and restrained appropriately before the aircraft leaves the scene. Always follow local protocols.

If training or a callout indicates its use, the TEMS unit leader will prearrange air medical transportation by disclosing the global positioning system (GPS) coordinates of the nearest landing zone (LZ), if possible. Once they are placed on standby, most air medical programs strive to be off the ground and flying

Safety

In the United States each year there are multiple air medical evacuation crashes and deaths. There is a theoretical risk of a crash each time an aircraft flies. If a patient is stable and can be transported by ground, then air medical evacuation should not be called.

Medical Gear

Air medical assets or boat assets are considerations that should be preplanned in certain regions to transport the patient to the hospital. Through careful preplanning, the TEMS unit can react to any situation.

within 3 minutes of the word "go" from the requesting units. Preidentifying the exact location of the LZ of the callout is an ideal way to confidentially inform a select few people that an air medical transport may be needed.

Before an air medical transport is activated, the scene must be as controlled as possible. If it cannot be guaranteed that the air medical transport will not be fired upon, then the use of the air transport should be discussed among the incident commander, the TEMS leader, the pilot, and air medical transport personnel. A risk/benefit analysis should be performed and alternative modes of transportation (ie, ground ambulance), level of care needed, and transport times should be considered. The lives of the air medical crew should not be risked unnecessarily.

Preparing a Landing Zone

The TEMS unit must be capable of preparing a safe LZ, with approach and departure paths free of all obstacles. As a TMP, you should be well integrated with the local air medical services and should follow all appropriate procedures and communication policies. You must know how to safely approach, load, unload, and safely leave a helicopter LZ.

A good helicopter LZ should consist of an area that is relatively flat, has no hills or depressions, and is sized appropriately for the helicopter. Most civilian air medical units recommend securing a landing area 100 feet × 100 feet square if daylight conditions exist with no obstructions. A larger area is indicated if night landings are involved. To prepare an LZ, follow these steps:

1. Designate a landing zone officer (LZO) to communicate with the air medical crew via radio and hand signals **Figure 16-18**. This person must not be distracted during flight operations and should not have patient care responsibilities or security duties when the helicopter is approaching or departing.

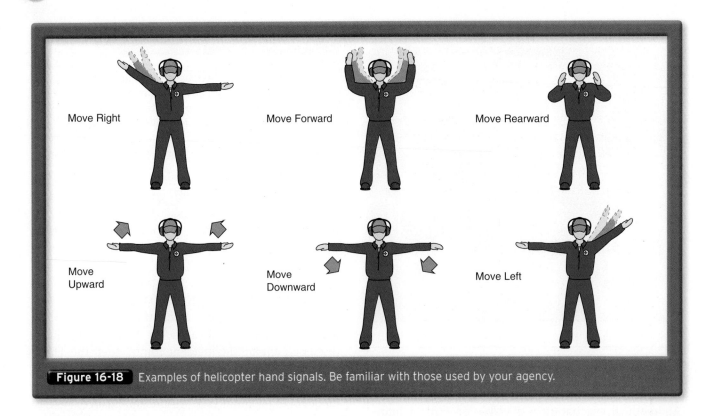

Figure 16-18 Examples of helicopter hand signals. Be familiar with those used by your agency.

2. Choose an LZ. It must be away from the rifle and pistol range of the suspect if the suspect is still at large. It should be away from towers, power lines, and any terrain features that could cause a crash. It must be at least 100 feet × 100 feet, flat, firm, and free of all obstacles, including pieces of trash or debris that may fly and hurt the helicopter or others nearby.

3. The LZO must be visible and identifiable from the air (ie, wearing an orange vest and using a flashlight). He or she should report wind speed, direction, and any hazards to the pilot by radio.

4. Illuminate and mark the LZ with nonflammable lights. Flares are hazardous as they may create grass fires and increase the risk of fire. Be sure that no bright lights are pointed directly toward the helicopter.

5. As the helicopter approaches, the LZO will stand with his or her back to the wind with hands raised above his or her head. The LZO must move out of the rotor wash area (high-speed windy area directly under the horizontal rotating helicopter blades), but maintain eye contact with the pilot. The helicopter pilot will circle the LZ once or twice, and may opt for a different LZ if conditions are not good.

6. No one should approach the helicopter unless directed by the crew.

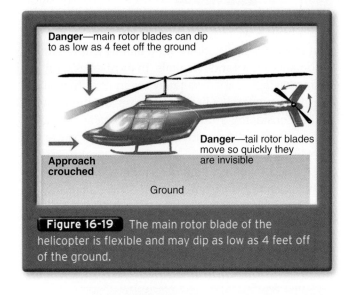

Figure 16-19 The main rotor blade of the helicopter is flexible and may dip as low as 4 feet off of the ground.

7. Only after being directed by the pilot(s) or medical helicopter crew, approach (and leave) the helicopter at a 90-degree angle from the doors. Crouching down may be useful, especially if the ground is uneven. The main rotor blade of the helicopter is flexible and may dip as low as 4 feet off of the ground **Figure 16-19**. Stay in the pilot's view. Avoid the front and back of the helicopter. The main rotors actually are lower to the ground in the front. The

back of the helicopter often has a rear rotor blade that is nearly invisible. Decapitation and other head injuries are not uncommon. Wear eye and ear protection, as some winds generated may be in excess of 170 mph.

8. Follow instructions from the crew when assisting with loading. Secure any loose items. Keep objects below shoulder level. Depart as a group.

9. As the helicopter departs, the LZO will keep the area clear and report hazards to the pilot.

Immediate Response Team

Sean McKay is a former fire fighter, paramedic, and TEMS team leader and is an experienced trainer and educator. He developed a new concept for TEMS, the immediate response team, similar to the fire department's rapid intervention team. The immediate response team carries a variety of specialized tools, such as bolt cutters, small sledgehammers, Halligan tools (crowbars), circular saws, ropes, collapsible stretchers, and drag harnesses, to create new entry and exit points to access and extract patients. This includes the capability of lowering or raising patients for vertical extraction **Figure 16-20**.

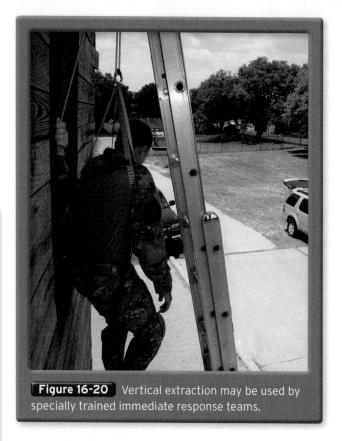

Figure 16-20 Vertical extraction may be used by specially trained immediate response teams.

Ready for Review

- Extraction is the process of moving the patient from the point of injury to a point of relative safety (ie, hard cover) where medical care can be provided.

- Some situations may allow a downed SWAT officer to perform immediate self-care and self-extraction, while other situations will require one or more SWAT officer and/or TMP to complete the extraction.

- Evacuation is ideally performed by TMPs who can initiate or continue to provide the appropriate level of medical care needed to maintain patient stabilization, including possibly dragging or carrying the patient from the initial hard cover to a patient collection point.

- In self-extraction, a SWAT officer who is struck by a bullet or blast fragment will ideally continue and finish the fight by securing the scene immediately around himself or herself by neutralizing threats, and then moving to a point of hard cover. Once behind hard cover, the wounded SWAT officer can assess and self-treat any injuries using the IFAK.

- Manual evacuation techniques include one- and two-rescuer drags, stretcher drags, thrown-rope drags, and one- and two-rescuer carries.

- The immediate action drill for a downed SWAT officer is discussed before the mission. Included in the discussion is whether to press forward with the assault or to hold in place and bring the TMPs forward, or to extract the downed SWAT officer as an entire team and withdraw from the mission.

- Communication with civilian EMS should be seamless in order to provide optimal patient care.

- The TEMS unit leader will arrange for air medical evacuation if it is required. As a TMP, you must know how to safely approach, load, unload, and leave a helicopter landing site.

Vital Vocabulary

__casualty collection point (CCP)__ The point outside of the outer perimeter where civilian EMS meet the patient and TMPs to initiate transportation to an appropriate local hospital.

__extraction__ The process of moving the patient from the point of injury to a point of relative safety.

__extrication__ The process of safely disentangling a patient who is trapped in a motor vehicle crash, building collapse, or explosion debris.

__evacuation__ Timely, efficient movement of patients from hard cover to transportation.

Ballistic, Blast, and Less-Lethal Weapons Injuries

OBJECTIVES

- Describe the factors that affect the severity of gunshot wounds.

- Describe the signs of a ballistic injury.

- List the ballistic injury locations that indicate the patient has a load-and-go injury.

- Describe how to remove a ballistic vest from a downed SWAT officer.

- List the four mechanisms of a blast injury.

- Describe the potential blast injuries that may occur if an explosive is detonated in the tactical environment.

- Describe how to remove the protective gear from a law enforcement bomb technician.

- Describe how to manage injuries from less-lethal weapons.

Introduction

As a tactical medical provider (TMP), you need to understand the potential injuries that patients may have based on the type of projectile and mechanism that caused the injury. In the tactical environment, your responsibility is to stabilize the patient for evacuation. Often the only definitive treatment for ballistic and blast injuries is surgery. These surgical repairs can be as simple as suturing a bleeding wound or as extensive as a complete bowel resection. The goal is to keep the patient alive by stabilizing the patient's circulation, airway, and breathing so the patient can be evacuated and transported to a hospital. You are the vital link in getting the patient from the tactical environment to the operating room alive.

On the other end of the spectrum, you may be required to assess and manage injuries from less-lethal weapons. A brief summary on the types of potential injuries that may occur from less-lethal weapons is presented in this chapter.

Ballistics

One of the greatest threats to law enforcement is a suspect who has a firearm and is willing to use it **Figure 17-1**. As a TMP, you must know the effects of firearms by having a thorough understanding of ballistics. Ballistics is the study of projectiles and/or firearms. **External ballistics** refers to the study of the **velocity** and trajectory of a projectile from the weapon to the target. External ballistics is very complex and is an area that is highly studied. This chapter focuses on the effects of **internal ballistics** or the effects of projectiles on human tissue **Figure 17-2**.

The **kinetic energy** of a projectile is the energy of motion. This energy is transferred to anything that comes in contact with the projectile. This chapter discusses the effects of transferred kinetic energy on solid and hollow organs, bones, and soft tissue. The mass of the projectiles can vary greatly. The differences in mass and velocity have a profound effect on the damage inflicted by the projectile on the human body. As a bullet enters and passes through the body, some of the kinetic energy that it possesses is transferred to the surrounding tissue. This creates a temporary

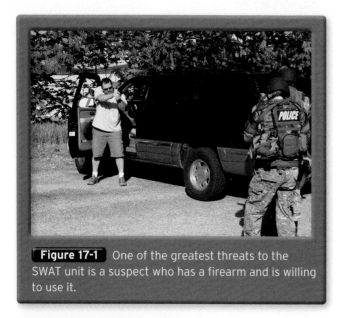

Figure 17-1 One of the greatest threats to the SWAT unit is a suspect who has a firearm and is willing to use it.

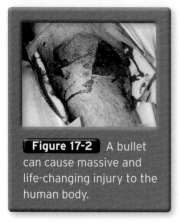

Figure 17-2 A bullet can cause massive and life-changing injury to the human body.

cavity at the point in which the most kinetic energy is released and transferred. The temporary cavity exists for milliseconds. If the bullet begins to tumble or breaks up, it slows down dramatically and transfers a larger amount of kinetic energy into the surrounding tissue. A wound channel and small permanent cavity remain after the bullet passes through the tissue.

The severity of a wound depends on several factors:

- **Bullet caliber (size).** The larger the bullet, the larger the ballistic wound.
- **Design and shape of the bullet.** Some bullets have soft tips that will expand upon striking the target, while others have an actual hollowed-out tip (hollow points) that are designed to mushroom on impact. A full metal jacket becomes unsteady upon striking the body, causing the bullet to tumble and pass through tissue sideways, causing devastating injury.
- **Weight of the bullet.** The kinetic energy of a bullet is proportional to its weight. The actual original weight of a bullet may change once the tissue is struck if the core of the bullet separates from the outer jacket or if the bullet breaks apart. If

a bullet can retain its weight, then the depth of penetration will be maximal.

- **Velocity.** The faster the bullet, the greater the kinetic energy.
- **Type of tissue struck or impact.** Ballistic wounds to the brain or heart may be instantly fatal.
- **Fragmentation of the bullet.** If the bullet wobbles as it spins (a motion known as yaw), tumbles, and breaks up into fragments, then the fragments will cause a greater amount of damage.

Pistols and shotguns have the slowest muzzle velocities, ranging from 800 feet per second to around 1,600 feet per second. These bullets generally have less energy and penetration than high-power rifle ammunition. Most of the damage caused by these slower rounds is from crushing and lacerating soft tissue. Ballistic wounds and the complications from ballistic wounds resulting from pistol and shotgun fire may manifest in a variety of ways:

- Simple penetrating wounds **Figure 17-3**
- Through-and-through penetrating wounds with disproportionately large exit wounds
- Fractures, amputations, and massive soft-tissue injuries when extremities are involved
- Eviscerations of body cavities
- Massive soft-tissue and internal organ injuries **Figure 17-4**
- Severe blood loss, shock, and death

Medium-velocity cartridges cause most of their damage by cavitation. **Cavitation** causes a temporary cavity that forms when the pressure wave from the bullet stretches the skin and tissue outward. The skin

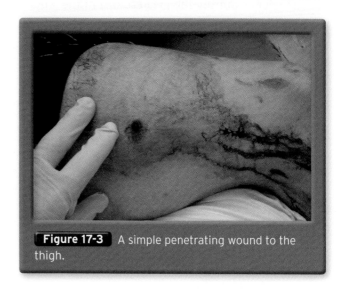

Figure 17-3 A simple penetrating wound to the thigh.

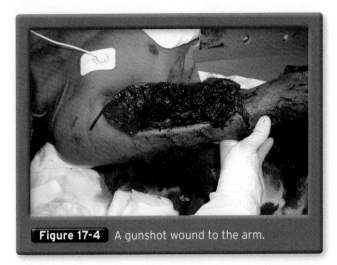

Figure 17-4 A gunshot wound to the arm.

and tissue can quickly return to their normal position but are often damaged. This can cause contusions to solid organs or rupture hollow organs. Large areas of hematomas can also form in the permanent cavity and from bleeding arteries.

Any high-velocity cartridge (rifle round) can cause **shock waves** in the soft tissue. These bullets cause the same type of crush injury and lacerations as the slower velocity bullets, but with increased cavitation. High-velocity cartridges can also cause a shock wave and hydrostatic energy that precedes the bullet. A shock wave is highly effective in stretching tissue but the effect lasts for only a few milliseconds.

Compare the cavitation of the full metal jacketed round versus the heavier hunting-type round from a shotgun. The full metal jacketed round penetrates much deeper before slowing down due to tumbling. At the point where the bullet slows, it releases most of its kinetic energy, putting the greatest area of the wound deep below the surface tissue.

The heavier hunting round is a slower projectile that still penetrates deeply through the tissue, but the greatest area of cavitation is near the skin or initial contact surface. The shotgun round has most of its destructive effects near the surface due to its less concentrated mass and slower velocity. Its penetration is also significantly less than the higher velocity solid bullets. However, this does not diminish the lethal effects of shotgun rounds at a close range. Remember, any well-placed bullet can be fatal.

Types of Ballistic Wounds

Gunshot wounds can be classified based on the range from the muzzle of the gun to the target. The five classifications are contact wounds, close-range wounds, near-contact wounds, intermediate-range wounds, and distant wounds:

Controversy

This topic is controversial, but for TMPs an essential skill set is to know the relative power and types of injuries that can occur from the various firearms that may be seen in the field. The bottom line is that even a .22-caliber rimfire 40-grain bullet can kill, and yet a powerful .30-06 rifle 185-grain bullet wound may be survivable depending on the location of the body that is involved and the volume and type of tissue destroyed. An additional consideration is penetration capability through a ballistic vest or helmet. A .44 Magnum bullet weighing 240 grains fired from a handgun may be stopped by a Level III vest, but a smaller diameter, lighter weight, and higher velocity .223-caliber or 5.56-mm bullet weighing 55 grains fired from an AR-15 or M-16/M-4 carbine (rifle) can penetrate this same vest.

- **Contact wounds.** These wounds occur when the muzzle is held against the body at the time it is fired. Contact wounds may have soot near the entrance wounds, torn edges around the wound, or bruising from the muzzle striking the skin.
- **Close-range wounds.** These wounds occur when the muzzle is approximately 6 to 12 inches away from the skin. There may be soot on the patient's skin or clothing from the gunpowder and blast.
- **Near-contact wounds.** These wounds have powder tattooing, powder soot, and sometimes seared blackened skin.
- **Intermediate-range wounds.** These wounds have numerous reddish-brown to orange-red small stippling markings around the entrance wound.
- **Distant wounds.** The only evidence of these wounds is often the wound itself.

Assessment and Management of Ballistic Injuries

If you witness a ballistic injury, first call for help while all threats are being abolished. Your first priority is your own safety and that of your unit. Once the scene is secure and you and the patient are in a point of relative safety, begin to assess the CAB 'N. Quickly expose and observe the location of the wound(s), approximate size of the wound(s), and the number of wound(s).

The signs of a ballistic wound include bleeding wounds and nearby clothing with powder stippling (small black marks from embedded burned gunpowder particles), soot marks, powder burns (actual burn markings from burning gunpowder), or powder tattooing (black marks from gunpowder smoke) **Figure 17-5**. Classic entry wounds are beveled inward with relatively smooth edges, while exit wounds have torn edges **Figure 17-6**. Ballistic wounds may be penetrating or perforating. Penetrating wounds have an entrance hole but no exit. Perforating wounds enter and exit the target. It is not necessary to try and determine if a wound is an entrance or exit wound. What matters is the location, size, and number of wounds.

Small-caliber, low-velocity ballistic wounds may leave little external evidence and be difficult to locate or detect due to the relatively low energy and smaller amount of tissue damage. The only sign of these wounds may be a slight tear in clothing or small area of bleeding. Be suspicious of any blood spots on the patient's clothing.

If the patient suffers a ballistic wound to the head, neck, or torso, you should consider this a life-threatening, load-and-go situation **Figure 17-7**. Bullets often travel long distances in the human body and may bounce off of hard bony surfaces; the exact organ(s) injured can never be determined accurately based on a rapid physical examination in the tactical environment. Always assume the worst—stop severe hemorrhage, secure the airway, ensure adequate breathing, and evacuate and transport the patient rapidly. The patient with normal vital signs may decompensate and he or she may die within minutes. Differentiating between lethal and nonlethal ballistic injuries is very difficult in the field. Assume that all nonextremity penetrating and perforating trauma are potentially lethal until proven otherwise. Always load and go.

If you accompany the patient during transport, perform a secondary assessment to ensure that there are no additional wounds. Monitor the patient's airway and breathing and take advanced measures if appropriate and per local protocols (see Chapter 14, "Advanced Airway Management," and Chapter 18, "Torso Injuries"). Monitor the patient for shock and treat appropriately per local protocols (see Chapter 15, "Shock Management").

For ballistic wounds in the extremities, stabilizing care is essential. If a TMP cannot reach a downed SWAT officer due to continued threats, the SWAT officer will

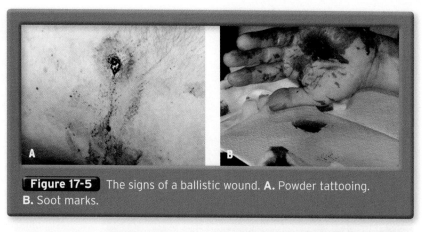

Figure 17-5 The signs of a ballistic wound. **A.** Powder tattooing. **B.** Soot marks.

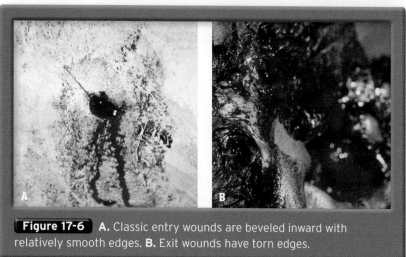

Figure 17-6 **A.** Classic entry wounds are beveled inward with relatively smooth edges. **B.** Exit wounds have torn edges.

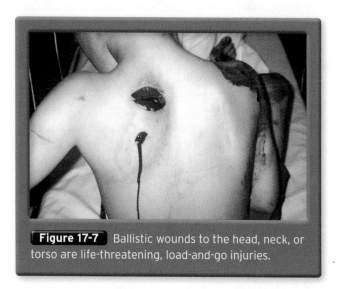

Figure 17-7 Ballistic wounds to the head, neck, or torso are life-threatening, load-and-go injuries.

apply a tourniquet if possible. If a patient is behind hard cover, then the TMP will assess the patient's circulation to determine if a tourniquet is required to stop significant bleeding. If any questions about the severity of bleeding exist, then err on the side of caution and apply a tourniquet. If the bleeding is minor, apply

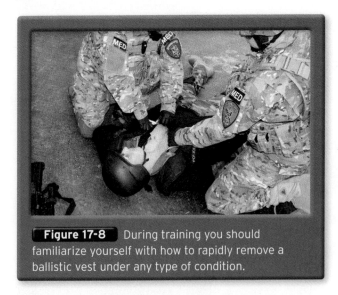

Figure 17-8 During training you should familiarize yourself with how to rapidly remove a ballistic vest under any type of condition.

direct pressure and a compression dressing. Secure the patient's airway, ensure breathing, evacuate the patient, and transport the patient to the hospital.

Ballistic Vest Removal

Treating the injured SWAT officer who is wearing a ballistic vest presents a unique challenge. During training you should familiarize yourself with the equipment in use in your jurisdiction and know how to remove it rapidly in all light conditions **Figure 17-8**. Routine training and immediate action drills for downed SWAT officers should enable you to determine the most effective way to rapidly remove ballistic vests and begin treatment.

In the tactical environment you must not remove the patient's ballistic vest until all threats have been abolished or the patient has been removed from the immediate danger of ballistic injury. If a patient has been extracted to hard cover, then rapidly loosen the vest and rapidly palpate and inspect under the vest for signs of bleeding—do not remove the vest. You may detect a blunt trauma injury with pain upon palpation and edema from a hematoma. This is not an unusual finding following a bullet strike to body armor.

At the Scene

The appearance of an entrance wound will vary based on the angle of the weapon, the distance of the weapon from the patient, ballistic protection, the patient's clothing, and other factors. Look for any bleeding including blood spots on clothing. This may be the only sign of a gunshot wound.

At the Scene

When inspecting a ballistic wound, you may have difficulty determining which are the entry wounds and which are the exit wounds due to many factors including the elastic nature of skin and tissue. During documentation, a basic description of the wounds should be provided. Do not attempt to guess if the wound was an entrance or exit wound. Conflicting police data and patient medical records can negatively impact a criminal case. Simply state how the wound and clothing appeared. Use the correct terminology, such as powder burns and stippling. For example, "Proximal thigh penetrating trauma, with a soot collar ring around the irregular 1-cm hole that is located approximately 20 cm above the left knee."

If the ballistic vest is struck by bullets or heavily contaminated with blood, it is usually used as evidence and eventually discarded, so you should not hesitate to cut the straps if this is the fastest way to remove the vest. Ideally, a SWAT officer will assist in removing the ballistic vest while you continue the patient assessment and management. Do not attempt to cut the ballistic material with scissors—scissors will not cut through this material.

Blast Injuries

Although most commonly associated with military conflict, blast injuries have occurred during SWAT callouts. People who are injured in explosions may be injured by any of four different mechanisms **Figure 17-9**:

- **Primary blast injuries**. These injuries are due entirely to the blast itself; that is, damage to the body is caused by the pressure wave generated by the explosion. When the victim is close to the blast, the blast wave causes disruption of major blood vessels and the rupture of major organs as the blast wave travels through the body.
- **Secondary blast injuries**. Damage to the body results from being struck by flying debris, such as shrapnel from the device or from glass or splinters that have been set in motion by the explosion. Objects are propelled by the force of the blast and strike the victim, causing injury. These objects can travel great distances and be propelled at

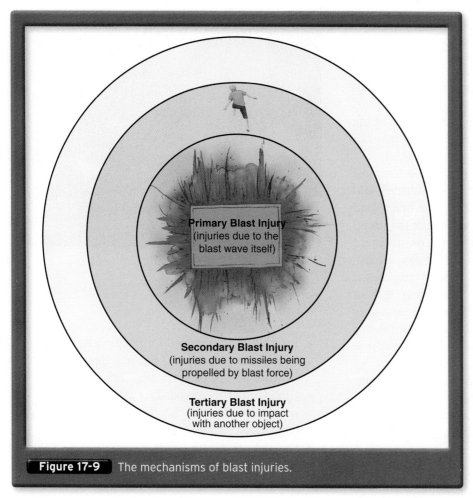

Figure 17-9 The mechanisms of blast injuries.

Primary Blast Injury
(injuries due to the
blast wave itself)

Secondary Blast Injury
(injuries due to missiles being
propelled by blast force)

Tertiary Blast Injury
(injuries due to impact
with another object)

Tissues at Risk

Organs that contain air, such as the middle ear, lung, and gastrointestinal tract, are the most susceptible to pressure changes. The junction between tissues of different densities and exposed areas such as head and neck tissues are prone to injury as well. The ear is the organ system that is most sensitive to blast injuries. The **tympanic membrane** in the ear detects minor changes in pressure and will rupture at pressures of 5 to 7 pounds per square inch (psi) above atmospheric pressure. Thus, the tympanic membranes are a sensitive indicator that you can use to help determine the possible presence of other blast injuries. The patient may complain of ringing in the ears, pain in the ears, and some loss of hearing, and blood may be visible in the ear canal. Dislocation of structural components of the ear may occur. Permanent hearing loss is possible.

tremendous speeds, up to nearly 3,000 mph for conventional military explosives.

- **Tertiary blast injuries.** These injuries occur when the patient is hurled by the force of the explosion against a stationary object. A "blast wind" also causes the patient's body to be hurled or thrown, causing further injury. This physical displacement of the body is also referred to as ground shock when the body impacts the ground. In some cases wind injuries can amputate limbs.
- **Miscellaneous (quaternary) blast injuries.** These injuries include burns from hot gases or fires started by the blast, respiratory injury from inhaling toxic gases, and crush injury from the collapse of buildings, among others.

Most patients who survive an explosion will have some combination of the four types of injury mentioned. The discussion in this chapter is limited to primary blast injuries because these injuries are the ones that are most easily overlooked.

Pulmonary blast injuries are defined as pulmonary trauma (consisting of contusions and hemorrhages to the lungs) that results from short-range exposure to the detonation of explosives. When the explosion occurs in an open space, the patient's side that was toward the explosion is usually injured, but the injury can be bilateral when the victim is located in a confined space and the blast wave reflects against the walls. The patient may complain of tightness or pain in the chest, may cough up blood, and may have tachypnea or other signs of respiratory distress. Pneumothorax and tension pneumothorax are common injuries and may require emergency decompression (which is covered in the Chapter 18, "Torso Injuries") in the field for your patient to survive. Pulmonary edema may ensue rapidly. If there is any reason to suspect lung injury in a blast victim (even just the presence of a ruptured eardrum), administer oxygen if possible. If possible, avoid giving oxygen under positive pressure or infusing excessive IV fluids.

Solid organs are relatively protected from shock wave injury but may be injured by secondary missiles or a hurled body. Hollow organs, however, may be injured by similar mechanisms as lung tissue. Petechiae (pinpoint hemorrhages that show up on the skin) to large hematomas (large areas of brusing) are initial signs of a primary blast injury. Perforation or rupture of the bowel and colon is a risk, although the patient may not show signs of this injury for several hours.

Neurologic injuries and head trauma are the most common causes of death from blast injuries. Subarachnoid (beneath the arachnoid layer covering the brain) and subdural (beneath the outermost covering of the brain) hematomas are often seen. Permanent or transient neurologic deficits may be secondary to concussion, intracerebral bleeding, or air embolism from lung-related injuries. Instant but transient unconsciousness, with or without retrograde amnesia, may be initiated not only by head trauma but also by cardiovascular problems. Bradycardia and hypotension are common after an intense pressure wave from an explosion.

Extremity injuries, including traumatic amputations, are common. Other injuries are often associated with tertiary blasts such as fractures, internal bleeding, abrasions, contusions, and other blunt trauma injuries. Patients with traumatic amputation by post-blast wind are likely to sustain fatal injuries secondary to the blast.

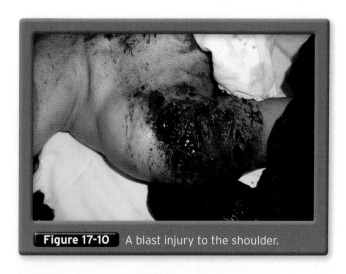

Figure 17-10   A blast injury to the shoulder.

Assessment and Management of Blast Injuries

If you witness the detonation of an explosive device, call for help while all threats are abolished. Secondary devices are a real threat and have injured and killed emergency medical responders in previous incidents throughout the world. You may only begin to approach patients once the scene is safe.

Blast injuries may not be obvious at first. As weapons increasingly take advantage of the physical properties of blast waves, be aware that a blast injury may be present in a patient whose only visible injuries are blunt trauma (bruising), penetrating trauma (bleeding, open wounds), or burns. Bleeding, loss of hearing, and ringing of the ears may be subtle signs of a blast injury, and you should continue to search for further injuries **Figure 17-10** . Remember, air-filled organs such as lungs, intestines, and inner ears are susceptible to blast injuries.

The care for blast injuries revolves around:

- Stabilizing the airway (see Chapter 13, "Basic Airway Management," and Chapter 14, "Advanced Airway Management")

- Breathing (be on guard for pneumothorax, hemothorax, flail chest, and pulmonary contusion) (see Chapter 18, "Torso Injuries")
- Circulation (be on guard for hemorrhage and shock) (see Chapter 12, "Controlling Bleeding," and Chapter 15, "Shock Management")
- Evacuation and transport is accomplished in a timely manner with stabilizing care being constantly provided.

Law Enforcement Bomb Technician

If an explosive device has been discovered, the bomb squad will be called to the scene. If an explosion occurs, you need to know how to remove the protective gear of the law enforcement bomb technician so you can assess and manage this patient. The removal process for the common SRS 5 MED ENG bomb suit, which is used extensively by FBI-certified bomb squads, is difficult and must be practiced. It is imperative that you are familiar with the equipment that is in use by the agencies that you support.

The typical law enforcement bomb technician uses a 90-lb bomb suit that requires a good deal of knowledge and strength to properly apply and remove **Figure 17-11** . These Kevlar-based, thick, heavy ballistic suits have unique neck protection assemblies, leg and groin armor, and a special air-cooled helmet with a thick, clear face shield with electrically blown air to keep the wearer cool. These garments are donned in an overlapping manner (with an assistant helping) and are designed to help protect the wearer from an explosion. They cannot be removed easily by cutting with scissors.

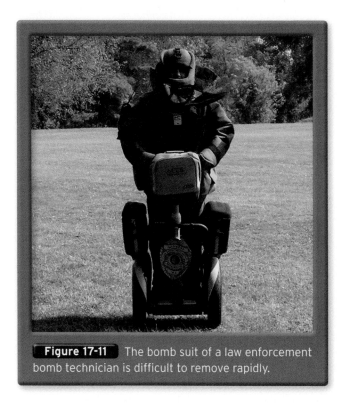

Figure 17-11 The bomb suit of a law enforcement bomb technician is difficult to remove rapidly.

When assessing a law enforcement bomb technician in a bomb suit, keep in mind these tips:

- You or your partner should stabilize the neck in a neutral, in-line position. Maintain manual in-line support throughout the assessment and management process.
- Assess the patient's airway and breathing once the clear face shield is removed. Support the patient's airway and breathing as necessary.
- After opening the suit, if you find significant bleeding from the arm(s) or leg(s), immediately apply a tourniquet.
- A team of up to six personnel may be needed to lift the law enforcement bomb technician onto a backboard or stretcher. Some agencies may use a flexible stretcher, depending on the bomb suit, and a TMP to provide manual in-line support and spinal immobilization.

Less-Lethal Weapons Injuries

Less-lethal weapons often cause minimal injury. You should manage injuries from less-lethal weapons per your agency's policies and protocols. If you are in doubt as to whether to have an injured suspect transported,

you should contact the tactical operations leader and/or the TEMS medical director.

Before assessing a suspect, hostage, or bystander, ensure that all threats are abolished. The suspect should be handcuffed by SWAT officers and thoroughly searched. If you do not witness a search for weapons, perform a search of the patient yourself. After the search, assess and manage the patient's CAB 'N.

Close-Range Impact Weapons

Close-range impact weapons, including batons, can cause contusions, soft-tissue swelling, abrasions, large lacerations, fractures, head injuries, and abdominal organ injuries. If the patient complains of abdominal pain or if there are signs of a head injury, have the patient immediately transported to the hospital for further evaluation and care. For closed soft-tissue injuries, follow the RICE mnemonic (Rest, Ice, Compression, Elevation), and for open soft-tissue injuries, stop the bleeding and dress the wound (see Chapter 21, "Soft-Tissue Injuries"). For fractures, consider splinting the injured extremity (see Chapter 20, "Extremity Injuries").

Extended-Range Impact Projectiles

Extended-range impact projectiles have the potential to cause life-threatening injuries if used at ranges closer than the manufacturer's recommended ranges or if the head, neck, or groin is struck. Most manufacturers recommend standing a minimum of 15 to 20 feet away from the intended target. Closer ranges may result in serious injuries, including the penetration of the bean bag into the body. If the bean bag or other projectile has penetrated the body, treat the projectile as an impaled object, stabilize the object, and have the patient transported to the hospital (see Chapter 21, "Soft-Tissue

At the Scene

If a TASER is used on a suspect, follow your agency's local protocols on the removal of the TASER darts. The protocols should address who is authorized to remove TASER darts and assess the suspect. Some agencies allow TMPs to remove the darts while others may require a mandatory evaluation at a hospital and the removal of the darts by a physician. When feasible, photograph the darts prior to removal to provide a visual record in the patient care report. If the darts are in a sensitive area such as the face, neck, breast, or genitalia, then the darts should be removed by a physician.

Injuries"). If the patient has contusions to the head, neck, chest, abdomen, torso, or genitals, the patient should be transported immediately to the hospital for further evaluation due to the risk of a fatal injury.

Noise-Flash Distraction Devices

Noise-flash distraction devices (NFDDs) are powerful explosive devices that can cause traumatic amputations, penetrating wounds, and burns. Fingers have been amputated and burns have occurred in the past due to unintentional discharge of these devices. Any injuries that are produced directly by these devices should be treated as blast injuries; stabilize the patient and have the patient transported to the hospital rapidly.

Less-Lethal Chemical Agents

After the release of less-lethal chemical agents (oleoresin capsicum [OC] spray, phenacyl chloride [CN], and 2-chlorobenzalmalononitrile [CS] tear gas), unprotected mucous membranes and eyes can become very irritated. If the patient's mucous membranes or eyes are red and inflamed, irrigate with water or normal saline. Adding sodium bicarbonate may hasten the rate of recovery. Brush the patient's skin off to remove any CS or CN particles.

Severe allergic reactions causing difficulty breathing are possible. Treat airway difficulties such as bronchospasm (wheezing) from a severe allergic reaction or asthma with medications per local protocols. Have the patient transported to a hospital for further evaluation and treatment.

Compressed-Air Technology

Compressed-air technology is used to launch plastic-coated .68-caliber projectiles with OC or pelargonyl vanilyamide (PAVA) capsaicin II. There are two potential effects: irritation from the chemical agent and the pain upon impact if the projectile hits the body. This impact can cause serious injury if the projectile hits the head, throat, or groin. If the patient complains of irritation, flush the skin and eyes with water. If the patient has a traumatic injury to the head, neck, or groin area or is wheezing, then have the patient transported immediately to the hospital. Fatal injuries have been reported from impacts to the eye with subsequent head trauma.

Ready for Review

- A thorough understanding of ballistics will enable you to better assess and manage ballistic injuries in the tactical environment.

- The severity of wounds depends on several factors:
  - Bullet caliber
  - Design and shape of the bullet
  - Weight of the bullet
  - Velocity
  - Type of tissue struck or impacted
  - Fragmentation of the bullet

- The signs of a ballistic wound include bleeding wounds and nearby clothing with powder stippling, powder burns, or powder tattooing.

- It is not necessary to try to determine if a wound is an entrance or exit wound. What matters is the location, size, and number of wounds.

- Ballistic wounds to the head, neck, or torso are load-and-go injuries.

- The four mechanisms of blast injury are: primary blast injuries, secondary blast injuries, tertiary blast injuries, and miscellaneous (quaternary) blast injuries.

- For blast injuries, evacuation and transport is accomplished in a timely manner with stabilizing care being constantly provided.

- Manage any injuries from less-lethal weapons per your agency's policies and protocols.

Vital Vocabulary

cavitation A temporary cavity that forms from the pressure wake from a bullet that stretches the skin and other tissues outward.

external ballistics The study of projectiles in the phase between the weapon and the intended target. This includes velocity, trajectory, and many other factors.

internal ballistics The study of projectiles and their effect on human tissue.

kinetic energy The energy of motion; this energy is transferred to anything that the projectile comes in contact with.

pulmonary blast injuries Pulmonary trauma resulting from short-range exposure to the detonation of high explosives.

shock waves Waves of pressure from muzzle velocities above 2,000 fps that precede the bullet and compress the tissue ahead of and around the bullet. Shock waves can reach pressures above 200 atmospheres.

tympanic membrane The eardrum; a thin, semitransparent membrane in the middle ear that transmits sound vibrations to the internal ear by means of the auditory ossicles.

velocity The rate of change of position or speed. Commonly measured in meters per second (m/s) or feet per second (fps).

Torso Injuries

Introduction

Given the location of the heart, lungs, and great blood vessels within the thoracic cavity, there is high potential for serious injury when the chest is injured by blunt or penetrating trauma. Any injury that interferes with the body's mechanics of normal breathing must be treated without delay to minimize or prevent permanent damage to tissues that depend on a continuous supply of oxygen. Internal bleeding is another major problem associated with chest injuries. Penetrating wounds to the thorax can result in blood from the thoracic organs or major blood vessels collecting in the thoracic cavity, compressing the lungs or heart. This may also occur when an open penetrating wound allows air to collect in the chest and prevents the lungs from expanding. Your ability to act quickly to care for patients with these injuries can be the difference between a successful outcome and death.

Extending from the diaphragm to the pelvis, the abdomen is another major body cavity that contains organs of the digestive, urinary, endocrine, and genitourinary systems. Although any of these organs can be injured, some organs are better protected than others. In civilian traumatic emergencies, unrecognized injuries to the abdomen are a leading cause of traumatic death. Maintain a high index of suspicion if there is a mechanism of injury (MOI) that suggests abdominal injury.

Load-and-Go Injuries to the Chest

In the tactical environment, the MOI is often known because injuries are witnessed either by a SWAT officer or a nearby TMP. Whether the patient is a neutralized armed suspect or a downed SWAT officer in full gear who was stabbed by a suspect, all threats must be abolished before you can provide stabilizing care **Figure 18-1** . Once the scene is safe or the patient has been brought to you at a site of relative safety, you will expose the patient's chest during the circulation phase of Call-A-CAB 'N Go to check for the presence of potentially life-threatening injuries to the front and back of the patient's body **Table 18-1** . You only have time to initiate stabilizing care (stop the bleeding, maintain an open airway, support breathing), while expediting rapid evacuation to an ALS ground or air ambulance to transport the patient to the hospital.

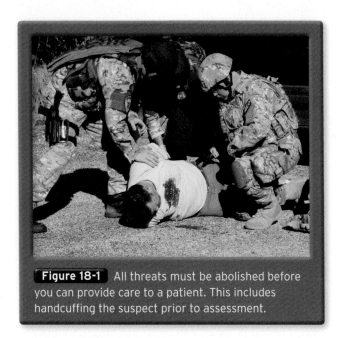

Figure 18-1 All threats must be abolished before you can provide care to a patient. This includes handcuffing the suspect prior to assessment.

Table 18-1	Load-and-Go Injuries to the Chest

- Penetrating trauma (knife, bullet, shrapnel) to the chest or torso
- Major blunt trauma to the chest
- Open pneumothorax
- Tension pneumothorax
- Flail chest

Penetrating Wounds and Major Blunt Trauma to the Chest

Due to improvements in ballistic vest design and more frequent use, the incidence of penetrating chest trauma to law enforcement officers has decreased. However, occasionally a bullet or a knife does penetrate the chest. There may be little or no bleeding from a small caliber bullet or a tiny 3-mm piece of shrapnel, yet the SWAT officer could die within minutes if that object struck a large blood vessel or vital organ such as the heart **Figure 18-2**. Although damage to the tissues usually occurs instantly, the signs and symptoms associated with the trauma may take time to develop as the damaged vessels continue to bleed.

Blunt trauma can cause chest contusions and fractured ribs. Fractured ribs in turn can damage the lungs and result in life-threatening complications such as pneumothorax, hemothorax, or tension pneumothorax. When blunt trauma occurs to the chest, the patient may have multiple rib fractures, flail chest, pulmonary contusions, and cardiac contusions even though there may be no visible injuries. Be sure to keep these complications in mind.

Important signs and symptoms of chest injury include:

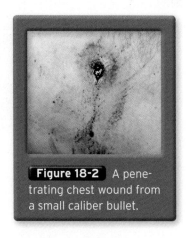

Figure 18-2 A penetrating chest wound from a small caliber bullet.

- Pain at the site of injury
- Pain localized at the site of injury that is aggravated by or increased with breathing
- Bruising to the chest wall
- Crepitus with palpation of the chest
- Puncture wounds
- Dyspnea (difficulty breathing, shortness of breath)
- Hemoptysis (coughing up blood)
- Failure of one or both sides of the chest to expand normally with inspiration
- Rapid, weak pulse and low blood pressure
- Cyanosis around the lips or fingernails

While you are assessing a downed SWAT officer's circulation, expose the chest by loosening or removing the ballistic vest if it is safe to do so. Lift the patient's arms and search the armpits and lateral chest, as these are not fully protected by ballistic armor. If there is any possibility of further gunfire or shrapnel, replace the SWAT officer's ballistic vest as quickly as possible after your rapid inspection for wounds. If the suspect is down and there are no known or suspected threats, ask SWAT officers to assist you in fully removing the downed SWAT officer's gear and ballistic vest.

Always inspect the patient's chest rapidly but thoroughly in the tactical environment **Figure 18-3**. When you are rapidly examining the exposed chest, look for shallow and difficult breathing, a cut or small hole with blood, bruising, cyanosis, or signs of shock. Look and listen for holes with air and blood being sucked in and out of the chest wall, indicating an open pneumothorax that needs to be sealed (discussed in detail later in the chapter). Look at both sides of the chest, log rolling the patient onto his or her side to inspect the back. If both sides of the chest have been punctured by a bullet or knife, then both lungs may be collapsed. Control any bleeding with direct pressure and a compression dressing.

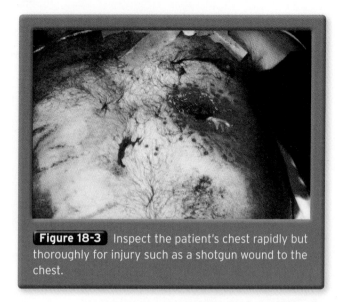

Figure 18-3 Inspect the patient's chest rapidly but thoroughly for injury such as a shotgun wound to the chest.

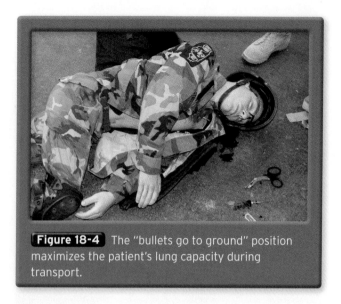

Figure 18-4 The "bullets go to ground" position maximizes the patient's lung capacity during transport.

Penetrating objects embedded in the patient should not be removed. Stabilize the object in place to minimize movement until it can be removed by surgeons at the hospital.

Next, ensure that your patient maintains a patent airway. If the patient is talking, then the patient has a patent airway. When available and if needed, use high-flow oxygen by mask or nasal cannula to maintain good oxygenation.

Check the patient's breathing. If needed, support the patient's ventilations with a bag-mask device or through more advanced methods such as intubation. Finally, perform a rapid neurologic exam. A penetrating chest injury is a load-and-go injury, so rapidly evacuate the patient to an ALS-level ambulance.

Patients with penetrating injuries to one side of the chest should be positioned on the stretcher on their side with the injured side of the chest toward the ground without blocking any chest seals, known as the "bullets to the ground position" **Figure 18-4** . This will increase the blood flow through the good lung (the only lung likely still working). This position also lessens the risk of aspiration from vomiting.

If you are permitted to accompany the patient during transport, perform a secondary assessment if time and conditions allow, ideally exposing and examining the entire body for additional wounds. Occasionally a patient with additional gunshot wounds may report no other pain or symptoms and, during a rapid examination in the tactical environment, you may miss a small nonbleeding wound from a shotgun, shrapnel, or knife that is a half-inch in size.

An IV (or two) should be started and fluid administered per your local protocols. Be aware that over-infusing IV fluids can cause clotting factors in the blood to be diluted and other coagulation problems, along with an elevated blood pressure that worsens internal bleeding. IV administration will usually not begin until the patient is on the way to the hospital; however, if there is a delay in the extraction or transport of the patient, then an IV may be started in the tactical environment if the TMP has the appropriate level of training.

During transport, continually reassess and monitor the patient to ensure that a penetrating wound has not become a tension pneumothorax. Monitor the patient for potential complications including pneumothorax, hemothorax, pulmonary contusion, myocardial contusion, and cardiac tamponade.

Complications of Penetrating Wounds and Major Blunt Trauma to the Chest

Pneumothorax

In any chest injury, damage to the heart, lungs, great vessels, and other organs in the chest can be complicated by the accumulation of air in the pleural space. This is a dangerous condition called a **pneumothorax** (commonly called a collapsed lung). In this condition, air enters through a hole in the chest wall or the surface of the lung as the patient attempts to breathe, causing the lung on that side to collapse **Figure 18-5** . As a result, any blood that passes through the collapsed portion of the lung is not oxygenated, and hypoxia can develop. If the lung is collapsed past 30% to 40%, you may hear diminished breath sounds on that side of the chest. Absent breath sounds are a significant finding in chest trauma and may indicate the development of a tension

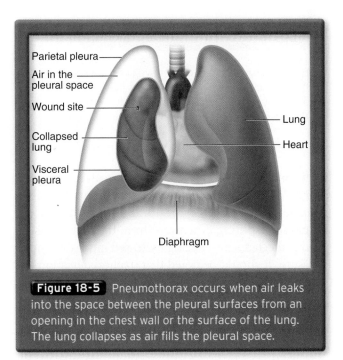

Figure 18-5 Pneumothorax occurs when air leaks into the space between the pleural surfaces from an opening in the chest wall or the surface of the lung. The lung collapses as air fills the pleural space.

Labels in figure: Parietal pleura, Air in the pleural space, Wound site, Collapsed lung, Visceral pleura, Diaphragm, Lung, Heart

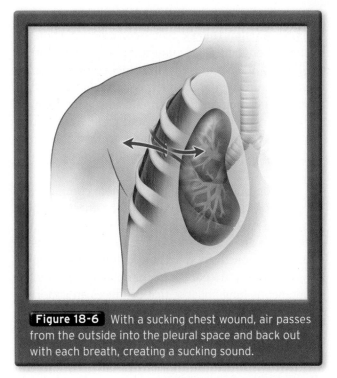

Figure 18-6 With a sucking chest wound, air passes from the outside into the pleural space and back out with each breath, creating a sucking sound.

pneumothorax, discussed later. Depending on the size of the hole and the rate at which air fills the cavity, the lung may collapse in a few seconds or a few hours. In the uncommon situation when a large enough hole is made in the chest wall, you may actually hear a sucking sound as the patient inhales and the sound of rushing air as he or she exhales. For this reason an **open pneumothorax** is also called a **sucking chest wound** **Figure 18-6**. In the tactical environment, an open pneumothorax is caused by a penetrating thoracic injury such as a shotgun blast at close range or a large knife wound. Fortunately, most gunshot wounds to the chest result in bullet holes that are too small to create an open pneumothorax.

During exhalation, you may see blood and air bubbling at the site of the chest wound. Due to the decreased ability to oxygenate and ventilate, the patient will experience tachycardia, tachypnea, and restlessness.

An open pneumothorax is a load-and-go emergency requiring immediate stabilizing medical care and evacuation to emergency transport. Stabilizing care of an open pneumothorax consists of placing an occlusive dressing or a commercial chest seal over the hole that will prevent air from entering the chest, but still allow air to easily exit the pleural space through the chest hole. This will allow air in the chest to escape and decrease the likelihood of the formation of a tension pneumothorax (discussed later in this chapter).

The application of an occlusive dressing or commercial dressing may be performed en route to the hospital or in the tactical environment if the evacuation is delayed. To seal an open pneumothorax, follow these steps:

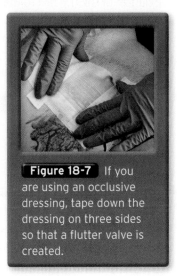

Figure 18-7 If you are using an occlusive dressing, tape down the dressing on three sides so that a flutter valve is created.

1. Ensure proper PPE for yourself and any SWAT officer or TMP nearby.
2. Prepare your equipment.
3. Clean the area around the wound. Avoid wiping or allowing any foreign debris into the wound.
4. If you are using a commercial chest seal, follow the manufacturer's directions. Ideally the contact adhesive will keep the seal in place. If not, consider using additional tape and/or dressings to keep the chest seal in position.
5. If you are using an occlusive dressing, tape down the dressing on three sides so that a flutter valve is created **Figure 18-7**. Follow your local protocols when applying and sealing an occlusive dressing.
6. Watch for the development of a tension pneumothorax or an inadequate seal as well as the need for needle decompression or assisted ventilation.

Tension Pneumothorax

Tension pneumothorax can occur when there is significant ongoing air accumulation in the pleural space **Figure 18-8** . This air gradually increases the pressure in the chest, causing the complete collapse of the affected lung and pushing the mediastinum (the central part of the chest containing the heart and great vessels) into the opposite pleural cavity. This prevents blood from returning through the venae cavae to the heart and can cause shock and cardiac arrest.

Tension pneumothorax occurs more commonly as a result of a closed, blunt injury to the chest in which a fractured rib lacerates a lung or bronchus. It may also occur with an open chest injury when the occlusive dressing is applied incorrectly or malfunctions, trapping air in the pleural space. Any penetrating wound or spontaneous lung collapse that produces an abnormal passageway for gas exchange into the pleural space may produce a tension pneumothorax.

The common signs and symptoms of tension pneumothorax include increasing respiratory distress, altered levels of consciousness, distended neck veins, deviation of the trachea to the side of the chest opposite the tension pneumothorax, tachycardia, low blood pressure, cyanosis, and decreased breath sounds on the side of the pneumothorax. Some of these signs and symptoms may be difficult to assess in the tactical

Medical Gear

Athletic SWAT officers often have chest walls with thick musculature, so short needles may not be long enough to reach the pleural cavity. TMPs with ALS training should carry 3.5-inch or longer over-the-needle catheters.

environment. You may encounter greater resistance when ventilating the patient with a bag-mask device. Another sign is a tight, rigid abdomen due to the diaphragm shifting downward from the high pressure on the affected side, causing increased intra-abdominal pressure. It should be noted that tracheal deviation is a late sign and rarely seen.

Treating a tension pneumothorax requires the use of ALS procedures. If you do not have the necessary ALS training to perform these skills, call for a TMP who does. A needle decompression is required to relieve the building pressure within the thoracic cavity. This procedure may be performed in the tactical environment to stabilize the patient for evacuation or during transport.

To perform a needle decompression, follow these steps:

1. Prepare and assemble the necessary equipment.
2. Identify the landmarks and decide where to place the needle.
3. Use alcohol, Betadine, or another agent to prep the site.
4. Select the appropriate site: midclavicular, second intercostal space, above the third rib; or, less commonly, at the midaxillary line, above the fifth or sixth rib. Go over the rib to avoid the neurovascular bundle located under each rib that contains the intercostal artery, vein, and nerve **Figure 18-9** .
5. Select the largest appropriate needle and plastic catheter. Attach it to a syringe with a few milliliters of saline so the bubbles are visible when aspirating during the insertion.
6. Insert the needle at a 90-degree angle over the

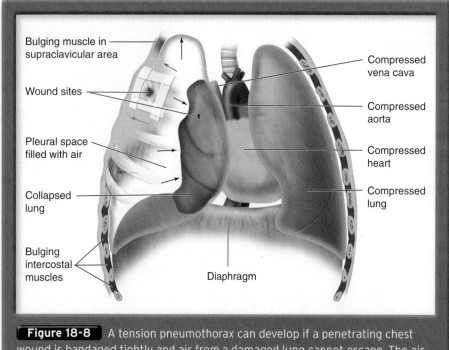

Bulging muscle in supraclavicular area

Wound sites

Pleural space filled with air

Collapsed lung

Bulging intercostal muscles

Compressed vena cava

Compressed aorta

Compressed heart

Compressed lung

Diaphragm

Figure 18-8   A tension pneumothorax can develop if a penetrating chest wound is bandaged tightly and air from a damaged lung cannot escape. The air then accumulates in the pleural space, eventually causing compression of the heart and great vessels.

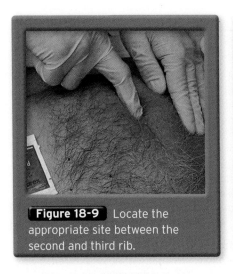

Figure 18-9 Locate the appropriate site between the second and third rib.

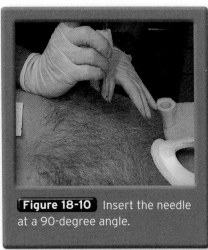

Figure 18-10 Insert the needle at a 90-degree angle.

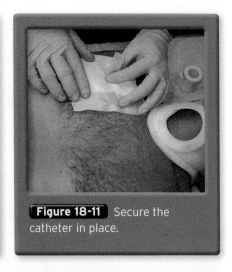

Figure 18-11 Secure the catheter in place.

rib, directed slightly laterally laterally away from the heart **Figure 18-10**.

7. Listen for a rush of air or look for bubbles in the syringe; allow the high-pressure air within the chest to escape and neutralize the pressure.
8. Advance the catheter over the needle and secure it in place **Figure 18-11**.
9. Use a one-way flutter valve or commercial device such as the Asherman chest seal. This will prevent or minimize reentry of air into the pleural space.
10. Dispose of the needles and all other sharps in a sharps container.
11. During transport, closely monitor the patient's vital signs, oxygen saturation, and lung compliance.
12. Be prepared to repeat decompression if the catheter becomes kinked/bent, becomes clogged with blood, or otherwise malfunctions.
13. Consider bilateral emergency needle decompressions per your local protocols if the tension pneumothorax is not decompressed.
14. Notify the trauma team and/or emergency physician upon arrival of this injury and treatment rendered.

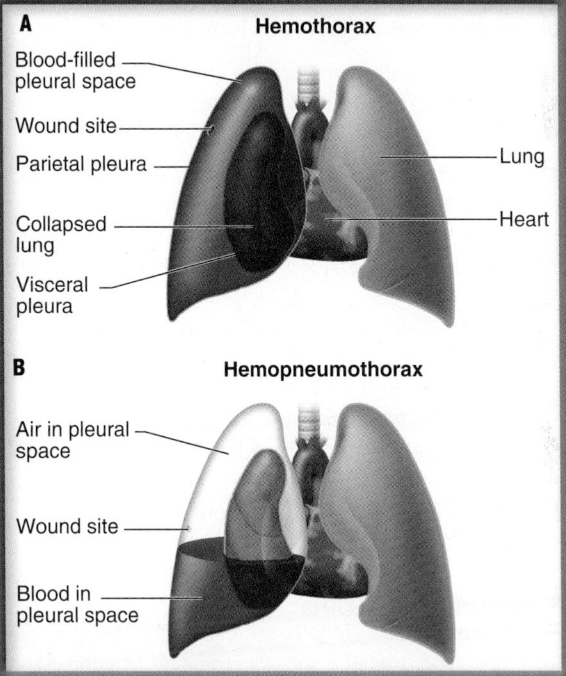

Figure 18-12 **A.** A hemothorax is a collection of blood in the pleural space produced by bleeding within the chest. **B.** When both blood and air are present, the condition is a hemopneumothorax.

Special Populations

In pediatric patients, if there is penetration of the chest wall below the nipples, or below the scapula, anticipate abdominal injury as well as tension pneumothorax. While gathering medical intelligence, if you discover that infants or children are involved in the callout, include a 14- or 16-gauge over-the-needle catheter and a 30-mL syringe in case you need to perform a needle thoracostomy.

Hemothorax

In blunt and penetrating chest injuries, blood can collect in the pleural space from bleeding vessels from the rib cage, lungs, heart, or great vessels resulting in **hemothorax** **Figure 18-12A**. If the patient has signs and symptoms of shock, increased respiratory distress, and decreased breath sounds on the affected side during the secondary assessment, these are indications that the thorax has blood present and that the lung may be

Chest Tube Insertion

Patients with a pneumothorax, tension pneumothorax, hemothorax, or hemopneumothorax ultimately may need a chest tube inserted. A chest tube is a flexible plastic tube that is inserted through the side of the chest into the pleural space. It is used to remove air, blood, pus, or other fluids from the pleural cavity. Patient survival is improved once the lung has the room to properly ventilate.

In some systems a TEMS unit physician may place a chest tube if transportation is not available, if evacuation is delayed for other reasons, or if a patient's condition is deteriorating despite all other measures. The majority of TMPs are not authorized to perform this procedure. However, TMPs may gain an awareness of the essential facts about this procedure and how to possibly assist a physician if permitted by local protocols.

The procedure for insertion of a chest tube begins with collecting the needed equipment (often packaged together as a "tray" or chest tube kit):

- Standard precaution equipment, including sterile gloves
- Scalpel
- Chest tube(s): 36F to 40F for adults, smaller sizes for pediatrics
- Kelly clamps, size large (one curved and one straight)
- Suturing material—size 2-0 silk on a straight needle is preferable (× 4)
- Chlorhexidine 2% or Betadine skin prep
- A local anesthetic if the patient is awake
- A fluid collection device with a one-way valve that allows air and blood to flow out of the chest into a chest seal or other device; if not available, an indwelling urinary catheter bag with a one-way valve may be used
- Sterile petroleum jelly occlusive dressing
- Tape and dressing supplies to cover the chest tube insertion site
- Mechanical suction device to generate negative pressure in order to withdraw air and blood from inside the pleural space

To insert the chest tube, the medical provider first selects the appropriate site: the midaxillary over the fifth rib (under the armpit). The equipment for the procedure is arranged. The indwelling catheter bag or the collection device is connected to the distal end of the one-way valve with a rubber band. The site is cleansed with the appropriate aseptic technique. The area of insertion is anesthetized if the patient is conscious and time permits. The distal end of the chest tube is clamped with a large clamp (such as a Kelly clamp) and the proximal end of the tube is clamped with a curved clamp.

A transverse incision is made about 1 inch over the fifth rib in the midaxillary line. If the patient has fractured ribs at that location, then the midclavicular line is used. The medical provider tunnels over the fifth rib with a large curved clamp, pushing through the pleural tissue in a controlled matter so as to not accidently puncture the heart or liver, spreads the clamp, and leaves it in place **Figure 18-13**. If sterile gloves are without contamination, then the medical provider places one small finger inside the chest and palpates to verify that the chest wall pleural tissue is punctured and the tube can be placed inside the pleural space.

The medical provider grasps the clamp attached to the end of the chest tube and advances it through the space created by the first clamp, directing it posteriorly and upwards toward the top of the chest **Figure 18-14**. The upper clamp is removed and the tube is advanced to the predetermined mark indicated on the tube, at least 5 cm beyond the last hole.

An assistant holds the outer portion of the chest tube and connects the collection device, then removes the distal clamp and applies suction. The medical provider sutures and ties the tube in place and closes the wound with suture material **Figure 18-15**. The depth of the tube is documented in the patient's record and the tube is marked with a felt-tip permanent marker as a reference point where it enters the skin. The insertion site is covered with an occlusive petroleum-gauze dressing and reinforced on all connections with tape.

displaced or compressed by this blood. In the tactical setting, it may be too noisy or chaotic to detect breath sounds using a stethoscope. Because the bleeding is typically caused by significant trauma within the chest cavity, there is virtually no practical way to control the bleeding in the prehospital setting. The only medical provider who can fully treat this condition is a surgeon.

If both air and blood are present in the pleural space, this is called a **hemopneumothorax** **Figure 18-12B**. Again, because the injury has occurred within the

walls of the chest, the treatment involves providing rapid transport to the nearest facility capable of performing surgery. If the bleeding is massive, it can shift the mediastinum; therefore, you should closely watch these patients for the development of tension hemothorax or tension hemopneumothorax.

Managing a hemothorax requires the use of ALS procedure. If you do not have the ALS training to perform these skills, call for a TMP or evacuate the patient to a civilian EMS ambulance staffed by an ALS-level crew.

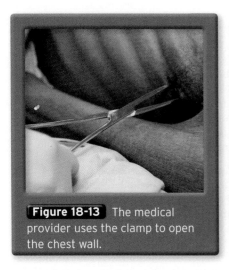

Figure 18-13 The medical provider uses the clamp to open the chest wall.

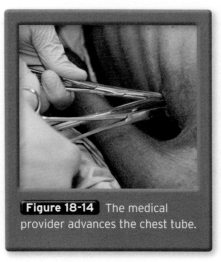

Figure 18-14 The medical provider advances the chest tube.

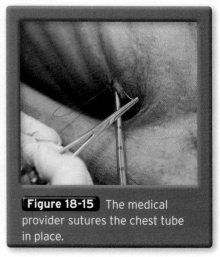

Figure 18-15 The medical provider sutures the chest tube in place.

If you are permitted to accompany the patient during transport, apply high-flow oxygen to the patient and start an IV per the permissive hypotension principles (keep the blood pressure at 90 mm Hg systolic or lower). Monitor the patient for signs of tension pneumothorax.

Pericardial Tamponade

Pericardial tamponade usually occurs from a penetrating injury to the tissues near the heart or to the heart muscle itself. It can also be caused by blunt force to the chest **Figure 18-16** . Pericardial tamponade occurs when the protective membrane around the heart, the pericardial sac, fills with blood or fluid, perhaps from a torn or lacerated coronary artery or vein. As the fluid volume increases, the heart is less able to fill with blood. As a result, the heart cannot pump an adequate amount of blood and the patient experiences a decrease in systemic blood flow.

Signs and symptoms of pericardial tamponade include the presence of a penetrating wound near the heart or over the heart, shock, and distention of the jugular veins. This is a load-and-go injury. Stabilize the patient's circulation, airway, and breathing and rapidly evacuate the patient to an ALS-level ambulance.

If you are permitted to accompany the patient during transport, you may hear faint or muffled heart tones with a stethoscope during the secondary assessment. There is often a narrowed pulse pressure (smaller difference between systolic and diastolic blood pressure). The cardiac monitor in the ambulance will often show pulseless electrical activity (PEA) with a sinus tachycardia of 120 to 150 beats per minute and rarely may show electrical alternans (alternating big and small QRS complexes on the cardiac monitor) every other heartbeat. **Beck's triad** is a collection of three signs associated with pericardial tamponade: low blood pressure; jugular venous distention; and distant, muffled heart sounds.

The treatment of a patient with pericardial tamponade begins by ensuring adequate oxygen delivery and establishing IV access. The patient should be transported rapidly to a trauma center for **pericardiocentesis**.

If the patient goes into cardiac arrest during transport, begin CPR with chest compressions per local protocols. The chest compressions may have a desired

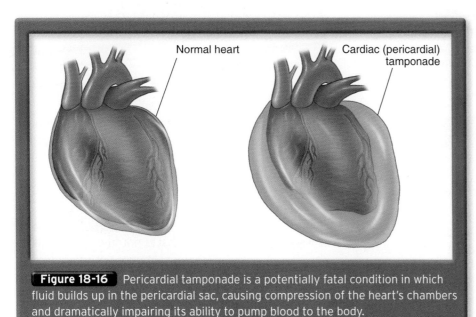

Figure 18-16 Pericardial tamponade is a potentially fatal condition in which fluid builds up in the pericardial sac, causing compression of the heart's chambers and dramatically impairing its ability to pump blood to the body.

Normal heart

Cardiac (pericardial) tamponade

Pericardiocentesis

In certain regions, a physician may be permitted by the medical director to perform pericardiocentesis. Knowing the general technique may enable the entire TEMS unit to assist in an emergency pericardiocentesis. As always, follow your local protocols.

The equipment needed for this procedure includes:

- PPE including eye protection, mask to cover mouth and nose, and gloves
- A cardiac monitor and defibrillator are highly desirable but are not mandatory.
- Pericardiocentesis kit including a large-bore plastic catheter
- 50-mL Luer lock syringe
- Chlorhexidine 2%, Betadine, or alcohol pads
- Sterile towels, drapes, sterile gloves, and other items for aseptic technique are ideal.
- If available, use of prehospital ultrasound imaging is diagnostic and can help determine the best insertion point for the pericardiocentesis. If possible, the entire procedure is performed under ultrasound guidance.

This emergency procedure will likely be performed in the back of a moving ambulance on a patient with a knife or gunshot wound near the mid-chest who has recently been injured and has lost his or her pulse. The medical provider will prepare the equipment and obtain baseline vital signs, including pulse oximetry. The patient is placed into a supine position, with the head of the stretcher elevated 20 to 30 degrees as tolerated. The medical provider premedicates the patient per local protocol or online medical control. All providers don masks, gowns, hair covers, and sterile gloves. The site is cleansed with appropriate aseptic technique and, if possible, the area is draped.

The medical provider identifies the needle entry site. It is preferable to insert the needle at the left parasternal site at the fourth interspace or insert directly below the xiphoid—approximately 1 cm left of midline. If an ultrasound image is visualized of the left parasternal view of the heart, then this point of skin is the ideal place to insert the needle as it has a lower complication rate and a higher procedure success rate. The area is infiltrated with 1% lidocaine into the skin and deeper tissues if the patient is conscious.

The medical provider attaches the large needle to the 30- or 60-cc syringe, and with 2 to 3 mL of air in the syringe inserts the needle into the skin and advances the needle tip about 1 cm toward the heart, then ejects the potential skin plug out of the large needle with the 3 mL of air. The left parasternal approach should be downwards toward the pericardial fluid. The subxiphoid approach should be done at a 30-degree angle directed toward the left shoulder blade **Figure 18-17**.

The medical provider gently aspirates while inserting the needle **Figure 18-18**. Some resistance may be felt as the needle enters the pericardial sac. *If the needle is advanced too far, the myocardium will become irritated. The needle may vibrate with the pulse. The needle should be pulled back slightly until fluid can be aspirated.* If blood is withdrawn and placed in an open container, it usually does not clot unless the rate of bleeding is significant. A sample can be placed into the collection container and transported with the patient.

A TMP may continue chest compressions and routine CPR until immediately before the actual needle is introduced. CPR ceases during the actual procedure. After 30 seconds of attempted aspiration, the medical provider may stop the procedure briefly for a minute of CPR by the TMP.

The medical provider may administer medications per protocol or online medical control. The patient is reassessed and monitored for postprocedure complications during the remaining travel time to the hospital.

Medical Gear

Portable Ultrasound

Although not currently in widespread use, a portable ultrasound is a useful diagnostic instrument. A portable ultrasound can be used to help diagnose intra-abdominal bleeding, cardiac tamponade, hemothorax, pneumothorax, and tension pneumothorax. In the future, this useful tool may be used more often in the tactical environment to aid in rapid assessment as the price and physical size of the portable units decrease.

effect of squeezing out pericardial fluid and blood, allowing increased cardiac filling and an improved blood pressure during transport.

Flail Chest

Flail chest occurs when three or more adjacent ribs are fractured in at least two places **Figure 18-19**. The result is a segment of chest wall that is not in continuity with the thorax. The flail segment moves with paradoxical (opposite) motion relative to the rest of the chest wall. When the patient inhales, the flail chest section will

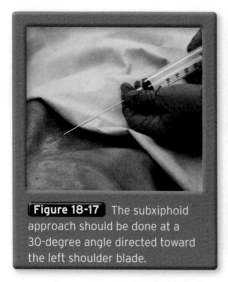

Figure 18-17 The subxiphoid approach should be done at a 30-degree angle directed toward the left shoulder blade.

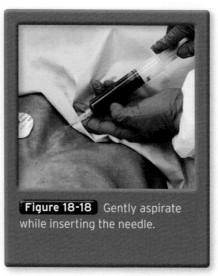

Figure 18-18 Gently aspirate while inserting the needle.

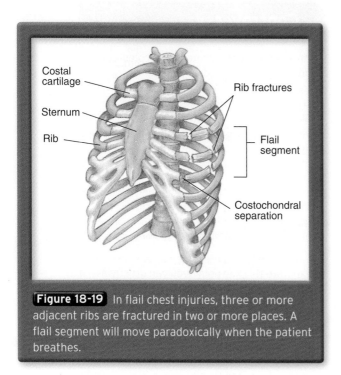

Costal cartilage

Sternum

Rib

Rib fractures

Flail segment

Costochondral separation

Figure 18-19 In flail chest injuries, three or more adjacent ribs are fractured in two or more places. A flail segment will move paradoxically when the patient breathes.

movement of chest wall due to increased pain with breathing), shallow breathing, agitation/anxiety (hypoxia) or lethargy (due to hypercarbia, a buildup of excess carbon dioxide), tachycardia, and cyanosis (bluish skin).

After stabilizing the patient's circulation and airway, assess the patient's ability to breathe. Consider placing your hand over the injured chest area to assess and minimize the movement of the chest wall by preventing it from moving in and out. Simply press gently and stabilize the flail segment to decrease the pain of breathing and encourage the patient to take slow, deep breaths. Stabilizing the moving section decreases pain and increases the efficiency of breathing. If you have ALS training and it is permitted under local protocols, consider administering pain medication. Once the patient is stabilized, rapidly evacuate the patient to an ALS-level ambulance.

If you are permitted to accompany the patient during transport to the hospital, perform a rapid secondary assessment. Initiate IV fluids to maintain permissive hypotension. Monitor oxygen saturation, vital signs, and cardiac rhythm. Be alert for development of tension pneumothorax, hemothorax, or respiratory failure secondary to a pulmonary contusion associated with the flail chest.

For large flail chest segments (five or more ribs adjacent, each fractured in two places), if the patient's breathing is significantly compromised by an underlying pulmonary contusion and other injuries, consider assisting ventilations by using a bag-mask device during spontaneous inspirations and consider providing CPAP (continuous positive airway pressure) mask assistance.

Pulmonary Contusion

Pulmonary contusion (bruising of the lung) is a serious chest injury produced by blunt and penetrating trauma **Figure 18-20** . Examples include major trauma from a motor vehicle collision, blast injury from close proximity to an explosion, and high-velocity gunshot wounds. Severe pulmonary contusions should always be suspected in patients with a flail chest. Pulmonary contusion is a potentially lethal chest injury, as the pulmonary alveoli of the bruised lung tissue become filled with blood and fluid accumulates in the injured area, leaving the patient hypoxic. Hypoxia and carbon dioxide retention lead to respiratory distress, dyspnea, tachypnea, agitation, and

become a depression while the remainder of the chest wall expands as normal.

The blunt trauma force necessary to produce this injury also will often bruise and damage the underlying lung tissue, and this pulmonary contusion may also contribute to hypoxia. Patients with flail chest are at risk for development of hemothorax or pneumothorax and may be in marked respiratory distress. In addition, pain from movement of the chest wall injury exacerbates the already impaired respirations from the paradoxical motion and the underlying lung contusion.

The signs and symptoms of flail chest include complaints of pain, splinting (limited voluntary

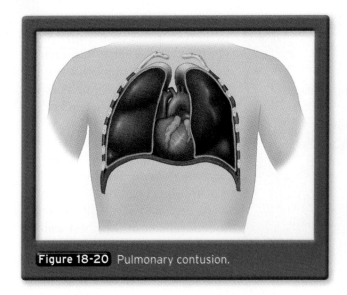

Figure 18-20   Pulmonary contusion.

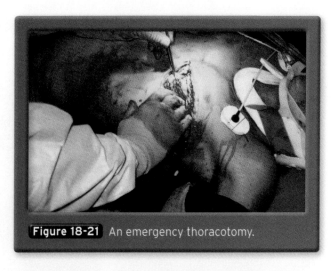

Figure 18-21   An emergency thoracotomy.

restlessness. Complications may include pneumonia and pulmonary infarct (tissue death). The patient may present with hemoptysis (coughing up blood) or paradoxical motion of the chest. You may hear wheezes, crackles, or rales. After stabilizing the patient's circulation and airway, consider providing ventilatory assistance with a bag-mask device or advanced airway measures such as intubation. Rapidly evacuate the patient to an ALS-level ambulance for transport to the hospital.

Myocardial Contusion

Blunt trauma to the chest may injure the heart itself, causing **myocardial contusion**, or bruising of the heart muscle. You should suspect myocardial contusion in all cases of severe blunt injury to the chest. Check the patient's pulse carefully and note any irregularities (from abnormal rhythms or arrhythmias). There is no specific prehospital treatment for this condition, but the patient is at risk for lethal arrhythmias (rare) and worsening cardiovascular status. After stabilizing the patient's circulation, airway, and breathing, rapidly evacuate the patient to an ALS-level ambulance.

If you are permitted to accompany the patient during transport, perform a secondary assessment and note any deterioration in blood pressure because this can be a direct result of the injury to the myocardium. Often the patient's signs and symptoms can mimic a heart attack where the patient may complain of chest pain or discomfort that is similar in nature to cardiac symptoms. You should utilize an ECG to determine the patient's heart rhythm and continuously monitor the patient's cardiac activity. Prehospital ultrasound, if available, can show the overall cardiac activity, heart wall motion defects, and possible presence of pericardial

Controversy

An emergency thoracotomy is a complex medical procedure performed by emergency physicians and trauma surgeons in the hospital. In essence, the chest is opened up so the surgeon can stop the internal hemorrhaging by repairing the heart or major blood vessels   Figure 18-21 . This procedure is dependent upon having multiple highly trained and certified medical providers and the proper specialized and sterilized medical equipment. It is *rarely* performed in the prehospital setting. Although controversial, there are some TEMS units who choose to carry the necessary equipment and remain prepared to perform an emergency thoracotomy in the field.

This procedure is presented briefly below to further illustrate this key point: you can greatly assist in the care of a downed SWAT officer by removing the downed SWAT officer's ballistic vests, equipment, and exposing the chest completely during transport to the hospital. This will save precious moments in the emergency department. By removing all gear and exposing the patient's chest, an emergency thoracotomy can be performed immediately if indicated.

During an emergency thoracotomy the patient is intubated, the physician uses a scalpel and scissors to slice open the left side of the chest, exposes the heart and lungs, then uses rib spreaders to enlarge the opening. The physician then cuts open the pericardium vertically and exposes the heart. Simultaneously, an open heart massage is provided while major bleeds in the heart or large blood vessels are found and repaired. If the patient develops a spontaneous heartbeat and blood pressure, then the patient will be taken to the operating room for further repair and closure of the chest. If not, then the patient is pronounced dead after a reasonable amount of effort.

Table 18-2	Load-and-Go Injuries to the Torso

- Penetrating wound to the abdomen, pelvis, or buttocks
- Tender, distended abdomen
- Pelvic instability

tamponade. Follow local protocols for management of arrhythmia should one develop.

Load-and-Go Injuries to the Abdomen

Abdominal trauma can occur from blunt and penetrating trauma. In the tactical environment, blunt trauma most often occurs from assaults, falls, motor vehicle collisions, or explosions. Penetrating trauma to the abdomen can be caused by many different objects such as knives, bullets, or improvised weapons (shanks, screwdrivers). Patients can die within minutes if one of the major blood vessels is struck. Patients can hemorrhage internally more than 2000 mL without any major external signs other than pain and mild distention of the abdomen, and can die within 10 to 20 minutes. Therefore, if the patient has any sign of a penetrating wound to the torso (abdomen, pelvis, or buttocks), this is a load-and-go indication Table 18-2 . A SWAT officer with a gunshot wound to the aorta may initially be awake, talking, and walking, but within 10 minutes may be in shock and soon dead.

Blunt Trauma

Blunt trauma to the abdomen results from compression or deceleration forces and can often lead to a **closed abdominal injury**—one in which soft-tissue damage occurs inside the body but the skin remains intact. When assessing the abdominal cavity in a patient who has received blunt trauma, consider three common MOIs: shearing, crushing, and compression.

In the rapid deceleration of a patient during a motor vehicle crash or fall from a height, a shearing force can be created as the internal organs continue their forward motion. This will cause hollow, solid, and visceral organs and vascular structures to tear, especially at their points of attachment to the abdominal wall. Organs that shear or tear include the liver, kidneys, small and large intestines, and spleen. In motor vehicle collisions, this MOI has been described as the third collision (eg, first, the car into the wall; then the patient into the steering column; and third, the internal organs into the patient's inner rib cage).

Crush injuries are the result of external factors at the time of impact; they differ from deceleration injuries occurring before impact. When abdominal contents are crushed between the anterior abdominal wall and the spinal column (or other structures in the rear), crushing occurs. Solid organs like the kidneys, liver, and spleen are at the greatest risk of injury from this mechanism. Direct application of crushing forces to the abdomen would come from things like the dashboard or front hood of a car (in a vehicle collision) or from falling objects.

The last MOI to consider is a compression injury resulting from a direct blow or external compression from a fixed object (such as a lap belt). These compression forces will deform hollow organs, increasing the pressure within the abdominal cavity. This dramatic change in abdominal pressure can cause a rupture of the small intestine or diaphragm. Rupture of organs can lead to uncontrollable hemorrhage.

Any patient with abdominal pain after a significant MOI should be considered a load-and-go patient, especially if signs of shock are noted. During your rapid assessment of the patient's circulation, airway, breathing, and neurologic status, you may also find an absence of peripheral and central pulses, tachycardia, pale and moist skin, and an altered level of consciousness. Rapidly evacuate the patient to an ALS-level ambulance for transport.

If you are permitted to accompany the patient during transport, perform a rapid secondary assessment. Provide supplemental oxygen by nonrebreathing mask and treat for shock. The biggest concern in patients with closed abdominal injuries is that you cannot know the true extent of the injury. For this reason, the patient requires expedient transport to the nearest and highest level of care available, primarily a trauma center with a surgeon.

Penetrating Trauma

Penetrating trauma results from gunshot or stab wounds Figure 18-22 . Penetrating trauma causes an **open abdominal injury**—one in which a break in the surface of the skin or mucous membrane exposes deeper tissue to potential contamination. In general, gunshot wounds cause more

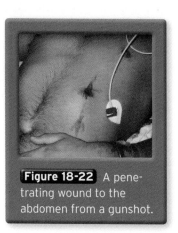

Figure 18-22 A penetrating wound to the abdomen from a gunshot.

injury than stab wounds because bullets travel deeper into the body and have more kinetic energy. Gunshot wounds most commonly involve injury to the small bowel, colon, liver, and vascular structures; the extent of injury is less predictable than for stab wounds because gunshot wounds depend mostly on the characteristics of the weapon and the bullet. In penetrating trauma from stab wounds, the liver, small bowel, diaphragm, and colon are the organs most frequently injured.

The extent of damage from a penetrating injury depends on which area of the body is injured, the mechanism of injury, and the amount of kinetic energy imparted to the involved tissues over a given time period. The permanent injury as well as the temporary injury from the track of the projectile can be considerable with high-velocity penetrations. The velocity delivered during penetrating trauma is typically divided into three levels: low velocity, such as from a knife, bayonet, or ice pick; medium velocity, such as from a handgun, 9-mm gun, or shotgun; and high velocity, such as from a high-powered sporting rifle or military assault rifle (M-16, AK-74). Projectile velocity is only one of many factors that can affect the seriousness of an injury.

Ballistics affect abdominal trauma greatly. Shrapnel wounds may be low, medium, or high velocity, depending on the distance of the patient from the blast. Consider the trajectory and distance of the bullet. The bullet may pass through numerous structures in various body locations. For example, penetrating trauma in the gluteal area is associated with significant intra-abdominal trauma in up to 50% of the cases. Penetrating wounds to the perineum, buttocks, and the genitalia should be treated as an abdominal wound—a load-and-go injury.

With stab wounds the patient may not initially appear to be in shock. The path of the penetrating object may not be apparent from the wound location. The path also depends on the position of the person at the point of injury (ie, inhaling versus exhaling). This could cause the injury to be an abdominal, lung, or heart injury. A stab wound to the chest may

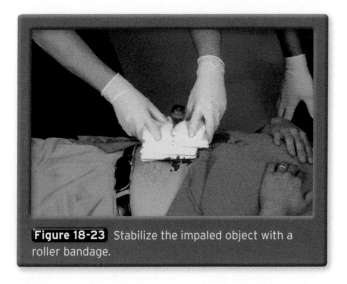

Figure 18-23 Stabilize the impaled object with a roller bandage.

also penetrate the abdomen. You must be aware of the possibility of intra-abdominal bleeding with hypovolemic shock. Remember, never remove an impaled object! Stabilize the object in place with a roller bandage **Figure 18-23** .

Patients with penetrating injuries to the abdomen generally have obvious wounds and external bleeding; however, large amounts of external bleeding may not be present. The extent of internal injury and organ systems involved cannot accurately be determined by examination of the external wound. Some penetrating injuries go no deeper than the abdominal wall, but the severity of the injury often cannot be determined in the tactical environment. Only a surgeon can accurately assess the damage. Therefore, as you care for a patient with this type of wound, you should assume that the object has penetrated the peritoneum, entered the abdominal cavity, and possibly injured one or more organs, even if there are no immediate obvious signs.

If major blood vessels are cut or solid organs are lacerated, bleeding may be rapid and severe. Other signs of intra-abdominal injuries may develop slowly, particularly in penetrating wounds to hollow organs.

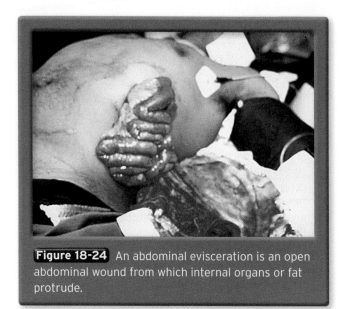

Figure 18-24 An abdominal evisceration is an open abdominal wound from which internal organs or fat protrude.

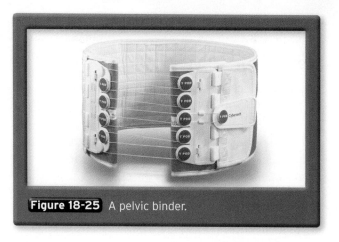

Figure 18-25 A pelvic binder.

If possible, perform a secondary assessment. Transport the patient to the highest level trauma center possible.

Pelvic Fracture

The pelvis is made up of large bones that have fused to form a solid, supportive framework. The pelvis is quite strong, and significant force is required to cause fracture. Common causes of pelvic fracture include pedestrian-versus-motor vehicle accidents, motor vehicle crashes, and falls from heights.

Because of the force involved, the presence of a pelvic fracture should alert you to the possibility of other injuries, such as internal hemorrhage, spinal injuries, and other organ injury. Signs and symptoms include tenderness, crepitus, instability during palpation, uneven length of the legs, deformity, bruising, blood at the urinary opening, and swelling of the lower abdomen and pelvis.

Pelvic fractures are a load-and-go injury. Avoid all excessive movement. Manage the patient for shock and stabilize the pelvis rapidly with a tightly wrapped sheet or commercial pelvic binder **Figure 18-25**. Rapidly evacuate the patient to an ALS-level ambulance for transport. If you are permitted to accompany the patient, treat the patient for shock per local protocols.

When you are assessing the patient's circulation, expose the patient's entire torso if it is tactically safe to do so. Inspect the patient's back and sides for exit wounds and apply a sterile dressing to all open wounds. If the penetrating object is still in place, apply a stabilizing bandage around it to control external bleeding and to minimize movement of the object during evacuation.

If a severe laceration has led to an abdominal evisceration, the organs should be covered with a large, clean, clear plastic-wrap or a moistened sterile dressing or cloth to help preserve moisture and prevent the bowel wall and other organs from drying out **Figure 18-24**. Do not attempt to push the organs or small bowel back inside the abdomen as this may cause further trauma and contamination. Any gross contamination from nearby rocks, dirt, or grass should be rapidly washed away with normal saline if possible prior to covering exposed organs, but do not delay rapid evacuation to transport. After stabilizing the circulation, airway, and breathing, rapidly evacuate the patient to an ALS-level ambulance. If you are permitted to accompany the patient during transport, provide high-flow oxygen and treat for shock.

Ready for Review

- Immediately treat any injury to the chest that interferes with the mechanical process of normal breathing.

- Load-and-go injuries to the chest include:
  - Penetrating trauma to the chest or torso
  - Major blunt trauma to the chest
  - Open pneumothorax
  - Tension pneumothorax
  - Flail chest

- There may be little or no bleeding from a small caliber bullet or a tiny 3-mm piece of shrapnel, yet the wounded SWAT officer could die within minutes if that tiny object struck a large blood vessel or vital organ such as the heart.

- Blunt trauma can cause chest contusions and fractured ribs. The ribs may be suddenly forced inwards, causing blunt or penetrating injury to the lungs.

- After the patient is stabilized and evacuated to emergency transport, the patient should be monitored for potential complications, including pneumothorax, tension pneumothorax, hemothorax, hemopneumothorax, pericardial tamponade, pulmonary contusion, and myocardial contusion.

- A pneumothorax is a dangerous condition in which air accumulates in the pleural space of the lung.

- An open pneumothorax can be caused by a penetrating injury to the chest and requires sealing.

- A tension pneumothorax requires a needle decompression. TMPs with ALS training should carry 3.5-inch or longer over-the-needle catheters

to properly puncture the often thick chest wall of the SWAT officer.

- Monitor the patient with signs of a hemothorax for signs of a tension pneumothorax during transport.

- A patient with signs of pericardial tamponade should be rapidly transported to a trauma center. Advanced medical care will include pericardiocentesis, emergency surgery, or possibly an emergency thoracotomy if the patient's pulse is lost.

- Patients with flail chest are at risk for development of hemothorax or pneumothorax.

- A pulmonary contusion may lead to hypoxia.

- If a lethal arrhythmia develops in a patient with a myocardial contusion during transport, manage per local protocols.

- The biggest concern in patients with closed abdominal injuries is the fact that you do not know what the true extent of the injury is. Because of this, the patient requires expedient transport to the nearest and highest level of care available, primarily a trauma center with a surgeon. In the tactical environment, any patient with abdominal pain after a significant MOI should be considered a load-and-go emergency.

- Gunshot wounds most commonly involve injury to the small bowel, colon, liver, and vascular structures; the extent of injury is less predictable than for an injury caused by stab wounds because gunshot wounds depend mostly on the characteristics of the weapon and the bullet. In penetrating trauma from stab wounds, the liver, small bowel, diaphragm, and colon are the organs most frequently injured.

- Due to the severe force needed to fracture the pelvis, be alert for other injuries.

Vital Vocabulary

Beck's triad The combination of narrowed pulse pressure, muffled heart tones, and jugular vein distention associated with cardiac tamponade; usually resulting from penetrating chest trauma.

closed abdominal injury An injury in which there is soft-tissue damage inside the body but the skin remains intact.

flail chest A condition in which two or more ribs are fractured in two or more places or in association with a fracture of the sternum so that a segment of the chest wall is effectively detached from the rest of the thoracic cage.

hemopneumothorax The accumulation of blood and air in the pleural space of the chest.

hemothorax A collection of blood in the pleural cavity.

myocardial contusion A bruise of the heart muscle.

open abdominal injury An injury in which there is a break in the surface of the skin or mucous membrane, exposing deeper tissue to potential contamination.

open pneumothorax An injury that extends from the surface of the skin into the peritoneal cavity. It may be associated with internal organ damage and creates the potential for contamination of the deeper tissues.

pericardial tamponade Impairment of diastolic filling of the right ventricle as a result of significant amounts of fluid in the pericardial sac surrounding the heart, leading to a decrease in the cardiac output.

pericardiocentesis A procedure in which a needle is introduced into the pericardial sac to remove fluid and relieve a pericardial tamponade.

pneumothorax Partial or complete accumulation of air in the pleural space.

pulmonary contusion Severe blunt injury to a lung resulting in swelling and bleeding within the lung tissue itself.

sucking chest wound An open or penetrating chest wall wound through which air passes during inspiration and expiration, creating a sucking sound. See also open pneumothorax.

tension pneumothorax A life-threatening collection of air within the pleural space; the volume and pressure have both collapsed the involved lung and caused a shift of the mediastinal structures to the opposite side.

Head, Neck, and Spine Injuries

OBJECTIVES

- List examples of load-and-go injuries to the head, neck, and spine.
- Describe the stabilizing care provided to a patient with a head injury in the tactical environment.
- Describe the stabilizing care provided to a patient with a neck injury in the tactical environment.
- Describe the stabilizing care provided to a patient with a spinal injury in the tactical environment.
- Describe the treatment of an eye injury in the tactical environment.
- Describe the treatment of a nasal injury in the tactical environment.
- Describe the treatment of an ear injury in the tactical environment.
- Describe the treatment of mouth and dental injuries in the tactical environment.

Introduction

As a tactical medical provider (TMP), one of your key goals is to determine if your patient has a load-and-go injury that requires immediate evacuation to transport. The head, neck, and spine have many vital organs and functions, as well as a high density of sensitive structures that are susceptible to trauma. Injuries to these structures can be life threatening but are often survivable with rapid medical care. A discussion follows on the treatment of injuries to the senses—eye, nose, ear, mouth, and dental injuries.

Load-and-Go Injuries to the Head, Neck, and Spine

In the tactical environment, the mechanism of injury (MOI) is often known because the injury is witnessed. Life-threatening injuries to the head, neck, and spine may occur due to a penetrating wound from a suspect's weapon or a blunt trauma such as a motor vehicle crash. Whether the patient is a suspect in a motor vehicle crash or a downed SWAT officer, all threats must be abolished before you can provide stabilizing care. Once the scene is safe or the patient has been brought to you, you will need to assess the patient's CAB 'N (circulation, airway, breathing, and neurologic exam) to check for the presence of potentially life-threatening injuries **Table 19-1**. You only have time to initiate stabilizing care while expediting rapid evacuation to an ALS ground or air ambulance.

Table 19-1	Load-and-Go Injuries to the Head, Neck, and Spine

- Penetrating wounds to the head, neck, and torso
- Head injury with unconsciousness, unequal pupils, or decreasing level of consciousness
- Blunt trauma to the larynx or trachea

Head

A head injury is a traumatic insult to the head that may result in injury to soft tissue, bony structures, or the brain. When head injuries are fatal, the cause is most often associated with injury to the brain. The brain can be injured directly by a penetrating object, such as a bullet, knife, or other sharp object. More commonly, brain injuries occur indirectly as a result of external forces exerted on the skull. Consider the most common cause of brain injury, the motor vehicle crash. When the passenger's head hits the windshield, the brain continues to move forward until it comes to an abrupt stop by striking the inside of the skull. This rapid deceleration results in compression injury (or bruising) to the anterior portion of the brain along with the stretching or tearing of the posterior portion of the brain **Figure 19-1**. As the brain strikes the front of the skull, the body begins its backward movement. The head falls back against the headrest and/or seat, and the brain slams into the rear of the skull. This type of front-and-rear injury is known as a **coup-contrecoup injury**. The same type of injury may occur on opposite sides of the brain in a lateral collision.

The injured brain starts to swell, initially because of cerebral vasodilation and capillary leakage. An increase in cerebral fluid (cerebral edema) then contributes to further brain swelling. However, **cerebral edema** may not develop until several hours following the initial injury.

Cerebral edema is aggravated by low oxygen levels in the blood and improved by high levels. In fact, the brain consumes more oxygen than any other organ in the body. For this reason you must make sure that the airway is open and that adequate ventilations are given to any patient with a head injury. This is especially true if the patient is unconscious. Do not wait for cyanosis or other obvious signs of hypoxia to develop.

It is not uncommon for the patient with a head injury to have a convulsion or seizure. This is the result of excessive excitability of the brain caused by direct injury or the accumulation of fluid within the brain (edema). You should be prepared to manage seizures in all patients who have had a head injury because the brain may have sustained an injury as well. Other effects of cerebral edema and increased intracranial pressure may be increased blood pressure, decreased pulse rate, and irregular respirations—known as **Cushing's reflex**.

Following a head injury, any patient who exhibits one or more of these signs or symptoms has potentially sustained a very serious underlying brain injury:

- Lacerations, contusions, or hematomas to the scalp
- Soft area or depression on palpation
- Visible fractures or deformities of the skull
- Decreased mentation
- Irregular breathing pattern
- Elevated blood pressure
- Bradycardia
- Ecchymosis about the eyes or behind the ear over the mastoid process
- Clear or pink CSF leakage from a scalp wound, the nose, or the ear
- Failure of the pupils to respond to light
- Unequal pupil size **Figure 19-2**

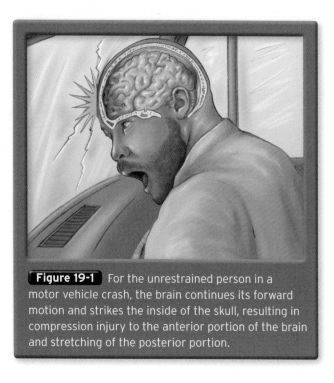

Figure 19-1 For the unrestrained person in a motor vehicle crash, the brain continues its forward motion and strikes the inside of the skull, resulting in compression injury to the anterior portion of the brain and stretching of the posterior portion.

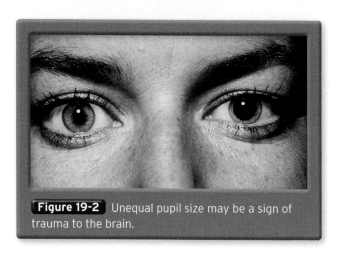

Figure 19-2 Unequal pupil size may be a sign of trauma to the brain.

Safety

The majority of SWAT officers wear ballistic helmets, which decreases the incidence of scalp injuries and other head trauma. TMPs should work with command to ensure that protective gear is worn at training as well as during callouts to protect SWAT officers' heads.

- Loss of sensation and/or motor function
- A period of unconsciousness
- Amnesia
- Seizures
- Numbness or tingling in the extremities
- Irregular respirations
- Dizziness
- Visual complaints
- Combative or other abnormal behavior
- Nausea or vomiting

A scalp laceration is a sign that you should examine the patient more closely for gunshot wounds and determine if there are mechanisms that may indicate a deeper injury such as a ricocheted bullet fragment (small cut, deep penetration into the brain) or a hard fall onto a pointed edge of a desk (with underlying open skull fracture). A scalp laceration from a broken glass window should be assumed to contain shards of glass and should be treated appropriately. The human scalp is highly vascular; any abrasions or lacerations tend to bleed heavily and may be difficult to stop **Figure 19-3**. See Chapter 21, "Soft-Tissue Injuries," for more information about treating lacerations.

Safety

Criminals with firearms will aim for vital areas of the SWAT officer's body that are not protected by ballistic gear—the neck and face.

Stabilization of Head Injuries

After calling for help and abolishing all threats, rapidly assess and stabilize the patient's airway. Patients with a traumatic head injury need oxygen immediately. If the patient is hypoxic or has an altered mental status, use the jaw-thrust maneuver to open the airway, take measures to maintain a patent airway through an oral airway or provide intubation. Assist with ventilation and provide

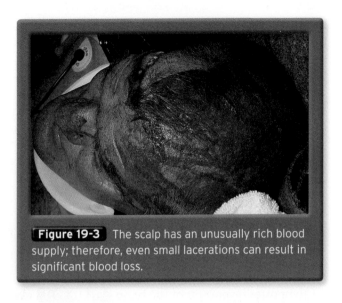

Figure 19-3 The scalp has an unusually rich blood supply; therefore, even small lacerations can result in significant blood loss.

high-flow oxygen via a nonrebreathing mask as soon as possible. Consider the need for spinal immobilization based on the MOI.

Penetrating injuries to the head may produce copious bleeding. Head wounds should be treated gingerly because compression of underlying skull fractures and bone fragments can injure blood vessels and brain tissue. Apply sterile dressings, and if the brain is exposed, then apply gentle pressure to any arterial bleeding that is significant. Otherwise, gently lay moistened sterile 4″ × 4″ gauze dressings in place and cover the exposed brain tissue.

Monitor the patient's airway and treat for any airway obstruction from swelling, blood, or secretions. If the patient deteriorates, recheck the patient's airway, breathing, or circulation. Be prepared to turn the patient onto one side and suction if the patient vomits.

Avoid hyperventilation in the tactical environment unless it is indicated, such as in cases of very recent signs of impending cerebral herniation including posturing, pupillary abnormalities, or sudden neurologic deterioration in a patient with the presence of normal blood pressure and good oxygenation. Hyperventilation for adults is 20 breaths per minute. If too large of a tidal volume is used (ie, squeezing the bag too deeply), then this will also hyperventilate the patient due to the increased tidal volume of air.

If the patient has a seizure, maintain the patient's airway with manual airway positioning. Use suction to clear any secretions or vomitus. Protect the patient from his or her surroundings by moving harmful objects out of the way. Never attempt to restrain a patient having a seizure.

Once the patient's circulation, airway, and breathing are stabilized, evacuate the patient as rapidly as possible. Ensure transport to the hospital by an ALS unit and make sure there is early notification of the medical director and the receiving hospital. If you are permitted to accompany the patient during transport, perform a rapid secondary assessment while en route. If possible, calculate the patient's Glasgow Coma Scale score. Reassess the patient's vital signs every 5 minutes while en route.

Elevate the head of the backboard 30 degrees if the patient's systolic blood pressure is greater than 100 mm Hg to decrease the amount of brain swelling. If the blood pressure is less than 100 mm Hg, then leave the patient flat.

Hypotension worsens traumatic brain injury. Do not withhold fluid administration in hypotensive head injury patients. Start an IV and infuse lactated Ringer's or normal saline as indicated per your local protocols. If the patient is hypotensive, administer a fluid challenge (500 mL IV fluid wide open). Reassess the patient and repeat if the patient's blood pressure is less than 100 mm Hg for adults. Consider the use of vasopressors such as dopamine or NeoSynephrine per your local protocols if the hypotension is not due to hypovolemia.

Neck

The critical structures running through the neck are relatively unprotected and therefore susceptible to many types of injuries. In addition to critical airway and vascular structures, the possibility of unstable cervical spine and cord injury must always be considered. Special airway considerations in the presence of neck injury include bleeding into the airway, expanding hematomas causing airway obstruction, and tracheal disruption.

Any penetrating neck trauma, no matter how small, should be treated as a potentially lethal wound and is a load-and-go emergency, especially if there is any associated swelling in the neck, active bleeding at the wound site, or a pulseless upper extremity. After a knife or gunshot wound, the carotid artery can bleed severely and can cause airway obstruction due to severe neck swelling and pressure on the trachea within a few minutes of injury **Figure 19-4**. In fact, injury to the carotid arteries and jugular veins can produce rapid exsanguination (bleeding to death) or embolization of air (air sucked into the veinous circulation). Many of the serious complications of these injuries do not occur for days to weeks and involve blood clots that lead to neurologic problems.

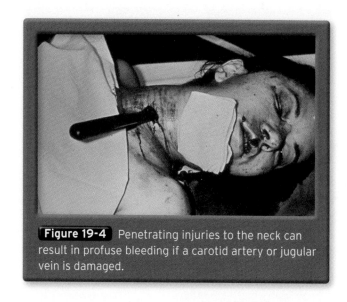

Figure 19-4 Penetrating injuries to the neck can result in profuse bleeding if a carotid artery or jugular vein is damaged.

A variety of life-threatening injuries can result if the structures of the front of the neck are crushed against the cervical spine following blunt trauma or if they are penetrated by a sharp object. The larynx and its supporting structures (ie, hyoid bone, thyroid cartilage) may be fractured and the trachea may be separated from the larynx. Many blunt injuries to the larynx and trachea are not apparent upon inspection; because they are not as obvious and dramatic as penetrating neck injuries, they can be easily overlooked. Maintain a high index of suspicion and carefully assess the airway of any patient who has suffered blunt trauma to the neck, such as striking a steering wheel or strangulation. Signs of larynx and trachea injury include bruising, redness, tenderness, dysphonia (inability to speak), dyspnea (shortness of breath), stridor (high-pitched wheezing), and swelling. Significant injuries to the larynx or trachea pose an immediate risk of airway compromise due to disruption of the normal passage of air **Figure 19-5**, soft-tissue swelling, or aspiration of blood into the lungs.

At the Scene

Criminals often learn to "aim for the triangle," otherwise known as the "white triangle of death." The white triangle refers to the collar of a white undershirt that shows from under the uniform. This triangle is located just above the ballistic vest, thus leaving the ballistic vest wearer vulnerable to a life-threatening injury.

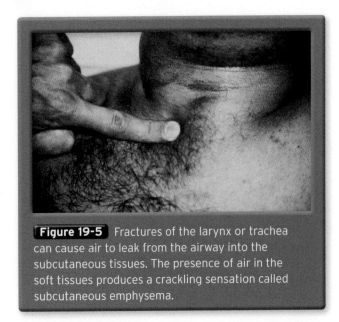

Figure 19-5 Fractures of the larynx or trachea can cause air to leak from the airway into the subcutaneous tissues. The presence of air in the soft tissues produces a crackling sensation called subcutaneous emphysema.

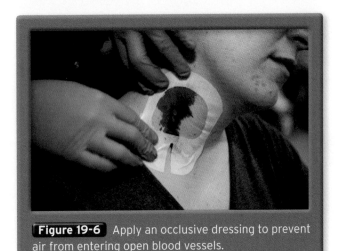

Figure 19-6 Apply an occlusive dressing to prevent air from entering open blood vessels.

Stabilization of Neck Injuries

Penetrating injuries to the neck may produce copious bleeding and may interfere with breathing. Control any external bleeding with firm direct pressure and monitor the patient for airway obstruction due to a major hematoma or a trachea filling with blood. If the carotid artery or other major artery is bleeding heavily, place direct pressure on the site with firm localized pressure over a small bandage to occlude it. Open injuries to the neck should be sealed with an occlusive dressing to prevent air from entering open blood vessels and causing an air embolus to the brain, heart, or lungs **Figure 19-6**.

You may also apply a sterile dressing to the neck and hold it in place when you wrap an elastic dressing around the neck and shoulder, crossing over to the opposite axilla so the compression is firm and consistent but not overly constricting.

Stabilize any impaled objects by placing bulky, damp dressings around them. Only impaled objects that obstruct the airway should be removed in the tactical environment; leave all others in place.

Be prepared to support the patient's respirations with a bag-mask device. Use suction to remove any airway obstructions caused by blood or secretions. Secure the airway with endotracheal intubation if indicated and appropriate. Endotracheal intubation may be extremely challenging, if not impossible, owing to distortion of the normal anatomic structures of the upper airway. If basic and advanced techniques to secure the patient's airway are unsuccessful or impossible, a surgical or needle cricothyrotomy may be your only means of establishing a patent airway and ensuring adequate oxygenation and ventilation. Follow your local protocols on advanced airway management.

Once the patient's circulation, airway, and breathing are stabilized, extricate and evacuate the patient as rapidly as possible. Ensure transport to the hospital by an ALS unit and notify the medical director and the receiving hospital. If you are permitted to accompany the patient, perform a rapid secondary assessment and reassess the patient's vital signs every 5 minutes while en route.

Controversy

The placement of a cervical collar in penetrating neck injuries may hinder observation of the neck during transport and therefore hide potentially life-threatening physical changes.

Spine

Injuries to the spine commonly result from MOIs involving high kinetic energy, including falls, motor vehicle accidents, forceful blows to the head or neck, penetrating trauma, and explosions. Any neurovascular impairment and spinal deformity indicate the likelihood of spinal injuries. Any patient with neck or back pain in the presence of a significant MOI should be assumed to have a possible spinal cord injury until proven otherwise.

Other signs and symptoms of spinal injury include an obvious deformity that is locally tender as you gently palpate the spine; numbness, weakness, or tingling in the extremities; and soft-tissue injuries in the spinal region. Patients with severe spinal injury may lose sensation or experience paralysis below the suspected level of injury or be incontinent (loss of urinary or bowel control). Obvious injury to the head and neck increases the likelihood of serious injury to the cervical spine.

Stabilization of Spinal Injury

Pay special attention to the condition of the patient's skin while you are assessing the patient's circulation. Spinal cord injury may cause loss of vascular tone, which results in vasodilation, so the distal points on the extremities may appear more warm and red initially, presenting as warm, flushed, and dry skin. Hold the patient's head still in a neutral, in-line position **Figure 19-7**. Open and maintain the patient's airway with the jaw-thrust maneuver if needed. Insert an oral airway or intubate the patient if needed to maintain the airway. Have a suctioning unit available and continuously monitor the airway (rate and depth of respiration, ability to talk).

Next, perform the rapid neurologic examination. Assess and record any pain on palpation of the spine, any motor or sensory neurologic deficits in any extremity, abnormal arm or leg position, incontinence,

altered mental status, ptosis (droopy eyelid), and/or priapism (sustained erection due to spinal cord injury) **Figure 19-8**.

Monitor and treat for shock. Patients with spinal cord injury are usually very upset about their sudden inability to move their arms and legs, so you should provide appropriate psychological support.

Prepare the patient for extrication by applying an appropriately sized rigid cervical collar and fully immobilize the spine on a backboard. This may require some improvisation in the tactical environment, such as using a door as an emergency backboard. If a true spinal cord injury is present or suspected and the TMP is unable to provide full spinal immobilization, you should make every effort to bring in civilian EMS with full spinal immobilization gear and a stretcher to ensure appropriate extrication and evacuation.

Any unnecessary movement of the spine could worsen the patient's outcome. To transfer a supine patient with a spinal cord injury, a six-plus-person lift onto a rigid long spine board may be performed. A six-plus-person lift is recommended due to the size of many SWAT officers and the heavy weight of their ballistic gear and equipment. The heavy weight of the ballistic gear and equipment can cause forward momentum during the log roll movement and thus cause potentially damaging motion to the spine. If there are only two to three TMPs or SWAT officers available, then consider using a scoop stretcher **Figure 19-9**.

To perform the six-plus-person lift, follow these steps:

1. Three or more persons line up on the right side of the patient.
2. Three or more persons line up on the left side of the patient.

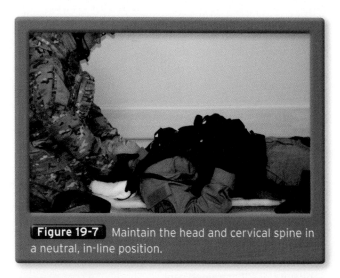

Figure 19-7 Maintain the head and cervical spine in a neutral, in-line position.

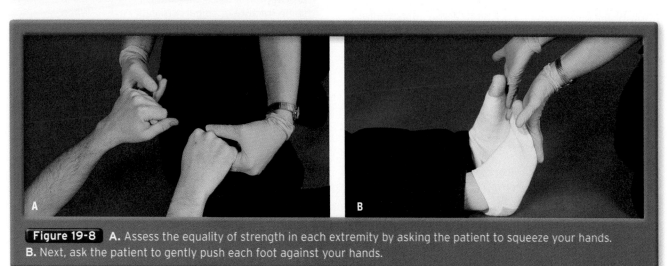

Figure 19-8 **A.** Assess the equality of strength in each extremity by asking the patient to squeeze your hands. **B.** Next, ask the patient to gently push each foot against your hands.

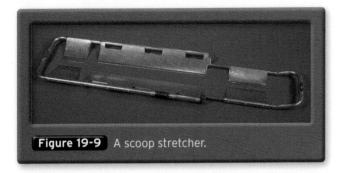

Figure 19-9 A scoop stretcher.

3. The group is directed by a leader at the head of the patient.
4. On the leader's count of three, the patient's neck and head are supported and the body is lifted by the clothing or belt/vest from the ground onto the backboard.

If the patient is prone (face-down), use the log roll technique to transfer the patient directly onto a rigid long spine board. Movement of the patient from the prone to the supine position should be done with a minimum of four people, with one designated to maintain the in-line stabilization of the patient's head and neck. All movement should be carefully coordinated to avoid having the head, neck, and torso move independently. With each movement, the chances of a secondary injury to the patient increase. Remove all bulky equipment and gear from the sides of the gear vest and from any thigh holsters prior to log rolling a SWAT officer in order to minimize spine movement and potential secondary injury.

Once the patient is on a backboard, protect the patient's spine and paralyzed limbs by securing the patient to the backboard, using a cervical collar and head blocks to minimize movement. Ensure transport by an ALS unit and notify the medical director and the appropriate level receiving hospital. If you are permitted to accompany the patient, perform a rapid secondary assessment while en route. Reassess the patient's vital signs every 5 minutes while en route.

Special Populations

It is difficult to find a cervical collar that really fits an infant or toddler. When a properly sized collar is not available, stabilize the child's spine on a backboard with padding to prevent movement.

At the Scene

Emergency medicine in the tactical environment does not often involve cervical spine (c-spine) precautions. That being said, however, when you approach a patient, the possibility of spinal injury should always be considered. In the tactical environment, most injuries due to penetrating trauma do not involve the spinal cord. Even for direct gunshot wounds to the neck, the incidence of spinal cord injuries is rare, and when there is injury, it tends to be complete. Penetrating trauma rarely causes unstable spinal injuries; therefore, the emphasis is placed on controlling life-threatening bleeding, supporting airway and breathing, and minimizing time in the inner perimeter.

Monitor for signs of neurogenic shock, including bradycardia (slow pulse) and low blood pressure. Neurogenic shock is caused by vasodilation of blood vessels, decreased pulse, and decreased respiratory rate. Follow your local protocols to treat neurogenic shock. Many EMS systems will authorize the use of large volumes of IV normal saline in order to "fill up" the increased vascular volume. More severe cases of vasodilation may eventually require doses of IV vasopressors such as Neosynephrine or dopamine medications to increase peripheral blood vessel vascular tone and help to reverse the vasodilation-associated neurogenic shock. Always follow local protocols.

Medical Gear

Removal of body armor and vests must be accomplished with proper spinal immobilization precautions if any significant likelihood of a spine fracture or spinal cord injury exists. When appropriate and behind hard cover, remove the body armor by loosening, cutting, or unstrapping the Velcro tabs and buckles that keep the vest and helmet in place, and then gently log roll the patient to the side while keeping the spine immobilized and supported with the assistance of fellow SWAT officers. Gently pull and slide the body armor off of the body and utilize appropriate spine boards and cervical collars to then transport the patient as per your local protocols. If the decision is made to move the patient in the position in which he or she was found, you may use the six-plus-person lift to lift the patient onto a backboard with spinal motion restriction.

Medical Gear

The modern level III vests used by a majority of the SWAT units are approximately one half to three quarters of an inch thick. For a SWAT officer who is lying on his or her back, this will elevate the chest the same distance, plus another quarter to half inch from the underlying ventilated rib shirt and uniform. The head and neck will be extended a slight distance to the rear when lying supine on a spinal board. Therefore, if a neutral position is to be achieved, carefully place a small towel under the patient's head **Figure 19-10**.

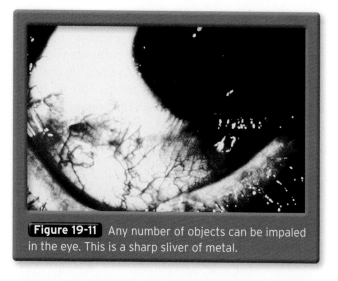

Figure 19-11 Any number of objects can be impaled in the eye. This is a sharp sliver of metal.

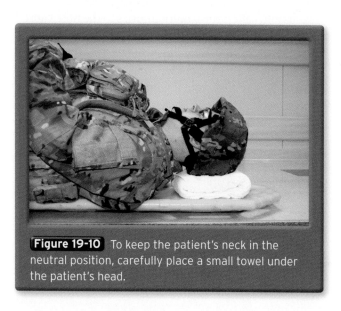

Figure 19-10 To keep the patient's neck in the neutral position, carefully place a small towel under the patient's head.

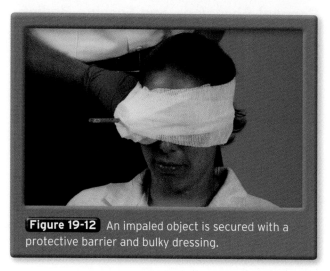

Figure 19-12 An impaled object is secured with a protective barrier and bulky dressing.

Treat-Then-Transport Injuries

Eye

Eye injuries are common in the tactical environment. Prevention of eye injuries is the ultimate goal. Protective eye goggles or shielding should be utilized whenever the possibility of projectiles, chemical splash, or body fluids is a threat. In the event that an eye injury occurs, ophthalmologic evaluation should be sought as soon as possible.

Penetrating Eye Injury or Ruptured Globe

High-velocity shrapnel and other objects have the potential to penetrate the eye. Larger punctures are usually evident and may lead to a ruptured eyeball or globe. However, smaller foreign bodies are difficult to locate and a missed diagnosis of a penetrating foreign body has a potentially disastrous outcome. If an object has punctured and impaled the eyeball, you should not remove the impaled object, and do not irrigate the eye or use eye drops **Figure 19-11**. You or a fellow SWAT officer should remain with the visually impaired patient at all times for guidance and reassurance. Stabilize the object with a bulky dressing, cover the unaffected eye, and have the patient transported to a hospital **Figure 19-12**. If you are permitted to accompany the patient during transport, follow your local protocols per administering pain medication.

Chemical Burns

Chemical burns, usually caused by acid or alkaline solutions, require immediate care. Immediately irrigate the affected eye using copious amounts of sterile saline

Figure 19-13 . Use of clean, chlorinated water from a faucet or garden hose is acceptable if sterile saline is not available. Irrigation should continue while the patient is en route to the hospital (preferably one with an ophthalmologist). Position the patient on his or her side so the affected eye is on the bottom. This will ensure that any contaminated water does not irritate the unaffected eye.

The eyes are irrigated by pouring water slowly into the patient's eye while holding open the eyelids. Avoid any rubbing or physical contact with the eye area. If the chemical was a strong base or alkali (high pH), then prolonged irrigation and an urgent ophthalmology consultation are required as these injuries have a very poor prognosis and often lead to blindness **Figure 19-14** .

Corneal Abrasions and Foreign Bodies

SWAT officers often train or maneuver in dusty and unclean environments and therefore are at risk of getting foreign bodies in, and sustaining abrasions of, the cornea. Due to the sensitivity of the eye, even a tiny, 1-mm piece of dust or foreign body can disable and render a SWAT officer ineffective. If a simple piece of dirt or debris is possibly in the eye, briefly examine and gently remove it with irrigation, a soft cotton swab, or another appropriate instrument **Figure 19-15** . Gently irrigate the eye with sterile normal saline (500 to 1000 mL) and reevaluate the eye. If reasonable attempts to remove the foreign body are unsuccessful or if significant injury is suspected, then cover the affected eye and have the patient transported to an ophthalmologist.

Ear

Injuries to the ear are caused by a variety of mechanisms, from insects to infections. Trauma to the ear can cause bleeding between the cartilage and its vascular supply, causing the cartilage to die. This dead cartilage can fibrose and leads to cauliflower ear (scarred tissue that has the appearance of a cauliflower). For minor trauma, provide standard wound care (see Chapter 21, "Soft-Tissue Injuries"). Complicated cases such as an entrapped foreign body or ear infection should be referred to an ear, nose, and throat (ENT) doctor for follow-up. Loss of hearing will necessitate the removal of a SWAT officer from the unit. Preventing hearing loss is discussed in Chapter 27, "Preventive Medicine."

Nose

The nose often takes the brunt of deliberate physical assaults and car crashes. Blunt injuries to the nose caused by a fist or a dashboard may be associated with fractures and soft-tissue injuries of the face, head injuries, and/or injuries to the cervical spine.

The patient may note the immediate change in nasal appearance that accompanies a significantly displaced nasal fracture. Epistaxis (nosebleed) may also indicate the presence of a fracture. The nose must be inspected

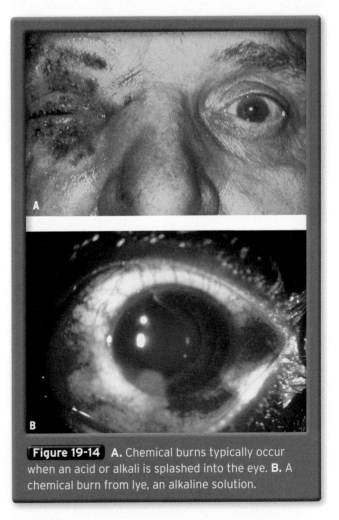

Figure 19-14 **A.** Chemical burns typically occur when an acid or alkali is splashed into the eye. **B.** A chemical burn from lye, an alkaline solution.

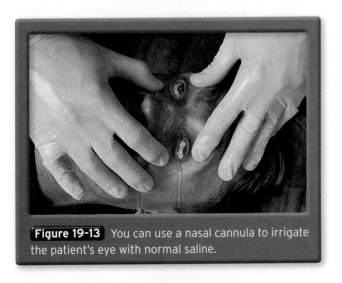

Figure 19-13 You can use a nasal cannula to irrigate the patient's eye with normal saline.

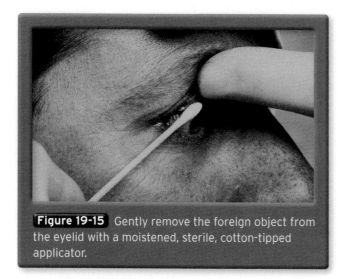

Figure 19-15 Gently remove the foreign object from the eyelid with a moistened, sterile, cotton-tipped applicator.

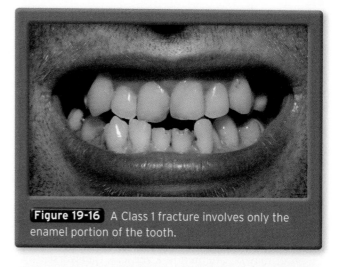

Figure 19-16 A Class 1 fracture involves only the enamel portion of the tooth.

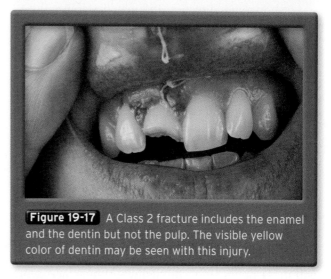

Figure 19-17 A Class 2 fracture includes the enamel and the dentin but not the pulp. The visible yellow color of dentin may be seen with this injury.

both internally and externally for lacerations, significant bruising, and hematomas, which all strongly suggest a fracture. A septal hematoma needs to be identified and drained urgently to prevent cartilage necrosis and a "saddle-nose" deformity (the nose appears to collapse in the middle). Nasal fractures are frequently accompanied by face and eyelid swelling, bruising, and pain. Swelling can interfere with the nose as an air passage. Gently pinch the nostrils together to stop any bleeding. Apply a cold pack and have the patient see his or her personal care physician.

Oral Injuries

Mouth

Lacerations of the lip may occur with tooth fractures and may be cleaned and covered with sterile gauze dressing or even repaired by a physician or dental surgeon at the scene if they are properly trained and equipped. The vast majority of lacerations and bleeding can be dressed initially with trauma pack dressings (4″ × 4″ or 6″ × 6″) with slight pressure provided by tape, followed by referral to the hospital for repair. Lacerations and tears within the oral cavity such as on the inner cheek, gums, lips, and tongue require a physician evaluation but often do not require any suturing or specific care. These can also be dressed with gauze. The easiest way to manage these injuries is to place the gauze between the teeth and the laceration using the natural pressure of the muscles within the lips and cheeks to apply direct pressure on the laceration while against the gauze. Although the face and mouth may bleed profusely, pack dressings are usually sufficient enough to stabilize the wound during transport from the field to the emergency department or a secondary treatment facility (eg, a dental surgeon's office).

Dental

Trauma to the mouth, lips, or teeth can occur at any time during training or callouts, so you need to have a basic understanding of common dental emergencies. You should know how to provide temporary care as well as how to contact a dentist or dental surgeon.

The four-class system for identifying broken teeth is as follows:

- **Class 1 dental fractures**. Involve only the enamel portion of the tooth **Figure 19-16**. The fracture edge may be rough but only minimal pain will be present. The SWAT officer may remain on duty and seek dental care later at his or her discretion.
- **Class 2 dental fractures**. Include the enamel and the dentin but not the pulp. The visible yellow color of dentin may be seen with this injury **Figure 19-17**. The tooth will also be more sensitive to contact with water or air. The SWAT officer can also remain in action after sustaining this injury but should seek dental care as soon

as possible after the callout has ended due to the pain and increased risk of infection.

- **Class 3 dental fractures**. Include the enamel, the dentin, and extends into the pulp chamber **Figure 19-18**. Much more pain will be present than with a Class 2 fracture as the nerves are very close and sensitive. The tooth may bleed as the artery nurturing the tooth may be injured. Bleeding should be locally controlled with pressure and pain controlled with the application of a topical pain reliver. Follow local protocols. If the pain is adequately controlled, the SWAT officer may remain on duty, but should seek a dental consultation as soon as possible.
- **Class 4 dental fractures**. Fractures of the tooth's root may be oriented in a vertical, transverse, or horizontal direction and may destabilize the tooth. The SWAT officer with a Class 4 fracture should be taken out of service and sent for immediate dental care.

Dental Alignment Injuries

A tooth may also sustain alignment injuries in its bony (alveolar) socket. These include luxation and avulsion injuries.

Luxation Injuries In a **luxation injury**, the tooth is displaced within the socket usually as a result of a direct blow to the front of the mouth. A luxation injury may only be minimally painful and the tooth may appear misaligned. If the displacement is 2 mm or less, the tooth may be gently repositioned. A diet of soft foods only and a dental consult within 24 hours are recommended. Immediate dental consultation is required to treat a serious luxation injury.

Gentle repositioning and buddy splinting of the tooth with super glue (cyanoacrylate glue) or Dermabond may be performed by TMPs who are physicians, experienced nurses, or physician's assistants, using caution not to allow the lip to contact the wet glue. Follow local protocols. Place the tooth in position, dry the tooth surface, and while protecting the area, gently and accurately place the adhesive on the loose tooth and both adjacent teeth, using a sufficient but not excessive amount.

Tooth Avulsion Tooth avulsion represents the complete loss of a tooth. Tooth avulsion is a dental emergency! Do not scrape, scrub, or disinfect the tooth. Gently cleanse the tooth with normal saline to remove debris. Do not clean the tooth socket unless gross contamination is present.

If you are permitted to do so by local protocols, replace the tooth into its socket and have the SWAT officer bite down on a sterile gauze pad over the replaced tooth to help push it deeper back to its original position and depth as best possible. Administration of pain medication per your level of training and local protocols may be beneficial because this procedure is painful. If that is not possible, place the tooth into a sterile, plastic, sealed container bathed in sterile saline or cold milk. Do not transport a dry tooth or store it in tap water as either may damage the tooth. The patient should be taken to a dental surgeon as soon as possible **Figure 19-19**.

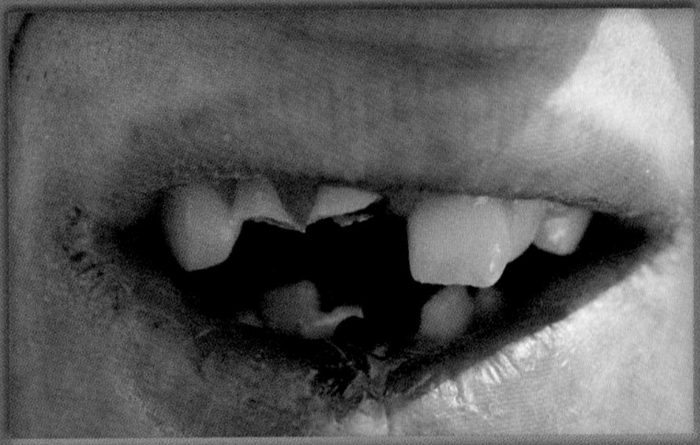

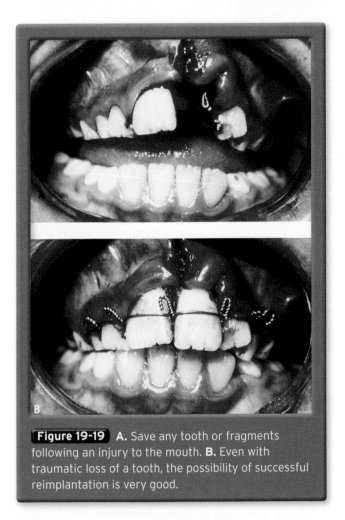

Figure 19-19 **A.** Save any tooth or fragments following an injury to the mouth. **B.** Even with traumatic loss of a tooth, the possibility of successful reimplantation is very good.

Figure 19-18 A Class 3 fracture includes the enamel, the dentin, and the pulp chamber.

Ready for Review

- As a TMP, one of your key goals is to determine if a patient has a load-and-go injury to the head, neck, or spine.

- Head injuries require the immediate assessment and stabilization of the airway.

- Due to the damage to the structures of the airway caused by trauma to the neck, advanced airway skills may be required in order to maintain a patent airway.

- To place a downed SWAT officer on a rigid backboard, a six-plus-person lift is recommended due to the size of many SWAT officers and the heavy weight of their ballistic gear and equipment.

- Eye injuries are common in the tactical environment. Protective eye goggles or shielding should be utilized whenever the possibility of projectiles, chemical splash, or body fluids is a threat.

- In the event that an eye injury occurs, ophthalmologic evaluation should be sought as soon as possible.

- Blunt injuries to the nose caused by a fist or a dashboard may be associated with fractures and soft-tissue injuries of the face, head injuries, and/or injuries to the cervical spine.

- A SWAT officer may remain on the scene for a minor tooth fracture. If the tooth is broken or knocked out, then the patient should be transported to a dental surgeon.

Vital Vocabulary

cerebral edema Swelling of the brain.

Class 1 dental fracture A fracture to the tooth that involves only the enamel portion of the tooth.

Class 2 dental fracture A fracture to the tooth that includes the enamel and the dentin but not the pulp.

Class 3 dental fracture A fracture to the tooth that includes the enamel, the dentin, and the pulp chamber.

Class 4 dental fracture A fracture to the tooth that involves the root and may destabilize the tooth.

coup-contrecoup injury Dual impacting of the brain into the skull; coup injury occurs at the point of impact; contrecoup injury occurs on the opposite side of impact, as the brain rebounds.

Cushing's reflex The combination of a slowing pulse, rising blood pressure, and erratic respiratory patterns; a grave sign for patients with head trauma.

luxation injury The tooth is displaced within the socket, usually as a result of a direct blow to the front of the mouth.

OBJECTIVES

- List examples of load-and-go injuries to the extremities.

- Describe the stabilizing care provided to a patient with an amputation in the tactical environment.

- List the items that can be used to make an improvised splint for a femur fracture in the tactical environment.

- Demonstrate splinting a fractured femur in the tactical environment.

- Describe the specialized care required for a patient with an entrapped or crushed extremity in the tactical environment.

- Describe the stabilizing care provided to a patient with an open fracture in the tactical environment.

- Demonstrate applying a SAM splint to an extremity with a closed fracture.

- Describe the treatment of strains and sprains in the tactical environment.

- Describe the treatment of a dislocation in the tactical environment.

Introduction

Extremity injuries range from potentially life threatening (femur fracture) to the inconvenient (sprained ankle). This chapter discusses which injuries are load-and-go emergencies and which injuries can be treated at the scene. Because some standard splints may not be available to you during a callout, how to improvise a lifesaving splint is also discussed.

Load-and-Go Injuries to the Extremities

In the tactical environment, the mechanism of injury (MOI) is often known because injuries are witnessed. If a penetrating wound or blunt trauma to an extremity occurs, expose the patient's extremity during the circulation phase of Call-A-CAB 'N Go to check for the presence of potentially life-threatening injuries, such as uncontrolled hemorrhage **Table 20-1** . You only have time to initiate stabilizing care (stop the bleeding, maintain an open airway, support breathing), while expediting rapid evacuation to an ALS ground or air ambulance.

Amputation

An **amputation** is the separation of a body part from the remainder of the body **Figure 20-1** . Amputations can be life threatening and are often disabling. With an amputation, bleeding will often be severe initially and a tourniquet is the best option to control the bleeding, especially if the amputation occurs above the knee or elbow. The tourniquet should be placed as close to the actual amputation site as possible in order to save as much tissue as possible.

Table 20-1	Load-and-Go Injuries to the Extremities
· Amputation	
· Penetrating or blunt trauma to the extremities with major uncontrolled hemorrhage	
· Femur fractures	
· Open fractures	

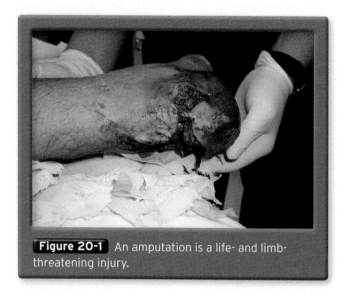

Figure 20-1 An amputation is a life- and limb-threatening injury.

Stabilizing Care for an Amputation

Apply pressure to the stump to control bleeding and cover the stump with a damp, sterile dressing and elastic wrap. Wrap the dressing tight enough to apply reasonable, uniform pressure across the entire stump. A damp, sterile dressing is needed to prevent the internal tissues from being exposed to the air and drying out Figure 20-2 . This can be accomplished by using sterile 4″ × 4″ gauze covered by a dressing and wrapped with an elastic wrap.

Make every attempt to locate the amputated part and transport it with the patient for possible reattachment Figure 20-3 . If located, the amputated part should be grossly decontaminated (wash off the dirt). A moist saline dressing should be placed over the exposed muscle, tendon, and nerve tissue. The amputated part should be placed into a plastic bag and placed in a mixture of ice and water. Do not put the plastic bag into a container of ice alone because this may damage the tissue beyond repair.

Once the patient's CAB (circulation, airway, and breathing) is stabilized, the patient should be transported by an ALS crew to a trauma center—if possible, a center that has microsurgery capabilities. If you accompany the patient during transport, perform a secondary assessment and monitor the patient for signs of shock.

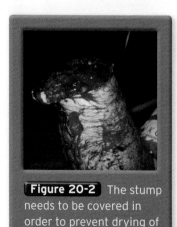

Figure 20-2 The stump needs to be covered in order to prevent drying of the exposed tissues.

At the Scene

A downed SWAT officer who is alone will self-apply a tourniquet to control the severe initial bleeding from an amputation, if possible. That tourniquet should remain in place during extrication and evacuation.

Femur Fractures

The femur is the largest bone in the body, surrounded by some of the body's strongest muscles. When the femur is broken, the muscles contract, causing sharp bone ends to override and damage soft tissue. More importantly, the slack muscle provides a large space for the collection of blood. Generally, femur fractures account for the loss of at least 1 L of blood from the circulation. A patient with bilateral femur fractures can hemorrhage a total of 3 L of blood—a grave life threat. The signs and symptoms of a femur fracture include pain, swelling, deformity, rigidity, shortening, contusions, guarding, and crepitus (air under the skin that produces a crackling sound on palpation; also, grinding sensation of two broken bones rubbing together).

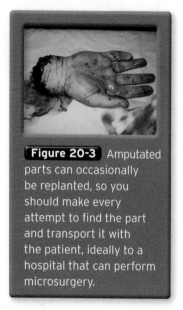

Figure 20-3 Amputated parts can occasionally be replanted, so you should make every attempt to find the part and transport it with the patient, ideally to a hospital that can perform microsurgery.

Stabilizing Care of a Femur Fracture

To stabilize the patient's circulation, you must splint the femur fracture. Femur fractures are ideally treated with a traction splint. The traction splint pulls the slack muscles taut again, controlling the bleeding. Applying a traction splint is difficult in the tactical environment because this type of splint is bulky and often not carried into a callout. There are compact traction splint kits available, such as the Kendrick splint, that can be carried in a backpack or in a SWAT unit vehicle Figure 20-4 . Traction splints should be applied as soon as possible to control bleeding and provide comfort.

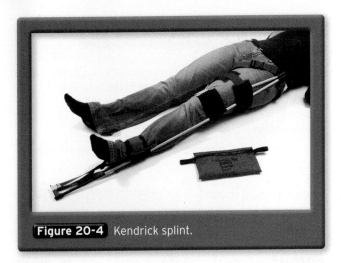

Figure 20-4 Kendrick splint.

If a traction splint is unavailable, splints may be improvised from such items as:

- Boards
- Poles
- Tree limbs
- Cardboard
- Broomsticks

Swathes or a combination of swathes and slings can also be used to immobilize an extremity with an anatomic splint using the uninjured leg to immobilize (to some extent) the fractured leg.

To apply an improvised splint, follow these steps:

1. Ensure that the splints are long enough to immobilize the knee.

2. If possible, use at least four ties (two above and two below the fracture) to secure the splints. The ties should be nonslip knots and should be tied away from the body on the splint.

3. Pad the splints where they touch any bony prominences to prevent excessive pressure to the area.

4. Check the circulation distal to the fractured femur. Note any pale, white, or bluish-gray color of the skin that may indicate impaired circulation. Assess the patient's capillary refill. Check the temperature of the injured extremity. Use your hand (ungloved portion) to compare the temperature of the injured side with the uninjured side of the body. The body area below the injury may be cooler to the touch, indicating poor circulation.

5. Apply the splint in place.

6. If the femur is severely deformed or distal circulation is compromised, align the long bones to their proper anatomic position. Before attempting realignment, consider administering pain medications per your training level and your local protocols. Use the least amount of force necessary. Grasp the foot or hand at the end of the injured limb firmly; once you start pulling, you should not stop until the limb is fully splinted. Always apply the direction of traction along the long axis of the limb. Imagine where the normal, uninjured limb would lie, and pull gently along the line of that imaginary limb until the injured limb is in approximately that position **Figure 20-5**. Grasping the foot and the initial pull of traction usually causes some discomfort as the bone fragments move. It helps if a second person can support the injured limb directly under the site of the fracture. This initial discomfort quickly subsides and you can then apply further gentle traction. However, if the patient strongly resists the traction or if it causes more pain that persists, you must stop and splint the limb in the deformed position. Only attempt to realign the fracture twice. If you are unsuccessful, splint the femur as is.

7. Place one splint on each side of the leg. If possible, make sure that the splints reach beyond the knee.

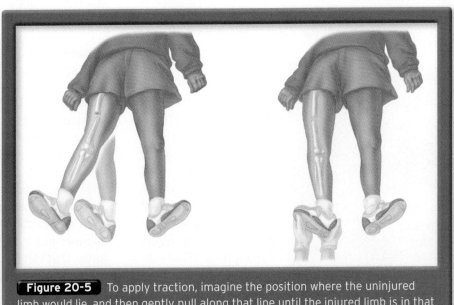

Figure 20-5 To apply traction, imagine the position where the uninjured limb would lie, and then gently pull along that line until the injured limb is in that position. Do not release traction once you have applied it.

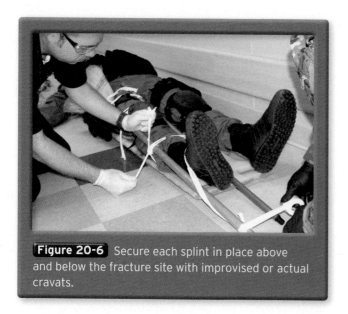

Figure 20-6 Secure each splint in place above and below the fracture site with improvised or actual cravats.

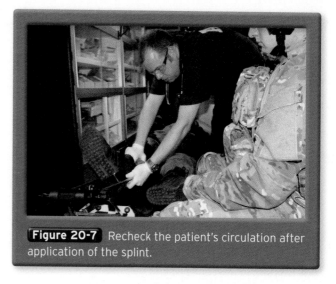

Figure 20-7 Recheck the patient's circulation after application of the splint.

8. Tie the splints. Secure each splint in place above and below the fracture site with improvised or actual cravats. Improvised cravats, such as strips of cloth, belts, or whatever else you have, may be used. With minimal motion to the injured areas, tie the splints with the bandages. Push the cravats through and under the natural body curvatures (spaces) and then gently position the cravats and tie in place. Use nonslip knots. Tie all knots on the splint on the outside of the patient **Figure 20-6**. Do not tie cravats directly over a suspected fracture/dislocation site.

9. Check the splint for tightness. Check to be sure that bandages are tight enough to securely hold splinting materials in place, but not so tight that circulation is impaired.

10. Recheck the patient's circulation and watch for swelling of the lower leg (possible compartment syndrome) after application of the splint **Figure 20-7**. A swathe is applied to an injured leg by wrapping the swathe(s) around both legs and securing it on the uninjured side.

11. Evacuate the patient to a civilian EMS ambulance or aircraft for transport.

If you were unable to apply a traction splint in the tactical environment, remove the improvised splint and apply a traction splint prior to transport. Check the circulation distal to the fractured extremity, then place the splint next to the uninjured leg to determine the proper length. The traction splint should extend 6 to 10 inches beyond the foot. Support and stabilize the leg to minimize movement while another TMP applies the ankle hitch. When the hitch is secure, the second TMP will apply gentle longitudinal traction using enough force to realign the extremity. You can then place the splint into position and connect the upper attachment point of the splint and then the ankle hitch. After applying the splint, reassess the patient's circulation before securing the patient and splint for transport.

The patient should be transported to a trauma center by an ALS level crew. If you accompany the patient during transport, perform a secondary assessment. Ensure that proper traction of the femur is maintained and monitor the patient's neurovascular status. Check the pulses, color, temperature, neurologic function, and capillary refill of the extremity distal to the fracture frequently. Elevate the injured extremity as much as possible. Apply ice-water packs to reduce pain and swelling, alternating between on and off every 20 minutes. Avoid placing ice directly onto the skin. Monitor for and take steps to prevent shock.

Open Fractures

In an open fracture the skin over the bone is broken, increasing the chances of infection, which can lead to sepsis and death **Figure 20-8**. Open fractures typically result from high-energy injuries, and thus have the potential for more blood loss than closed fractures.

Stabilizing Care for an Open Fracture

Arrange for immediate evacuation of any patient with an open fracture. To stabilize the patient for evacuation, brush and flush away any debris and control any external bleeding by applying sterile dressings over the wound and bone. The bandage should be secure enough to control bleeding without restricting circulation distal to the injury. Monitor bandage tightness by assessing the circulation, sensation, and movement distal to the bandage. Swelling from fractures and internal

Entrapped or Crushed Extremities

The increase in terrorist activities has increased the likelihood that you may encounter an entrapped or crushed extremity. You should know what the appropriate medical care is for patients who have extremities compressed under heavy building debris or heavy machinery. However, you should not attempt to provide this care unless you have the proper training and authorization from your medical director. The bottom line for care of entrapped extremities is this: Improper extrication can result in the sudden death of a patient simply by lifting the heavy object off of the trapped extremity.

If a victim is pinned beneath heavy wreckage or building materials, immediately call for help. You will need a properly trained rescue team and equipment. Do not attempt to extricate the victim if you do not have the proper training in search and rescue or ALS techniques or the proper extrication and medical equipment. Just as you would not run into a hazardous materials incident without the proper protection and training, you cannot run toward a debris field without the proper equipment and training. Becoming a victim will not help anyone. Communicate with the victim(s) and let them know that help is on the way.

Victims whose limbs are entrapped by heavy debris or objects are at risk of developing crush syndrome. **Crush syndrome** occurs because of a prolonged compressive force that impairs muscle metabolism and circulation following the extrication or release of an entrapped limb. This condition also occurs in patients who have been lying on an extremity for an extended period (4 to 6 hours of compression).

After a muscle is compressed for 4 to 6 hours, the muscle cells begin to die and release their contents into the localized vasculature. When the force compressing the region is released, blood flow is reestablished and the material from the cells that was released into the local vasculature quickly returns to the systemic vasculature. The primary substances that are of concern are lactic acid, potassium, and **myoglobin**. In particular, the return of myoglobin is likely to result in decreased blood pH, **hyperkalemia**, and renal dysfunction (**rhabdomyolysis** and acute renal failure). Crush syndrome is known as the "smiling death" because extricated patients are often smiling until the released potassium reaches their heart and sudden death ensues.

Working with the search and rescue team, the goal is to prevent the complications that occur in the body once an entrapped limb is released. Patient management should always be performed by properly trained medical professionals according to local protocols.

First, apply high-flow oxygen to the patient and get an IV started. Immediately prior to rescue, 2 L or more of normal saline (*not* potassium-containing lactated Ringer's solution) should be infused and 1 mEq/kg of sodium bicarbonate should be given. Just before the weight is removed, consider placing one or two tourniquets above the injury. The patient should be on a heart monitor when the body part is released, and if signs of elevated potassium are seen (increased height of the "T" wave, hyperacute T waves), then calcium gluconate should also be given as often as every 5 minutes as a slow IV push. If IV or intraosseous access cannot be obtained, a tourniquet should be applied proximal to the entrapment to slow down the release of myoglobin and potassium and the entry of fluid into the muscle mass. The tourniquet may later be released slowly at the hospital or during transport if the transport time is extended.

Once an indwelling catheter is placed, fluids should be given to maintain output of 200 to 300 mL/h. Bicarbonate should be given to keep urine pH greater than 6.5. This can be done by adding 3 amps to a liter of D_5W to maintain an isotonic solution. Mannitol is the diuretic of choice. It is an osmotic diuretic, reducing swelling of the damaged muscle, and it serves as an intravascular volume expander. It also dilates and flushes the renal tubules. Mannitol also is a free-radical scavenger that reduces direct damage. Loop diuretics (furosemide) should be avoided because they acidify the urine.

Rapid transportation to an appropriate medical facility by an ALS crew is a critical component to maximize the survival of the patient and the crushed limb(s). Check and record the presence or absence of distal pulses and motor and sensory functions. Monitor for compartment syndrome. Continue to administer IV fluids as indicated during transport and administer appropriate pain medications as needed and per local protocols.

bleeding may cause bandages to become too tight. If bleeding cannot be controlled, apply a tourniquet. Once the bleeding is controlled, evacuate the patient and rapidly transport, preferably with an ALS crew. If you accompany the patient during transport, perform a secondary assessment, looking for additional signs of trauma. Medications may be administered to control the patient's high level of pain per local protocols. Watch for signs of sepsis, such as tachycardia, low blood pressure, and warm skin around the wound.

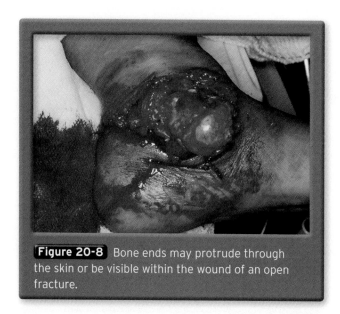

Figure 20-8 Bone ends may protrude through the skin or be visible within the wound of an open fracture.

Complications of Extremity Injuries

Compartment Syndrome

In **compartment syndrome**, bleeding or swelling occurs within the fibrous fascia tissue that divides each extremity into compartments and exceeds the amount of space available, thus impairing circulation and causing pain. The most common anatomic locations for compartment syndrome are the forearms and legs. However, any extremity and the buttocks can develop compartment syndrome. Compartment syndrome usually develops over a period of hours and is most frequently discovered during the secondary assessment during transport.

Causes of compartment syndrome include recent trauma and long-term use of bandages, splints, casts, and pneumatic anti-shock garments (PASGs) that are applied too tightly and restrict circulation. A number of internal factors can also increase the amount of material within a compartment. For example, bleeding within a compartment may occur because of a fracture, dislocation, or crush injury. A common misconception is that open fractures are safe from compartment syndrome.

The signs and symptoms of compartment syndrome initially present as pain out of proportion with the evident injury, sometimes described as burning and paresthesia (numbness and tingling) over the compartment site. Additional signs include tension of a muscle when not in use, loss of distal sensation or pulses, and extreme pain on extension or voluntary movement. The presence of pulses does not rule out compartment syndrome. The signs are commonly referred to as the six Ps—Pain, Pallor, Pulselessness, Paresthesia, Paralysis, and Pressure.

Sometimes a seventh P is included—Poikilothermia (ie, affected extremities may be cold).

The goal is to deliver the patient to an emergency facility as soon as possible. Extremity muscles can still die in the presence of good distal pulses, as there are multiple compartments in each arm and leg. Elevate the extremity to heart level (not above), place ice-water packs over the extremity, and open or loosen constrictive dressings and splint material.

Treat-Then-Transport Injuries

Closed Fractures

Closed fractures to the forearm, humerus, or tibia are not load-and-go injuries. In a closed fracture, the skin over the bone remains intact, thus reducing the probability of infection. The signs and symptoms of closed fractures include pain, swelling, deformity, rigidity, shortening, rotation, angulation, ecchymosis, guarding, and crepitus **Figure 20-9** .

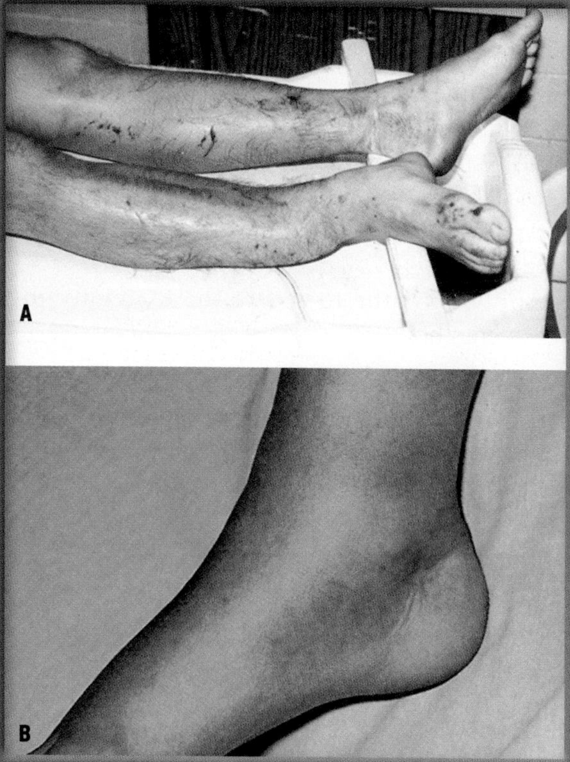

Figure 20-9 **A.** Obvious deformity is a sign of a fracture. **B.** Fractures almost always have associated bruising into the surrounding tissue.

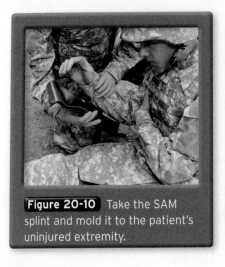

Figure 20-10 Take the SAM splint and mold it to the patient's uninjured extremity.

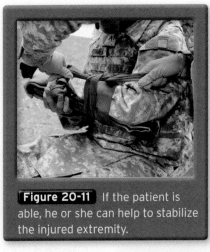

Figure 20-11 If the patient is able, he or she can help to stabilize the injured extremity.

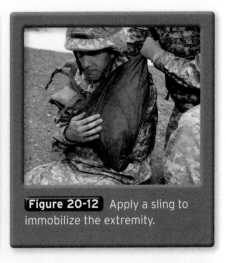

Figure 20-12 Apply a sling to immobilize the extremity.

Management of Closed Fractures

Because closed fractures to the forearm, humerus, or tibia are not load-and-go injuries, you have the time to apply a SAM splint prior to evacuation and transport. A SAM splint may be molded to fit the extremity and can be useful in the tactical environment. To apply a SAM splint, follow these steps:

1. Have the patient apply self-stabilization techniques to immobilize the injured extremity, if possible.
2. Mold the SAM splint to the patient's uninjured extremity **Figure 20-10**.
3. Splint the injured extremity with the molded SAM splint and then secure the injured extremity to the SAM splint. If the patient is able, he or she can help to stabilize the injured extremity **Figure 20-11**.
4. Apply a sling to immobilize the extremity **Figure 20-12**.
5. Apply a swathe to secure the extremity to the patient's body.

Do not evacuate the patient until the extremity fracture is completely immobilized through splinting. Since this is not a load-and-go injury, the patient should be able to wait until the callout is resolved and the civilian EMS crew can evacuate him or her on a stretcher or litter. If appropriate, administer pain medication per local protocols while awaiting evacuation. If you accompany the patient during transport, perform a secondary assessment and monitor for shock.

Sprain

A **sprain** is a stretching or tearing injury to ligaments and soft tissues that support a joint. Signs include pain or pressure at joint, pain upon movement, swelling, tenderness, possible loss of movement, discoloration, or

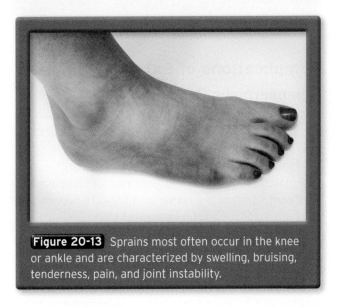

Figure 20-13 Sprains most often occur in the knee or ankle and are characterized by swelling, bruising, tenderness, pain, and joint instability.

strains **Figure 20-13**. Sprains can be caused by a forcible overstretching or tearing of a muscle or tendon. Additional signs are pain, lameness or stiffness (sometimes involving knotting of muscles), moderate swelling at the place of injury, discoloration, and a possible loss of strength in the affected area. If significant muscle tearing is present, a distinct gap will be felt at the site.

While the intensity may vary, pain, bruising, and swelling are common to all three categories of sprains—mild, moderate, and severe. A ligament is stretched in a mild sprain, but there is no joint loosening. A moderate sprain partially tears the ligament, producing joint instability and some swelling. A severe sprain produces excruciating pain at the moment of injury, as ligaments tear completely or separate from the bone. A complete tear of the ligaments may make the joint unstable and potentially nonfunctional.

A sprain is caused by direct or indirect trauma (a fall, a blow to the body, etc) that knocks a joint out of position and overstretches the supporting ligaments; in severe cases, the ligaments may be ruptured. In the tactical environment, this injury often occurs when a SWAT officer lands on an outstretched arm, jumps and lands on the side of the foot, runs on an uneven surface, or attempts to restrain a physically combative suspect.

Strain

A **strain** is a twist, pull, or tear of a muscle and/or the fibrous cords of tissue that attach muscles to the bone, the tendon. A direct blow to the body, overstretching, or excessive muscle contraction can cause an acute strain. Chronic strains are the result of overuse—prolonged, repetitive movement of muscles and tendons. Inadequate rest breaks during intensive training can lead to a strain. Tendons can be partially injured or strained, and in severe cases can completely tear or rupture. The biceps and Achilles tendons are the two tendons that are most commonly ruptured in the tactical environment.

SWAT officers also often experience:

- **Back strain.** When the muscles or the tendons that support the spine are twisted, pulled, or torn, the result is a back strain. Heavy lifting, violent altercations, or dragging a downed SWAT officer can cause this injury.
- **Hamstring muscle strain.** A hamstring muscle strain is a tear or stretch of a major muscle or its tendon in the back of the thigh. The injury can sideline a SWAT officer for up to 6 months. The likely cause is muscle strength imbalance between the hamstrings and the muscles in the front of the thigh, the quadriceps. Kicking in a door, running, or leaping can pull a hamstring. Hamstring injuries tend to be recurring.

Strains are associated with pain, muscle spasm, muscle weakness, swelling, inflammation, and cramping. With a mild strain, the muscle or tendon is stretched or pulled slightly. Some muscle function will be lost with a moderate strain, where the muscle or tendon is overstretched and slightly torn. In severe strains, the muscle and/or tendon is partially or completely ruptured, which usually incapacitates the SWAT officer.

Treatment of Sprains and Strains

Most sprains and strains do not require transport to the hospital. However, it is difficult to differentiate between a severe sprain and a fracture, so err on the side of caution and transport for further evaluation.

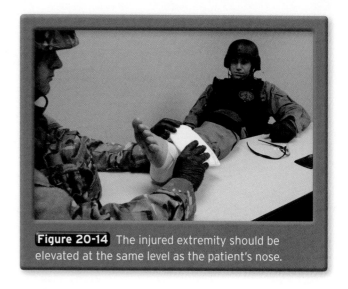

Figure 20-14 The injured extremity should be elevated at the same level as the patient's nose.

For mild to moderate sprains and strains, refer the patient to a physician to further evaluate the injury and establish a treatment and rehabilitation plan. Some moderate sprains or strains may require surgery followed by months of physical therapy. Mild sprains and strains may require rehabilitation exercises and activity modification during recovery. Good rehabilitation is critical to avoid the possibility of further or permanent disability.

With the majority of sprains and strains, the injured patient needs to follow the mnemonic "RICE" while waiting to see a personal physician. This consists of Rest, Ice, Compression, and Elevation. Ensure that the injured patient does not walk on or use the injured extremity if swelling or pain is present. Tell the patient, "If it hurts, don't do it." A cool pack should be applied to the injury site, alternating on and off every 20 minutes for the first 24 to 48 hours. The injured extremity should be elevated above the level of the heart to decrease swelling. Advise the patient to keep the injured extremity at the same level as his or her nose **Figure 20-14**. Nonconstricting compression with an elastic bandage will help decrease the swelling and improve healing. Compression bandages should not be worn while there is swelling. After 2 days of RICE, apply heat to the injured site, which brings more blood to the area and speeds healing.

Dislocations

When a bone displaces from a joint, the condition is called a dislocation **Figure 20-15**. When a body part exceeds its normal range of motion, a dislocation can occur. Until proven otherwise, all dislocations should be assumed to be coupled with a fracture. Although

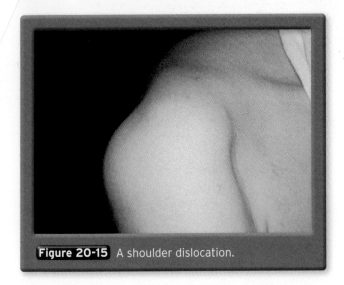

Figure 20-15 A shoulder dislocation.

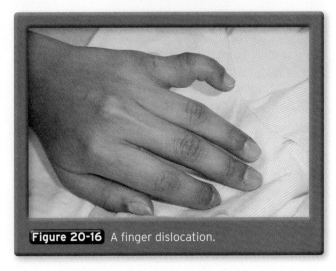

Figure 20-16 A finger dislocation.

joint dislocations are not life threatening, they are true emergencies due to the potential for neurovascular compromise that could lead to amputation if not appropriately treated. Consider administering pain medications as permitted by your level of training and local protocols. The signs and symptoms of a dislocation include pain, swelling, distorted anatomy, shortening, ecchymosis, guarding or being "locked," and being unable to move **Figure 20-16**.

Only attempt to reduce a dislocation if you are properly trained and if local protocols or your medical director permit you. Attempts to realign or reduce dislocations can lead to more damage. Splint the joint in the position of comfort with an appropriate splint while maintaining circulation. Reassess pulses distal to the injury site after application of the splint. Have the patient transported to the hospital for further evaluation and care.

Ready for Review

- Extremity injuries encountered in the tactical environment can range from inconvenient to life threatening.

- Load-and-go injuries include amputations, femur fractures, and open fractures.

- Initial bleeding with an amputation may be severe. In the tactical environment, a tourniquet is the best option to control the bleeding.

- Sharp bone ends can damage soft tissue when the femur is broken. If possible, use a traction splint to control bleeding and provide comfort.

- An open fracture puts the body at risk for infection that could lead to sepsis or death. Open fractures are a surgical emergency and require immediate evacuation and transport.

- The goal of treating compartment syndrome is to deliver the patient to an emergency facility before the extremity is pulseless.

- Closed fractures to the forearm, humerus, or tibia are not load-and-go injuries. Apply a SAM splint prior to evacuation and transport.

- A sprain is a stretching or tearing injury to ligaments and soft tissues that support a joint. Sprains can be categorized as mild, moderate, or severe.

- A strain is a twist, pull, or tear of a muscle or tendon. The biceps, Achilles tendon, back muscles, and hamstrings are common strains in the tactical environment.

- A dislocation is a condition in which a bone displaces from a joint. Dislocations are emergencies due to the potential for neurovascular compromise. Only attempt to reduce a dislocation if you are appropriately trained and authorized to do so.

Vital Vocabulary

amputation An injury in which part of the body is completely severed.

compartment syndrome Swelling in a confined space that produces dangerous pressure; may cut off blood flow or damage sensitive tissue; frequently seen in fractures below the elbow or knee in children.

crush syndrome Significant metabolic derangement that develops when crushed extremities or body parts remain trapped for prolonged periods. This can lead to renal failure and death.

hyperkalemia An abnormally high level of potassium in the blood.

myoglobin An oxygen-carrying protein present in high concentrations of the cardiac and skeletal muscles.

rhabdomyolysis The destruction of muscle tissue leading to a release of potassium and myoglobin, which then accumulate in the blood and urine and impair filtration; occurs often with crush injuries.

sprain A joint injury involving damage to supporting ligaments and sometimes partial or temporary dislocation of bone ends.

strain Stretching or tearing of a muscle; also called a muscle pull.

Soft-Tissue Injuries

OBJECTIVES

- Describe the stabilizing care provided to a patient with a major thermal burn injury.

- Describe the stabilizing care provided to a patient with a major electrical burn injury.

- Describe the treatment of a closed soft-tissue injury in the tactical environment.

- Describe the treatment of an abrasion in the tactical environment.

- Describe the treatment of a laceration in the tactical environment.

- Describe the treatment of an avulsion in the tactical environment.

- Describe the treatment of a bite wound in the tactical environment.

- Describe the treatment of a splinter in the tactical environment.

- Describe the treatment of fungal skin diseases in the tactical environment.

- Describe the treatment of contact dermatitis in the tactical environment.

- Describe the treatment of a subungual hematoma in the tactical environment.

- Describe the treatment of a blister in the tactical environment.

Introduction

The skin is our first line of defense against external forces and infection. Although it is relatively tough, skin is still quite susceptible to injury. Injuries to soft tissues range from simple bruises and abrasions to burns. Minor injuries such as a simple laceration require little care and will heal with time. Electrical burns are load-and-go injuries that require stabilizing care and rapid transport in order to increase the chance of patient survival. This chapter covers the spectrum of soft-tissue injuries.

Load-and-Go Injuries

In the tactical environment, the mechanism of injury (MOI) is often known because the injury is witnessed. When major thermal or chemical burns occur, you only have time to initiate stabilizing care (stop the burning, stabilize circulation, maintain an open airway, support breathing), while expediting rapid evacuation to an ALS ground or air ambulance **Table 21-1**.

Thermal Burns

Thermal burns in the tactical environment are rare, but they may occur from diversionary devices, booby traps, explosions, or fires. Some of the chemical munitions used by SWAT units generate a considerable amount of heat, and when used in a house where a suspect is hiding, these munitions may accidentally start a fire. This is why many SWAT units have firefighters standing by when chemical munitions are used.

To determine if the burn is a load-and-go injury, you need to determine the depth, size, and severity of the burn.

Table 21-1   Load-and-Go Injuries
• Full-thickness burns larger than 10% body surface area
• Subdermal burns
• Electrical burns

Burn Depth

Superficial burns, or first-degree burns, involve only the epidermis and are usually the result of ultraviolet light exposure (sunburn) or minor flash burns. The skin is red but not blistered; healing will usually occur without scarring in approximately 7 days. This is not a load-and-go injury.

Partial-thickness burns, or second-degree burns, are subdivided into superficial and deep burns. In **superficial partial-thickness burns** (superficial second-degree burns), the epidermis and part of the dermis are involved, but the deeper layers of the dermis are spared, including the sweat glands, sebaceous glands, and hair follicles. These burns are typically caused by minimal contact with flame. Blisters form, and the injured skin is red and painful to touch. These burns do not typically require skin grafting unless they are extensive and occur on areas of the body with thin skin such as the face, hands, genitals, and feet. Superficial partial-thickness burns will heal in 14 to 21 days. The extent of the scarring depends on the extent of the burn. **Deep partial-thickness burns** (deep second-degree burns) are most often the result of steam, hot oil, or flames, and involve the deeper layers of the dermis. They may be difficult to distinguish from full-thickness burns. The skin is blistered but not charred and is painful to touch. Healing takes 21 days or more and may require surgical skin grafts. Scarring may be moderate and depends on the extent and location of the burn.

Full-thickness burns, or third-degree burns, involve the entire thickness of the dermis down to the subcutaneous fat. All epidermal and dermal structures including nerve endings in the burned area are destroyed, resulting in a bloodless, pale, painless, leathery charred area of skin. Full-thickness burns will not heal spontaneously, and surgical skin grafting is usually necessary. Full-thickness burns result in significant scarring and long-term management. Full-thickness burns larger than 10% of body surface area (BSA)—especially in a patient with unstable vital signs—are a load-and-go injury requiring transportation to a burn center when feasible.

Subdermal burns, or fourth-degree burns, involve all layers of skin and dermis down to the deep structures of muscle and bone, larger blood vessels, and nerves. These injuries are severe and life threatening—a load-and-go injury. Like larger full-thickness burns, they will not heal spontaneously and require surgical intervention.

Superficial, partial-thickness, full-thickness, and subdermal burns are shown in **Figure 21-1**.

Burn Size

The depth of the burn is only one factor determining its severity; the size of the burn is also a determining factor. Numerous methods are available to estimate the BSA involved in a burn. The **rule of nines**, the most common formula, is based on the fact that large regions of the adult body can be divided into areas that represent roughly 9% of the total BSA or multiples of 9% **Figure 21-2**. The **Lund and Browder chart** **Figure 21-3** may also be used to determine the size of the burn.

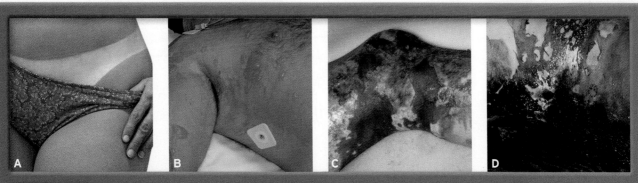

Figure 21-1   Classification of burns. **A.** Superficial (first-degree) burns involve only the epidermis. **B.** Partial-thickness (second-degree) burns involve some of the dermis but do not destroy the entire thickness of the skin. The skin is mottled, white to red, and often blistered. **C.** Full-thickness (third-degree) burns extend through all layers of the skin and may involve subcutaneous tissue and muscle. The skin is dry, leathery, and often white or charred. **D.** Subdermal (fourth-degree) burns involve deep structures such as muscle, bone, large blood vessels, and nerves.

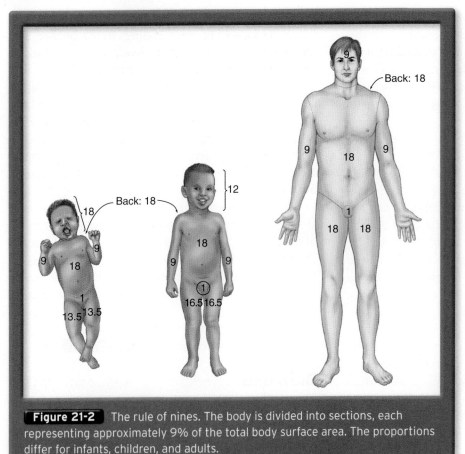

Figure 21-2 The rule of nines. The body is divided into sections, each representing approximately 9% of the total body surface area. The proportions differ for infants, children, and adults.

Burn Severity

The American Burn Association classifies burns into three primary categories—major, moderate, and minor. Major burn injuries include:

1. Partial-thickness burns involving more than 25% of BSA in adults or 20% of BSA in children younger than 10 years and adults older than 50 years
2. Full-thickness burns involving more than 10% of BSA
3. Burns involving the face, eyes, ears, hands, feet, or perineum that may result in functional or cosmetic impairment
4. Burns caused by caustic chemical agents
5. High-voltage electrical injury
6. Burns complicated by inhalation injury or major trauma
7. Burns sustained by high-risk patients (eg, patients with

Region	%
Head	
Neck	
Ant. Trunk	
Post. Trunk	
Right arm	
Left arm	
Buttocks	
Genitalia	
Right leg	
Left leg	
Total burn	

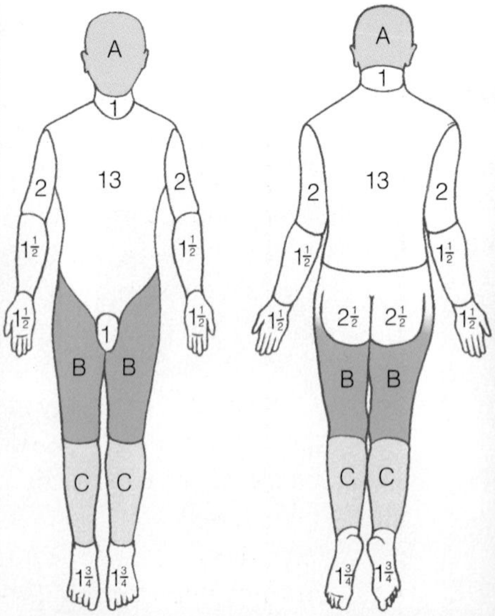

Relative percentages of body surface area affected by growth

Age (years)	A ($\frac{1}{2}$ of head)	B ($\frac{1}{2}$ of one thigh)	C ($\frac{1}{2}$ of one leg)
0	$9\frac{1}{2}$	$2\frac{3}{4}$	$2\frac{1}{2}$
1	$8\frac{1}{2}$	$3\frac{1}{4}$	$2\frac{1}{2}$
5	$6\frac{1}{2}$	4	$2\frac{3}{4}$
10	$5\frac{1}{2}$	$4\frac{1}{4}$	3
15	$4\frac{1}{2}$	$4\frac{1}{2}$	$3\frac{1}{4}$
Adult	$3\frac{1}{2}$	$4\frac{3}{4}$	3

Figure 21-3 The Lund and Browder chart.
Adapted from Lund CC, Browder NC. *Surg Gynecol Obstet*. 1944;79:352-358.

debilitating diseases such as diabetes or congestive heart failure)

8. Circumferential burns resulting in swelling with respiratory compromise or decreased circulation to the extremities.

Moderate burn injuries include the following (note that this list excludes high-voltage injury):

1. Partial-thickness burns of 15% to 25% of BSA in adults or more than 10% to 20% of BSA in children and older adults

2. Full-thickness burns involving 2% to 10% BSA that do not present a serious threat to functional or cosmetic impairment of the eyes, ears, face, hands, feet, or perineum

Minor burn injuries include:

1. Partial-thickness burns involving less than 15% BSA in adults or 10% of BSA in children and older adults

2. Full-thickness burns involving less than 2% BSA that do not present a serious threat of functional or cosmetic risk to the eyes, ears, face, hands, feet, or perineum

Stabilizing Care for a Thermal Burn Injury

After all threats have been abolished, the goal in stabilizing patients with burns is to stop the burning process, assess and stabilize circulation, airway, and breathing (CAB), and provide rapid transport. Follow standard precautions. Because a burn destroys the patient's protective skin layer and body fluid exposure is present, always wear gloves and handle patients carefully with clean gloves and equipment.

Move the patient away from the burning area. If any clothing is on fire, wrap the patient in a blanket or follow specific guidelines outlined by your local fire department protocol to put out the flames, then remove any smoldering clothing and/or jewelry. Do not pull

Special Populations

Burns to children are generally considered more serious than burns to adults. This is because infants and children have more surface area relative to total body mass, which means greater fluid and heat loss. In addition, children do not tolerate burns as well as adults do. Children are also more likely to go into shock, develop hypothermia, and experience airway problems because of differences associated with their age and anatomy.

away clothing that is melted and attached to burned skin. Loose clothing may be gently cut away to expose the patient's skin. Complete removal of burned clothing will be performed later at the burn center.

Any burned skin that is still hot should be cooled to body temperature using clean water. Follow your local protocols. If the burned area is fairly small (less than 15% BSA), immerse the area in cool, sterile water or saline solution, or cover with a clean, wet, cool dressing. This stops the burning and relieves pain. Prolonged immersion, however, may increase the risk of infection and hypothermia. For this reason, you should not keep the affected part submersed in water for more than 10 minutes. If the burning has stopped before you reach the patient and the burn areas are at body temperature, do not immerse the affected part at all. As an alternative to immersion, the burned area can be irrigated until the burning stops, followed by the application of a sterile dressing.

Once the skin is no longer burning and is back to body temperature, rapidly estimate the burn's severity, then cover the burned area with a dry, sterile dressing to prevent further contamination. Sterile gauze is best if the area is not too large. You may cover larger areas with a clean, white sheet. Most importantly, do not put anything else on the burned area. Never use ointments, lotions, or antiseptics of any kind. In addition, do not intentionally break any blisters.

Provide high-flow oxygen as soon as possible or provide assisted ventilations with a bag-mask device as needed. More fire victims die of smoke inhalation than of skin burns. A patient who has inhaled smoke or fumes may have soot on the face and within the nostrils, and may develop airway problems such as stridor and difficulty breathing. Therefore, you should provide high-flow oxygen as soon as possible. Keep in mind that a patient who appears to be breathing well at first may rapidly develop severe respiratory distress. Therefore, continually assess the airway for possible problems and if indicated then arrange for appropriate airway intervention and possible intubation.

Check for traumatic injuries that may be more immediately life threatening. Most patients who have been burned have normal vital signs and can communicate initially, which will make your rapid assessment easier.

Treat the patient for shock. An extensive burn can produce hypothermia (loss of body heat) due to evaporative heat loss and other factors. Prevent further heat loss by covering the patient with warm blankets.

Provide rapid evacuation to ALS-level transport. Do not delay transport to do a prolonged assessment or to apply coverings to burns on a load-and-go patient. If you are permitted to accompany the patient during transport, consider direct transportation to a burn center if the patient is stable and does not need to go to the nearest hospital immediately. Contact the medical director for clarification and recommendations.

Many critical burn patients will ultimately require intubation, even though they were talking and in no distress in the tactical environment. Although it is obviously preferable to have such patients intubated in a controlled environment with a full complement of anesthesia agents, a few patients will absolutely require an emergency advanced airway during transport. Due to the potential internal injuries to the burn patient's airway, the most experienced intubator should manage the patient's airway.

A large-bore IV catheter should be inserted as early as possible in any patient who has been severely burned. If a delay of more than 4 hours occurs in starting IV fluids in burn patients, then the mortality rate is higher. Start a large-bore IV catheter into a large vein and give lactated Ringer's solution or normal saline. You can use the burned extremity for the IV site if you cannot find another site—an IV line in a burned upper extremity is still preferable to an IV line in a lower extremity.

The ideal amount of fluid to infuse will depend on several factors, including whether the patient was burned during a blast. If the patient has burns due to an explosion, follow the principles of permissive hypotension and your local protocols.

If no blast injuries are involved, the approximate amount of fluid the burn patient will need may be calculated by using the **Parkland formula**, which recommends resuscitation with lactated Ringer's solution (normal saline is an acceptable substitute) of 4 mL/kg/%BSA burned; half this amount should be given over the first 8 hours (from the time of injury), one fourth of the total amount should be given over the second 8 hours, and one fourth of the total amount should be given over the third 8 hours. All calculations are determined from the time of the injury, and therefore fluid boluses may be necessary to correct deficits in fluid resuscitation, either due to a delay in presentation or because of under-resuscitation. It may also be necessary to administer fluids more aggressively if the patient is in shock with unstable vital signs.

Any patient with burns should receive aggressive pain management according to your local protocols. Assess the patient's pain before administering any analgesia. Reassessment should be completed using the same scale (for example, 1 to 10) every 5 minutes. Burn patients may require higher than usual doses of pain medications to achieve relief. Their metabolic rate may

USAISR Rule of Ten

The United States Army's Tactical Combat Casualty Care (TCCC) guidelines have introduced a new fluid resuscitation formula for patients with burns. This formula has been adopted by some TEMS units. As always, follow your local protocols.

The United States Army Institute of Surgical Research (USAISR) Rule of Ten states that if the patient has burns over 20% of his or her body, you should begin fluid resuscitation promptly via an IV or IO. The following formula is used to calculate the initial fluid rate for adults weighing 40 to 80 kg (88 to 176 lb):

Percentage of the total body surface area burned (% TBSA) × 10 mL/hr

For every 10 kg (22 lb) above 80 kg (176 lb), increase the initial fluid rate by 100 mL/hr.

be accelerated, which creates the need for higher than normal doses of analgesics. Consult your local protocols or contact medical control for guidance in administering analgesics.

Electrical Burns

Electrical injuries are possible during tactical missions and training **Figure 21-4**. When searching rooms, attics, and basements of old or abandoned buildings, SWAT officers may come in direct contact with exposed electrical wiring. Contact an electrical company representative if you suspect that any high-voltage threat remains.

Electrical burns may produce devastating internal injuries with little external evidence **Figure 21-5**. The entrance wound can be quite small, but the exit wound can be extensive and deep **Figure 21-6**. This is a load-and-go injury. The degree of tissue injury is related

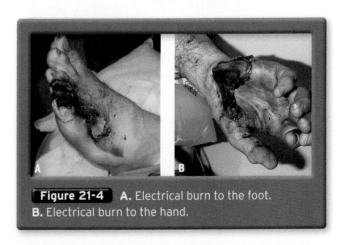

Figure 21-4   **A.** Electrical burn to the foot. **B.** Electrical burn to the hand.

to the resistance of the body tissues, the intensity of current that passes through the victim, and the duration of exposure.

When a person comes in contact with an electrical source, the amount of current delivered to the inside of the body depends to some extent on the resistance of the skin. Wet, thin, clean skin offers less resistance than dry, thick, dirty skin; thus a moist inner surface of the forearm will have much less resistance than a dry, calloused palm. As electric current travels from the contact site into the body, it is converted to heat, which follows the current flow—usually along blood vessels and nerves—causing extensive damage to the tissues in its path. The greater the current flow, the greater the heat generated. When the voltage is low (< 1000 volts, as in household sources), the current follows the path of least resistance, generally along blood vessels, nerves, and muscles. When the voltage is high (as from high-tension lines), the current takes the shortest path.

Alternating current is considerably more dangerous than direct current because the alternations cause repetitive muscle contractions that may "freeze" the victim to the conductor until the current source is turned off. Furthermore, alternating current is more likely than direct current to induce ventricular fibrillation. The path of current flow is also significant. Current moving from one hand to the other is particularly dangerous because it may flow across the heart; a current of only 0.1 amp to the heart can cause ventricular fibrillation.

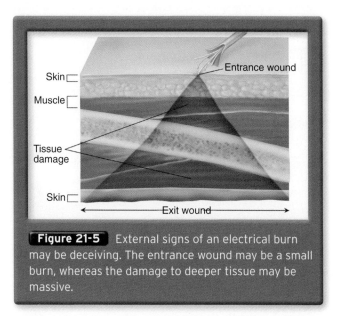

Figure 21-5 External signs of an electrical burn may be deceiving. The entrance wound may be a small burn, whereas the damage to deeper tissue may be massive.

Stabilizing Care for an Electrical Burn

The first priority at the scene of an electrical injury is to protect yourself and bystanders from becoming the next victims. Do *not* use a rope, wooden pole, or any other object to try to dislodge the patient from the current source. Do *not* try to cut the wire. Do *not* go anywhere near a high-tension line.

Many parts of the electrical grid are protected by automatically resetting breakers. In everyday situations, such as when the wind blows a branch into wires, it is desirable to have the breaker reset after a few minutes to avoid power outages. As a consequence, a downed wire that looks "dead" can jump back to life, perhaps several times. There is only one safe way to deal with a downed high-voltage wire: Call the electric company. Wait until a qualified person has shut off the power before you approach the patient. This can be a traumatic

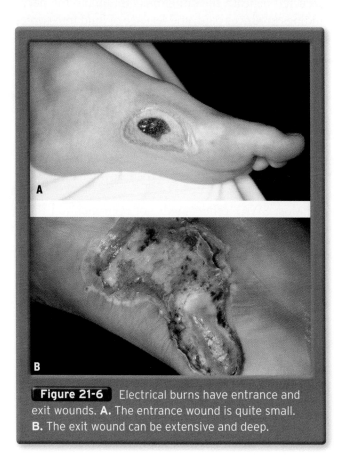

Figure 21-6 Electrical burns have entrance and exit wounds. **A.** The entrance wound is quite small. **B.** The exit wound can be extensive and deep.

Safety

Many training sites include old houses that are about to be torn down and donated to the town or city for training. Prior to training, command should work with the fire department to ensure that there are no electrical hazards. During the medical threat assessment prior to training, ensure that the training site has been inspected for any electrical hazards.

event for TMPs, who will feel helpless waiting for the power to be shut down while a possibly critical patient lies on the ground nearby. But remember—*rescuers die in these situations*. You can help the greatest number of people by being cautious and safe in this circumstance.

Once the electric hazard has been neutralized, focus first on the patient's airway. Open the airway using the jaw-thrust maneuver, keeping in mind the possibility of cervical spine injury. Start CPR as indicated, and attach the monitor or AED to identify and treat ventricular fibrillation. If the patient is not in cardiac arrest, arrhythmias remain a risk.

Make careful note of the patient's state of consciousness. Try to determine the path the current has taken through the body by looking for entrance and exit wounds and by carefully palpating the skin and soft tissues. When deep tissues have been seriously damaged by heat, the surrounding muscle may swell and become rock-hard. Thus, a rigid abdomen or rigid extremity may indicate a serious internal injury. Be alert for fractures or dislocations, and check the distal pulses in all four extremities.

Once the airway, breathing, and circulation have been stabilized, rapidly evacuate the patient to ALS-level transportation. Contact medical control for advice in making a transport decision or regarding the need to use air medical evacuation directly to the burn center.

If you are permitted to accompany the patient during transport, start an IV and provide fluid therapy for the care of a burn injury. Contact medical control about administering medications to manage extreme pain. Provide oxygen and manage the patient for impending shock. These patients are usually very anxious, so be sure to talk with them calmly and explain how you plan to obtain the best care for them.

Treat-Then-Transport Injuries

Injuries to soft tissues range from simple bruises and abrasions to serious lacerations. Soft-tissue injury may result in loss of soft tissue, exposing deep structures such as blood vessels, nerves, and bones. In all instances of soft-tissue injury, you must control bleeding, prevent further contamination to decrease the risk of infection, and protect the wound from further damage.

Closed Wounds

In a **closed wound**, soft tissues beneath the skin surface are damaged, but there is no break in the epidermis. The

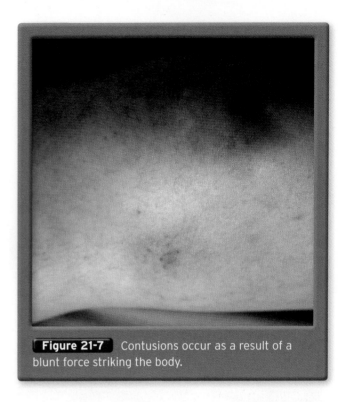

Figure 21-7 Contusions occur as a result of a blunt force striking the body.

characteristic closed wound is a **contusion** **Figure 21-7**. In a contusion (bruise), the skin is intact but damage has occurred beneath the epidermis. Trauma to the nerve endings produces pain, and leakage of fluid into spaces between the damaged cells produces swelling (edema). If small blood vessels in the dermis are disrupted, then blood will flow into the tissue and a black-and-blue mark (ecchymosis) will cover the injured area; if large blood vessels are torn beneath the contused area, a hematoma—a collection of blood beneath the skin—will be evident as a lump with a bluish discoloration. As the body heals, the appearance will change from purple to brown to green to yellow and then slowly fade away to normal skin color.

Most SWAT officers will not even mention these injuries. For those SWAT officers who do, utilize the standard RICE (rest, ice, compression with elastic bandage, and elevation to the same height as the nose) treatment for the first 24 to 48 hours. The cold packs should be a mixture of ice and water and should not be placed directly on the skin. The cold pack should be applied for 20 minutes, and then removed for 20 minutes. Warn the patient against sleeping with compression bandages on, as swelling and constriction may occur overnight, resulting in possible tissue damage. After 36 to 48 hours, the patient may apply moist heat occasionally during the day to facilitate increased blood flow to the area and to speed healing.

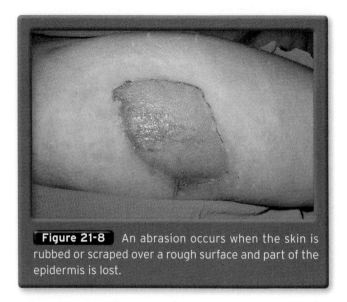

Figure 21-8 An abrasion occurs when the skin is rubbed or scraped over a rough surface and part of the epidermis is lost.

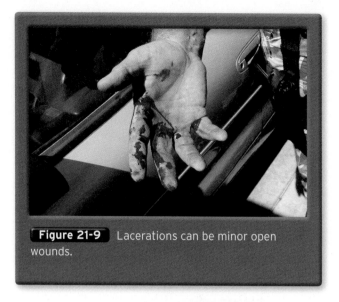

Figure 21-9 Lacerations can be minor open wounds.

Open Wounds

An **open wound** is characterized by a disruption in the skin. Open wounds are potentially much more serious than closed wounds for two reasons. First, they are vulnerable to infection. An open wound is contaminated with microorganisms. Whether the **contamination** produces infection depends in large measure on how the wound is managed. Second, open wounds have a greater potential for serious blood loss (see Chapter 12, "Controlling Bleeding"). Certain wounds, such as grossly contaminated wounds and bite wounds, are at higher risk for serious complications and therefore should always be evaluated by a physician.

Abrasions

An **abrasion** is a superficial wound that occurs when the skin is rubbed or scraped over a rough surface and part of the epidermis is lost 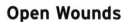. So-called brush burns or mat burns are good examples of abrasions. Abrasions typically ooze small amounts of blood and may be quite painful. They may also be contaminated with dirt and debris—for example, from "road rash" caused by sliding on the pavement. Because the skin has been disrupted, infection is a danger. If a small foreign body such as a rock or a stick remains embedded in the wound, the chance of a serious infection is much higher.

Follow standard precautions. For small abrasions with no foreign matter embedded in the wound, provide simple and safe cleansing of the skin to remove germs and dirt particles. Apply direct pressure with a sterile dressing to stop any bleeding that will likely be caused. Once the bleeding has stopped, apply a topical antibacterial ointment such as bacitracin to the wound. A bandage or appropriately sized dressing should be placed over the ointment. Once the mission or training is complete, the SWAT officer should seek follow-up care with a physician to ensure that the wound heals properly without infection.

Do not try to pick out foreign matter embedded in the wound. Simply irrigate the site copiously and then cover the wound with a dry, sterile dressing. Patients with debris embedded in their wound require transport to a hospital for further treatment.

Lacerations

A **laceration** is a cut inflicted by a sharp instrument such as a knife or razor blade that produces a clean or jagged incision through the skin surface and underlying structures **Figure 21-9**. Sometimes the term laceration is reserved for jagged or irregular cuts, and **incision** is used to refer to a clean (linear) cut. Incisions tend to heal better than lacerations because of their relatively even wound margins. The seriousness of a laceration will depend on its depth and the structures that have been

Safety

SWAT officers with abrasions or lacerations should have their tetanus vaccination history checked. If the SWAT officer has a contaminated wound and it has been more than 5 years since receiving a vaccination, or if the SWAT officer has a minor laceration and it has been more than 10 years since receiving a vaccination, then a tetanus vaccine booster shot is required. Inform the SWAT officer that he or she needs to see his or her physician or the public health department within a day or two to be vaccinated appropriately.

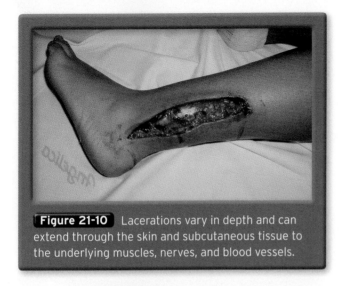

Figure 21-10 Lacerations vary in depth and can extend through the skin and subcutaneous tissue to the underlying muscles, nerves, and blood vessels.

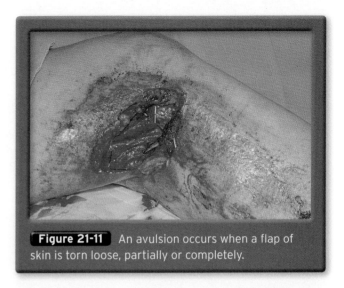

Figure 21-11 An avulsion occurs when a flap of skin is torn loose, partially or completely.

damaged **Figure 21-10** . Lacerations may be the source of significant bleeding if they disrupt the wall of a blood vessel, particularly in regions of the body where major arteries lie close to the surface (as in the wrist). The first priority in treating a laceration is to control bleeding, initially by applying direct manual pressure over the wound. Laceration of a major artery can be fatal due to the severe bleeding that can occur (see Chapter 12, "Controlling Bleeding").

Before you begin caring for the patient, protect yourself by following standard precautions. Apply a dry, sterile dressing over the entire wound. Apply pressure to the dressing with your gloved hand. Maintain the pressure and secure the dressing with a roller bandage. If bleeding continues or recurs, leave the original dressing in place. Apply a second dressing on top of the first and secure it with another roller bandage. Evacuate the patient to transport the patient to an emergency department for wound closure. If bleeding continues or recurs, apply a tourniquet to an extremity above the level of the wound.

Avulsions

An **avulsion** occurs when a flap of skin is torn loose, partially or completely **Figure 21-11** . Depending on where the avulsion occurs, it may or may not be accompanied by profuse bleeding. The principal danger in this type of injury—besides blood loss and contamination—is loss of the blood supply to the avulsed flap. If the part of the flap that connects it to the body (the pedicle) is folded back or kinked, circulation to the flap will be compromised and that piece of skin will die if the circulation is not restored quickly.

In treating a partially avulsed piece of skin that is fairly small, quickly irrigate any dirt or debris out of the wound and then gently fold the skin flap back onto the wound so that it is more or less normally aligned. Hold the flap in place with a dry, sterile compression dressing. Larger avulsion lacerations will need to be repaired with sutures or staples at the local emergency department. Transport the patient to the hospital for further care.

Splinters

Splinters are actually small puncture or penetrating wounds. Small foreign bodies such as splinters may be removed as soon as it is convenient, per local protocols. Most splinters can be removed with an 18-gauge needle or a #11 scalpel blade. Once removed, the splinter should be inspected. If it appears some of the splinter has broken off and may still be in the wound, the patient should be transported to the hospital for a follow-up examination and care. Surgical exploration may be needed to complete the removal and to prevent infection.

Bite Wounds

SWAT officers are at risk for both dog bites and human bites, both of which are high-risk wounds. Suspects often keep pit bulls and other aggressive dogs around to scare off enemies **Figure 21-12** . All bite wounds have a high potential for developing serious infections or abscesses.

Because the mouth is warm and constantly moist, it offers a hospitable environment for the growth of bacteria. Injection of human saliva into tissue can result in significant infection. Rabies is a serious infection that can develop from the bite of an infected animal (such as wild raccoons, dogs, and cats).

All animal and human bites should be evaluated by a physician. A patient with a bite wound may develop a severe infection such as cellulitis (bacterial skin

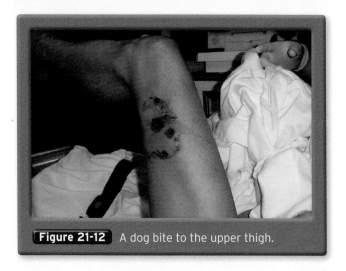

Figure 21-12 A dog bite to the upper thigh.

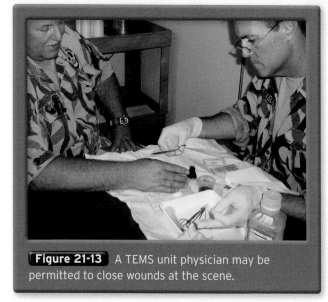

Figure 21-13 A TEMS unit physician may be permitted to close wounds at the scene.

Advanced Wound Management

According to protocols, TEMS unit physicians or other advanced medical personnel may be permitted to close wounds at the scene **Figure 21-13**. Common sense and the requirements of the mission must be factored into the decision of where and when the wound should be closed. Some minor wounds may be safely closed at the scene using:

- **Steri-strips.** Steri-strips look like adhesive tape and are noninvasive, rapid, and easy to apply. These are made in ⅛-inch, ¼-inch, and ½-inch wide strips of adhesive, fiber-reinforced plastic material.

- **Cyanoacrylic glue.** This "tissue glue" may be used to close simple wounds on areas of the body such as the face, areas not adjacent to a joint, and areas not likely to be bumped or rubbed. The glued laceration should be kept as dry as possible, and may only get wet for the briefest amount of time (less than 5-7 minutes) in the shower for the next several days. The glue falls off in 8 to 10 days.

- **Staples.** Many lacerations of the scalp, torso, arms, and legs are simple incisions and are amenable to repair using staples. Staples are usually composed of stainless-steel metal, and once they are placed, they very securely hold the wound edges. The advantage of using staples is that a large laceration can be closed much more quickly than when compared to using sutures **Figure 21-14**. The only disadvantage of staples is that there might be a slightly larger scar than with sutures, as each staple puncture may leave a very small scar marking. Therefore, staples are not to be used in areas where cosmetic appearance is important.

- **Sutures.** Laceration repair by using surgical sutures is a common practice that in the United States is typically performed by physicians. In the military, and increasingly in the private sector, physician assistants and advanced medical personnel are using sutures to close wounds in the skin.

Advanced wound management includes knowing which wounds require closure. If a simple laceration is present without deep involvement, foreign body, fracture, or cut tendon, then cleansing followed by use of Polysporin, bacitracin, or other antibiotic ointment and a sterile dry dressing will enhance healing. If there is a more significant laceration into the deep dermis layer (subcutaneous fat is visible), then closure with steri-strips, staples, sutures, or skin adhesive should be considered.

To close a wound using advanced closure techniques, the medical provider inspects the wound and performs a distal neurovascular examination. Then the medical provider decides how best to repair the laceration. A local or regional block anesthesia is used to numb the laceration area. The wound is cleansed.

Using good light, a final thorough inspection is performed, looking for foreign bodies and contamination. Any foreign material is removed, significant bleeding is stopped, and the wound is irrigated with a sterile normal saline solution.

If sutures are used, then the simple interrupted vertical mattress-style suture is the technique that is often used for a good cosmetic result. After the repair is complete, the patient is educated on wound care, dressing changes, and complications to watch for such as wound infections.

Sutures should be kept in place on the trunk and extremities for approximately 10 days and on the face for 5 days. Sutures are removed by a medical provider in a sterile environment. Steri-strips may be placed across the wound after suture removal to ensure that the wound remains closed.

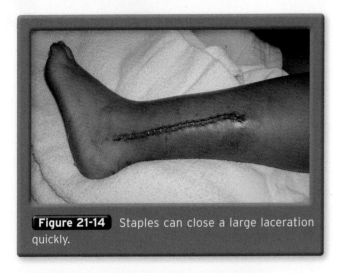

Figure 21-14 Staples can close a large laceration quickly.

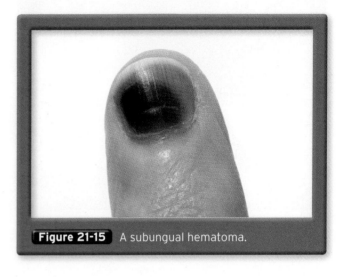

Figure 21-15 A subungual hematoma.

Safety

SWAT officers and TMPs should use caution when around unfamiliar animals. Rabies-infected animals may be encountered at inner-city locations as well as rural areas, including skunks, foxes, raccoons, and bats. Some dogs are also infected with rabies if they are wild dogs or if their owners ignore the laws mandating rabies vaccination. Any person with a bite wound from an animal species known to carry rabies, or a domestic dog or cat whose immunization status is unknown or not immunized, should undergo a careful rabies evaluation. If a SWAT officer is bitten by an animal, the animal should either be kept in a secure place for observation (10-12 days) or put down so its brain can be sent to a diagnostic lab to screen for the rabies virus.

infection), abscess (pus in a sac), or sepsis and should be admitted to the hospital for IV antibiotics and possibly surgery. With small animal bites, the patient is also at risk for rabies and will need to receive postexposure treatment. Bring the SWAT officer's medical record with you for the hospital physician to consult. Place a dry, sterile dressing over the wound and promptly transport the patient to an emergency department. In severe cases, pain control measures may be indicated. Follow local protocols.

Subungual Hematoma

A **subungual hematoma** is a sudden compression injury to a fingernail or toenail that can result in injury of the nail bed with a purple-colored blood collection under the nail **Figure 21-15**. If subungual hematomas are not

treated early, this condition may cause more pain and possible complications. If the subungual hematoma does not spontaneously bleed and drain, it will remain painful for several weeks and ultimately lead to the loss of the fingernail. These injuries are treated by **trephination**, creating a small hole in the nail at the deepest point of the blood collection. This is a physician-level procedure but is sometimes performed by nurses and paramedics. Always follow your local protocols.

To perform trephination, clean the nail with a small alcohol wipe or povidone-iodine (eg, Betadine) and then trephinate the nail. The preferred method is to use a handheld battery-powered cautery to burn a hole in the nail, but this specialized piece of medical equipment is rarely available at the scene. The tip of a paper clip may be heated in a flame to sterilize it. A cold pack is placed on the nail bed to numb it before the procedure. Once the tip is red-hot, it is placed against the nail to burn a hole over the middle of the purple hematoma. An alternative method is to use a small drill, 18-gauge needle, or the point of a #11 scalpel blade to gently drill a hole in the nail.

If the subungual hematoma contains a thick blood clot, it may not drain completely from a single hole and a second or third trephination may be necessary. Following drainage of the blood, a small amount of antibacterial ointment should be applied and then a Band-Aid. The nail often falls off within several weeks and can take 3 to 6 months to grow back.

Fungal Skin Diseases

Fungal infections are common on the feet and the body. Fungal infections may be itchy. Occasionally there is tenderness and inflammation. Superficial fungal infections are most commonly acquired from humans, but may also be acquired from the soil and animals.

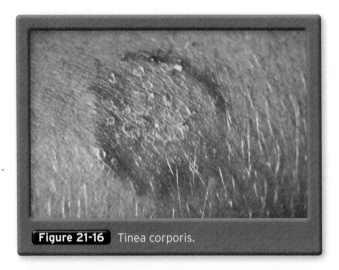

Figure 21-16 Tinea corporis.

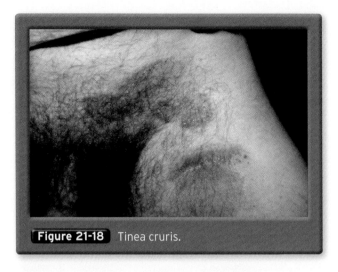

Figure 21-18 Tinea cruris.

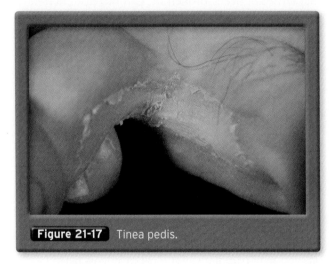

Figure 21-17 Tinea pedis.

Safety

Methicillin-resistant *Staphylococcus aureus* (MRSA) skin infections have become increasingly more common in the past few years. This bacterial infection is resistant to treatment by multiple classes of antibiotics, making the infection difficult to control. MRSA can cause cellulitis, abscesses, wound infections, pneumonia, and septic shock. Signs and symptoms include an area of redness, warmth, tenderness, and fever. MRSA is spread through direct contact with a contaminated patient, so take standard precautions and isolate the patient from the rest of the SWAT unit. Contact medical control for further instruction.

Superficial skin infections are named according to their anatomic location:

- Body (**tinea corporis**), also known as ringworm **Figure 21-16**. Usually appears in a ring shape that looks as though a worm is under the skin. Ringworm is not due to an actual worm. Intense inflammation with or without a pus-filled lesion may be present.
- Feet (**tinea pedis**), also known as athlete's foot **Figure 21-17**. Infections typically begin in the webbed spaces of the toes and may later involve the bottom surface of the foot. These lesions may become dry, scaly, cracked, and bloody.
- Groin (**tinea cruris**), also known as jock itch **Figure 21-18**. Typically a ringed lesion extends from the skin fold between the scrotum and upper thigh. One or both sides may be affected. It may be extremely itchy and may produce pain on walking or running (due to friction).

These minor fungal skin diseases usually do not interfere with training or a mission; however, during a long deployment in a hot humid environment, the discomfort associated with fungal rashes can be an irritating distraction. Advise the SWAT officer to keep the involved skin dry and clean and to change all socks and clothing often. Refer the SWAT officer to a personal care physician to obtain a prescribed antifungal cream. The symptoms of itching, redness, and irritation are improved when steroid cream is used. A more serious infection may require oral antifungal medicines and referral to a dermatologist.

Contact Dermatitis

Contact dermatitis is a skin inflammation caused by exposure to irritants (eg, poison ivy, poison oak) or allergens (eg, certain soaps, medications, gun-cleaning oils). One of the most frequent disorders that arises

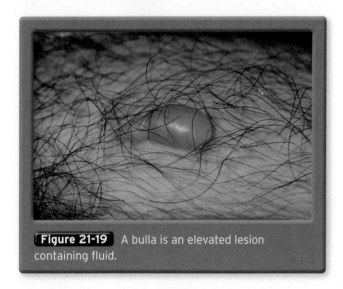

Figure 21-19 A bulla is an elevated lesion containing fluid.

during callouts is dermatitis caused by contact with environmental or work-related materials. Education about the cause of the contact dermatitis is important, especially if there is a lot of poison ivy nearby that should be avoided.

Examples of agents that may cause contact dermatitis include:

- Plants: poison oak, ivy, or sumac
- Industrial agents, dyes
- Rubber and latex
- Perfumes, personal hygiene products
- Jewelry metals (copper, silver, nickel)

Signs and symptoms of contact dermatitis include a rash that is red and itchy, or more severe swelling with **bullae** **Figure 21-19**. With poison oak, ivy, or sumac, linear streaks are characteristic. The fluid inside the vesicle or bulla is not infectious. Pruritus (itching) and vesiculation (small clear clusters of blisters) are common. Typically the dermatitis is limited to the site of contact but may later spread. Bullae may rupture, ooze, and crust. Secondary bacterial infections may occur. As

inflammation subsides, scaling and some temporary thickening of the skin can occur. Continued exposure to the causative agent may perpetuate the dermatitis. Counsel the patient not to scratch the rash because of the risk of it spreading. Refer the patient to his or her personal care physician for prescribed medications, including oral steroids, oral antihistamines, and topical steroid cream.

If the SWAT officer must remain on scene to complete the mission, the administration of sedating antihistamines or any medication that causes drowsiness is not permitted.

Friction Blisters

Long patrols, strenuous exertion, and wearing boots that have not been "broken in" can increase friction to parts of the foot (usually the heel) and cause blisters. The pain and discomfort associated with blisters can make a SWAT officer ineffective. The best treatment is prevention. During training, remind SWAT officers to properly break in new boots, stop activity at the earliest discomfort, and use a doughnut of moleskin around the sensitive spot to minimize blister formation.

When treating blisters, the skin should be left intact unless it is in a place where it will obviously rupture (eg, the heel or sole of the foot). In these cases, make a small hole at the edge of the blister with a sterilized pin, needle, or scalpel blade. Press gently to remove the fluid. Place a large piece of moleskin or a sterile dressing over the blister. If the top of the blister is partially ripped off, you may trim it away if local protocols permit you. Clean the area and cover it with some povidone-iodine or bacitracin ointment and a self-adhesive dressing. Instruct the patient to keep the feet and blister clean for the duration of training or the mission, since the wound is susceptible to infection. The patient should be referred to a personal care physician for a follow-up examination and care.

Ready for Review

- To determine if the burn injury is a load-and-go injury, you need to determine its depth, size, and severity.

- Burns are classified as superficial, partial-thickness, full-thickness, or subdermal burns based on severity of depth involved.

- To provide stabilizing care for thermal burns:

  - Use standard precautions to protect yourself from potentially contaminated body fluid and to protect the patient from potential infection.
  - Ensure you have cooled the burned area to prevent further cellular damage.
  - Remove jewelry or constrictive clothing; never attempt to remove any material that may have melted into the burned skin.
  - Ensure an open and clear airway. Provide high-flow oxygen as soon as possible or provide assisted ventilations with a bag-mask device as needed.
  - Place sterile dressings over the burned area(s); prevent hypothermia by covering the patient with a clean blanket. Provide rapid evacuation to transport.

- The first priority at the scene of an electrical injury is to protect yourself from becoming the next victim. Do not approach the patient until all threats are abolished.

- For open wounds to the soft tissues, stop the bleeding, provide a dressing, and transport for additional care if there is debris in the wound or the wound will not stop bleeding.

- Small animal and human bites can lead to serious infection and must be evaluated by a physician. Small animals can carry rabies.

Vital Vocabulary

abrasion Loss or damage of the superficial layer of skin as a result of a body part rubbing or scraping across a rough or hard surface.

avulsion An injury in which soft tissue either is torn completely loose or is hanging as a flap.

bulla An elevated lesion containing fluid.

closed wound Wound in which damage occurs beneath the skin or mucous membrane but the surface remains intact.

contact dermatitis Skin inflammation caused by exposure to irritants or allergens.

contamination The presence of infective organisms or foreign bodies such as dirt, gravel, or metal.

contusion A bruise from an injury that causes bleeding beneath the skin without breaking the skin.

deep partial-thickness burn A burn in which the skin is blistered but not charred and is painful to the touch, usually the result of steam, oil, or flames and involving the deeper layers of the dermis.

full-thickness burn A burn that affects all skin layers and may affect the subcutaneous layers, muscle, bone, and internal organs, leaving the area dry, leathery, and white, dark brown, or charred; traditionally called a third-degree burn.

incision A sharp, smooth cut.

laceration A jagged open wound.

Lund and Browder chart A detailed version of the rule of nines chart that takes into consideration the changes in body surface area brought on by growth.

open wound Wound in which there is a break in the surface of the skin, exposing deeper tissue to potential contamination.

Parkland formula A formula that recommends giving 4 mL of lactated Ringer's solution or normal saline for each kilogram of body weight, multiplied by the percentage of body surface area burned; sometimes used to calculate fluid needs during lengthy transport times.

partial-thickness burn A burn affecting the epidermis and some portion of the dermis but not the subcutaneous tissue characterized by blisters and skin that is white to red, moist, and mottled; traditionally called a second-degree burn.

rule of nines A system that assigns percentages to sections of the body, allowing calculation of the amount of skin surface involved in the burn area.

subdermal burn A severe, life-threatening burn involving the deep structures of muscle, bone, larger blood vessels, and nerves; also called a fourth-degree burn.

subungual hematoma An accumulation of blood underneath the fingernail or toenail, usually due to a compression force that causes bleeding under the nail; usually treated using the trephination technique.

superficial burn A burn affecting only the epidermis, characterized by skin that is red but not blistered or actually burned through; traditionally called a first-degree burn.

superficial partial-thickness burn A burn involving the epidermis and part of the dermis but the deeper layers of the dermis are not involved; also called a second-degree burn.

tinea corporis Also called ringworm; a plaque with well-defined and usually raised margins.

tinea cruris Also called jock itch; a ringed lesion that extends from the skin fold between the scrotum and upper thigh.

tinea pedis Also called athlete's foot; a common superficial fungal infection.

trephination Creation of a small hole to relieve pressure.

Environmental Emergencies

OBJECTIVES

- List the five different ways a body can lose heat and the ways heat loss or gain can be modified.
- Describe the risk factors for developing hypothermia in the tactical environment.
- Describe the stabilizing care provided to the patient with hypothermia.
- Describe local cold injuries and their underlying causes.
- List the risk factors of developing a local cold injury.
- Describe the stabilizing care provided to the patient with a local cold injury.
- List the three types of illness caused by heat exposure.
- Describe the stabilizing care provided to the patient with heat cramps.
- Describe the stabilizing care provided to the patient with heat exhaustion.
- Describe the stabilizing care provided to the patient with heatstroke.
- Describe the stabilizing care provided to the patient who has sustained a lightning strike.
- Describe the stabilizing care provided to the patient who has been bitten by a black widow spider.
- Describe the stabilizing care provided to the patient who has been bitten by a brown recluse spider.
- Describe the stabilizing care provided to the patient who has been stung by a hymenoptera.
- Describe the stabilizing care provided to the patient with an anaphylactic reaction.
- Describe the stabilizing care provided to the patient who has been bitten by a pit viper.
- Describe the stabilizing care provided to the patient who has been bitten by a coral snake.
- Describe the stabilizing care provided to the patient who has been stung by a scorpion.
- Describe the stabilizing care provided to the patient who has been bitten by a tick.

Introduction

SWAT operations are rarely conducted in ideal conditions. Heat and cold can both overwhelm the body's temperature-regulating mechanisms, including sweating and radiating body heat into the atmosphere. As a tactical medical provider (TMP), you can save lives by preventing environmental emergencies from occurring, and recognizing and responding properly to these emergencies. In this chapter you will learn how the body regulates core temperature and the ways in which body heat is lost to or gained from the environment. The various types of heat- and cold-related emergencies are described, including how to diagnose and treat hypothermia, frostbite, and hyperthermia. Other environmental emergencies include injuries caused by lightning and by envenomation from bites and stings.

Cold Exposure

Normal body temperature must be maintained within a very narrow range for the body's chemistry to work efficiently. If the body is exposed to cold environments, these mechanisms may be overwhelmed. Cold exposure may cause injury to individual parts of the body, such as the feet, hands, ears, or nose, or to the body as a whole. When the core body temperature falls, **hypothermia** occurs.

Because heat always travels from a warmer place to a cooler place, the body tends to lose heat to the environment. The body can also gain heat from the environment. Both can occur in five ways:

- **Conduction** is the direct transfer of heat from a part of the body to a colder object by direct contact, such as when a warm hand touches cold metal or ice, or is immersed in water with a temperature of less than 98°F (37°C). Heat passes directly from the body to the colder object. Heat can also be gained if the substance being touched is warm.
- **Convection** occurs when heat is transferred to circulating air, such as when cool air moves across the body surface. A person standing outside in windy winter weather and wearing lightweight clothing is losing heat to the environment, mostly by convection.
- **Evaporation** is the conversion of any liquid to a gas, a process that requires energy, or heat. Evaporation is the natural mechanism by which sweating cools the body. SWAT officers who run vigorously

in a cool environment may sweat and feel warm at first, but later, when they are no longer active and their sweat evaporates, they can become exceedingly cold and develop hypothermia.

- **Radiation** is the transfer of heat by radiant energy. Radiant energy is a type of invisible light that transfers heat. The body can lose heat by radiation, such as when a person stands in a cold room. Heat can also be gained by radiation, for example, when a person stands by a fire or in bright sunlight.
- **Respiration** causes body heat to be lost as warm air in the lungs is exhaled into the atmosphere and cooler air is inhaled. In warm climates, the air temperature can be well above body temperature, causing an individual to gain heat with each breath.

Hypothermia

Hypothermia literally means "low temperature." It is diagnosed when the **core temperature** of the body—the temperature of the heart, lungs, and vital organs—falls below 95°F (35°C). Normal body temperature is 98.6°F (37°C). The body can usually tolerate a drop in core temperature of a few degrees. However, below this critical point, the body loses the ability to regulate its temperature and to generate body heat (muscles stop shivering). Progressive loss of body heat then begins unless the patient is moved to warmer conditions.

To protect itself against heat loss, the body normally constricts blood vessels in the skin; this results in the characteristic appearance of blue lips and/or fingertips. As a secondary precaution against heat loss, the body tends to create additional heat by shivering, which is the active contraction of many muscles to generate heat. As cold exposure worsens and these mechanisms are overwhelmed, many body functions begin to slow down. Eventually the functioning of key organs, such as the heart, is impaired. Untreated, this can lead to death.

Hypothermia can develop quickly, for example when a SWAT officer slips and falls down into a shallow ice-cold creek and remains on the frozen ground during

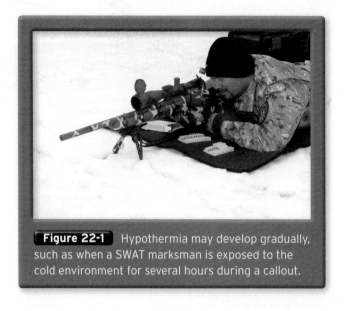

Figure 22-1 Hypothermia may develop gradually, such as when a SWAT marksman is exposed to the cold environment for several hours during a callout.

a long standoff. It may occur gradually, such as when a marksman is exposed to the cold environment for several hours while stationed on a roof **Figure 22-1**. The temperature does not have to be below freezing for hypothermia to occur. If a SWAT officer becomes wet from sweating, it is possible for hypothermia to occur even when the temperature is 50°F (10°C).

Signs and Symptoms

Signs and symptoms of hypothermia generally become progressively more severe as the core temperature falls. Hypothermia generally progresses through four general stages, as shown in **Table 22-1**. Although there is no clear distinction among the stages, the different signs and symptoms of each will help you estimate the severity of the problem.

To assess the patient's general temperature, pull back on your glove and place the back of your hand directly on the patient's skin **Figure 22-2**. If the skin feels cool, the patient is likely experiencing a generalized cold emergency.

Safety

In cold weather with minimal wind, radiation of body heat is one of the most significant methods of heat loss, especially from an exposed head and neck.

Special Populations

Like all heat- and cold-related injuries, hypothermia is more common among the geriatric and pediatric populations, who are less able to adjust to temperature extremes. These populations are less able to physically move to less harsh conditions, have less ability to modify their environment, and may be taking medications that affect temperature-regulation mechanisms.

Table 22-1	Characteristics of Systemic Hypothermia			
Core Temperature	90°F to 95°F (32°C to 35°C)	89°F to 92°F (32°C to 33°C)	80°F to 88°F (32°C to 33°C)	< 80°F (< 27°C)
Signs and symptoms	Shivering, foot stamping	Loss of coordination, muscle stiffness	Coma	Apparent death
Cardiorespiratory response	Constricted blood vessels, rapid breathing	Slowing respirations, slow pulse	Weak pulse, arrhythmias, very slow respirations	Cardiac arrest
Level of consciousness	Withdrawn	Confused, lethargic, sleepy	Unresponsive	Unresponsive

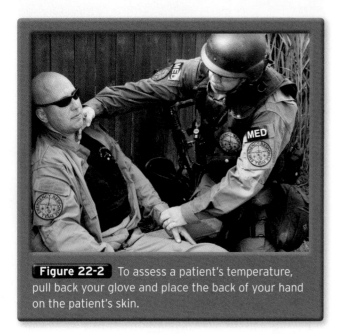

Figure 22-2 To assess a patient's temperature, pull back your glove and place the back of your hand on the patient's skin.

Medical Gear

If you work in a cold environment, you may carry a hypothermia thermometer, which registers lower core temperatures. It must be inserted in the rectum for an accurate reading. Regular thermometers will not register the temperature of a patient who has significant hypothermia.

As the core temperature drops toward 85°F (29°C), the patient becomes lethargic, usually losing interest in continuing to fight the cold. The patient's level of consciousness decreases; the confusion associated with hypothermia may cause the patient to remove his or her own clothes. Poor coordination and memory loss follow, along with reduced or complete loss of sensation to touch, mood changes, and impaired judgment. The patient becomes less communicative, experiences joint or muscle stiffness, and has trouble speaking. The muscles eventually become rigid, and the patient begins to appear stiff or rigid.

If the temperature continues to fall to 80°F (27°C), vital signs slow; the pulse becomes weaker, and respirations become slow and shallow or become absent. Cardiac arrhythmias may occur as the blood pressure decreases or disappears.

Mild hypothermia occurs when the core temperature is between 90°F and 95°F (32°C and 35°C). The patient is usually alert and shivering in an attempt to generate more heat through muscular activity. The patient may jump up and down and stamp his or her feet. Pulse rate and respirations are usually rapid. The skin in light-skinned individuals can be red, but may eventually appear pale, then cyanotic. Individuals in a cold environment may have blue lips or fingertips because of the body's constriction of blood vessels at the skin to retain heat.

More severe hypothermia occurs when the core temperature is less than 90°F (32°C). Shivering stops and muscular activity decreases. At first, small, fine muscle activity such as coordinated finger motion ceases. Eventually, as the temperature falls further, all muscle activity stops.

Safety

During the hectic pace of a SWAT callout, it is often difficult to detect the subtle signs of a SWAT officer who is in an early cold emergency. During a prolonged callout, each SWAT officer should be assessed for a cold emergency in the rehabilitation station.

At a core temperature of less than 80°F (27°C), all cardiorespiratory activity may cease, pupillary reaction is slow, and the patient may appear dead.

Never assume that a cold, pulseless patient is dead. Patients may survive even severe hypothermia in the right circumstances if proper emergency measures are carried out.

Assessment and Stabilizing Care

Cold emergencies may be discovered when the SWAT officer returns to the tactical operations center, during an evaluation at the rehabilitation station, or when a SWAT officer notes the signs and symptoms in a fellow officer. Whether the patient is a SWAT officer in a rehabilitation station or a hostage who has been held in an unheated room during a long standoff, you will begin your assessment once the scene is safe or the patient has been brought to you at a point of relative safety. You will assess the patient's CAB 'N (circulation, airway, breathing, and neurologic exam) to check for the presence of potentially life-threatening injuries. When assessing the patient's circulation, if you cannot feel a radial pulse, gently palpate for a carotid pulse and wait 30 to 45 seconds before you decide that the patient is pulseless. Physicians disagree about performing cardiopulmonary resuscitation (CPR) on a patient with hypothermia who appears to be pulseless. Such a patient actually may be in a kind of "metabolic ice box," having achieved a metabolic balance that CPR may upset. Even a pulse rate of 1 or 2 beats/min indicates cardiac activity, and cardiac activity may spontaneously recover once the body core is warmed. However, there is evidence that CPR, when correctly done, will increase blood flow to the critical parts of the body. For this reason some authorities recommend starting CPR on a patient with hypothermia and no pulse. The American Heart Association recommends that CPR be started if the patient has no detectable pulse or breathing. Again, for a patient with hypothermia, this may require a prolonged pulse check.

Perfusion will be compromised based on the degree of cold the patient is experiencing. Your assessment of the patient's skin will not be helpful in determining shock. Assume that shock is present and treat it appropriately. Bleeding may be difficult to find because of the slow-moving circulation and thick clothing. If there is a mechanism of injury that suggests the potential for bleeding, look for it.

When assessing the patient's airway, take into account the physiologic changes that occur as a result of hypothermia. Ensure that the patient has an adequate airway and is breathing. If your patient's breathing is slow or shallow, ventilation with a bag-mask device may be necessary. If warmed and humidified oxygen is available, use it.

Always make sure to handle the patient gently so that you do not cause any pain or further injury to the skin. Do not massage the extremities. Do not allow the patient to eat; to use any stimulants such as coffee, tea, or cola; or to smoke or chew tobacco.

Even mild degrees of hypothermia can have serious consequences and complications, including cardiac arrhythmia and blood-clotting abnormalities. Therefore, all patients with hypothermia require rapid evacuation and transport for evaluation and treatment. Assess the scene for the safest way to evacuate your patient from the cold environment (see Chapter 16, "Extraction and Evacuation"). Work quickly, safely, and gently. Rough handling of a hypothermic patient may cause a cold, slow, weak heart to fibrillate and the patient to lose any pulse that may have existed. To prevent further damage to the feet, do not allow the patient who has suspected frostbite on the toes or feet to walk.

If transportation is delayed, protect the patient from further heat loss. Move the patient out of the wind and away from contact with any object that will conduct heat away from the body. Remember that most body heat is lost around the head and neck. Remove any wet clothing, and place dry blankets over and under the patient **Figure 22-3**.

Rapidly evacuate the patient to ALS-level transport. If you are permitted to accompany the patient during transport, perform a rapid secondary assessment. General care of the patient during transport is directed at preventing further heat loss and rewarming. Remove wet clothing and prevent further heat loss by covering the head and body. If the patient is conscious, alert, and shivering, place heat packs in the groin, axillary,

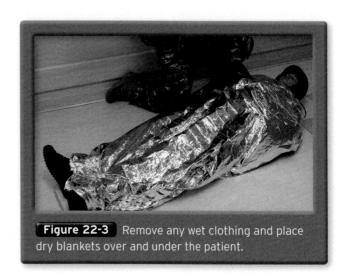

Figure 22-3   Remove any wet clothing and place dry blankets over and under the patient.

and cervical regions, being careful not to cause burns. Remember to handle the patient gently to decrease the risk of ventricular fibrillation. Follow your local protocols for treating moderate or severe hypothermia. If the patient does not have a pulse or is not breathing, provide resuscitation per local protocols.

Local Cold Injuries

Most injuries from the cold are localized to the extremities or exposed parts of the body, such as the tips of the ears, nose, upper cheek, and tips of the fingers or toes **Figure 22-4**. Local freezing injuries fall under the general heading of frostbite. **Frostbite** is an ischemic injury that is classified as superficial or deep depending on whether tissue loss occurs.

A very mild form of frostbite, sometimes called frostnip, comes on slowly and generally is not painful, so the victim tends to be unaware of its occurrence. Frostnip is easily treated by placing a warm hand firmly over the chilled nose or ear, or, when the fingers are frostnipped, by placing the fingers into the armpits. The return of warmth to a frostnipped area is usually signaled by some redness and tingling. Windmilling involves rapidly making a large circle with your hand, starting with your hand next to your side, raising it backward and up until you are reaching straight up, and moving it rapidly down frontward **Figure 22-5**. This technique forces blood into the cold hand.

Deeper degrees of frostbite involve freezing of tissues and can occur only in ambient temperatures well below the freezing point. Cells are composed chiefly of water, so when they are subjected to low enough temperatures, the water within them turns into ice crystals, which can damage or destroy the cells.

Risk Factors for Frostbite

Several factors predispose a person to frostbite:

- Going out on a cold, windy day without gloves or a hat.
- Impeding the circulation to the extremities:
  - Wearing tight gloves and shoes and too many socks.
  - Lacing boots very tightly and remaining in a cramped position for a while.
  - Wearing plastic boots that do not expand. Preferably, boots should be lined with felt, which will expand when wet.
  - Smoking and drinking caffeine, which constricts arteries.

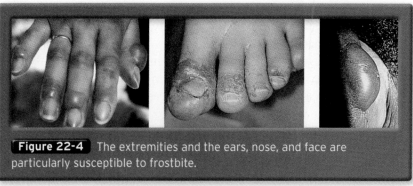

Figure 22-4   The extremities and the ears, nose, and face are particularly susceptible to frostbite.

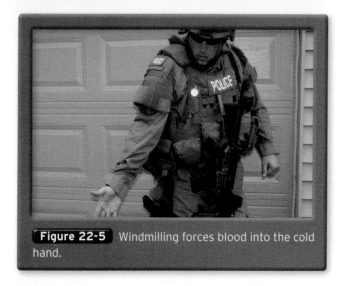

Figure 22-5   Windmilling forces blood into the cold hand.

- Drinking alcohol, which causes lapses in judgment, and peripheral blood vessels to dilate, resulting in greater heat loss and higher chance of hypothermia.
- Going out in the cold when tired, dehydrated, or hungry.
- Coming in direct contact with cold objects and exposure to water.
- Not staying hydrated, which would otherwise promote increased blood flow.
- Allowing oneself to become thoroughly chilled. Generalized hypothermia is the most effective way to sustain local cold injury.

To avoid getting frostbite, avoid all of the preceding behaviors. Note the wind chill factor, and always cover your face when you are outside for a long time. Utilizing four layers of clothing will help to prevent a local cold injury (see Chapter 4, "Equipment of the Tactical Medical Provider"). Keep your feet dry and warm, cover your neck, visit the rehabilitation station to warm up, and choose clothing carefully for cold weather operations.

Trench Foot

<u>Trench foot</u> involves a process similar to frostbite but can occur at temperatures as high as 60°F (16°C). It is caused by prolonged exposure to cool, wet conditions. The mechanism of injury can be explained by conduction: Wet feet lose heat 25 times faster than dry feet. Vasoconstriction and an ischemic cascade similar to that seen in frostbite then set in. Prevention—keeping the feet dry and warm—is the best treatment. Carry multiple pairs of clean, dry socks and, whenever your feet become wet, change your socks and dry your boots as well as possible.

Superficial Frostbite

The most common symptom of frostbite is an altered sensation: numbness, tingling, or burning. The skin typically appears white and waxy. Because it is frozen, the skin is firm to palpation, but the underlying tissues remain soft. Once thawing occurs, the injured area turns cyanotic, and the patient experiences a hot, stinging sensation. Edema occurs in the frostbitten area. Dull or throbbing pain may persist for days or weeks after the injury.

The care of superficial frostbite differs significantly from that of deep frostbite, so it is very important to distinguish between the two. Usually it is difficult to determine the depth of the injury when you first see it—even a shallow frostbite injury can appear to be frozen solid. If the tissues beneath the skin are soft when you press down on the skin surface, the frostbite is probably superficial. If not, or if there is any doubt, treat the injury as deep frostbite.

Mild cold injuries are generally managed by a combination of dressing properly, rest, food, and limiting exposure to the cold. Once you have determined that the patient has superficial frostbite, get the patient out of the cold. Take the patient someplace warm indoors or into a heated ambulance so the body can stop hoarding its warm blood in the core and send some to the periphery where it is urgently needed. Wrap the patient in blankets and wrap the patient's head and neck in warm clothing or blankets. Have the patient lie down or sit in a warm environment, and encourage shivering to increase the body temperature. Give the patient hot beverages, but avoid coffee, tea, chocolate, or caffeinated drinks.

Rewarm the injured part with body heat if the frostbite appears to be superficial. If an ear, nose, or foot is frostbitten, apply firm, steady pressure against the area with a warm hand. If a hand is frostbitten, have the patient insert the hand into the armpit and hold it there without moving. Do not try to rewarm a frostbitten part with radiant or dry heat as the skin is numb and cannot accurately detect when the heat is too damaging to the skin. Do not rub or massage the frostbitten area; massage will cause further damage to injured tissues. If blisters form, do not puncture them but rather cover them with a dry, sterile dressing and protect the area from further injury. Rapidly evacuate the patient to transport and transport the patient to the hospital with the injured area elevated and protected from the cold.

Deep Frostbite

Deep frostbite usually involves the hands or the feet and rarely involves exposed ears and noses. A frozen extremity looks white, yellow-white, or mottled blue-white, and it is hard and cold and lacks sensation **Figure 22-6** . The major tissue damage occurs not from the freezing of the tissues, but rather when the tissues thaw out, particularly if thawing occurs gradually. When tissues thaw slowly, partial refreezing of melted water may occur. Because these new ice crystals tend to be much larger than those formed during the original freeze, they cause even greater tissue damage. As thawing occurs, the injured area turns purple and becomes excruciatingly painful as the frozen nerve endings rewake. Gangrene (permanent cell death) may set in within a few days, requiring possible amputation of all or part of the injured limb **Figure 22-7** .

If there is no chance that the frostbitten extremity will refreeze during evacuation or transport, then initiate steps to thaw the extremity. However, if severe conditions require the patient with frostbitten feet to walk during evacuation, or if there is a chance of exposure to freezing temperatures during evacuation, then do not attempt to rewarm the frostbitten extremity. It is extremely important to not thaw the frostbite areas if there is any chance of a refreezing injury during evacuation or transportation. Once the patient is in the

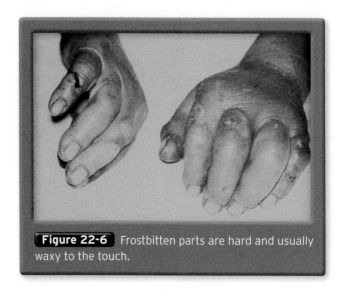

Figure 22-6 Frostbitten parts are hard and usually waxy to the touch.

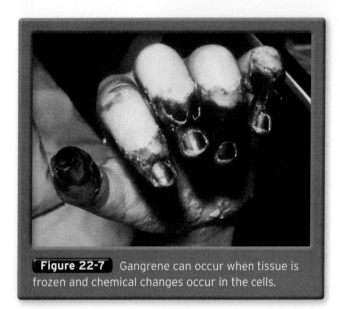

Figure 22-7 Gangrene can occur when tissue is frozen and chemical changes occur in the cells.

ambulance, the patient's injured extremity should be padded to protect the tissues from further trauma and kept away from the heater or any other sources of dry heat. Do not massage the extremity. The cells are full of ice crystals, and massaging the extremity will cause the ice crystals to damage tissue cells.

If the evacuation or transport will be delayed, contact medical control to discuss field rewarming. If you are permitted, rewarm the injured extremity before and, if possible, during transport. To do so, you will need a warm water bath—a large, clean container in which the extremity can be immersed without touching the container's side or bottom. Water should be heated in a second container and then stirred into the water bath until the temperature of the bath is between 104°F (40°C) and 108°F (42°C). While the water is heating, an intravenous analgesia such as fentanyl or morphine may be administered by an ALS-level provider if local protocols allow. The patient will experience very severe pain as the limb thaws, so mitigating the pain will make the patient more comfortable.

When the water bath has reached the appropriate temperature, gently immerse the injured extremity. Keep a thermometer in the water. When the water temperature falls below 104°F (40°C), temporarily remove the injured extremity from the bath while you add more hot water to the container. Stir the water around and keep adding more hot water until the bath is again in the appropriate temperature range; then reimmerse the injured extremity.

The rewarming procedure typically takes 15 to 30 minutes. It is complete when the frozen area is warm to the touch and is deep red or bluish (and remains red when you remove the limb from the water bath). While

rewarming is in progress, the patient should be kept warm, preferably indoors, with insulated clothing and blankets. Do not permit the patient to smoke or to drink caffeinated beverages, because nicotine and caffeine cause vasoconstriction, which decreases the blood flow to the injured area. Once rewarming is complete, clean and dry the injured extremity and apply sterile dressings very gently. Use sterile gauze to separate frostbitten fingers and toes. Rapidly transport the patient to the hospital.

Heat Exposure

Normal body temperature is 98.6°F (37°C). Complicated regulatory mechanisms keep this internal temperature constant, regardless of the **ambient temperature**—the temperature of the surrounding environment. In a hot environment or during vigorous physical activity, the body will try to rid itself of the excess heat. The two most efficient methods are sweating (and evaporation of the sweat with the use of fans and air conditioning) and dilation of the skin's blood vessels, which brings blood to the skin surface to increase the rate of heat radiation. In addition, a person who becomes overheated can remove clothing and try to find a cooler environment.

Ordinarily, the heat-regulating mechanisms of the body work very well and individuals are able to tolerate significant temperature changes. When the body is exposed to more heat energy than it loses or it generates more heat than it can lose, hyperthermia results. **Hyperthermia** is a high core temperature, usually 101°F (38.3°C) or higher.

Illness occurs when the body's heat-regulating mechanisms are overwhelmed. High ambient temperature can reduce the body's ability to lose heat by radiation; high humidity reduces the ability to lose heat through evaporation. A lack of acclimation to the heat is a risk factor. Another risk factor is vigorous exercise, during which the body can lose more than 1 L of sweat per hour, causing loss of fluid and electrolytes.

Safety

Keeping yourself hydrated while on duty is very important, especially during periods of heavy exertion or when working in the heat. Drink at least 3 L of water a day and more when exertion or heat is involved. The color of urine (usually darker with dehydration) and frequency of urination correlate directly with the body's fluid level.

Illness from heat exposure can take the following forms:

- Heat cramps
- Heat exhaustion
- Heatstroke

All three forms of heat illness may be present in the same patient because untreated heat exhaustion may progress to heatstroke. Heatstroke is a life-threatening emergency.

Heat Cramps

Heat cramps are acute and involuntary muscle pains, usually in the lower extremities, the abdomen, or both, that occur because of profuse sweating and subsequent sodium losses in sweat. Heat cramps may occur during training or during a long callout in hot weather conditions, and may be severe enough to interfere with a SWAT officer's performance. Three factors contribute to heat cramps: salt depletion, dehydration, and muscle fatigue. Heat cramps most often afflict people in good physical condition—for example, SWAT officers, athletes, military personnel, and manual laborers. Usually a person exerting himself or herself in a hot environment will become thirsty and increase fluid intake. But if the person is not acclimated and is sweating heavily, he or she is losing fluids and salt through the skin. If the person drinks plain water, he or she will not replace sweat sodium losses.

Heat cramps usually start suddenly during strenuous and/or prolonged physical activity. They may be mild, characterized by only slight abdominal cramping and tingling in the extremities. More often, however, they present with severe, incapacitating pain in the extremities and abdomen. The patient may become nauseated but will remain alert. The pulse is generally rapid, the skin is pale and moist, and the skin temperature feels normal.

Treatment of heat cramps aims to eliminate the exposure to hot weather conditions and to restore lost salt and water to the body. Remove the patient from the hot environment, including sunlight, a source of radiant heat gain. Loosen any tight clothing. If possible, administer high-flow oxygen. Rest the cramping muscles.

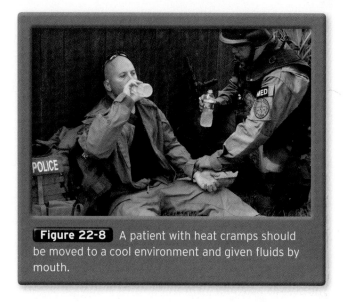

Figure 22-8 A patient with heat cramps should be moved to a cool environment and given fluids by mouth.

Have the patient sit or lie down until the cramps subside. Replace fluids by mouth **Figure 22-8**. Use water or a diluted (half-strength) balanced electrolyte solution, such as Gatorade. In most cases, plain water is the most useful. Do not give salt tablets or solutions that have a high salt concentration. The patient already has an adequate amount of electrolytes circulating; they are just not distributed properly. With adequate rest and fluid replacement, the body will adjust the distribution of electrolytes, and the cramps will disappear. Cool the patient with a warm (not cold) water spray and add convection to the cooling method by manually or mechanically fanning the patient.

When the heat cramps are gone, the patient may resume activity. For example, a SWAT officer can return to duty once the heat cramps have disappeared. However, heavy sweating may cause the cramps to recur. The best preventive and treatment strategy is hydration by drinking sufficient quantities of water and electrolytes.

If the cramps do not go away after these measures, transport the patient to the hospital. If you are uncertain about the cause of the patient's cramps or you note anything out of the ordinary, contact medical control or transport the patient to the hospital.

At the Scene

An excellent drink for SWAT officers is 1 part orange juice with 1 part water added to ice. This drink should be served during training and at the rehabilitation center during callouts.

Heat Exhaustion

Heat exhaustion is a clinical syndrome thought to represent a milder form of heat illness on a continuum leading to heatstroke. Its hallmarks are volume depletion and heat stress. Classically, two forms are described: water depleted and sodium depleted. Water-depleted heat exhaustion occurs primarily in active SWAT officers or athletes who do not adequately replace fluids in a hot environment. Sodium-depleted heat exhaustion may take hours or days to develop and results from huge sodium losses from sweating, when efforts to hydrate replace only water, not sodium.

Symptoms of heat exhaustion include headache, fatigue, dizziness, nausea, vomiting, and abdominal cramping. The patient is usually sweating profusely, and the skin is pale and clammy. He or she may be slightly disoriented. The heart rate is elevated. Respirations are fast and shallow. The temperature may be normal or slightly elevated (up to 104°F [40°C]).

The treatment of heat exhaustion is aimed at removing the patient from exposure to heat and repairing the derangement in fluid and electrolyte balance. Remove any excessive layers of clothing, particularly around the head and neck. Move the patient promptly from the hot environment, preferably into the back of an air-conditioned ambulance. If outdoors, move out of the sun. Give the patient oxygen if possible. Splash the patient with warm water if his or her body temperature is elevated. Cold water will cause vasoconstriction and decrease the heat exchange with the skin's surface. Encourage the patient to lie down and elevate the legs. Loosen any tight clothing and fan the patient for cooling.

If the patient is fully alert, encourage him or her to sit up and slowly drink up to 1 liter of water, as long as nausea does not develop. Never force fluids by mouth on a patient who is not fully alert, or allow drinking while supine, because the patient could aspirate the fluid into the lungs. Transport the patient on his or her side if you think the patient may be nauseated and ready to vomit, but make certain that the patient is secured.

In most cases these measures will reverse the symptoms, causing the patient to feel better within 30 minutes. But you should prepare to transport the patient to the hospital for more aggressive treatment, such as IV fluid therapy and close monitoring, especially in the following circumstances:

- The symptoms do not clear up promptly.
- The level of consciousness decreases.
- The body temperature remains elevated.
- The person is very young, older, or has an underlying medical condition, such as diabetes or cardiovascular disease.

At the Scene

During a prolonged callout, you should note the temperature and behavior of SWAT officers during breaks at the rehabilitation station. Remind SWAT officers on the signs and symptoms so that they can monitor each other for signs of heat exhaustion and heatstroke.

Heatstroke

Heatstroke, the least common but most serious illness caused by heat exposure, occurs when the body is subjected to more heat than it can handle and normal mechanisms for getting rid of the excess heat are overwhelmed. The body temperature then rises rapidly to the level at which tissues are destroyed. Untreated heatstroke always results in death.

Heatstroke can develop in patients during vigorous physical activity (exertional heatstroke) or when they are inside a hot, closed, poorly ventilated, humid space such as a small house or apartment that is not air conditioned (classic heatstroke). Many patients with heatstroke have hot, dry, flushed skin because their sweating mechanism has been overwhelmed. However, early in the course of exertional heatstroke, the skin may be moist or wet. Keep in mind that a patient can have heatstroke even if he or she is still sweating. The body temperature rises rapidly in patients with heatstroke. It may rise to 106°F (41°C) or more. As the body core temperature rises, the patient's level of consciousness falls, resulting in unconsciousness.

Often the first sign of heatstroke is a change in behavior. However, the patient then becomes unresponsive very quickly and seizures may occur. The pulse is usually rapid and strong at first, but as the patient becomes increasingly unresponsive, the pulse becomes weaker and the blood pressure falls. The respiratory rate increases as the body is attempting to compensate. One of the telltale signs you should be acutely aware of is when your patient ceases to perspire, which means the body has lost its thermoregulatory mechanisms. If you are perspiring in the environment, your patient should also be perspiring.

Assessment and Stabilizing Care of Heatstroke

The signs and symptoms of heatstroke are often observed when the SWAT officer is in the rehabilitation station. Whether the patient is a SWAT officer in a rehabilitation station or a hostage who has been held in an overheated room during a long standoff, you will begin your assessment once the scene is safe or the patient has been brought to you in a point of relative safety. Assess the patient's CAB 'N (circulation, airway, breathing, and neurologic exam) to check for the presence of potentially life-threatening injuries. Circulation is assessed by palpating a pulse. If it is adequate, assess the patient for perfusion and bleeding. Assess the patient's skin condition and temperature. The skin condition is highly variable. Most patients will have hot, dry skin in the field. Treat the patient aggressively for shock by removing the patient from the heat.

Assess the patient's airway and breathing and treat any life-threatening problems found. Unless the patient is unresponsive, the airway should be patent. Nausea and vomiting, however, may occur with some heat problems. Position the patient to protect the airway as necessary. Breathing may be fast depending on the patient's core temperature but should otherwise be adequate. If your patient is unresponsive, insert an airway and provide bag-mask device ventilations initially; consider advanced airway options according to your local protocols. If your patient has any signs of heatstroke (high temperature; red, dry skin; altered mental status; tachycardia; poor perfusion), evacuate to ALS-level transport without delay.

Once the patient is in a cool environment, strip the patient to underclothing. Monitor the rectal temperature every 10 minutes. Cooling efforts should continue until the rectal temperature has fallen to about 102°F (39°C). Cool the patient as rapidly as possible by the most expeditious means available. Spray the patient with tepid water while fanning constantly to promote rapid evaporation. The ambulance should carry a portable fan during the summer months for this purpose. Apply ice packs to the patient's neck, groin, and armpits to aid in cooling from evaporative techniques **Figure 22-9**. Consider ice-water–soaked towels and massage of body tissue in cases of prolonged transport or delayed evacuation.

Pay close attention to the patient's airway status; watch for seizures and monitor the patient's core body temperature to avoid overcooling. Once the patient reaches the core body temperature of about 102°F

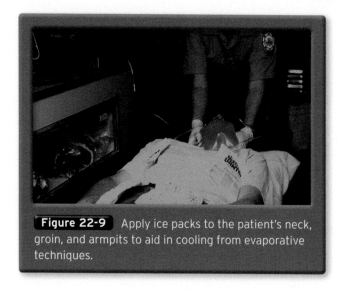

Figure 22-9 Apply ice packs to the patient's neck, groin, and armpits to aid in cooling from evaporative techniques.

(39°C), moderate the air conditioning and pause to allow the skin to dry. If cooling efforts are continued too long, then the core temperature may become too low, causing hypothermia and complications.

If you are permitted to accompany the patient during transport, start an IV line, give normal saline, and check the blood glucose level. Many of these patients may be volume depleted and may require a significant amount of IV normal saline for rehydration. In addition to boluses of normal saline, advanced TMPs should consider starting an isotonic IV containing dextrose (glucose) in order to prevent the development of hypoglycemia, especially in pediatric patients, if permitted by local protocols. Remember that cooling promotes vasoconstriction that can raise the blood pressure. Monitor the patient's cardiac rhythm. Be prepared to treat seizures with common antiseizure medicines (lorazepam, midazolam, or diazepam) per local protocols.

Lightning

According to the National Weather Service, there are an estimated 25 million cloud-to-ground lightning flashes in the United States each year. On average, lightning kills between 60 and 70 people per year in the United States based on documented cases. Although documented lightning injuries in the United States average about 300 per year, undocumented lightning injuries are likely much higher. Lightning is the third most common cause of death from isolated environmental phenomena.

The fact that SWAT units train outdoors during all kinds of weather and may be forced to establish a perimeter around a suspect's barricaded home during a storm raises the chances of SWAT officers being struck by lightning. Any type of activity that exposes the SWAT officer to a large, open area increases the risk of being struck by lightning.

Whether or not lightning injures or kills depends on whether a person is in the path of the lightning discharge. The current associated with the lightning discharge travels along the ground. Although some persons are injured or killed by a direct lightning strike, many individuals are struck indirectly when standing near an object that has been struck by lightning, such as a tree (splash effect).

The cardiovascular and nervous systems are most commonly injured during a lightning strike; therefore, respiratory or cardiac arrest is the most common cause of lightning-related deaths. The tissue damage caused by lightning is different from that caused by other electrical injuries (ie, high-voltage power line injuries) because the tissue damage pathway usually occurs over the skin, rather than through it. During your assessment, you should look for not only the entrance wound, but also the exit wound. The exit wound does not necessarily occur on the same side of the body. Many lightning strike victims will have no signs of injury, except for a few reddish streaks on the skin. Additionally, because the duration of a lightning strike is short, any skin burns are usually superficial; full-thickness (third-degree) burns are rare. Lightning injuries are categorized as being mild, moderate, or severe:

- **Mild**. Loss of consciousness, amnesia, confusion, tingling, and other nonspecific signs and symptoms. Burns, if present, are typically superficial.
- **Moderate**. Seizures, respiratory arrest, cardiac standstill (asystole) that spontaneously resolves, and superficial burns.
- **Severe**. Cardiopulmonary arrest.

Stabilizing Care

Your safety takes priority. Take measures to protect yourself from being struck by lightning, especially if the thunderstorm is still in progress. Contrary to popular belief, lightning can, and does, strike in the same place twice. The patient(s) should be extracted to a place of safety, preferably a dry, sheltered area.

If you are in an open area and adequate shelter is not available, it is important to recognize the signs of an impending lightning strike and take immediate action to protect yourself. If you suddenly feel a tingling sensation or your hair stands on end, the area around you has become charged—a sure sign of an imminent lightning strike. Make yourself as small a target as possible by

---

At the Scene

If there are multiple victims in cardiopulmonary arrest after a lightning strike, then multiple rescuers may begin CPR in the hopes that the victim's heart will stabilize itself while the rescuer assists the victim to breathe until additional resources arrive on scene.

---

squatting down into a ball, close to but not touching the ground except for your feet. If you are standing near a tree or other tall object, move away as fast as possible, preferably to a low-lying area. Lightning has an affinity for objects that project from the ground (ie, trees, fences, buildings).

The process of triaging multiple victims of a lightning strike is different than the conventional triage methods used during a mass-casualty incident. When a person is struck by lightning and respiratory or cardiac arrest occurs, it occurs immediately and the victim(s) will collapse to the ground and be unresponsive after a few seconds of brief seizure-like activity. Those who are conscious and moving purposefully following a lightning strike are much less likely to develop delayed respiratory or cardiac arrest; most of these persons will survive. Therefore, you should focus your efforts on those who are lying still in respiratory or cardiac arrest. This process, called **reverse triage**, differs from conventional triage, where such patients would ordinarily be classified as deceased.

When a person is struck by lightning, it causes massive direct current shock, with the patient experiencing massive muscle spasms (tetany) that can result in fractures of long bones and spinal vertebrae. Therefore you should manually stabilize the patient's head in a neutral, in-line position and open the airway with the jaw-thrust maneuver. If the patient is in respiratory arrest with a pulse, begin immediate bag-mask device ventilations with 100% oxygen if possible while sending other rescuers to get an AED. If there are no pulses detected in the patient, then attach an AED as soon as possible and provide immediate defibrillation if indicated. If severe bleeding is present, control it immediately.

Provide full spinal stabilization and evacuate the patient to transport to the closest appropriate facility. If you are permitted to accompany the patient during transport, then perform CPR and ventilations if indicated. If additional EMS staff is present and can perform CPR and ventilations, then start an IV and perform a secondary assessment. Address other injuries (ie, splint fractures, dress and bandage burns) and provide continuous monitoring while en route to the hospital.

Bites and Envenomations

This section discusses bites and stings from spiders, hymenoptera (bees/wasps), snakes, scorpions, and ticks.

Spider Bites

Spiders are numerous and widespread in the United States. Many species of spiders bite. However, only two, the female black widow spider and the brown recluse spider, are able to deliver serious, even life-threatening bites. When you care for a patient who has had some type of bite, be alert to the possibility that the spider or similar spiders may be in the area. Remember that your safety is paramount.

Black Widow Spider

The female black widow spider (*Latrodectus*) is fairly large, measuring approximately 2 inches long with its legs extended. It is usually black and has a distinctive, bright red-orange marking in the shape of an hourglass on the bottom of its abdomen **Figure 22-10**. The female black widow spider is larger and more toxic than the male. Black widow spiders are found in every state except Alaska. They prefer dry, dim places around buildings, in woodpiles, and among debris.

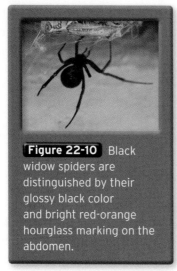

Figure 22-10 Black widow spiders are distinguished by their glossy black color and bright red-orange hourglass marking on the abdomen.

The bite of the black widow spider is sometimes overlooked. If the site becomes numb right away, the patient may not even recall being bitten. However, most black widow spider bites cause localized pain and other symptoms, including agonizing muscle spasms. In some cases, a bite on the abdomen causes muscle spasms so severe that the patient may be thought to have an acute abdominal condition. The main danger with this type of bite, however, is that the black widow's venom is poisonous to nerve tissues (neurotoxic). Other systemic symptoms include dizziness, sweating, nausea, vomiting, and rashes. Tightness in the chest and difficulty breathing develop within 24 hours, as well as severe cramps, with board-like rigidity of the abdominal muscles. Generally, these signs and symptoms subside over 48 hours.

If necessary, a physician can administer a specific **antivenin**, a serum containing antibodies that counteract the venom, but because of a high incidence of side effects, its use is reserved for very severe bites, for the aged or very feeble, and for children younger than 5 years. In children, these bites can be fatal. The severe muscle spasms are usually treated in the hospital with IV benzodiazepines such as diazepam (Valium) or lorazepam (Ativan).

In general, care for a black widow spider bite in the tactical environment consists of stabilizing the patient's airway and breathing. Rapidly evacuate the patient to emergency transport. Provide high-flow supplemental oxygen. If you are permitted to accompany the patient and have the appropriate level of training, establish vascular access. Manage pain in cramping muscles by giving opioids or benzodiazepines per local protocol. Provide wound care (see Chapter 21, "Soft-Tissue Injuries").

Brown Recluse Spider

The brown recluse spider (*Loxosceles*) is dull brown and, at 1 inch, smaller than the black widow **Figure 22-11**. The short-haired body has a violin-shaped mark, brown to yellow in color, on its back. Although the brown recluse spider lives mostly in the southern and central parts of the country, it may be found throughout the continental United States. The spider takes its name from the fact that it tends to live in dark areas—reclusive in corners of old, unused buildings, under rocks, and in woodpiles. In cooler areas, it moves indoors to closets, drawers, cellars, and old piles of clothing.

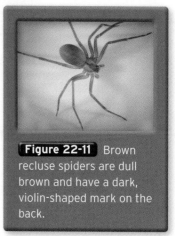

Figure 22-11 Brown recluse spiders are dull brown and have a dark, violin-shaped mark on the back.

In contrast to the venom of the black widow spider, the venom of the brown recluse spider is not neurotoxic but cytotoxic; that is, it causes severe local tissue damage. Typically, the bite is not painful at first but becomes so within hours. The area becomes swollen and tender, developing a pale, mottled, cyanotic center and possibly a small blister **Figure 22-12**. Over the next several days, a scab of dead skin, fat, and debris forms and digs down into the skin, producing a large ulcer. The development of a skin ulcer can take up to a week. If a SWAT officer is bitten by a brown recluse spider, the SWAT officer usually will not see the spider, but will feel a small pinprick

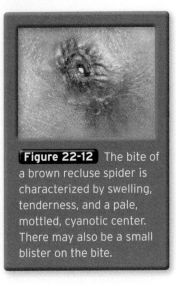

Figure 22-12 The bite of a brown recluse spider is characterized by swelling, tenderness, and a pale, mottled, cyanotic center. There may also be a small blister on the bite.

sensation. Often patients do not complain of any signs or symptoms until 12 to 24 hours after the spider bite. Refer the patient to his or her primary care physician for further assessment and care. Continued reevaluation by a physician over the following weeks will monitor for signs of serious infection, muscle involvement, and other complications.

It is rare to evacuate or rapidly transport a patient for a brown recluse spider bite. If a brown recluse spider bite does cause systemic symptoms and signs, support the patient's airway, breathing, and circulation during transportation to the emergency department.

Hymenoptera Stings

Typically **hymenoptera** (bees, wasps, ants, and yellow jackets) stings are painful but are not a medical emergency **Figure 22-13**. If the patient is allergic to the venom, then **anaphylaxis** and death may occur. The signs and symptoms of anaphylaxis are flushed skin, dizziness or fainting, hypotension, difficulty breathing usually associated with reactive airway sounds such as wheezes, or, in severe cases, diminished or absent breath sounds. The patient can also have swelling to the throat and tongue. This is a dire emergency and can be fatal if not recognized and treated quickly. The patient may develop hives (urticaria) near the site of envenomation or centrally on the body. If untreated, such an anaphylactic reaction can proceed rapidly to death. In fact, more than two thirds of patients who die of anaphylaxis do so within the first half hour, so speed on your part is essential.

Treatment of a hymenoptera sting without anaphylaxis focuses primarily on pain relief and reducing the risk of infection. First, determine whether the stinger and venom sac are still attached to the skin as may occur in honeybee stings. All other hymenoptera do not leave

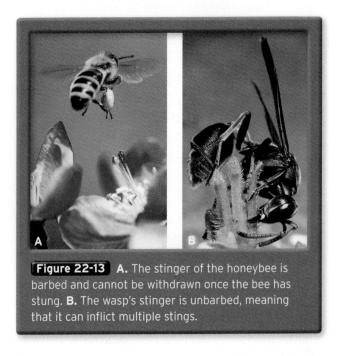

Figure 22-13 **A.** The stinger of the honeybee is barbed and cannot be withdrawn once the bee has stung. **B.** The wasp's stinger is unbarbed, meaning that it can inflict multiple stings.

their stingers imbedded. If so, use a firm-edged item such as a credit card or scalpel blade to gently scrape the stinger and venom sac from the wound. Do not try to pluck the stinger out with your fingertips, tweezers, or forceps. If you squeeze the stinger or the venom sac, you will pump more venom into the wound! After removing the stinger, clean the wound thoroughly with soap and water or an antiseptic solution such as povidone-iodine. Apply cold packs to the site for pain relief.

If the patient is known to have an allergy to bee stings, he or she might carry a commercial bee-sting kit such as an EpiPen auto-injector or a Twinject auto-injector that contains a standard syringe of epinephrine for intramuscular injection **Figure 22-14**. To help administer the epinephrine from the EpiPen auto-injector or a Twinject auto-injector, first follow standard precautions, and ensure that the medication belongs to this patient, is not discolored, and the expiration date has not passed.

To assist a patient with an auto-injector, remove the auto-injector's safety cap and quickly wipe the thigh with antiseptic. Place the tip of the auto-injector against the lateral part of the thigh. Push the auto-injector firmly against the thigh and hold it in place until all the medication has been injected. If the first dose does not significantly relieve symptoms within 10 minutes, then consider using a second auto-injector at a different site. Follow local protocols.

To assist a patient with a Twinject auto-injector, remove the injector from the container. Clean the administration site with an alcohol prep. Pull off the green cap "1" to expose a round red tip. Do not cover

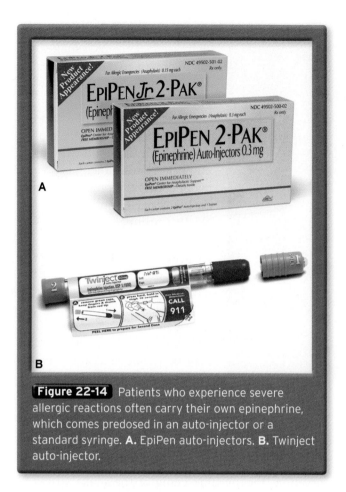

Figure 22-14 Patients who experience severe allergic reactions often carry their own epinephrine, which comes predosed in an auto-injector or a standard syringe. **A.** EpiPen auto-injectors. **B.** Twinject auto-injector.

Controversy

The MAST (Military Anti-Shock Trousers) is a pneumatic inflatable device that can be pumped up to increase pressure on the legs and pelvis, which increases the blood flow return to the heart and thus increases blood pressure. There have been cases reported of improved blood pressure with the use of MAST trousers. Follow your local protocols on the use of this device.

the rounded tip with your hand. Pull off the green cap "2." Place the round red tip against the lateral thigh. It can be administered outside of clothing if necessary. Once the needle has entered the skin, press hard for 10 seconds. Remove the Twinject and check to see that the needle is visible. If the needle is NOT visible, the dose was not administered and the above steps should be repeated. If symptoms recur or have not improved within 10 minutes, repeat the dose. Carefully unscrew and remove the red tip. Hold the blue plastic, pulling the syringe out of the barrel without touching the needle. Slide the yellow collar off the plunger without pulling on the plunger. Insert the needle into the skin on the lateral thigh and push the plunger down.

Because epinephrine constricts blood vessels, it may cause an increased pulse rate, anxiety, cardiac arrhythmias, tachycardia, pallor, dizziness, chest pain, headache, nausea, and vomiting. In a life-threatening situation, the administration of epinephrine outweighs the risk of side effects. Remember that patients who are not wheezing or who have no signs of respiratory compromise or hypotension should not be given epinephrine. After you have provided emergency care, evacuate the patient to transport. If you are permitted

to accompany the patient during transport, closely monitor the patient's vital signs and give high-flow, high-concentration oxygen.

Managing an Anaphylactic Reaction

An anaphylactic reaction is a life-threatening emergency and must be treated as such. This is a load-and-go patient who requires a high level of care. If you are not an ALS-level provider, consider calling for ALS assistance.

Psychological support is a crucial component of management. Anaphylaxis can progress rapidly and has the potential to be a life-threatening event. Patients will need reassurance as you perform the necessary interventions.

Maintain the patient's airway, breathing, and circulation, which may require aggressive airway management and supplemental oxygen administration. Evaluate the patient's ventilatory status and the need for bag-mask device assistance.

Maintain circulation by inserting at least one large-bore IV catheter to give an isotonic solution (lactated Ringer's or normal saline) at a wide-open rate. Ideally, you should place two IV lines en route. Administer epinephrine to stop the allergic reaction. With IV epinephrine, give adults 0.1 mg (1 mL of a 1:10,000 solution) over 3 to 5 minutes. An IV infusion of epinephrine should be considered at 1 to 4 µg/min (that is, 1 mg in 250 mL of saline = 4 µg/mL concentration). Patients who receive epinephrine must be monitored closely for adverse effects. Reassess the patient's vital signs frequently.

An antihistamine such as diphenhydramine (Benadryl) should be given to patients in anaphylactic shock after epinephrine. The typical dose for adults is 50 mg administered via the IM route or slowly via an IV push over 1 minute.

Corticosteroids do not have an immediate effect but are useful in preventing late-phase anaphylactic reactions and should be administered early in the treatment process. Common corticosteroids include

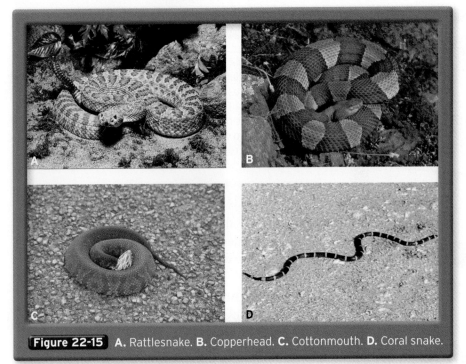

Figure 22-15 **A.** Rattlesnake. **B.** Copperhead. **C.** Cottonmouth. **D.** Coral snake.

methylprednisolone (Solu-Medrol), hydrocortisone (Solu-Cortef), and dexamethasone (Decadron).

Glucagon may also be indicated for an anaphylactic patient, especially if the patient does not respond to epinephrine or is taking a beta-blocker. The usual dose is 1 to 2 mg IM or IV every 5 minutes.

Vasopressors, such as dopamine or Levophed, should be considered if the patient does not respond to fluid administration to treat the hypotension.

Inhaled beta-adrenergic agents such as albuterol may also be included as part of the care regimen if bronchospasm is present. Follow your local medication administration protocols.

Snake Bites

In the United States, 40,000 to 50,000 snake bites are reported annually, with about 7000 caused by poisonous snakes. However, snake bite fatalities in the United States are extremely rare, about 15 per year for the entire country. Of the approximately 115 different species of snakes in the United States, only 19 are venomous. These include the rattlesnake (*Crotalus*), the copperhead (*Agkistrodon contortrix*), the cottonmouth, or water moccasin (*Agkistrodon piscivorus*), and the coral snakes (*Micrurus* and *Micruroides*) **Figure 22-15**. At least one of these poisonous species is found in every state except Alaska, Hawaii, and Maine. As a general rule, these snakes are timid. They usually do not bite unless provoked or accidentally injured, as when they are stepped on. There are a few exceptions to these

rules. Cottonmouths are often aggressive, and rattlesnakes are easily provoked. Coral snakes, in contrast, usually bite only when they are being handled.

Most snake bites occur between April and October, when the animals are active. Texas reports the largest number of bites. Other states with a major concentration of snake bites are Louisiana, Georgia, Oklahoma, North Carolina, Arkansas, West Virginia, and Mississippi. If you work in one of these areas, you should be thoroughly familiar with the emergency handling of snake bites. Remember, almost any time you are caring for a patient with a snake bite, another snake may be in the area and create a second victim—you. Therefore, use extreme caution.

In general, only one third of poisonous snake bites result in significant local or systemic injuries. Often, envenomation does not occur because the snake has recently struck another animal and exhausted its supply of venom for the time being or the snake struck in defense without injecting its venom. This is termed a "dry strike" or "dry bite."

With the exception of the coral snake, poisonous snakes native to the United States all have hollow fangs in the roof of the mouth that inject the poison from two sacs at the back of the head. The classic appearance of the poisonous snake bite, therefore, is two small puncture wounds, usually about 0.5 inch apart, with discoloration and swelling, and the patient usually reports pain surrounding the bite **Figure 22-16**. Nonpoisonous snakes can also bite, usually leaving a horseshoe of tooth marks. However, some poisonous snakes have teeth as well as fangs, making it impossible to say which kind is responsible for a given set of tooth marks. Conversely, fang marks are a clear indication of a poisonous snake bite.

Pit Vipers

Rattlesnakes, copperheads, and cottonmouths are all pit vipers, with triangular-shaped, flat heads **Figure 22-17**. They take their name from the small pits located just behind each nostril and in front of each eye. The pit is a heat-sensing organ that allows the snake to strike accurately at any warm target, especially in the dark when it cannot see through its vertical, slit-like pupils.

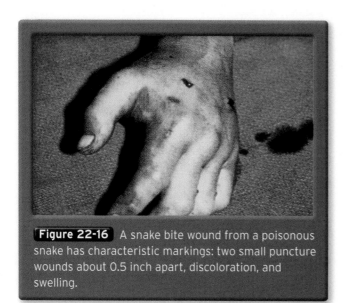

Figure 22-16 A snake bite wound from a poisonous snake has characteristic markings: two small puncture wounds about 0.5 inch apart, discoloration, and swelling.

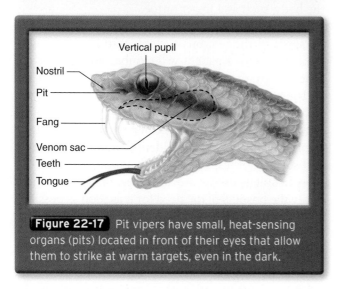

Vertical pupil
Nostril
Pit
Fang
Venom sac
Teeth
Tongue

Figure 22-17 Pit vipers have small, heat-sensing organs (pits) located in front of their eyes that allow them to strike at warm targets, even in the dark.

The fangs of the pit viper normally lie flat against the roof of the mouth and are hinged to swing back and forth as the mouth opens. When the snake is striking, the mouth opens wide and the fangs extend; in this way, the fangs penetrate whatever the mouth strikes. The fangs are actually special hollow teeth that act much like hypodermic needles. They are connected to a sac containing a reservoir of venom, which in turn is attached to a poison gland. The gland itself is a specially adapted salivary gland, which produces enzymes that digest and destroy tissue. The primary purpose of the venom is to kill small animals and to start the digestive process prior to their being eaten.

In the United States, the most common form of pit viper is the rattlesnake. Several different species of rattlesnake can be identified by the rattle on the tail. The rattle is composed of numerous layers of dried skin that were shed but failed to fall off, coming to rest against

a small knob on the end of the tail. Rattlesnakes have many patterns of color, often with a diamond pattern. They can grow to 6 feet or more in length.

Copperheads are smaller than rattlesnakes, usually 2 to 3 feet long, with a reddish coppery color crossed with brown or red bands. These snakes typically inhabit woodpiles and abandoned dwellings, often close to areas of habitation. Although they account for most of the venomous snake bites in the eastern United States, copperhead bites are almost never fatal; however, note that the venom can destroy extremities.

Cottonmouths grow to about 4 feet in length. Also called water moccasins, these snakes are olive or brown, with black cross-bands and a yellow undersurface. They are water snakes and have a particularly aggressive pattern of behavior. Although fatalities from these snake bites are rare, tissue destruction from the venom may be severe.

The signs of envenomation by a pit viper are severe burning pain at the site of the injury, followed by swelling and a bluish discoloration (ecchymosis) in light-skinned individuals that signals bleeding under the skin. These signs are evident within 5 to 10 minutes after the bite has occurred and spread over the next 36 hours. In addition to destroying tissues locally, the venom of the pit viper can also interfere with the body's clotting mechanism and cause bleeding at various distant sites. This toxin affects the entire nervous system. Other systemic signs, which may or may not occur, include weakness, nausea, vomiting, sweating, seizures, fainting, vision problems, changes in level of consciousness, and shock. If swelling has occurred, you should mark its edges on the skin. This will allow physicians to assess what has happened and when it happened with greater accuracy. If the patient has no local signs an hour after being bitten, it is safe to assume that envenomation did not take place.

The amount of toxin injected is related to the toxicity of the bite. A bite will affect children more than adults because there is less body mass to absorb the toxin. The same principle holds true for a small-statured adult.

Occasionally, a patient bitten by a snake will faint from fright. The patient will usually regain consciousness promptly when placed in a supine position. Do not confuse a fainting spell with shock. If shock occurs, it will happen much later.

In treating a snake bite from a pit viper, follow these steps to get the patient to the hospital in a timely manner:

1. Calm the patient; assure him or her that poisonous snake bites are rarely fatal. Place the patient in a supine position and explain that staying quiet will

slow the spread of any venom through the system. Determine the approximate time of the bite and document your time en route to a receiving facility. This time from onset to evaluation at the facility is one of the criteria used in grading the severity of the incident and in determining the amount of antivenin to be used.

2. Locate the bite area; clean it gently with soap and water or a mild antiseptic. Do not apply ice to the area. A constricting band may be applied 4 to 6 inches above the bite site if called for by your local protocols. You should be able to slide two fingers underneath the band. Some local protocols do not allow the use of a constricting band in treating snake bites because of the potential of the venom pooling into the localized bite area. This could potentially cause greater damage to the localized area.

3. If the bite occurred on an arm or leg, splint the extremity to decrease movement. If practical, the limb should be placed below the heart level to decrease venous return.

4. Be alert for vomiting, which may be a sign of anxiety rather than the toxin itself.

5. Do not give the patient anything by mouth.

6. If, as rarely happens, the patient was bitten on the trunk, keep him or her supine and quiet and transport as quickly as possible.

7. Monitor the patient's vital signs and mark the skin with a pen over the area that is swollen. Note if the swelling is spreading.

8. Treat the patient for signs of shock.

9. If the snake has been killed, as is often the case, be sure to bring it with you in a secure container so that physicians can identify it and administer the proper antivenin.

10. Notify the hospital that you are bringing in a patient who has a snake bite; if possible, describe the snake.

11. Rapidly evacuate the patient to transport to the hospital. All patients with a suspected snake bite should be taken to the emergency department, whether they show signs of envenomation or not.

If you are permitted to accompany the patient during transport, support the patient's airway and breathing as needed, place a sterile dressing over the suspected bite area, and immobilize the injury site. Treat the wound as you would any deep puncture wound to prevent infection (see Chapter 21, "Soft-Tissue Injuries").

If you work in an area where poisonous snakes are known to live, you should know your local protocol for handling snake bites. You should also know the address of the nearest facility where antivenin is available. This may be a nearby zoo, the local or public state health department, or a local community hospital.

Coral Snakes

The coral snake is a small reptile with a series of bright red, yellow, and black bands completely encircling the body. Many harmless snakes have similar coloring, but only the coral snake has red and yellow bands next to one another, as this helpful rhyme suggests: "Red on yellow will kill a fellow; red on black, venom will lack."

A rare creature that lives in most southern states and in the Southwest, the coral snake is a relative of the cobra. It has tiny fangs and injects the venom with its teeth by a chewing motion, leaving behind one or more puncture or scratch-like wounds. Because of its small mouth and teeth and limited jaw expansion, the coral snake usually bites its victims on a small part of the body, such as a finger or toe.

Coral snake venom is a powerful toxin that causes paralysis of the nervous system. Within a few hours of being bitten, a patient will exhibit bizarre behavior, followed by progressive paralysis of eye movements and respiration. Often, there are limited or no local symptoms.

Successful treatment, either emergency or long term, depends on positive identification of the snake and support of respiration. Antivenin is available, but most hospitals do not stock it. Therefore, you should notify the hospital of the need for it as soon as possible. The steps for emergency care of a coral snake bite are as follows:

1. Immediately quiet and reassure the patient.

2. Flush the area of the bite with 1 to 2 L of warm, soapy water to wash away any poison left on the surface of the skin. Do not apply ice to the region.

3. Splint the extremity to minimize movement and the spread of venom at the site.

4. Check the patient's vital signs and continue to monitor them.

5. Keep the patient warm to help prevent shock.

6. If possible, give supplemental oxygen if needed.

7. Rapidly evacuate the patient to transport promptly. Give advance notice that the patient has been bitten by a coral snake.

8. Give the patient nothing by mouth during transport.

Scorpion Stings

Scorpions are eight-legged arachnids from the biologic group Arachnida with a venom gland and a stinger at the end of their tail **Figure 22-18**. Scorpions are rare; they live primarily in the southwestern United States and in deserts. With one exception, a scorpion's sting is usually very painful but not dangerous, causing localized swelling and discoloration. The exception is the *Centruroides sculpturatus*. It is found naturally in Arizona and New Mexico, as well as parts of Texas, California, and

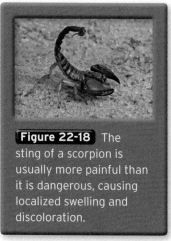

Figure 22-18 The sting of a scorpion is usually more painful than it is dangerous, causing localized swelling and discoloration.

Nevada. The venom of this particular species may produce a severe systemic reaction that brings about circulatory collapse, severe muscle contractions, excessive salivation, hypertension, convulsions, and cardiac failure. Antivenin is available but must be administered by a physician. If you suspect that the patient was stung by a *C. sculpturatus*, notify medical control as soon as possible. Support the patient's airway and breathing. Evacuate the patient to transport as rapidly as possible. If you are permitted to accompany the patient during transport and have the appropriate level of training, provide pain relief with analgesics per local protocols.

Tick Bites

Found most often on brush, shrubs, trees, sand dunes, or other animals, ticks usually attach themselves directly to the skin **Figure 22-19**. Only a fraction of an inch long, they can easily be mistaken for a freckle, especially since their bite is not painful. Indeed, the danger

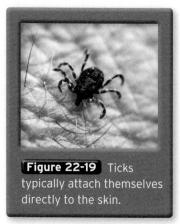

Figure 22-19 Ticks typically attach themselves directly to the skin.

with a tick bite is not from the bite itself, but from the infecting organisms that the tick carries. Ticks commonly carry two infectious diseases, Rocky Mountain spotted fever and Lyme disease. Both are spread through the tick's saliva, which is injected into the skin when the tick attaches itself.

Rocky Mountain spotted fever, which is not limited to the Rocky Mountains, occurs within 7 to 10 days after a bite by an infected tick. Its symptoms include nausea,

vomiting, headache, weakness, paralysis, and possibly cardiorespiratory collapse.

Lyme disease has received extensive publicity. Originally seen only in Connecticut, Lyme disease has now been reported in 35 states. It occurs most commonly in the Northeast, the Great Lake states, and the Pacific Northwest; New York State reports the largest number of cases. The first symptom, a rash that may spread to several parts of the body, begins about 3 days after the bite of an infected tick. The rash may eventually resemble a bull's-eye pattern in one third of patients **Figure 22-20**. After a few more days or weeks, painful swelling of the joints, particularly the knees, occurs. Lyme disease may be confused with rheumatoid arthritis and, like that disease, may result in permanent disability.

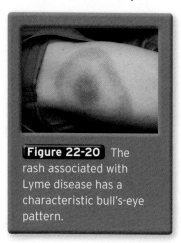

Figure 22-20 The rash associated with Lyme disease has a characteristic bull's-eye pattern.

However, if it is recognized and treated promptly with antibiotics, the patient may recover completely.

Tick bites occur most commonly during the summer months when people are outdoors in the woods or a field **Figure 22-21**. Transmission of the infection from the tick to a person takes at least 12 hours, so if you are called on to remove a tick you should allow yourself time to proceed carefully. Do not attempt to suffocate the tick with gasoline or Vaseline or burn it with a lighted match; you will only burn the patient. Instead, using fine tweezers, grasp the tick by the body and pull gently but firmly straight up so that the skin is tented. Hold this position until the tick releases. This method will usually remove the whole tick. Even if part of the tick is left embedded in the skin, the part containing the infecting organisms has been removed. Cleanse the area with disinfectant and

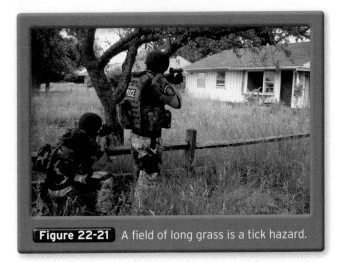

Figure 22-21 A field of long grass is a tick hazard.

High Altitude Deployment and Acute Mountain Sickness

SWAT units who deploy to mountainous regions and who are not acclimated to high altitude are at risk for developing several types of altitude sickness by traveling too high too quickly. Acute mountain sickness (AMS) is the most common altitude illness. AMS is not life threatening but will cut down on performance significantly if SWAT officers develop nausea, vomiting, dizziness, fatigue, malaise, and headache within 12 to 24 hours of arrival. Proper acclimatization takes 5 to 7 days that the SWAT unit may not have. A TEMS unit physician may administer acetazolamide (Diamox) 125 mg every 6 hours or the medication may be issued in advance by the medical director. Note: the 500-mg extended release form should be avoided due to the side effects such as drowsiness and nausea. If the SWAT officer continues to complain of a severe headache or has difficulty breathing, persistent shortness of breath, and a cough, then rapidly transport to the hospital for further evaluation and treatment by a physician.

save the tick in a glass jar or other container so that it can be identified. Do not handle the tick with your fingers. Provide any necessary supportive emergency care, and transport the patient to the hospital.

Poisonous Plants

Poison ivy, poison oak, and poison sumac can cause minor to severe itching and rash in those persons who have a skin sensitivity to these plants. All SWAT officers who will be hiking through fields or forests should be able to visually recognize and avoid these plants **Figure 22-22**. If the SWAT officer is exposed to an irritating plant, then you have about 20 minutes to wash the oil off before the skin reacts in a rash.

There are three principal medications used for treating rashes from poison ivy and other plants. These include steroid pills (prednisone) to decrease the inflammation, topical steroid creams (triamcinolone 0.1%), and diphenhydramine (Benadryl). Unfortunately, Benadryl also causes significant drowsiness and slowness

Medical Gear

If there is a possibility that a mission will take place on or near the water, all SWAT and TEMS personnel should be fitted with an appropriately sized and tested life vest. During training in a safe environment, double-check that the flotation devices will actually keep the fully equipped SWAT officer afloat with positive buoyancy.

of reflexes. Therefore, during live-fire training and callouts, this medication must be avoided. If itching is significant then a nonsedating antihistamine may be used. Follow local protocols.

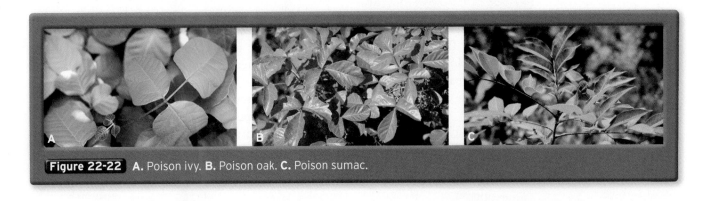

Figure 22-22 **A.** Poison ivy. **B.** Poison oak. **C.** Poison sumac.

Safety

If you work in a recreation area near lakes, rivers, or the ocean, you should have a prearranged plan for water rescue. This plan should include access to and cooperation with local personnel who are trained and skilled in water rescue; these personnel should help to develop the protocol for water rescue. Because the success of any water rescue depends on how rapidly the patient is removed from the water and ventilated, make sure you always have immediate access to personal flotation devices and other rescue equipment. Survival rates drastically decline the longer a victim is immersed. Cold water drowning survival rates are somewhat higher. Ventilation and CPR are crucial to the patient's survival.

You must ensure the safety of rescue personnel before a water rescue can begin. If the patient is conscious and still in the water, you should perform a water rescue. Remember the saying: "Reach, throw, and row, and only then go." This phrase sums up the basic rule of water rescue. First, try to reach for the patient. If that does not work, throw the patient a rope, a life preserver, or any floatable object that is available. Next, use a boat if one is available. Do not attempt a swimming rescue unless you are trained and experienced in the proper techniques. Even then, you should always wear a helmet and a personal flotation device. Too many well-meaning individuals have themselves become victims while attempting a swimming rescue.

Diving Injuries

Diving is performed by some SWAT officers in coastal cities and where rivers and lakes are nearby. Tactical diving teams can utilize underwater approaches to get close to the target objective in a stealthy manner, and can move close to allow observation of targets. Some tactical diving teams are also available for other missions such as underwater recovery and rescue. Many of these missions do not involve diving to depths where **decompression sickness** (the bends) is a risk, but there are some injuries that can affect divers even in as little as 10 to 20 feet of water. If your TEMS unit supports a tactical dive team, you should be capable of recognizing and providing stabilizing care for dive injuries including:

- Pneumothorax (air enters the pleural space and compresses the lungs)
- Pneumomediastinum (air enters the mediastinum)
- Air emboli (air enters the bloodstream and creates bubbles of air in the blood vessels)
- Decompression sickness

In addition, medical intelligence should note the location of the closest hyperbaric chamber.

Ready for Review

- The body's regulatory mechanisms normally maintain body temperature within a very narrow range around 98.6°F (37°C). Body temperature is regulated by heat loss to the atmosphere via conduction, convection, evaporation, radiation, and respiration.

- The key to treating hypothermic patients is to stabilize vital functions and prevent further heat loss. Patients who have moderate to severe hypothermia are at risk of developing lethal cardiac arrhythmias if they are moved harshly or suddenly jolted during extraction; therefore, use extreme caution during extraction and evacuation.

- Some patients without a pulse or spontaneous breathing may have been suddenly cooled by immersion in cold water and may still be viable with proper resuscitation and rewarming procedures. Do not consider a patient dead until he or she is "warm and dead."

- Local cold injuries include frostbite, frostnip, and trench foot. Frostbite is the most serious because tissues actually freeze. All patients with a local cold injury should be removed from the cold and protected from further exposure.

- Heat illness can take three forms: heat cramps, heat exhaustion, and heatstroke.

- Heat cramps are painful muscle spasms that occur with vigorous exercise. Treatment includes removing the patient from the heat, resting the affected muscles, and replacing lost fluids.

- Heat exhaustion is essentially a form of hypovolemic shock caused by dehydration. Symptoms include cold and clammy skin, weakness, headache, and rapid pulse. Body temperature can be high, and the patient may or may not still be sweating. Treatment includes removing the patient from the heat and treating for mild hypovolemic shock.

- Heatstroke is a life-threatening emergency, usually fatal if untreated. Patients with heatstroke are usually dry and will have high body temperatures. Changes in mental status are a hallmark of heatstroke and can include confusion, seizure, altered mental status, and coma. Rapid lowering of the body temperature in the field is critical.

- Poisonous spiders include the black widow spider and the brown recluse spider.

- Poisonous snakes include pit vipers and coral snakes.

- A person who has been bitten by a pit viper needs prompt transport; clean the bite area and keep the patient quiet to slow the spread of venom.

- Notify the hospital as soon as possible if a patient has been bitten by a coral snake; its venom can cause paralysis of the nervous system and most hospitals do not have appropriate antivenin on hand.

- Patients who have been bitten by ticks may be infected with Rocky Mountain spotted fever or Lyme disease and should see a doctor for antibiotic treatment within a day or two. Remove the tick using tweezers and save it for identification.

Vital Vocabulary

ambient temperature The temperature of the surrounding environment.

anaphylaxis An extreme, life-threatening systemic allergic reaction that may include shock and respiratory failure.

antivenin A serum that counteracts the effect of venom from an animal or insect.

conduction The loss of heat by direct contact (eg, when a body part comes into contact with a colder object).

convection The loss of body heat caused by air movement (eg, breeze blowing across the body).

core temperature The temperature of the central part of the body (eg, the heart, lungs, and vital organs).

decompression sickness A painful condition seen in divers who ascend too quickly, in which gas, especially nitrogen, forms bubbles in blood vessels and other tissues; also called "the bends."

evaporation Conversion of water or another fluid from a liquid to a gas.

frostbite Damage to tissues as the result of exposure to cold; frozen body parts.

heat cramps Painful muscle spasms usually associated with vigorous activity in a hot environment.

heat exhaustion A form of heat injury in which the body loses significant amounts of fluid and electrolytes because of heavy sweating; also called heat prostration or heat collapse.

heatstroke A life-threatening condition of severe hyperthermia caused by exposure to excessive natural or artificial heat, marked by warm, dry skin; severely altered mental status; and often irreversible coma.

hymenoptera A family of insects that includes bees, wasps, ants, and yellow jackets.

hyperthermia A condition in which the body's core temperature rises to 101°F (38.3°C) or more.

hypothermia A condition in which the body's core temperature falls below 95°F (35°C) after exposure to a cold environment.

radiation The transfer of heat to colder objects in the environment by radiant energy—for example, being warmed by a fire.

respiration The loss of body heat as warm air in the lungs is exhaled into the atmosphere and cooler air is inhaled.

reverse triage A triage process in which efforts are focused on those who are in respiratory and cardiac arrest, and different from conventional triage where such patients would be classified as deceased. Used in triaging multiple victims of a lightning strike.

trench foot Cold injury similar to frostbite caused by prolonged exposure to cool, wet conditions (up to 60°F [16°C]).

Medications in the Tactical Environment

Introduction

Only authorized medical personnel should dispense medication. Local EMS and TEMS unit protocols will designate who is authorized to directly dispense medication. Any medication that requires a physician's order or prescription should only be provided to patients if authorized by agency policy.

All TEMS unit personnel who are authorized to administer medications must be thoroughly familiar with the safe and effective use of all medications carried by the TEMS unit. If a civilian paramedic on a routine EMS call has a question about a medication, then medical control may be immediately consulted. This is not always true for the TEMS unit. Time or communications capability may not permit contact with medical control and some situations may require medication to be administered immediately. It is imperative that all TEMS unit personnel who are authorized to administer medication know and understand local protocols, including medication dosages, indications and contraindications, and side effects.

Medication Considerations

Local protocols should clearly delineate who is authorized to administer medication and under what circumstances, which medications are permitted to be used in the tactical environment, and how the medication should be administered. Medication indications and contraindications should also be discussed within local protocols. Before any medication is administered, a tactical patient assessment (Call A CAB 'N Go) and a secondary assessment should be completed.

Key considerations when preparing to use medications in the tactical environment include:

1. All serious signs and symptoms, regardless of whether they respond to medications, should be followed up with a thorough secondary assessment. For example, a SWAT officer with heartburn-like chest pain may be given an antacid. This SWAT officer should receive a thorough patient assessment to determine if there are additional signs and symptoms of a more serious condition, such as a heart attack.

2. Any medication that may alter the SWAT officer's mental status, cause drowsiness, or decrease performance should be avoided in SWAT officers who have ongoing tactical responsibilities.

The Five Rights of Medication Administration

Prior to giving any medication, verify the following five rights of medication administration:

1. **Right patient.** Verify the identity of the patient. Verify that the patient does not have any contraindications to the medication.
2. **Right medication.** Check to ensure that the medication you are about to administer is correct.
3. **Right dosage.** Check the pill size, tablet amount, or concentration for the medication to be administered.
4. **Right time.** Consider how long it will take to evacuate the patient to an ambulance for transport to a hospital and what other medications may be given at that time.
5. **Right route.** Confirm whether the medication should be given by the oral, intramuscular (IM), sublingual (SL), transdermal, intraosseous (IO), or intravenous (IV) route.

Medication Administration in the Tactical Environment

Over-the-Counter Medications

Over-the-counter (OTC) medications can be purchased without a prescription. OTC medications can ease many of the common ailments faced by SWAT officers, such as muscle ache or headache. The TEMS medical director and local protocols will dictate how and when OTC medications are made available. Some TEMS units may make OTC medications readily available for SWAT officers to self-administer by storing the OTC medications in a cabinet in the SWAT raid van, while other TEMS units may require an authorized TMP to administer the OTC medication to SWAT officers **Figure 23-1**. Follow your local protocols on administering OTC medications for minor ailments.

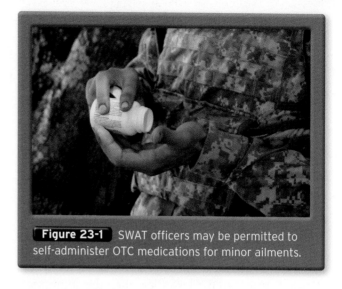

Figure 23-1 SWAT officers may be permitted to self-administer OTC medications for minor ailments.

Prescription Medications

Prescription medications may be administered to SWAT officers by authorized TMPs as indicated by local protocols. If a SWAT officer has a prescription from his or her primary care physician for a nonsedating medication that he or she takes on a daily basis, such as blood pressure medication, he or she may take it, provided it does not cause a decrease in performance or impaired mental status. It is the responsibility of each SWAT officer to ask his or her primary care physician if the prescribed medication can cause such problems, and if so, to avoid the medication. If there are any questions regarding the prescribed medication and its effect on the SWAT officer, then the TEMS medical director should consult with the primary care physician and work together to find the best solution for the SWAT officer.

During prolonged operations, if a SWAT officer forgets to bring any daily prescribed medications, such as an antihypertensive (high blood pressure) medication, then the TEMS unit leader may work with the SWAT officer's primary care physician or the TEMS medical director to obtain this medication for the SWAT officer due to the SWAT officer's medical condition.

Reporting the Use of Medications to Command Staff

During training and callouts, SWAT officers should be reminded that they should report to the TMP when they feel that they need to take an OTC or prescription medication. The reason for taking the medication (ie, headache or chest pain) may warrant a thorough patient assessment. The results of the patient assessment may lead to a referral to the SWAT officer's personal care physician or transport to the emergency room.

Some developing medical conditions such as muscle cramps or a toothache may actually interfere with the performance of the SWAT officer. These conditions should be reported to the command staff by the TMP and/or the SWAT officer, and a plan of action should then be decided upon. The SWAT unit's mission should not be compromised due to a medical condition.

Pain Medications

Efforts should be made to appropriately control a patient's pain, even in the hectic tactical environment. Early alleviation of pain will help to diminish suffering and may help to improve the patient's outcome. When a patient has a complaint or obvious signs of discomfort, such as the painful grimace of a SWAT officer with a gunshot wound to the lower leg, then the appropriate use of pain medicine may be indicated **Figure 23-2**. In addition to administering medications, provide comfort and reassurance to patients who are in pain. Minor contusions and small fractures may be adequately treated with acetaminophen or ibuprofen, whereas large displaced fractures or dislocations may require narcotic medications such as morphine or fentanyl to control the pain.

During the secondary assessment, discuss the patient's symptoms and level of pain. For example: On a scale of 1 to 10, with 10 being the most severe pain you can think of, how bad is your pain right now? Another method is to use a printed pain scale where the patient points to the line on the 1 to 10 scale that matches the patient's current level of pain.

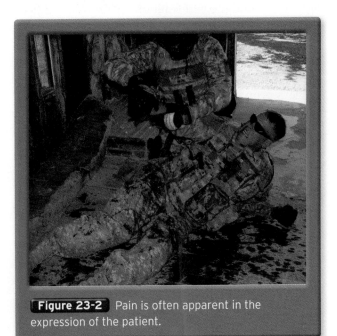

Figure 23-2 Pain is often apparent in the expression of the patient.

Medical Gear

A medication that has been used on the battlefield is the fentanyl lozenge (also known as a fentanyl lollipop). The fentanyl lozenge is basically a sweet lozenge on a small handheld stick containing 200 to 1600 µg of fentanyl (a type of morphine). On the battlefield, a soldier with a painful injury is provided this medication attached to the fingers with tape. The soldier is instructed to not bite or chew it, but to let it dissolve in his or her mouth. Once the pain is tolerable, the soldier is instructed to take it out of his or her mouth. If the soldier becomes less alert, then the relaxed muscles of the arm should work with gravity to pull the fentanyl lozenge out of the soldier's mouth. Patients given this medication must be reassessed every 15 minutes and monitored for respiratory depression.

If you determine that the patient does not have an underlying serious issue that requires transport to the hospital, then either provide or allow the patient to self-administer non-narcotic pain medications such as acetaminophen or ibuprofen. For more severe pain, the use of morphine, fentanyl, or other narcotic pain medicine should be considered according to local protocols. Pain medications are discussed in detail later in this chapter.

Antibiotics

If a SWAT unit is deploying for a short mission (2 to 3 hours) and completes the mission in that time frame, then a non-life-threatening wound such as a large knee abrasion may be initially cleansed and dressed in the field. Further care and need for antibiotics may be determined when the patient arrives at the emergency room. A prolonged or remote multihour or multiagency callout, however, may result in a delay in evacuation. In such cases, antibiotics may be administered for significant injuries with a high risk of infection, such as deep cuts into muscle and joints, large puncture wounds, and contaminated wounds. Follow local protocols on the antibiotics that may be administered.

Safety

Fentanyl lozenges are specially packaged in child-resistant packaging that requires scissors or a knife to open, and must absolutely be kept away from small children as they are so powerful that a child could easily be killed from respiratory cessation if he or she unintentionally obtains and eats one.

Pain Medications in the Tactical Environment

Meloxicam, Acetaminophen, and Ibuprofen

Indications

The pain medications meloxicam (Mobic), acetaminophen (Tylenol), and ibuprofen (Advil, Motrin) are used for mild to moderate pain in SWAT officers still able to continue the mission or training. These medications do not cause sedation.

Adverse Effects

Meloxicam and ibuprofen can cause gastrointestinal irritation and pain if given in high doses and if not given with food to buffer the potentially harsh effects on the stomach lining. Acetaminophen can cause liver damage if given at high doses for an extended period of time. This rarely occurs when the total daily dose is less than 4000 mg per day.

Route of Administration

Meloxicam may be administered to the patient orally 15 mg once a day. Ibuprofen may be administered orally 600 mg every 6 hours or 800 mg every 8 hours. The maximum total dosage of ibuprofen is 2400 mg per day. Acetaminophen may be given orally in 1000-mg to 1300-mg doses every 6 hours. Document every dose given. Instruct the patient what time he or she can take the next dose and the dosage amount if needed. If agency policy permits self-administration, tactical personnel must document similar information on a form that is kept with the OTC medication.

Morphine

Morphine is an excellent narcotic pain medication that is relatively inexpensive and can reliably be used to decrease pain.

Indications

You may need to administer morphine to injured patients who:

- Have serious injuries
- Are in severe pain
- Have a long evacuation time

Contraindications and Adverse Effects

Morphine has serious adverse effects and therefore should be administered cautiously to patients with head injuries. Administration of morphine may cause increased intracranial pressure (ICP) and may induce vomiting. Morphine also causes constriction of the pupils and inhibits pupillary reactions. Using pupillary response to assess the patient for a severe or worsening head injury is not reliable after the administration of morphine.

Although morphine is a powerful pain reliever, it can depress respiration. This rarely is a problem for those in severe pain because the pain itself usually blocks the respiratory effect of the morphine. For patients in less pain, the respiratory rate must be constantly monitored. These types of patients include:

- Upper airway obstruction
- Burns to the respiratory tract
- Wounds to the throat, nasal passages, oral cavity, or jaws
- Bronchial asthma
- Significant chest injuries
- Altered mental status (morphine may cause mental confusion and may interfere with making a proper assessment)
- Shock (morphine lowers the blood pressure, increasing the effects of shock)
- Known allergies to morphine

The side effects of morphine include:

- Sedation (morphine may cause considerable mental confusion and therefore should not be given to ambulatory patients or anyone who needs to remain mentally alert)

- Nausea, vomiting, and constipation
- Pruritus (itching) and skin flushing (red rash near the injection site)

Routes of Administration

Morphine comes in multiple strengths and may be administered in a variety of ways. The IV route is the preferred method of administration due to a more rapid pain relief response over the more traditional IM methods.

IV Morphine Dosage Many agencies utilize a morphine sulfate 2- to 6-mg slow IV push as needed for significant discomfort (more than 4 or 5 on a 10-point scale), which may be repeated if indicated every 5 minutes if the systolic blood pressure is more than 100 mm Hg, to a total dose of 10 mg or more. To make titration more accurate, morphine given by IV should be diluted in sterile water for injection or in normal saline (NaCl) prior to administration. Most adults will experience significant pain relief at a total dose of 10 to 20 mg, although higher doses may be required. In many agencies the medical director is often contacted once the dose reaches 15 mg and the patient is still in pain. Follow your local protocols.

Monitor the patient closely for any adverse effects. A common side effect is nausea and itching. These can be lessened if Benadryl (diphenhydramine) is given 25- to 50-mg slow IV push. Both morphine and Benadryl will cause the patient to become less alert.

IM Morphine Dosage Load the prefilled cartridge into the injector device (usually at a dose of 5 or 10 mg) **Figure 23-3** . If you are not giving the full 10-mg dose to the patient, place the unused portion into another syringe (if possible), properly label, and safely store this medication before administering the injection. The extra medicine will either be used for patient care within the next hour or two, or will be destroyed with a reliable witness documenting that it was properly discarded.

Never waste medical supplies if you do not have to while in the tactical environment.

Administer the injection to the patient. Document the injection site, amount, time given, and who administered it on the patient care report. Monitor the patient for adverse reactions. Prepare to give additional medication if the therapeutic goal is not reached. Aim to decrease the pain to a level of 4 or less.

Fentanyl

Indications

You may administer fentanyl to a patient who has serious pain and who is not allergic to the medication. Fentanyl is a narcotic that may be given by IV, SQ (subcutaneously), IM, by slow release skin patch, or orally via the fentanyl lollipop **Figure 23-4** . The benefit of a fentanyl lozenge is that it is lightweight, easy to carry, waterproof, durable, has a long shelf life, and is easily administered, even in a tactical environment.

Contraindications

Contraindications to administering fentanyl include allergy to the medication or any of its components. Exercise caution in giving it to a patient who has already been given morphine or a benzodiazepine, as the effects can be magnified. Fentanyl and any other narcotic medications increase the chance of respiratory depression and other adverse side effects, especially when given in combination.

Route of Administration

Oral administration via the fentanyl lozenge may be the most efficient route of administration in the tactical environment. Wear gloves when administering the fentanyl lozenge to avoid exposure to the medication. The fentanyl lozenges are produced in six different concentrations, ranging from 200 to 1600 µg. The 800-µg fentanyl lozenge is the most common dosage used in the tactical environment. Follow local dosage

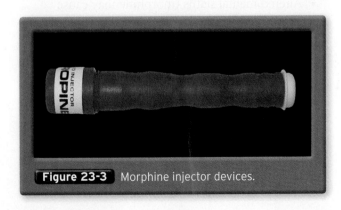

Figure 23-3 Morphine injector devices.

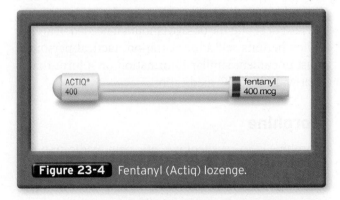

Figure 23-4 Fentanyl (Actiq) lozenge.

protocols. Instruct the patient that the lozenge must not be chewed or swallowed whole or it will be less effective. Ideally, absorption occurs when the lozenge dissolves over 15 minutes.

Reassess the patient every 15 minutes. Monitor for respiratory depression. If the patient goes into respiratory depression, administer Narcan per local protocols and provide ventilatory support. If nausea and vomiting occur, then consider administering Zofran or other antiemetic medication per local protocols.

Medication Storage

Narcotic abuse is prevalent in the United States and medication must be secured in a double-locked location that maintains the appropriate environmental conditions. All TEMS unit personnel who are authorized to administer narcotic medications are responsible for maintaining accountability for the narcotic through a logbook and must abide by all US Food and Drug Administration (FDA), Drug Enforcement Agency (DEA), and state-controlled substances regulations pertaining to the storage and administration of narcotics.

Keep the presence of narcotics in strict confidence so that the supply does not become the target of theft. If the narcotic supply is stolen or there is a discrepancy in the tracking log, then both the TEMS and EMS medical directors must be notified immediately.

Policies should be in place to drug test all personnel, both medical and law enforcement, who could have access to controlled substances and might have handled them inappropriately. Policies should take into account federal, state, and local statutes. If possible, consult with local employee assistance programs when creating agency policy.

Ready for Review

- Only authorized medical personnel should dispense medication. Always follow local protocols.

- Two key considerations when preparing to use medication in the tactical environment are:

  - All serious signs and symptoms, regardless of whether they respond to medications, should be followed up with a thorough secondary assessment.

  - Any medication that may alter a person's mental status, cause drowsiness, or decrease performance should be avoided in SWAT officers who have ongoing tactical responsibilities.

- Prior to giving any medication, verify the following five rights of medication administration:

  - Right patient
  - Right medication
  - Right dosage
  - Right time
  - Right route

- The TEMS medical director and local protocols will dictate how and when OTC medications are made available.

- If a SWAT officer has a prescription from his or her primary care physician for a nonsedating medication that will not decrease performance that he or she takes on a daily basis, such as blood pressure medication, he or she may take it with the approval of the TEMS medical director.

- During training and callouts, SWAT officers should be reminded that they should report to the TMP when they feel that they need to take an OTC or prescription medication. A policy for self-administration of OTC medication can be used in some circumstances.

- Efforts should be made to appropriately control a patient's pain, even in the hectic tactical environment. Early alleviation of pain will help to diminish suffering and may help to improve the patient's outcome.

- Narcotic abuse is prevalent in the United States and medications must be secured in a double-locked location that maintains the appropriate environmental conditions. Policies to identify and deal with law enforcement or medical personnel who inappropriately use controlled substances should be in place.

Vital Vocabulary

over-the-counter (OTC) medications Medications that do not require the authorization of a physician.

prescription medications Medications requiring the authorization of a physician.

Weapons of Mass Destruction

- Describe how the tactical medical provider (TMP) may maintain personal safety at a scene with weapons of mass destruction.

- List the four main classifications of chemical agents.

- Describe the effects of chemical agents on the patient and the stabilizing care the TMP can provide.

- List the three categories of biologic agents.

- Describe effects of biologic agents on the patient and the stabilizing care the TMP can provide.

- Discuss the sources of radiologic materials and dispersal devices.

- Describe the stabilizing care the TMP may provide to the patient exposed to radiation.

- Describe the protective measures against radiation exposure that can be taken by the TMP.

- Describe how the TMP may maintain personal safety at a scene with a suicide bomber.

Introduction

Since the September 11, 2001, attacks, public safety agencies in the United States have become keenly aware of the worldwide escalation of terrorist threats, which raises the risk of incidents involving unconventional weapons such as **weapons of mass destruction (WMDs)**. At this time, the most common type of terrorist attack throughout the world continues to be conventional weapons, mainly explosions from bombs and ballistic trauma from firearms. However, the risk of chemical, biologic, radiologic, and nuclear attacks exists, so SWAT and TEMS units must be prepared to respond to both conventional and unconventional threats.

Chemical, Biologic, Radiologic, and Nuclear Threats

The acronym **CBRN** stands for chemical, biologic, radiologic, and nuclear threats. SWAT and TEMS units responding to CBRN incidents should assume that they are deliberate, malicious acts intended to kill, sicken, and/or disrupt society. Evidence preservation and perpetrator apprehension are of great concern with CBRN incidents.

CBRN threats have several features in common: they are rare and sometimes difficult to identify, require specialized training to understand and mitigate, and are frightening to the general population. The threat of and actual use of these agents cause fear in the general population, which is the larger goal of the terrorist group. These agents may cause injuries and illnesses that are unusual and difficult to treat. Although the risk of a CBRN threat is rare, if utilized in a well-planned and coordinated fashion, CBRN agents could potentially kill thousands of innocent people and terrorize millions more.

Chemical Terrorism/Warfare

Chemical agents are manmade substances that can have devastating effects on living organisms. They can be produced in liquid, powder, or vapor form depending on the desired route of exposure and dissemination technique. Developed during World War I and further refined since then, these agents have caused injuries and death since being introduced on the battlefield, and have been used to terrorize civilian populations. These agents consist of the following types:

- Vesicants (blister agents)
- Respiratory agents (choking agents)
- Nerve agents
- Metabolic agents (blood agents)

Biologic Terrorism/Warfare

Biologic agents are organisms or toxins produced by organisms that cause disease. They are generally found in nature; for terrorist use, however, they are cultivated, synthesized, and mutated in a laboratory or may be stolen or acquired illegally from government stockpiles. The **weaponization** of biologic agents may be performed to artificially maximize the target population's exposure to the germ, thereby exposing the greatest number of people and achieving the desired result.

The primary types of biologic agents that you may come into contact with during a biologic event include:

- Viruses
- Bacteria
- Toxins

Nuclear/Radiologic Terrorism

There have been only two publicly known incidents involving the use of a nuclear device to target human populations. During World War II, the Japanese cities of Hiroshima and Nagasaki were devastated when the United States conducted atomic bombings of both cities. The destructive power demonstrated by the attacks ended World War II and has helped to serve as a deterrent to future nuclear war.

Several nations that hold close ties with terrorist groups (known as **state-sponsored terrorism**) have obtained some degree of nuclear capability. It is also possible for a terrorist to secure radioactive materials or waste to perpetrate an act of terror. These materials are far easier for the determined terrorist to acquire than a nuclear weapon. Radioactive materials, such as those in old X-ray machines, medical nuclear laboratories, research facilities, and industrial plants can be placed next to a stick of dynamite or other explosive to make a **radiologic dispersal device (RDD)**, also known as a "dirty bomb." Dirty bombs can also be made with biologic and chemical agents.

Scene Safety for the TMP

The best form of protection from a WMD agent is avoiding contact with the agent. The greatest threats you will face in a WMD attack are contamination and **cross-contamination**. Contamination with an agent occurs when you have direct contact with the WMD or are exposed to it. Cross-contamination occurs when you then come into contact with a person who has not yet been decontaminated.

Secondary Device or Event (Reassessing Scene Safety)

Terrorists have been known to plant additional explosives that are set to explode after the initial bomb. This type of **secondary device** is intended primarily to injure public safety personnel and to secure media coverage, because the media generally arrives on scene just after the initial response. Do not rely on others to secure your safety. It is your responsibility to constantly assess and reassess the scene. It is easy to overlook a suspicious package lying on the floor while you are treating patients. Stay alert. Something as subtle as a change in the wind direction during a gas attack or an increase in the number of contaminated patients can place you in danger. Never become so involved with the tasks that you are performing that you do not look around and make sure that the scene remains safe.

Chemical Weapons

Chemical agents are liquids or gases that are dispersed to kill or injure. Modern-day chemicals were first developed during WWI and WWII. During the Cold War many of these agents were perfected and stockpiled. Whereas the United States has long renounced the use of chemical weapons, many nations still develop and stockpile them. These agents are deadly and pose a threat if acquired or manufactured by terrorists.

Chemical weapons have several classifications. The properties or characteristics of an agent can be described

Safety

You are of no help to the public if you become a patient. More importantly, once you become a victim of the event, you place an additional burden on your fellow TMPs and responders who must treat you. After calling for help, ensure that all threats are abolished before you respond. Resist the urge to run in and help (do not develop tunnel vision). You may place your life in danger. Do not become a victim.

At the Scene

In a mass-casualty incident, it is important to communicate frequently with your patient. Remember that your patient is probably scared and does not know what is happening. By explaining to your patient any delays that are occurring, as well as the actions you are taking, the patient's fears may be alleviated.

It is also important to provide your patient with some type of protection when needed. Whether it is from building materials, backboards, or tarps, some type of material should be used to minimize the potential for further harm.

as liquid, gas, or solid material. **Persistency** and **volatility** are terms used to describe how long the agent will stay on a surface before it evaporates. Persistent or nonvolatile agents can remain on a surface for long periods of time, usually longer than 24 hours. Nonpersistent or volatile agents evaporate relatively quickly when left on a surface in the optimal temperature range. An agent that is described as highly persistent (such as VX, an oily liquid nerve agent) can remain in the environment for weeks to months, whereas an agent that is highly volatile (such as sarin, also a nerve agent) will turn from liquid to gas (evaporate) within minutes to seconds.

Route of exposure is a term used to describe how the agent enters the body. Chemical agents can have either a vapor or contact hazard. Agents with a **vapor hazard** enter the body through breathing in the vapors. Agents with a **contact hazard** (or skin hazard) give off very little or no vapor and enter the body through the skin.

Because chemical agents affect the patient's airway with severe consequences, the airway and breathing need to be stabilized before circulation.

Blister Agents

The primary route of exposure for blister agents is the skin (contact); however, if blister agents are left on the skin or clothing long enough, or if the victim is close to the source of exposure, they produce vapors that can enter the respiratory tract. Blister agents cause burnlike blisters that form on the victim's skin as well as in the respiratory tract (mouth, nose, throat, esophagus, and lungs). The blister agents consist of sulfur mustard (H), Lewisite (L), and phosgene oxime (CX) (the symbols H, L, and CX are military designations for these chemicals). The blister agents usually cause the most damage to damp or moist areas of the body, such as the armpits,

groin, eyes, and respiratory tract, where the chemical reaction is stronger.

Sulfur mustard (agent H) is a brownish-yellowish oily substance that is generally considered very persistent. When released, mustard has the distinct smell of garlic or mustard and is quickly absorbed into the skin and/ or mucous membranes (eyes, inside of nose, inside of the mouth). As the agent is absorbed into the skin and membranes, it begins an irreversible process of damage to the cells. Absorption through the skin or mucous membranes usually occurs within seconds, and damage to the underlying cells takes place within 1 to 2 minutes **Figure 24-1** . Severe blisters and irreversible damage occur if the victim is not decontaminated within 20 minutes. Unfortunately, the physical symptoms of pain or a burning sensation do not occur until after 20 minutes of exposure, and may take up to 4 hours. Mustard is considered a **mutagen**, which means that it mutates and damages the structures in cells and eventually cellular death occurs.

The patient will develop a progressive reddening of the affected area, which will gradually develop into large blisters. These blisters are very similar in shape and appearance to those associated with second-degree thermal burns. The fluid within the blisters does not contain any of the agent; however, the skin covering the area is considered to be contaminated until decontamination by trained personnel has been performed.

Mustard also attacks vulnerable cells within the bone marrow and depletes the body's ability to reproduce white blood cells. As with burns, the primary complication associated with vesicant blisters is secondary infection. If the patient does survive the initial direct injury from the agent, the depletion of the white blood cells leaves the patient with a decreased resistance to infections.

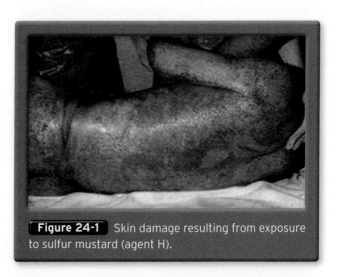

Figure 24-1 Skin damage resulting from exposure to sulfur mustard (agent H).

Although sulfur mustard is regarded as persistent, it does release enough vapors when dispersed to be inhaled. This creates upper and lower airway compromise. The result is damage to and swelling of the airways. The airway compromise makes the patient's condition far more serious.

Lewisite (L) and phosgene oxime (CX) produce blister wounds very similar to mustard. They are highly volatile and can produce serious illness and death. The onset of the symptoms is much faster than sulfur mustard, and these agents produce immediate intense pain and discomfort when contact is made. The patient may have a grayish discoloration at the contaminated site as tissue damage occurs following exposure. Exposure to the eye can be painful and result in temporary and permanent vision loss.

Vesicant Agent Treatment

There are no antidotes for mustard or CX exposure. British anti-Lewisite (BAL) is a partial treatment for Lewisite exposure. Use of BAL will decrease the internal effects of Lewisite, but it does not halt damage to the skin, eyes, or airway. It is not typically carried by TMPs or civilian EMS. You must ensure that the patient has been decontaminated before stabilizing the patient's airway, breathing, and circulation (ABCs). The patient may require prompt airway support if any agent has been inhaled, but this should not occur until after decontamination. IV access should be initiated as soon as possible by an ALS-level provider. Transport should be initiated as soon as possible. Generally, burn centers are best equipped to handle the wounds and subsequent infections produced by vesicants. Follow your local protocols when deciding what facility to transport the patient to.

Pulmonary Agents (Choking Agents)

Pulmonary agents are gases or vapors that cause immediate harm to persons exposed to them. The primary route of exposure for these agents is through the respiratory tract, which makes them an inhalation or vapor hazard. Once inside the lungs, they damage the lung tissue and fluid leaks into the lungs. Pulmonary edema (fluid in the lungs) develops in the patient, resulting in difficulty breathing. This class of chemical agents consists of chlorine (CL) and phosgene.

Chlorine (CL) was the first chemical agent ever used in warfare. It has a distinct odor of bleach and creates a green haze when released as a gas. Initially it produces airway irritation and a choking sensation. Each year, such mixtures overcome hundreds of people in their own home when they try to mix household cleaners. Chlorine is used extensively, and large storage tanks of this chemical are stored in nearly every community to add to water supplies in order to ensure cleanliness. It is transported extensively through our railway and highway transportation systems, and accidental and intentional releases can cause significant death and illness.

After the initial upper airway irritation, the patient may later experience the following signs/symptoms:

- Shortness of breath
- Chest tightness
- Bronchospasm
- Wheezing
- Hoarseness and stridor as the result of upper airway constriction
- Gasping and coughing

With serious exposure, patients may experience pulmonary edema, complete airway constriction, and death.

Phosgene should not be confused with phosgene oxime, the blistering agent. Phosgene has been produced for chemical warfare, but it is also a product of combustion such as might be produced in a fire at a textile factory or house, or from metalwork or burning Freon (a liquid chemical used in refrigeration). It is heavier than air and tends to settle in low-lying areas such as trenches and bunkers during warfare, and in basements and cellars during structure fires.

Phosgene is a very potent agent that has a delayed onset of symptoms, usually hours. Unlike CL, when phosgene enters the body it generally does not produce severe irritation that would possibly cause the victim to leave the area or hold his or her breath. In fact, the odor produced by the chemical is similar to that of freshly mown grass or hay. The result is that much more of the gas is allowed to enter the body unnoticed. The initial symptoms of a mild exposure may include the following signs/symptoms:

- Nausea
- Chest tightness
- Severe cough
- Dyspnea on exertion

The victim of a severe exposure may present with dyspnea at rest and excessive pulmonary edema (the patient will actually expel large amounts of fluid from the pulmonary edema in his or her lungs). The pulmonary edema experienced after a severe exposure produces such large amounts of fluid from the lungs that the patient may actually become hypovolemic and subsequently hypotensive.

Pulmonary Agent Treatment

The best initial treatment for any patient who has been exposed to a pulmonary agent is to remove the patient from the contaminated atmosphere. This should be done by trained personnel in the proper personal protective equipment (PPE). Aggressive management of the airway, breathing, and circulation should be initiated, paying particular attention to oxygenation, ventilation, and suctioning if required. Do not allow the patient to be active because this will worsen the condition much faster. There are no antidotes to counteract the pulmonary agents. Stabilizing the airway, breathing, and circulation (ABCs), allowing the patient to rest in a position of comfort with the head elevated, gaining IV access by an ALS provider, and initiating rapid transport are the primary goals.

Nerve Agents

The **nerve agents** are among the most deadly chemicals developed. Initially developed as insecticides, they were noted to be able to kill large numbers of people with small quantities. Nerve agents can cause cardiac arrest within seconds to minutes of exposure. These agents have been used successfully in warfare and to date represent the only type of chemical agent that has been used successfully in a large-scale terrorist act. Nerve agents, discovered while in search of a superior pesticide, are a class of chemical called organophosphates, which are found in modern household bug sprays, agricultural pesticides, and some industrial chemicals, at far lower strengths than military nerve agents.

G agents came from the early nerve agents, the G series, which were developed by German scientists (hence the G) in the period after WWI and into WWII. There are three G series agents commonly known, which are all designed with the same basic chemical structure with slight variations to produce different properties. The variations of these agents differ in their lethality and volatility. The following G agents are listed from high volatility to low volatility:

- **Sarin (GB)**. Highly volatile, colorless, and odorless liquid. It evaporates from liquid to gas within seconds to minutes at room temperature. Sarin is primarily a vapor hazard. This highly lethal agent is especially dangerous in enclosed environments such as office buildings, shopping malls, or subway cars. When this agent comes into contact with the skin, it is quickly absorbed. When sarin is absorbed into clothing, it later has the effect of **off-gassing**, which means that the vapors are continuously released over a period of time (like perfume). This renders the victim as well as the victim's clothing contaminated. On March 20, 1995, members of Aum Shinrikyo, a Japanese cult, released GB in the Tokyo subway. In the end, more than 5000 people sought medical care for exposure to sarin, and 12 people died. About 10% of the victims were EMS and other rescue workers, none of whom wore protective clothing, and most became cross-contaminated.

- **Soman (GD)**. Twice as persistent as sarin and five times as lethal. It has a fruity odor as a result of the type of alcohol used in the agent and generally has no color. This agent is both a contact and inhalation hazard that can enter the body through skin absorption and through the respiratory tract.

- **Tabun (GA)**. Approximately half as lethal as sarin and 36 times more persistent; under the proper conditions it will remain for several days. It also has a fruity smell and an appearance similar to sarin. The components used to manufacture GA are easy to acquire and the agent is easy to manufacture, which make it unique. GA is both a contact and inhalation hazard that can enter the body through skin absorption as well as through the respiratory tract.

- **V agent (VX)**. Clear oily agent that has no odor and looks like baby oil. V agent was developed by the British after World War II and has similar chemical properties to the G series agents. The difference is that VX is over 100 times more lethal than sarin and is extremely persistent **Figure 24-2**. In fact, VX is so persistent that given the proper conditions it will remain relatively unchanged for weeks to months. These properties make VX primarily a contact hazard, because it lets off very little vapor. It is easily absorbed into the skin and the oily residue that remains on the skin's surface is extremely difficult to decontaminate. This agent is so deadly that it only takes about one-half of a drop onto exposed human skin to cause death.

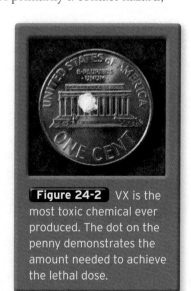

Figure 24-2 VX is the most toxic chemical ever produced. The dot on the penny demonstrates the amount needed to achieve the lethal dose.

Therefore it is critical to use protective clothing and other equipment to prevent exposure.

Nerve agents all produce similar symptoms but have varying routes of entry. Nerve agents differ slightly in lethal concentration or dose and also differ in their volatility. Some agents are designed to become a gas quickly (nonpersistent or highly volatile), whereas others remain liquid for a period of time (persistent or nonvolatile). Once the agent has entered the body through skin contact or through the respiratory system, the patient will begin to exhibit a pattern of predictable symptoms. Like all chemical agents, the severity of the symptoms will depend on the route of exposure and the amount of agent to which the patient was exposed. The resulting symptoms are described below using the military mnemonic SLUDGEM and the medical mnemonic DUMBELS. SLUDGEM/DUMBELS mnemonics are used to describe the symptoms of nerve agent exposure. The medical mnemonic is more useful to you because it lists the more dangerous symptoms associated with exposure to nerve agents.

There are only a handful of medical conditions that are associated with the bilateral pinpoint constricted pupils (miosis) seen with nerve agent exposure. Conditions such as a cerebrovascular accident, direct light to both eyes, and a drug overdose can all cause bilateral constricted pupils. You should therefore assess the patient for all of the SLUDGEM/DUMBELS signs and symptoms to determine whether the patient has been exposed to a nerve agent.

Miosis is the most common symptom of nerve agent exposure and can remain for days to weeks. This symptom, along with the others listed in Table 24-1, will help you recognize exposure to a nerve agent early. The seizures that are associated with nerve agent exposure are unlike those found in patients with a history of a seizure disorder. The patient will continue to seize until death or until treatment is given with a nerve agent antidote (Mark 1 or NAAK).

Nerve Agent Treatment

Fatalities from severe nerve agent exposure occur as a result of respiratory complications that lead to respiratory arrest. Once the patient has been decontaminated, the TMP should be prepared to treat these patients aggressively. You can greatly increase the patient's chances of survival simply by providing airway and ventilatory support. As with all emergencies, securing the ABCs is the best and most important treatment that you can provide. Often patients exposed to these agents will begin seizing and will not stop. These patients will

Table 24-1   Symptoms of Persons Exposed to Nerve Agents

Military Mnemonic: SLUDGEM	Medical Mnemonic: DUMBELS
Salivation, Sweating	Diarrhea
Lacrimation (excessive tearing)	Urination
Urination	Miosis (pinpoint pupils)
Defecation, Drooling, Diarrhea	Bradycardia, Bronchospasm (spasm of the bronchioles)
Gastric upset and cramps	Emesis (vomiting)
Emesis (vomiting)	Lacrimation (excessive tearing)
Muscle twitching/ Miosis (pinpoint pupils)	Seizures, Salivation, Sweating

require administration of nerve agent antidote kits in addition to support of the ABCs.

In terms of medical treatment for nerve agent exposure, the most common antidote kit used in treatment is the Mark 1 Nerve Agent Antidode Kit (NAAK). The Mark 1 contains two medications—2 mg of atropine and 600 mg of pralidoxime chloride (2-PAM)—in two separate auto-injectors. An updated version of the Mark 1 is the DuoDote auto-injector. The DuoDote contains 2.1 mg of atropine and 600 mg of 2-PAM and is delivered as a single dose through one needle.

In some regions, civilian EMS may carry Mark 1 or DuoDote kits on their ambulance. TMPs may be called on to administer one or both of the antidotes, to either themselves or their patients. These medications are delivered using the same technique as the EpiPen auto-injector; however, multiple doses may need to be administered, remembering that activated nerve agent antidote kits need to be disposed of properly in a sharps container. Some agencies may keep the needle with the patient during a mass-casualty incident. Always follow your local protocols.

Nerve agent antidotes interfere with the action of nerve agents by reversing some of the harmful effects, such as excessive secretion in the lungs. When nerve agents enter the body, they bind to an enzyme called acetylcholinesterase (AChE) and prevent it from working normally. Normally, the AChE enzyme quickly inactivates acetylcholine. Acetylcholine is a chemical signal that

Table 24-2   The Nerve Agents

Name	Military Designation	Odor	Special Features	Onset of Symptoms	Volatility	Route of Exposure
Tabun	GA	Fruity	Easy to manufacture	Immediate	Low	Both contact and vapor hazard
Sarin	GB	None (if pure) or strong	Will off-gas while on victim's clothing	Immediate	High	Primarily respiratory vapor hazard; extremely lethal if skin contact is made
Soman	GD	Fruity	Ages rapidly, making it difficult to treat	Immediate	Moderate	Contact with skin; minimal vapor hazard
V agent	VX	None	Most lethal chemical agent; difficult to decontaminate	Immediate	Very low	Contact with skin; no vapor hazard (unless aerosolized)

helps nerves to instruct the body to contract muscles and control functions such as secretion of saliva and mucus, urination, defecation, and other bodily functions. Nerve agent poisoning occurs when these toxic poisons bind to the AChE enzyme and keep it from working effectively, leading to an excessive buildup of acetylcholine. This results in overstimulation that causes a set of symptoms called "cholinergic syndrome," which includes the SLUDGEM/DUMBELS symptoms described earlier in the chapter. The excess acetylcholine causes muscle contractions, bronchospasm, excess secretions that result in hypoxia, urination, defecation, altered mental status, seizures, muscle paralysis, coma, and possibly death. The two main causes of death from nerve agents are from respiratory compromise and muscular paralysis.

The treatment for nerve agents is two medicines that effectively serve as "antidotes" to nerve agent exposure, and a third medicine to prevent or treat seizures. The first medicine, atropine, works by blocking one type of acetylcholine receptor so that the excess acetylcholine that is already in the nerve junction synapse will not cause overstimulation. Atropine is given in repeat doses until excessive oral and lung secretions cease. The second medication is pralidoxime (2-PAM), which works by partially blocking the binding of the nerve agent to the AChE enzyme. It also helps to reactivate the AChE enzyme. The third medication is diazepam (Valium), used to prevent seizures. Diazepam is also available in an auto-injector, called Convulsive Antidote for Nerve Agent (CANA), and may be used in severe exposure to prevent seizures from occurring. Diazepam may also be used to treat seizures, although seizures are very difficult to stop once triggered by nerve agents. Some nerve agents act very quickly and are irreversible, therefore it is important to use these antidotes quickly—within minutes—if needed. **Table 24-2** provides a quick reference and comparison of nerve agents.

Metabolic Agents (Cyanides)

Hydrogen cyanide (AC) and cyanogen chloride (CK) are both agents that affect the body's ability to use oxygen. **Cyanide** is a colorless gas that has an odor similar to almonds. The effects of the cyanides begin on the cellular level and are very rapidly seen at the organ system level. Beside the nerve agents, metabolic agents are the only chemical weapons known to kill within seconds to minutes. Unlike nerve agents, however, these deadly gases are commonly found in many industrial settings. Cyanides are produced in massive quantities throughout the United States every year for industrial uses such as gold and silver mining, photography, lethal injections, and plastics processing. They are often present in fires associated with textile or plastic factories or in house fires due to common construction materials. Cyanide is naturally found in the pits of many fruits in very low doses.

There is very little difference in the symptoms found between AC and CK. In low doses, these chemicals are associated with dizziness, lightheadedness, headache, and vomiting. Higher doses will produce symptoms that include the following:

- Shortness of breath and gasping respirations
- Tachypnea

- Flushed skin color
- Tachycardia
- Altered mental status
- Seizures
- Coma
- Apnea
- Cardiac arrest

The symptoms associated with the inhalation of a large amount of cyanide will all appear within several minutes. Death is likely unless the patient is treated promptly.

Cyanide Agent Treatment

Cyanide binds with the body's cells, preventing oxygen from being used. Several medications act as antidotes, but most TEMS units and EMS services do not carry them. Once trained personnel wearing the proper PPE have removed the patient from the source of exposure, even if there is no liquid contamination, all of the patient's clothes must be removed to prevent off-gassing in the ambulance. Trained and protected personnel must decontaminate any patients who may have been exposed to liquid contamination before you can initiate treatment. Then you should support the patient's ABCs. Mild effects of cyanide exposure will generally resolve by simply removing the victim from the source of contamination and administering supplemental oxygen. Severe exposure, however, will require aggressive oxygenation and perhaps intubation and ventilation with supplemental oxygen. The agent can easily be passed on from the patient to you through mouth-to-mouth or mouth-to-mask ventilations, so use proper caution.

Medical Gear

Chemical threats from terrorists require the use of basic protective gear such as respiratory protection (APR, PAPR), nitrile gloves, foot protection, a water-impermeable decontamination hooded suit, and tape to seal the wrists and ankles of the protective suit. The air-purifying respirator (APR) or powered-air purifying respirator (PAPR) should be equipped with specific filters that block chemical agents and particulate matter.

Many TEMS units acquire and use specific filters that effectively filter all biologic and nuclear dust particles (N-100) and also have special filter components that will absorb and neutralize the chemical agents mentioned previously as long as the concentration in the air is not overwhelmingly high.

Initiate ALS-level transport immediately. Cardiac monitoring and an intravenous line may be initiated. Follow local protocols on fluid and medication administration. If a cyanide antidote kit is carried on the ambulance, follow local protocols on its administration.

There are two different cyanide antidote kits available, including the Cyanide Antidote Kit (CAK) and the Cyanokit. The CAK contains amyl nitrite pearls, sodium nitrite, and sodium thiosulfate. The Cyanokit contains hydroxocobalamin, which combines with the cyanide in the body to form vitamin B-12 and is harmlessly cleared by the kidneys. Some studies suggest coadministration with sodium thiosulfate through a different IV line may improve treatment. There are adverse side effects of these medications and they should be administered according to the manufacturer's recommendations and your local protocols.

Table 24-3 summarizes the chemical agents. The odors of the particular chemicals are provided for informational purposes only. The sense of smell is a poor tool to use to determine whether there is a chemical agent present. Many persons are unable to smell the agents, and the odor could be derived from another source. This information is useful to you if you receive reports from victims who claimed to smell bleach or garlic, for example. You should never enter a potentially hazardous area and "smell" to determine whether a chemical agent is present.

Biologic Agents

Biologic agents pose many difficult issues when used as a WMD. Biologic agents can be almost completely undetectable. Biologic agents are grouped as viruses, bacteria, or neurotoxins and may be spread in various ways. **Dissemination** is the means by which a terrorist will spread the agent—for example, poisoning the water supply or aerosolizing the agent into the air or ventilation system of a building. A **disease vector** is an animal that once infected spreads disease to another animal. For example, the plague can be spread by infected rats and smallpox by infected persons. How easily the disease is able to spread from one human to another human is called **communicability**. In instances when communicability is high, such as with smallpox, the person is considered **contagious**.

Incubation describes the period of time between the person becoming exposed to the agent and when symptoms begin. The incubation period is especially important to understand. Although your patient may

Table 24-3 Chemical Agents

Name	Military Designation	Odor	Lethality	Onset of Symptoms	Volatility	Primary Route of Exposure
Nerve agents	Tabun (GA) Sarin (GB) Soman (GD) V agent (VX)	Fruity or none	Most lethal chemical agents; can kill within minutes; effects are reversible with antidotes	Immediate	Moderate (GA, GD) Very high (GB) Low (VX)	GA–both GB–vapor hazard GD–both VX–contact hazard
Vesicants	Mustard (H) Lewisite (L) Phosgene oxime (CX)	Garlic (H) Geranium (L)	Causes large blisters to form on victims; may severely damage upper airway if vapors are inhaled; severe, intense pain and grayish skin discoloration (L and CX)	Delayed (H) Immediate (L, CX)	Very low (H, L) Moderate (CX)	Primarily contact with some vapor hazard
Pulmonary agents	Chlorine (CL) Phosgene (CG)	Bleach (CL) Cut grass (CG)	Causes irritation, choking (CL); severe pulmonary edema (CG)	Immediate (CL) Delayed (CG)	Very high	Vapor hazard
Cyanide agents	Hydrogen cyanide (AC) Cyanogen chloride (CK)	Almonds (AC) Irritating (CK)	Highly lethal chemical gases; can kill within minutes; effects are reversible with antidotes	Immediate	Very high	Vapor hazard

not exhibit signs or symptoms, he or she may be contagious.

Because biologic agents affect the patient's airway with severe consequences, the airway and breathing are stabilized before circulation.

Viruses

Viruses are germs that require a living host to multiply and survive. A virus is a simple organism and cannot thrive outside of a host (living body). Once in the body, the virus invades healthy cells and replicates itself to spread through the host. As the virus spreads, so does the disease that it carries.

Viral agents that may be used during a biologic terrorist attack pose an extraordinary problem for health care providers, especially those in EMS. Although some viral agents do have vaccines, there is no treatment for a viral infection other than antiviral medications for some agents. Because of this characteristic, the following viruses have the potential to be used as terrorist agents.

Smallpox

Smallpox is a highly contagious disease. All forms of standard precautions must be used to prevent cross-contamination. Simply by wearing examination gloves, a HEPA-filtered respirator, and eye protection, you will greatly reduce your risk of contamination. The last natural case of smallpox in the world was seen in 1977. Before the rash and blisters appear, the patient will have a high fever and body aches and headaches. The patient's temperature is usually in the range of 101°F to 104°F (38°C to 40°C).

A quick way to differentiate the smallpox rash from other skin disorders is to observe the size, shape, and location of the lesions. In smallpox, all the lesions are identical in their development. In other skin disorders, the lesions will be in various stages of healing and development. Smallpox blisters also begin on the face and extremities and eventually move toward the chest and abdomen. The disease is in its most contagious phase when the blisters begin to form **Figure 24-3**.

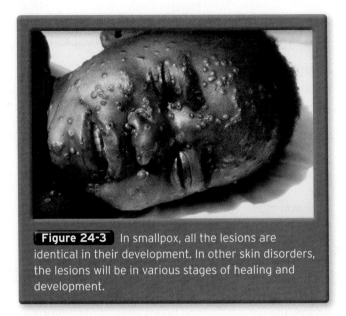

Figure 24-3 In smallpox, all the lesions are identical in their development. In other skin disorders, the lesions will be in various stages of healing and development.

Unprotected contact with these blisters will promote transmission of the disease. There is a vaccine to prevent smallpox; however, it has been linked to medical complications and in rare cases death **Table 24-4**. Should an outbreak occur, the US government has enough vaccine to vaccinate every person in the United States.

Viral Hemorrhagic Fevers

Viral hemorrhagic fevers (VHFs) consist of a group of diseases that include the Ebola, Rift Valley, and Yellow Fever viruses, among others. This group of viruses causes the blood in the body to seep out from the tissues and blood vessels **Figure 24-4**. Initially the patient will have flu-like symptoms, progressing to more serious symptoms such as internal and external hemorrhaging. Outbreaks are not uncommon in Africa and South America; outbreaks in the United States, however, are extremely rare. All standard precautions must be taken when treating these illnesses. Mortality rates can range from 5% to 90%, depending on the strain of virus, the victim's age and health condition, and the availability of a modern health care system **Table 24-5**.

Bacteria

Unlike viruses, **bacteria** do not require a host to multiply and survive. Bacteria are much more complex than viruses and can grow up to 100 times larger than the largest virus. Bacteria contain all the cellular structures of a normal cell and are completely self-sufficient. Most importantly, bacterial infections can be fought with antibiotics.

Most bacterial infections begin with flu-like symptoms, which can make it difficult to identify whether the cause is a biologic attack or if the patient just has a routine illness.

Table 24-4	Characteristics of Smallpox
Dissemination	Aerosolized for warfare or terrorist uses.
Communicability	High from infected individuals or items (such as blankets used by infected patients). Person-to-person transmission is possible.
Route of entry	Through inhalation of coughed droplets or direct skin contact with blisters.
Signs and symptoms	Severe fever, malaise, body aches, headaches, small blisters on the skin, bleeding of the skin and mucous membranes. Incubation period is 10 to 12 days and the duration of the illness is approximately 4 weeks.
Medical management	Standard precautions. There is no specific treatment for smallpox victims. Patients should be provided with supportive care (ABCs).

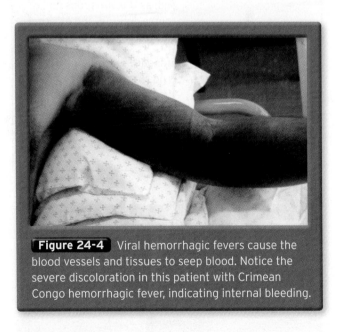

Figure 24-4 Viral hemorrhagic fevers cause the blood vessels and tissues to seep blood. Notice the severe discoloration in this patient with Crimean Congo hemorrhagic fever, indicating internal bleeding.

Inhalation and Cutaneous Anthrax (*Bacillus anthracis*)

Anthrax is a deadly bacterium that lies dormant in a spore (protective shell). When exposed to the optimal temperature and moisture, the germ will be released from the spore. The routes of entry for anthrax are inhalation, skin contact, or ingestion (food that contains spores) **Figure 24-5** .

The inhalational form, or pulmonary anthrax, is the most deadly and often presents as a severe upper respiratory infection. Pulmonary anthrax infections are associated with a 90% death rate if untreated. Antibiotics can be used to treat anthrax successfully. There is also a vaccine to prevent anthrax infections **Table 24-6** .

Plague (Bubonic/Pneumonic)

Of all the infectious diseases known to humans, none has killed as many as the plague. The 14th century plague that ravaged Asia, the Middle East, and Europe (the Black Death) killed an estimated 33 to 42 million people. In the early 19th century, almost 20 million people in India and China perished due to plague. Infected rodents and fleas carry the disease. When a person is either bitten by an infected flea or comes into contact with an infected rodent (or the waste of the rodent), the person can contract bubonic plague.

Bubonic plague infects the lymphatic system (a passive circulatory system in the body that bathes the tissues in lymph and works with the immune system). When this occurs, the patient's lymph nodes (area of the lymphatic system where infection-fighting cells are housed) become infected and grow. The glands of the nodes will grow large (up to the size of a tennis ball) and round, forming **buboes** **Figure 24-6** . If left untreated, the infection may spread

Table 24-5	Characteristics of Viral Hemorrhagic Fevers
Dissemination	Direct contact with an infected person's body fluids. It can also be aerosolized for use in an attack.
Communicability	Moderate from person to person or contaminated items.
Route of entry	Direct contact with an infected person's body fluids.
Signs and symptoms	Sudden onset of fever, weakness, muscle pain, headache, and sore throat. All of these symptoms are followed by vomiting and, as the virus runs its course, internal and external bleeding.
Medical management	Standard precautions. There is no specific treatment for viral hemorrhagic fever. Patients should be provided supportive care (ABCs) and treatment for shock, if present.

Table 24-6	Characteristics of Anthrax
Dissemination	Aerosol
Communicability	Only in the cutaneous form (rare)
Route of entry	Through inhalation of spore or skin contact with spore or direct contact with skin wound (cutaneous)
Signs and symptoms	Flu-like symptoms, fever, respiratory distress with tachycardia, shock, pulmonary edema, and respiratory failure after 3 to 5 days of flu-like symptoms
Medical management	Pulmonary/inhalation: Standard precautions, oxygen, ventilatory support if in pulmonary edema or respiratory failure, and transport. Cutaneous: Standard precautions, apply dry sterile dressing to prevent accidental contact with wound and fluids.

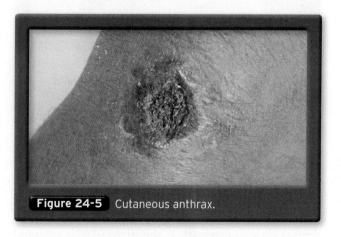
Figure 24-5 Cutaneous anthrax.

through the body, leading to sepsis and possibly death. This form of plague is not contagious and is not likely to be seen in a bioterrorist incident.

Pneumonic plague is a lung infection, also known as plague pneumonia, that results from inhalation of plague bacteria. This form of the disease is contagious and has a much higher death rate than the bubonic form. This form of plague is easier to disseminate (aerosolized), has a higher mortality rate, and is contagious **Table 24-7**.

Tularemia

Tularemia is an infection caused by the bacterium *Francisella tularensis*, and is common in wild rodents. It is transmitted to humans through contact with infected animal tissue or through ticks, biting flies, and mosquitoes. Symptoms include chills, fever, headache, muscle and joint pain, red spots that progress to a sore (ulcer), and if severe may include shortness of breath and weight loss. It could be released in an aerosol form, with symptoms occurring within 2 to 10 days of exposure. Treatment is with a course of antibiotics (streptomycin, gentamycin, or fluoroquinolones).

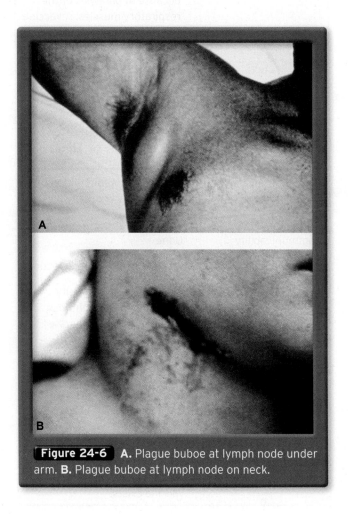

Figure 24-6 **A.** Plague buboe at lymph node under arm. **B.** Plague buboe at lymph node on neck.

Neurotoxins

Neurotoxins are the most deadly substances known to humans. The strongest neurotoxin is 15,000 times more lethal than VX and 100,000 times more lethal than sarin. These toxins are produced from plants, marine animals, molds, and bacteria. The route of entry for these toxins is through ingestion, inhalation from aerosols, or injection. Unlike viruses and bacteria, neurotoxins are not contagious. Although these biologic toxins have immense destructive potential, they have not been used successfully as a WMD.

Botulinum Toxin

The most potent neurotoxin is **botulinum**, which is produced by bacteria. When introduced into the body, this neurotoxin affects the nervous system's ability to

Table 24-7	Characteristics of Plague
Dissemination	Aerosol
Communicability	Bubonic: low, only from contact with fluid in buboe Pneumonic: high, from person to person
Route of entry	Ingestion, inhalation, or cutaneous
Signs and symptoms	Fever, headache, muscle pain and tenderness, pneumonia, shortness of breath, extreme lymph node pain and enlargement (bubonic)
Medical management	Standard precautions, ABCs, provide oxygen as soon as possible, and transport

Medical Gear

Typically, standard precautions are enough to prevent contamination from contagious biologic organisms. An important and reassuring fact is that the N-95 (also called a tuberculosis [TB] mask) and the even more effective N-100 APR mask are effective ways to decrease exposure to any contagious biologic germ or spore **Figure 24-7**. Along with standard precautions, these are sufficient to protect the TEMS and SWAT units from nearly all biologic terrorist agents.

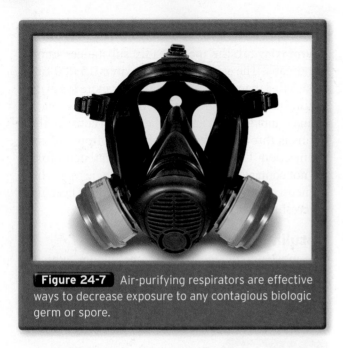

Figure 24-7 Air-purifying respirators are effective ways to decrease exposure to any contagious biologic germ or spore.

Table 24-8	Characteristics of Botulinum Toxin
Dissemination	Aerosol or food supply sabotage or injection
Communicability	None
Route of entry	Ingestion or gastrointestinal
Signs and symptoms	Dry mouth, intestinal obstruction, urinary retention, constipation, nausea and vomiting, abnormal pupil dilation, blurred vision, double vision, drooping eyelids, difficulty swallowing, difficulty speaking, and respiratory failure as the result of paralysis
Medical management	ABCs, provide oxygen as soon as possible, and transport. Ventilatory support during transport may be needed because of paralysis of the respiratory muscles. A vaccine is available.

function. Voluntary muscle control diminishes as the toxin spreads. Eventually the toxin causes muscle paralysis that begins at the head and face and travels downward throughout the body Table 24-8 .

Exposure is possible through ingestion from foodborne botulism or inhalation if weaponized. There is a specific botulism-immune globulin and antitoxin that can be given to help reverse the effects of exposure, and was included in the Strategic National Stockpile in 2007.

Other Biologic Toxins

Ricin

Although not as deadly as botulinum, **ricin** is still five times more lethal than VX. This toxin is derived from mash that is left from the castor bean Figure 24-8 . When introduced into the body, ricin causes pulmonary edema and respiratory and circulatory failure leading to death Table 24-9 .

The clinical picture depends on the route of exposure. The toxin is quite stable and extremely toxic by many routes of exposure, including

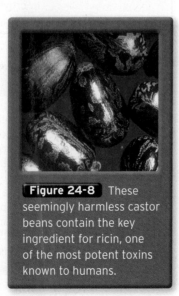

Figure 24-8 These seemingly harmless castor beans contain the key ingredient for ricin, one of the most potent toxins known to humans.

Table 24-9	Characteristics of Ricin
Dissemination	Aerosol or contamination of a food or water supply by sabotage
Communicability	None
Route of entry	Inhalation, ingestion, injection
Signs and symptoms	Inhaled: cough, difficulty breathing, chest tightness, nausea, muscle aches, pulmonary edema, and hypoxia Ingested: nausea and vomiting, internal bleeding, and death Injection: no signs except swelling at the injection site and death
Medical management	ABCs. No treatment or vaccine exists.

Table 24-10   Biologic Agents

Disease	Transmission Person to Person	Incubation Period	Duration of Illness	Lethality (approximate case fatality rates)
Inhalation anthrax	No	1 to 6 days	3 to 5 days (usually fatal if untreated)	High
Pneumonic plague	High	2 to 3 days	1 to 6 days (usually fatal)	High unless treated within 12 to 24 hours
Smallpox	High	7 to 17 days (average 12 days)	4 weeks	High to moderate
Viral hemorrhagic fevers	Moderate	4 to 21 days	Death between 7 and 16 days	High to moderate, depending on type of fever
Botulinum	No	1 to 5 days	Death in 24 to 72 hours; lasts months if patient does not die	High without respiratory support
Ricin	No	18 to 24 hours	Days; death within 10 to 12 days for ingestion	High

inhalation. It is likely that 1 to 3 mg of ricin can kill an adult, and the ingestion of one seed can most likely kill a child.

Although all parts of the castor bean are actually poisonous, it is the seeds that are the most toxic. Castor bean ingestion causes a rapid onset of nausea, vomiting, abdominal cramps, and severe diarrhea, followed by vascular collapse. Death usually occurs on the third day in the absence of appropriate medical intervention.

Ricin is least toxic by the oral route. This is probably a result of poor absorption in the gastrointestinal tract, some digestion in the gut, and, possibly, some expulsion of the agent as caused by the rapid onset of vomiting. Ingestion causes local hemorrhage and necrosis of the liver, spleen, kidney, and gastrointestinal tract. Signs and symptoms appear 4 to 8 hours after exposure.

Signs and symptoms of ricin ingestion include:

- Fever
- Chills
- Headache
- Muscle aches
- Nausea
- Vomiting
- Diarrhea
- Severe abdominal cramping
- Dehydration

Inhalation of ricin causes nonspecific weakness, cough, fever, hypothermia, and hypotension. Symptoms occur about 4 to 8 hours after inhalation, depending on the inhaled dose. The onset of profuse sweating some hours later signifies the termination of the symptoms.

Signs and symptoms of ricin inhalation include:

- Fever
- Chills
- Nausea
- Local irritation of eyes, nose, and throat
- Profuse sweating
- Headache
- Muscle aches
- Nonproductive cough
- Chest pain
- Dyspnea
- Cyanosis
- Convulsions

Table 24-10 summarizes the biologic agents.

Nuclear Weapons

What Is Radiation?

Ionizing radiation is energy that is emitted in the form of rays or particles. This energy can be found in radioactive

material, such as rocks and metals. Radioactive material is any material that emits radiation. This material is unstable, and over time will naturally decompose and stabilize itself by changing its structure in a natural process called **decay**. As the substance decays it gives off radiation until it stabilizes. The process of radioactive decay can take from as little as minutes to billions of years; meanwhile, the substance remains radioactive.

The energy that is emitted from a strong radiologic source is either **alpha radiation**, **beta radiation**, **gamma (X-rays)**, or **neutron radiation**. Alpha is the least harmful penetrating type of radiation and cannot travel fast or through most objects. In fact, a sheet of paper or the body's skin easily stops it. Beta radiation is slightly more penetrating than alpha and requires a layer of clothing to stop it. Gamma rays are far faster and stronger than alpha and beta rays. These rays easily penetrate through the human body and require either several inches of lead or concrete to prevent penetration. Neutron energy is the fastest moving and most powerful form of radiation. Neutrons easily penetrate through lead and require several feet of concrete to stop them **Figure 24-9**.

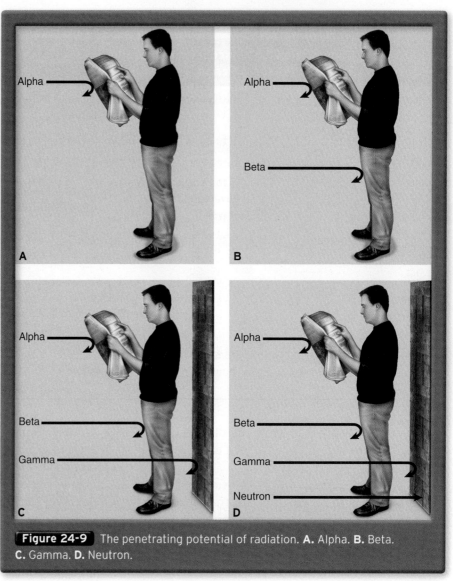

Figure 24-9 The penetrating potential of radiation. **A.** Alpha. **B.** Beta. **C.** Gamma. **D.** Neutron.

Sources of Radiologic Material

There are thousands of radioactive materials found on the earth. These materials are generally used for purposes that benefit humankind, such as medicine, killing germs in food (irradiating), construction work, and nuclear power plants. Once radiologic material has been used for its purpose, the material remaining is called radiologic waste. Radiologic waste remains radioactive but has no more usefulness. These materials can be found at the following locations:

- Hospitals
- Colleges and universities
- Chemical and industrial sites, and nuclear power plants

Not all radioactive material is tightly guarded, and the waste is often not guarded.

Nuclear Energy

Nuclear energy is harnessed and converted into electricity when energy is released by the splitting of radioactive atoms. The result is an immense amount of energy. Much of this energy takes the form of heat. This heat is used to boil water and then the steam is used to turn turbines attached to electric magnets that spin and thus transfer this energy into electricity. Nuclear material is used in medicine, weapons, naval vessels, and power plants. Fortunately, most of the nuclear power plants are protected by high-quality security systems and personnel to prevent theft and malicious intent to damage these systems.

Nuclear Weapons

The destructive energy of a nuclear explosion is unlike any other weapon, which is why nuclear weapons are kept in secure facilities throughout the world. Several nations with ties to terrorist organizations have attempted to build nuclear weapons, although they have not yet been sucessful.

The likelihood of a nuclear attack is remote. However, if a nuclear blast does occur within the United States, the challenges to nearby communities as well as the entire nation will be sizable.

A nuclear blast occurs when a nuclear weapon explodes, causing destruction over a wide area within seconds. The blast creates a large fireball and a mushroom cloud of dust and particles. The fireball produces temperatures up to millions of degrees, shock waves similar to a large earthquake, extremely bright flashes similar to lightning, and radiation of electromagnetic energy that causes fires, death, and radiation injury. The blast wave of compressed air and tremendous heat destroys everything within a quarter mile or greater, depending upon the size and type of bomb.

Few living creatures survive within the surrounding 0.5- to 1-mile area depending on the size and efficiency of the device. In the nuclear bombings that ended World War II, there were 135,000 deaths in Hiroshima and 64,000 in Nagasaki. A majority of these casualties occured within 1 mile of the blast center.

After the blast, there is nuclear fallout in at least a 50-mile radius. This radioactive substance causes long-term increased incidence of cancer and medical complications.

Radiologic Dispersion Device

A radiologic dispersion device (RDD) (also called a dirty bomb) is thought by experts to be more likely than a nuclear attack. An RDD is made by combining an explosive agent (eg, TNT, plastic explosives, homemade explosives) with radioactive materials that may have been stolen from a local source, such as a hospital (eg, X-ray machine). The initial explosion may cause a limited number of immediate deaths and injuries from the conventional explosion blast, while the radioactive material spreads, exposes, and contaminates survivors and any emergency responders with radioactive materials. Survivors will need to receive treatment for their blast injuries after receiving a thorough decontamination from the radioactive materials.

One of the main impacts of an RDD attack will be psychological. The general public is highly fearful of radiation. This invisible threat may cause panic and chaos when people learn that radiation has been released in their community. Many may call 9-1-1 and request EMS, or drive to and overwhelm local emergency departments. In the years following such an event, the sickness and cancer death rate in people exposed to radioactive particles will be higher than the national average. It is only through education, preparation, use of protective equipment, and use of radiation victim management principles that the area SWAT and TEMS units will be able to remain effective.

How Radiation Affects the Body

The effects of radiation exposure will vary depending on the amount of radiation that a person receives. Radiation exposure to the human body is measured in **rem**. A simple chest X-ray exposes the human body to about 0.03 to 0.05 rem. The average human exposure from background radiation is about 0.36 rem per year. Acute radiation syndrome can occur after exposure to about 30 to 70 rem. **Acute radiation syndrome** will mainly cause hematologic, central nervous system, and gastrointestinal changes. Many of these changes occur over several days and will not be apparent during contact with TEMS providers. Some common signs of acute radiation sickness are nausea, vomiting, and diarrhea. Additional injuries will occur with a nuclear blast, such as thermal and blast trauma, trauma from flying objects, and eye injuries.

Response

The response to an incident involving radiation victims—either through an RDD blast or a nuclear explosion—involve the same principles. Scene safety is the initial concern. The primary goal is to avoid ingesting, inhaling, or becoming contaminated by radioactive dust or particles. Radiation exposure from gamma and X-rays must also be minimized. Ideally, any public safety professionals involved will each have and use an individual personal radiation dosimeter **Figure 24-10**. Several newer designs are able to not only sound an alarm if radiation is detected, but also count and keep track of the cumulative radiation exposure. In general, once the radiation dosimeter has shown that a responder has been exposed to 100 millirems (Roentgen equivalent man) of radiation, then the responder should move away from the radioactive source(s) and limit further exposure for that day.

If a responder is not required to be near the blast scene, the responder should avoid the radiation and minimize contact with people who are contaminated with radioactive dust. If radioactive particles are inhaled

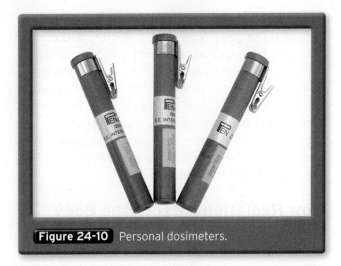

Figure 24-10 Personal dosimeters.

or otherwise ingested into the human body, the radiation will substantially increase the chance for ionizing damage to a person's cellular DNA by gamma radiation, neutron particles, or alpha and beta particles. Ionizing damage causes cellular DNA to be damaged and mutated, which can lead to cancer and other illness.

In the case of an RDD, measures can be used to decrease exposure to radioactive materials. Use of eye goggles and N-95 face mask protection (or APR) can shield or stop radioactive dust particles, thus minimizing exposure to radioactivity. Other measures include rotating staff and aggressive radiation decontamination. Your agency should have policies and procedures in place to deal with such an event.

Medical Management

Being exposed to a radiation source does not make a patient contaminated or radioactive. However, when patients have a radioactive source on their body (such as debris from a dirty bomb), they are contaminated and must be decontaminated prior to stabilizing care. Once the patient is decontaminated and there is no threat to you, you may begin to stabilize the ABCs and treat the patient for any burns or trauma.

Suicide Bombings

Explosive devices can be used as WMDs. A lethal delivery device is the suicide bomber (or homicidal bomber), a person who is willing to die in order to kill others, often to further a cause. The suicide bomber's goal is typically to make a political, ideological, or religious statement.

The fact that the suicide bomber is killed eliminates the need for an escape plan.

In a suicidal attack, bombs are usually carried on the person or in a vehicle. This type of bomb can be used for a specific target or in a random attack. This form of attack does not consider innocent bystanders; more carnage will often result in greater media coverage and greater fear in the target population.

Suicide bombs are limited in size and complexity, since most are worn on the body, often as a vest or belt. Loose or baggy clothing may be worn over the bomb to conceal it. However, the bomb may be detectable under the clothing as bulges, or in clothing that appears inappropriate for the environment (long coat in the summer) or wearer.

Some terrorist organizations have used sophisticated high-yield explosives, whereas others simply use homemade explosives such as pipe bombs. Suicide bombers frequently add shrapnel in the form of metal sheets, marbles, ball bearings, nuts, bolts, or nails. The need to conceal the bomb limits the amount of explosive that can be carried. However, as much as 30 pounds of explosive material can be worn on the body or carried in a briefcase or backpack. Even small amounts of explosives can kill multiple people in a heavily occupied location.

Vehicles can carry very large amounts of explosives, in the range of hundreds to thousands of pounds. For example, in the 1995 Oklahoma City bombing, a building was destroyed by a blast from a mix of improvised explosives (ammonium nitrate/nitromethane/blasting caps) in a rental truck. The 1993 World Trade Center bombing was a 1500-pound urea nitrate/hydrogen gas-enhanced device placed in a vehicle that killed six people and injured more than 1000.

Secondary devices or a second suicide bomber are threats that should be taken into account during a suicide bomber attack. A secondary device is a second bomb or other explosive device that is designed to inflict further damage and kill responders such as police, EMS, and firefighters. These can be hidden bombs, vehicle bombs, or other devices.

Response

The most effective way to prevent vehicle bombings is to exclude unknown vehicles from target areas identified by local emergency response agencies prior to any incidents. An IED discovered in a vehicle should prompt all public safety personnel to evacuate the scene perimeter (from 5000 to 7000 feet away) until the explosive is defused or moved by explosive ordnance disposal (EOD) personnel.

If a SWAT unit is called to the scene of a blast, the immediate concern is to neutralize other suspicious vehicles and other explosives at the scene, at the same time searching for active shooters or other terrorists who may be nearby. EMS and firefighter response will search for and treat victims, but they will not likely be allowed into the area until it has been deemed safe. TMPs will be integral in the early stabilization of victims (see Chapter 17, "Ballistic, Blast, and Less-Lethal Weapons Injuries") and interfacing with EMS and firefighters on patient care when they are allowed into the scene.

Safety

The risk of secondary explosions at a suicide bombing incident is great. Be wary of any approaching person(s) who do not seem to fit in. Arriving ambulances, EMTs, and other rescue personnel who do not have recognizable vehicles or have unusual uniforms should be considered highly suspicious and immediate action should be taken. Women also pose a risk—a large explosive charge can be disguised as a pregnant belly. A sudden or uncharacteristic movement, rapid approach by unauthorized vehicles, or anything that seems out of place should warrant immediate attention and action, including rapid movement to a safe zone and neutralization of the threat by SWAT personnel.

Ready for Review

- CBRN incidents are responded to under the assumption that they are deliberate, malicious acts with the intention to kill, sicken, and/or disrupt society. Evidence preservation and perpetrator apprehension are of great concern with CBRN incidents.

- A secondary device may be set to explode as public safety personnel and the media respond to the scene. Constantly assess and reassess the scene for safety.

- Chemical agents are manmade substances that can have devastating effects on living organisms.

- The route of exposure is how the agent enters the body.

- Biologic agents are organisms that cause disease.

- Biologic agents include viruses such as smallpox and viral hemorrhagic fevers; bacteria such as anthrax and plague; and neurotoxins such as botulinum toxin and ricin.

- Nuclear or radiologic weapons can create a massive amount of destruction.

- Ionizing radiation is energy that can enter the human body and cause damage.

Vital Vocabulary

acute radiation syndrome The clinical course that usually begins within hours of exposure to a radiation source. Symptoms include nausea, vomiting, diarrhea, fatigue, fever, and headache. The long-term symptoms are dose-related and hematophoietic and gastrointestinal.

alpha radiation Type of energy that is emitted from a strong radiologic source; it is the least harmful penetrating type of radiation and cannot travel fast or through most objects.

anthrax A deadly bacterium (*Bacillus anthracis*) that lies dormant in a spore (protective shell); the germ is released from the spore when exposed to the optimal temperature and moisture. The route of entry is inhalation, cutaneous, or gastrointestinal (from consuming food that contains spores).

bacteria Microorganisms that reproduce by binary fission. These single-cell creatures reproduce rapidly. Some can form spores (encysted variants) when environmental conditions are harsh.

beta radiation Type of energy that is emitted from a strong radiologic source, is slightly more penetrating than alpha, and requires a layer of clothing stop it.

botulinum Produced by bacteria, this is a very potent neurotoxin. When introduced into the body, this neurotoxin affects the nervous system's ability to function and causes botulism.

buboes Enlarged lymph nodes (up to the size of tennis balls) that were characteristic of people infected with the bubonic plague.

bubonic plague An epidemic that spread throughout Europe in the Middle Ages, causing over 25 million deaths, also called the Black Death, transmitted by infected fleas and characterized by acute malaise, fever, and the formation of tender, enlarged, inflamed lymph nodes that appear as lesions, called buboes.

CBRN Acronym that stands for chemical, biologic, radiologic, and nuclear threats.

chlorine (CL) The first chemical agent ever used in warfare. It has a distinct odor of bleach and creates a green haze when released as a gas. Initially it produces upper airway irritation and a choking sensation.

communicability Describes how easily a disease spreads from one human to another human.

contact hazard A hazardous agent that gives off very little or no vapors; the skin is the primary route for this type of chemical to enter the body; also called a skin hazard.

contagious A person infected with a disease that is highly communicable.

cross-contamination Occurs when a person is contaminated by an agent as a result of coming into contact with another contaminated person.

cyanide Agent that affects the body's ability to use oxygen. It is a colorless gas that has an odor similar to almonds. The effects begin on the cellular level and are very rapidly seen at the organ system level.

decay A natural process in which a material that is unstable attempts to stabilize itself by changing its structure.

disease vector An animal that spreads a disease, once infected, to another animal.

dissemination The means with which a terrorist will spread an agent, for example, by poisoning the water supply or aerosolizing the agent into the air or ventilation system of a building.

G agents Early nerve agents that were developed by German scientists in the period after WWI and into WWII. There are three such agents: sarin, soman, and tabun.

gamma (X-rays) Type of energy that is emitted from a strong radiologic source that is far faster and stronger than alpha and beta rays. These rays easily penetrate through the human body and require either several inches of lead or concrete to prevent penetration.

incubation The period of time from a person being exposed to a disease to the time when symptoms begin.

ionizing radiation Energy that is emitted in the form of rays or particles.

Lewisite (L) A blistering agent that has a rapid onset of symptoms and produces immediate intense pain and discomfort on contact.

mutagen A substance that mutates, damages, and changes the structure of the DNA in the body's cells.

nerve agents A class of chemical called organophosphates; they function by blocking an essential enzyme in the nervous system, which causes the body's organs to become overstimulated and burn out.

neurotoxins Biologic agents that are the most deadly substances known to humans; they include botulinum toxin and ricin.

neutron radiation Type of energy that is emitted from a strong radiologic source; neutron energy is the fastest moving and most powerful form of radiation. Neutrons easily penetrate through lead, and require several feet of concrete to stop them.

off-gassing The emitting of an agent after exposure, for example from a person's clothing that has been exposed to the agent.

persistency Term used to describe how long a chemical agent will stay on a surface before it evaporates.

phosgene A pulmonary agent that is a product of combustion, such as might be produced in a fire at a textile factory or house, or from metalworking or burning Freon.

phosgene oxime (CX) A blistering agent that has a rapid onset of symptoms and produces immediate intense pain and discomfort on contact.

pneumonic plague A lung infection, also known as plague pneumonia that is the result of inhalation of plague bacteria.

radioactive material Any material that emits radiation.

radiologic dispersal device (RDD) Any container that is designed to disperse radioactive material.

rem A unit of measure that quantifies the amount of radiation exposure to the human body.

ricin Neurotoxin derived from mash that is left from the castor bean; causes pulmonary edema and respiratory and circulatory failure, leading to death.

route of exposure Manner by which a toxic substance enters the body.

sarin (GB) A nerve agent that is one of the G agents; a highly volatile, colorless and odorless liquid that turns from liquid to gas within seconds to minutes at room temperature.

secondary device An additional explosive used by terrorists, set to explode after the initial bomb.

smallpox A highly contagious disease; it is most contagious when blisters begin to form.

soman (GD) A nerve agent that is one of the G agents; twice as persistent as sarin and five times as lethal; it has a fruity odor, as a result of the type of alcohol used in the agent, and is both a contact and inhalation hazard that can enter the body through skin absorption and through the respiratory tract.

state-sponsored terrorism Terrorism that is funded and/or supported by nations that hold close ties with terrorist groups.

sulfur mustard (agent H) A blister agent; it is a brownish-yellowish oily substance that is generally considered very persistent; has the distinct smell of garlic or mustard and, when released, it is quickly absorbed into the skin and/or mucous membranes and begins an irreversible process of damaging the cells.

tabun (GA) A nerve agent that is one of the G agents; is 36 times more persistent than sarin and approximately half as lethal; has a fruity smell and is unique because the components used to manufacture the agent are easy to acquire and the agent is easy to manufacture.

tularemia An infection caused by a bacterium called *Francisella tularensis*; common in wild rodents.

V agent (VX) One of the G agents; it is a clear, oily agent that has no odor and looks like baby oil; over 100 times more lethal than sarin and is extremely persistent.

vapor hazard An agent that enters the body through the respiratory tract.

viral hemorrhagic fevers (VHFs) A group of diseases that include the Ebola, Rift Valley, and Yellow Fever viruses among others. This group of viruses causes the blood in the body to seep out from the tissues and blood vessels.

viruses Germs that require a living host to multiply and survive.

volatility Term used to describe how long a chemical agent will stay on a surface before it evaporates.

weaponization The creation of a weapon from a biologic agent generally found in nature and that causes disease; the agent is cultivated, synthesized, and/ or mutated to maximize the target population's exposure to the germ.

weapons of mass destruction (WMDs) Any agent designed to bring about mass death, casualties, and/ or massive damage to property and infrastructure (bridges, tunnels, airports, and seaports).

Hazardous Materials and Clandestine Drug Labs

OBJECTIVES

- Describe the levels of personal protective equipment for a hazardous materials incident that the tactical medical provider may utilize.

- Describe the precautions that the tactical medical provider should take when responding to a clandestine drug lab.

- Describe how to perform a rapid decontamination.

Introduction

As a tactical medical provider (TMP), you could potentially be involved in a **hazardous materials (hazmat) incident** that places you and the SWAT unit at direct risk of injury or death from dangerous toxic chemicals or agents. **Hazardous materials** are any materials that pose a risk of damage or injury to persons, property, or the environment if they are not properly controlled during handling, storage, manufacture, processing, packaging, use and disposal, or transportation. Due to the thousands of tons of chemicals used in and transported by industries in the United States each year, hazardous materials pose a risk to communities and public safety personnel.

In addition to the risks posed by industry, the increasing prevalence of clandestine drug labs that contain toxic and hazardous chemicals has significantly raised the risk of hazardous materials exposure to SWAT and TEMS units. Add to this the ever-present risk of a terrorist group intentionally creating a hazardous materials incident. Because of these factors, you need to be prepared, educated, and equipped to keep yourself and your units safe. Depending on local protocols and your previous level of hazardous materials training, you may be required to receive additional and advanced hazardous materials training and certification.

Hazardous Materials

A SWAT unit may encounter hazardous materials at any time. If a high-risk arrest or search warrant is known to involve a chemical factory, illegal methamphetamine lab, or warehouse with chemicals, the incident commander will contact the fire department and/or their hazardous materials unit for guidance and a possible response. If the threat of a hazardous materials incident is high enough, the tactical operations leader may decide to arrange for the hazardous materials unit to wait on standby a few blocks away before exercising the warrant or mission. In the event of a chemical spill or chemical release that results in the contamination of the SWAT officers, the Hazardous Materials Response Team can immediately respond, reducing harm and potentially saving lives.

Some hazardous materials incidents are discovered unexpectedly at the scene, such as a methamphetamine lab inside a farm building found during a hostage rescue. These situations require immediate action by the TEMS unit. Any exposed patients—from SWAT officers to hostages—need immediate decontamination. Because of these variables, you should have access to personal protective equipment for hazardous materials incidents, and your TEMS unit should have an emergency field-expedient decontamination plan in place with supplies at the ready. You must be prepared to perform rapid decontamination for every mission.

Classifications of Hazardous Materials

The National Fire Protection Association (NFPA) 704 Hazardous Materials Classification standard classifies hazardous materials according to health hazard or toxicity levels, fire hazard, chemical reactive hazard, and special hazards (such as radiation or acids) for fixed facilities that store hazardous materials. Toxicity protection levels are also classified according to the level of personal protection required. For your safety, you must know the type and degree of health, fire, and reactive hazard protection needed to operate safely near these substances.

Toxicity Level

Toxicity level measures the health risk that a substance poses to someone who comes into contact with it. There are five toxicity levels: 0, 1, 2, 3, and 4. The higher the number, the greater the toxicity, as follows:

- **Level 0** includes materials that would cause little, if any, health hazard if you came into contact with them.
- **Level 1** includes materials that would cause irritation on contact but only mild residual injury, even without treatment.
- **Level 2** includes materials that could cause temporary damage or residual injury unless prompt medical treatment is provided. Both Levels 1 and 2 are considered slightly hazardous

Table 25-1	Toxicity Levels of Hazardous Materials	
Level	Health Hazard	Protection Needed
0	Little or no hazard	None
1	Slightly hazardous	SCBA (Level C suit) only
2	Slightly hazardous	SCBA (Level C suit) only
3	Extremely hazardous	Full protection, with no exposed skin (Level A or B suit)
4	Minimal exposure causes death	Special hazmat gear (Level A suit)

but require use of **self-contained breathing apparatus (SCBA)** if you are going to come into contact with them.
- **Level 3** includes materials that are extremely hazardous to health. Contact with these materials requires full protective gear so that none of your skin surface is exposed.
- **Level 4** includes materials that are so hazardous that minimal contact will cause death. For Level 4 substances, you need specialized gear that is designed for protection against that particular hazard.

Note that all health hazard levels, with the exception of 0, require respiratory and chemical protective gear that is not standard on most ambulances. Use of this equipment requires specialized training. Table 25-1 further describes the five hazard classes.

Protective Equipment for Hazardous Materials Incidents

Remember that you may encounter hazardous materials on any tactical mission. A battery-acid booby trap or an explosion in a clandestine drug lab with armed felony suspects requires an immediate and appropriate response by the SWAT and TEMS units. For this reason, the personal protective equipment required to remain safe at a hazardous materials incident must always be available in the raid van or medical support vehicles Figure 25-1 .

Personal protective equipment (PPE) levels indicate the amount and type of protective gear that you need to prevent injury from a particular substance. PPE for hazardous materials is divided into four levels: A, B, C, and D. As a TMP, you will most likely use Levels C or D, while the fire fighter or an advanced TMP who is properly trained in hazardous materials operations may use Levels A or B.

- **Level A.** This is the highest and most protective level, usually worn by a fire fighter with specialized hazardous materials training who is part of a Hazardous Materials Response Team **Figure 25-2A**. Level A is fully encapsulated,

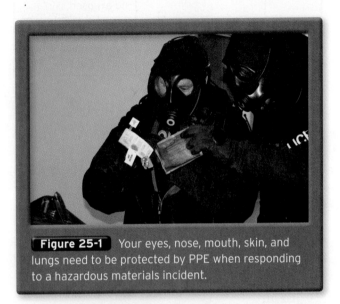

Figure 25-1 Your eyes, nose, mouth, skin, and lungs need to be protected by PPE when responding to a hazardous materials incident.

chemical-resistant protective clothing that provides full-body protection, as well as SCBA and special, sealed equipment. This equipment requires assistance to put on as well as take off.

- **Level B.** Level B and Level A both use supplied air, usually from a pressurized SCBA tank. Level B may involve supplied air from an air hose to a face mask, but this is rarely used in the out-of-hospital setting. Level B PPE is not fully sealed but uses nonencapsulated protective clothing that is sealed in all areas except for the periphery of the face area where the face mask is attached. Some clothing is designed to protect against a particular hazard **Figure 25-2B**. Usually, this clothing is made of material that will let only limited amounts of moisture and vapor pass through (nonpermeable) and will protect against most chemicals.

- **Level C.** Level C and Level D do not have supplied air, but instead utilize some type of filtered air face mask. Like Level B, Level C PPE uses nonpermeable clothing that is fully sealed except for the face area where the face mask is attached. Face masks range from a simple gas mask-style air-purifying respirator (APR), to a **powered air-purifying respirator (PAPR)** **Figure 25-2C**. A PAPR uses a battery-powered blower to pass outside air through a filter system and then into the mask or hood via a low-pressure hose. This

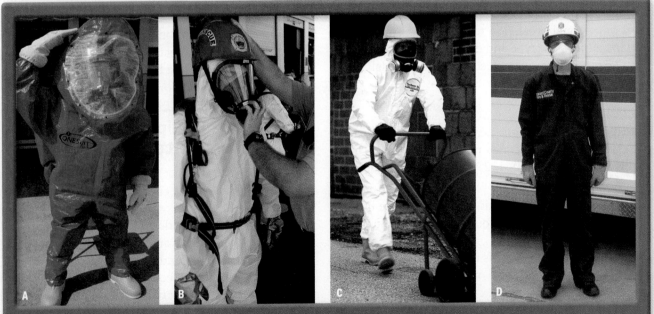

Figure 25-2 Four levels of protection. **A.** Level A protection. **B.** Level B protection. **C.** Level C protection. **D.** Level D protection. Most serious injuries and deaths from hazardous materials result from airway and breathing problems. Part C: Courtesy of the DuPont Company.

device is used by many SWAT and TEMS units and can deploy for as long as the batteries last (one lithium battery may last 8 hours or longer).

- **Level D.** Level D is commonly worn by health care workers and occupations that need to filter out dust or biologic particles, and consists of a protective waterproof or water-resistant overgarment such as coveralls, along with a HEPA N-95 or N-100 type facial mask **Figure 25-2D**.
- All levels of protection require the use of eye protection and gloves. Two pairs of chemical-resistant rubber gloves (nitrile or other type) are required for protection in case of a leak in the outer glove, as well as increasing safety when removing the contaminated clothing and equipment.

SWAT units have a choice of several types of protective uniforms for functioning in a hazardous materials environment. The standard breathable charcoal suit contains activated charcoal to absorb chemical contaminants while helping SWAT and TEMS units to remain cool and not overheat. The waterproof suit protects the skin of SWAT and TEMS officers from liquid contamination but tends to retain heat that could lead to heat injuries. Many SWAT units choose to wear a breathable charcoal suit made of camouflage cloth as it works well, is quiet (less crinkly noise with movement), is associated with less dehydration, and provides adequate protection for entries and SWAT operations.

This level of protection is worn over the standard uniform in cooler weather or by itself in warm weather. Ballistic vests and helmets are worn over the top of these uniforms. If SWAT or TEMS gear becomes contaminated, then it can later be decontaminated with special neutralizing chemicals and cleaning agents. Many SWAT units have developed the capability to deploy in Level B or Level C protection.

What should you, the TMP, wear into an environment with a high risk of hazardous materials exposure? The proper hazardous materials PPE for TEMS unit deployment should be a military-style APR (M-40 or equivalent) used with a proper filter (such as a chemical-biologic N-100 filter) or a PAPR with a waterproof butyl rubber hood and chemical-biologic

N-100 filter, in addition to a protective Level C chemical coverall-type suit with a hood. If you are going to be performing rapid decontamination with water, then a water-resistant or waterproof Level C uniform with sealed seams is preferred over the breathable charcoal suit. In addition, you should wear nitrile or other chemical-resistant gloves and boots that are sealed at the wrists and ankles with duct tape or other water-resistant tape.

SCBA and the Tactical Environment

If there is a known hazardous material in the area, then the medical threat assessment (MTA) should include arranging for the Hazardous Materials Response Team to be present to perform or assist with decontamination. The Hazardous Materials Response Team will bring their Level A and Level B PPE, which offers the most protection against highly toxic materials and vapors. The threat of toxic vapors requires the hazardous materials responder to use supplied air, wearing either an SCBA high-pressure air tank or an air-supply hose and mask. The pressure contained inside of the SCBA tank is often over 3,200 pounds per square inch (psi). Older style SCBA tanks essentially explode when struck by a bullet or metal fragment; newer tanks have composite layering that helps to prevent an explosion in the event of a rupture of the tank **Figure 25-3**. The risks of a tank explosion with likely death to the SCBA wearer and those nearby should be taken into consideration during the MTA.

In a majority of missions, simply wearing an APR with appropriate filters will provide adequate filtration protection. However, when breathing becomes difficult and it is unclear whether enough ambient oxygen is available, only TMPs with the proper training in SCBA use should don SCBA for the remainder of the mission. Fire departments and law enforcement clandestine drug laboratory entry teams typically carry oxygen concentration meters to check this. Follow local protocols on testing and working in these low-oxygen conditions.

Clandestine Drug Labs

Clandestine drug lab missions pose many unique considerations and threats and are increasing in number nationally. The threats posed by these illegal drug labs include the risks of explosion and burns by ether and other explosive chemicals used in the manufacture of

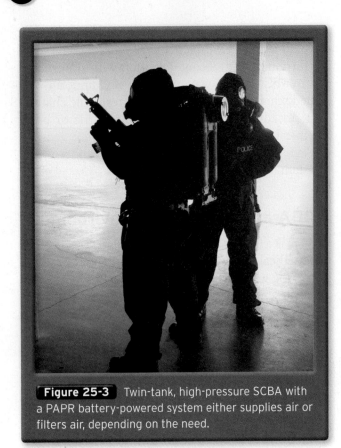

Figure 25-3 Twin-tank, high-pressure SCBA with a PAPR battery-powered system either supplies air or filters air, depending on the need.

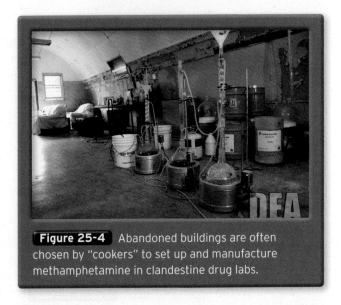

Figure 25-4 Abandoned buildings are often chosen by "cookers" to set up and manufacture methamphetamine in clandestine drug labs.

the drugs, as well as the direct toxic and carcinogenic (cancer-causing) effects of the precursors and byproducts of "cooking" methamphetamine. Over 10% of labs also contain booby traps and fully automatic weapons; unfortunately, children are often found on the premises **Figure 25-4**.

SWAT units are often aware of the existence of methamphetamine labs prior to a tactical raid; however, it is possible for a SWAT unit to serve a high-risk warrant or go to the site of an explosion and unexpectedly find a methamphetamine lab with dangerous chemicals inside the building.

Clandestine Drug Lab Considerations

Certain precautions should be taken when entering clandestine drug labs. These precautions include the following:

1. If in doubt about the contents of the building involved in a mission, the local Hazardous Materials Response Team should be contacted. TEMS and SWAT officers should bring and be ready to use the appropriate level hazardous materials PPE. Depending on local protocols and the training level of the SWAT and TEMS units, this may include the use of SCBA inside the building if there is a suspicion of low oxygen concentrations or overwhelming chemical vapor density.

2. TEMS units should prepare decontamination equipment prior to being activated, in the event that rapid field decontamination is necessary; this may include securing a nearby water outlet and hose.

3. Notify the appropriate authorities for their help and support. The fire department may be contacted to provide standby fire suppression and Hazardous Materials response if needed. The Drug Enforcement Administration (DEA) typically handles the interdiction, investigation, and cleanup of clandestine drug labs, and ideally should be notified in advance and involved as per local law enforcement agency policy.

4. Carefully clean your hands, equipment, and gear after the mission. SWAT officers should be monitored for compliance with required cleaning of all exposed SWAT gear, as well as for signs of hazardous materials exposure or illness.

5. Do not enter a clandestine drug lab unless it is absolutely necessary and you have the proper level of training. When entering a clandestine drug lab, Level A PPE is preferred but Level C protection may be all that is available. Follow your local protocols.

6. Do not touch, smell, or taste anything found at the clandestine drug lab site. No smoking, eating, or drinking should be done until after operations and cleanup. Your hands should not touch any unprotected skin.

7. Beware of booby traps outside and inside the clandestine drug lab. Watch carefully for trip wires that may detonate booby traps. Do not turn on

switches or open any refrigerator doors as sometimes these are wired to detonate explosives. Common improvised weapons include crude homemade pipe shotguns with trip wires, holes dug in the ground with sharp metal or wooden spikes at the bottom (pungi sticks), loose boards with nails pointing up, ceiling and refrigerator lights with gunpowder-filled bulbs, and even explosive flashlights. A high index of suspicion is mandatory when entering a clandestine drug lab.

8. If a SWAT officer is exposed to chemicals or body fluids, immediately perform a rapid field decontamination. Cleanse the SWAT officer by using a large amount of water to flush away any hazardous materials. If the SWAT officer is significantly symptomatic or was exposed to a potentially dangerous chemical, arrange for rapid transport to a hospital for further evaluation.

9. Clandestine drug labs are highly toxic. During the mission briefing, remind the SWAT unit that many of the chemicals on scene are known carcinogens and must be avoided.

Unfortunately, some clandestine drug labs have family members living within the building, including children. These children are at high risk for illness, chemical toxins on their clothing, toxins ingested or inhaled, and abuse and neglect. Child protective services should be contacted and brought to the scene. Rapid field decontamination of these children should occur as soon as practical, in a safe manner. New clothing that is not from within the contaminated building should be used to replace the children's clothes. Safely store the children's clothing for evidence collection. After decontamination, these children should be taken into protective custody and taken to an experienced physician who can evaluate them.

Rapid Decontamination

If the tactical callout is known in advance to involve a hazardous material, then involvement of the fire

Safety

Be prepared to provide adequate hydration to your SWAT officers before, during, and after the mission. Monitor the SWAT officers for heat exhaustion and heatstroke. Heatstroke can occur even in cool environments while wearing chemical-protective clothing and heavy tactical gear.

department and their Hazardous Materials Response Team or other appropriate agency to assist in decontamination is advisable. A formal decontamination shower and multiple personnel who work on a formal decontamination line should be on standby, ideally with access to warm water to treat contaminated personnel and patients.

An unexpected callout may thrust the SWAT unit into a challenging situation, such as a barricade scenario with unexpected toxic chemicals dispersed on the SWAT unit. This type of emergency will need to be handled with the use of **rapid decontamination**, which involves rapidly removing patients' clothing and washing them with high-volume, low-pressure water and perhaps soap if available. There is no formal decontamination line or personnel. One to two TMPs or designated fellow SWAT officers basically hose people down.

At a minimum, the TEMS unit should store a garden hose, fire hydrant adaptor, and wrench in the tactical vehicle to set up a rapid decontamination station at the nearest fire hydrant. A set of paper scrubs or disposable clothing will allow the decontaminated personnel to change into clean clothing. If time allows, a privacy screen or several large vehicles encircling the rapid decontamination stations will minimize exposure.

If a garden hose or hydrant is not available, intravenous fluid bags or another water source such as a water cooler, canteen, or Camelbak may be used to irrigate the eyes or small areas of exposure. In remote settings, water sources may be limited, requiring use of military-style decontamination with special activated charcoal and other neutralizing agents. The military trains their personnel to use a 5% chlorine bleach solution to remove hazardous materials from equipment and a 0.5% chlorine bleach solution to remove hazardous materials from the skin. In the absence of adequate water or bleach, there are several decontamination kits that use dry, inert powder (lime and magnesium oxide) and resins. These kits may have value depending on the expected threats.

Training

The Drug Enforcement Administration (DEA) offers a free, week-long clandestine drug lab awareness course at Camp Upshur, Quantico, Virginia, for appropriate personnel.

Ready for Review

- Your TEMS unit could be involved in a hazardous materials incident that places both the TEMS and SWAT units at direct risk of injury or death from dangerous toxic chemicals or agents.

- Depending on local protocols and your level of hazardous materials training, you may be required to receive additional and advanced hazardous materials training and certification.

- If the threat of a hazardous materials incident is high enough, then the tactical operations leader may decide to arrange for the Hazardous Materials Response Team to arrive and wait on standby a few blocks away before exercising the warrant or mission.

- The personal protective equipment required to remain safe at a hazardous materials incident must always be available in the raid van or TEMS support vehicles.

- As a TMP, you will most likely use Levels C or D PPE, while the fire fighter or an advanced TMP who is properly trained in hazardous materials operations may use Levels A or B.

- The threats posed by clandestine drug labs include the risks of an explosion and burns by ether and other explosive chemicals used in the manufacture of the drugs, as well as the direct toxic and carcinogenic (cancer-causing) effects of the precursors and byproducts of "cooking" methamphetamine.

- Rapid decontamination is required during an unexpected exposure to hazardous materials. Patients remove their clothing and are rapidly washed down with low-pressure water and perhaps soap if available.

Vital Vocabulary

hazardous materials Any substances that are toxic, poisonous, radioactive, flammable, cause infections, or explode resulting in illness, injury, or death due to exposure.

hazardous materials (hazmat) incident An incident in which a hazardous material is no longer properly contained and isolated.

personal protective equipment (PPE) levels Measures of the amount and type of protective equipment that an individual needs to avoid injury during contact with a hazardous material.

powered air-purifying respirator (PAPR) A battery-operated air filter device that supplies filtered air to the wearer and removes contaminants.

rapid decontamination The process of removing clothing and flushing victims with water in the field when a formal decontamination line is unavailable.

self-contained breathing apparatus (SCBA) Respirator with independent air supply used by fire fighters to enter toxic and otherwise dangerous atmospheres.

toxicity level Measure of the risk that a hazardous material poses to the health of an individual who comes into contact with it.

- Describe how to safely treat the restrained patient.
- Describe the signs and symptoms of a patient with excited delirium syndrome.
- Describe how an onsite screening examination of a suspect is performed.
- Describe how to assist in preserving the crime scene when providing patient care.
- Describe the role of the TMP in maintaining the chain of custody.

Challenges in Tactical Medicine

Introduction

In a perfect world all emergency medical care would be provided in a quiet, warm, dry, brightly lit environment with no threats. However, in the tactical environment, TMPs may be called on to assess and stabilize patients who are in restraints. Restraints are applied to decrease the patient's ability to cause physical harm to him- or herself or others. The TMP also may be called upon to preserve evidence at the crime scene while simultaneously providing care to a patient. This chapter covers the many challenges that you may face while providing care in the tactical environment.

Challenges of Treating the Restrained Patient

Thoroughly assessing patients who are in restraints in the tactical environment is a challenge. The restrained patient may be under arrest or may simply be in temporary custody while the patient's identity or involvement in the situation can be verified. Usually a suspect is restrained to some degree before the TMPs can approach and begin an assessment **Figure 26-1**.

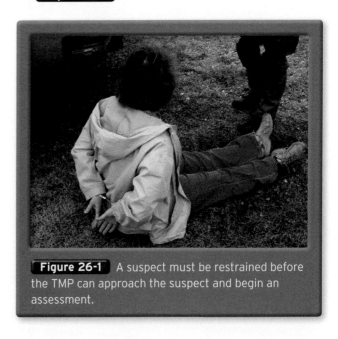

Figure 26-1 A suspect must be restrained before the TMP can approach the suspect and begin an assessment.

There are several types of physical restraints that may be used by SWAT officers. These include metal handcuffs that may be attached to each other by chain, hinge, metal bar, or rigid device. Chains designed to be worn at the waist can be attached to the handcuffs to limit motion of the arms. Legcuffs are metal restraints designed to be applied to the

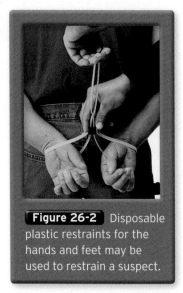

Figure 26-2 Disposable plastic restraints for the hands and feet may be used to restrain a suspect.

ankles. There are several types of disposable plastic restraints for hands and feet as well **Figure 26-2**. When a patient is in restraints, your ability to measure blood pressure or gain IV access may be limited.

A suspect who is cuffed with the hands in front has a greater ability to use his or her hands. When handcuffed with the hands behind the back, the suspect will usually have limited movement and be less capable of grabbing, striking, or hitting you. However, even a properly handcuffed suspect with hands locked behind the lower back remains a formidable threat and you must always remain wary of being kicked, headbutted, bitten, or spit on. Use of a face mask may be required if the suspect is spitting or threatening to spit. The suspect may have access to a key, paperclip, or other hidden device to unlock the handcuffs and may suddenly have both hands free to attack you. Stay fully alert and prepared. Do not let your situational awareness lapse simply because the suspect is handcuffed.

If handcuffs with ankle restraints have been attached, checked properly for clearance and circulation, and double-locked, then the restrained patient will not be able to intentionally or unintentionally tighten the cuffs and cut off circulation to the extremities. Work with SWAT officers to ensure that the cuffs are properly

Safety

Most law enforcement agencies have a use-of-force policy that provides guidelines regarding restraint techniques. Ideally, any resisting suspects are restrained by police using adequate and objectively reasonable force. When handcuffed, suspects should remain standing, sitting up, or lying on their side.

Safety

A dangling handcuff that is not closed can be a devastating weapon if the suspect swings it during the cuffing or uncuffing process.

applied and double-locked prior to your assessment. One method of checking the cuffs is to use the tip of your small finger to measure the gap between the cuff and the wrists or ankles. Your finger should barely fit between the locked cuff and the skin.

Along with placement of cuffs, a proper search of the suspect should always be performed, in particular searching for any hidden handcuff keys or a metal device such as a paper clip that could allow the suspect to unlock the handcuffs. As a general rule, it is a good idea for two people to assess a patient in custody using a contact and cover approach. With the TMP providing care, an armed SWAT officer or law enforcement officer can function as the covering officer and can raise an alarm or use force as appropriate, to restrain the suspect if an escape or attack is attempted. A handheld metal detector is useful, because some criminals will sew a small key or paperclip into a hem on their clothing, which makes it nearly impossible to feel **Figure 26-3**. Ideally, a SWAT officer or law enforcement officer will perform the search properly, while being assisted and watched by the TMP. You should assume that the patient is not fully searched unless you witness it. Remember that a suspect's pockets could contain needles and other sharps.

In order to properly assess and treat the restrained patient, the position of restraint is important. A patient should be carefully secured on his or her back with

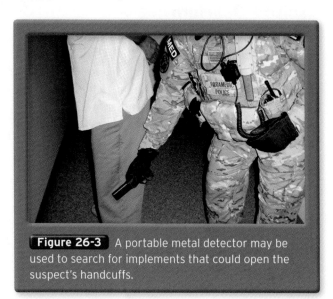

Figure 26-3 A portable metal detector may be used to search for implements that could open the suspect's handcuffs.

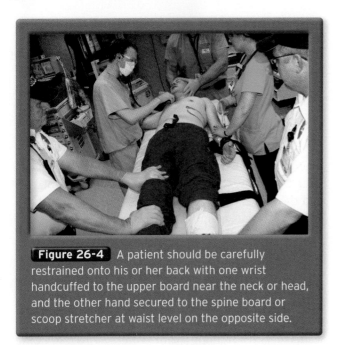

Figure 26-4 A patient should be carefully restrained onto his or her back with one wrist handcuffed to the upper board near the neck or head, and the other hand secured to the spine board or scoop stretcher at waist level on the opposite side.

one wrist handcuffed to the upper spine or scoop stretcher board near the neck or head, and the other hand secured to the spine board or scoop stretcher at waist level on the opposite side **Figure 26-4**. This keeps the patient from being able to sit up while still providing airway control and access to both limbs for IV access. Legs should be restrained to the board in the most effective manner possible, given the patient's condition. In the case of vomiting, the restrained patient can be quickly rolled onto his or her side. If possible, pad and position the patient, taking into consideration the condition of the patient, so that no damage occurs in the joints, the neurovascular structures, and the skin.

Excited Delirium

In October 2009, the American College of Emergency Physicians (ACEP) formally recognized **excited delirium syndrome (ExDS)** as a unique syndrome. This is important as it can now be recognized and more specifically treated. Further research is being performed and will lead to improved knowledge in prevention and proper treatment of patients with ExDS.

Classically, patients with ExDS are males below the age of 40 who are acutely intoxicated with stimulants. Patients with ExDS are at high risk of sudden, unexpected cardiac arrest and death. These patients may also have a history of mental illness and may be noncompliant with prescribed psychotherapeutic medications. A SWAT

Controversy

Treatment for ExDS remains mostly speculative and consensus-driven. Many experts feel that aggressive chemical sedation is a first-line intervention once physical control is obtained. Always follow your local protocols. These patients should be placed in the recovery position if possible. This allows better expansion of the diaphragm while still allowing control of the patient. This position also assists with airway control should the patient vomit.

unit may be called to the scene if a patient with ExDS exhibits disruptive, hyperaggressive, erratic behavior and appears disoriented. Patients with ExDS may be impervious to pain and extremely combative. Some will strip off all clothing and walk around in public. Additional symptoms of ExDS include a patient making nonsensical statements, constant activity, delirium, profuse sweating, rapid breathing, and failing to respond to a police presence.

These patients are extremely dangerous. Physical and chemical control measures usually do not work reliably, and electronic control devices may need to be used.

Once the subject is under control and physically restrained, disarmed, and searched, then ALS-level TMPs should begin to perform a tactical patient assessment. Assess and stabilize the CABs. Potentially harmful effects of overexertion and extreme muscle activity include hyperthermia, dehydration, and lactic acidosis. If the patient feels hot or has a fever, begin cooling measures (see Chapter 22, "Environmental Emergencies"). If the patient remains agitated, you must remain wary of the potential for further violence. Work with SWAT officers and law enforcement to evacuate and transport the

Suicide-by-Cop

The term suicide-by-cop is commonly used in the media. It describes a crisis situation during which an individual purposefully behaves in such a manner that law enforcement officers must use lethal force against the individual to protect themselves and the community. These incidents can cause mental trauma to those involved. A critical incident stress management (CISM) team may be contacted to provide group debriefings and work with law enforcement one-on-one.

patient with possible ExDS to the hospital for further evaluation and treatment. At least one SWAT officer or other law enforcement officer should accompany the patient with ExDS during transport and remain with the patient during the medical evaluation at the hospital.

If conditions permit, at least one ALS-level TMP should accompany the patient during transport to perform a secondary assessment and continue close observation and medical care. Patients with ExDS should remain restrained in a safe manner. Closely monitor the patient's vital signs, cardiac rhythm, and pulse oximetry. Administer supplemental oxygen. Obtain IV access if this can be done safely and obtain a glucose measurement. If the patient is hypoglycemic, treat according to local protocols. If your local protocols permit, consider chemical sedation. Several medications could be used, and one that is gaining favor recently is ketamine, a dissociative agent that is faster-acting than benzodiazepines and antipsychotics (Haldol), especially by the IM route. In addition, ketamine avoids respiratory depression (sometimes seen with benzodiazepines) and cardiac conduction effects such as QT prolongation (seen with antipsychotics). If the patient continues to be hyperthermic (feels hot or has a temperature of more than 101.5°F [38.6°C]) during transport, then cooling efforts should be continued. This may include cold packs on both sides of the axillae, groin, and neck, and spraying water on the skin and fanning the patient to maximize evaporative cooling **Figure 26-5**. Reassess the patient's vital signs every 5 minutes en route to the hospital.

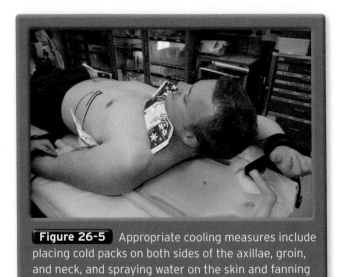

Figure 26-5 Appropriate cooling measures include placing cold packs on both sides of the axillae, groin, and neck, and spraying water on the skin and fanning the patient to maximize evaporative cooling.

On-Site Screening Exam for Suspects

There may be callouts where the mission is completed and the suspect is arrested without any force required, weapons deployed, or apparent injury sustained. If the suspect has a normal mental status, is medically stable, and has no complaints about his or her physical condition, then the suspect will likely be taken to a nearby jail and incarcerated according to local protocol. At the jail, the suspect will typically receive a preincarceration examination by medical staff. As the TMP, you do not need to be involved with the assessment of the suspect under these circumstances.

Local law enforcement protocol may mandate that all suspects are evaluated at the scene by TMPs or other medical personnel such as civilian EMS prior to transport to jail. Command staff may request that you perform a **screening examination** to evaluate the suspect on-site due to the suspect's complaints or obvious injuries. The screening examination follows the standard patient assessment process of checking the ABCs, taking a medical history, and performing a rapid physical examination. It is important to emphasize the difference between a screening examination and a clearance examination. A clearance examination is a much more thorough examination performed in a controlled setting by the custodial agency and not the TMP. The screening examination only checks for the presence of obvious conditions requiring immediate medical attention.

You must be aware of the health care capabilities of the nearby jail and hospitals at all hours. Depending on the situation and available resources, the screening examination will help determine whether further emergency care or psychiatric evaluation at the hospital should be arranged.

If the medical history, vital signs, and physical examination are essentially normal or reveal only minor medical issues, the TMP, if authorized to do so by local protocols, may declare the suspect medically stable. For minor injuries and illness (such as a sprained ankle), the TEMS unit, the local jail medical system, or the hospital emergency department may provide treatment. If the suspect has a significant medical problem such as a seizure disorder or has symptoms that may be serious (chest pain, severe abdominal pain, other) then the suspect should be taken by ambulance to the nearest, most appropriate hospital and accompanied by both a TMP and a SWAT officer. When in doubt, err on the side of being overcautious and proceed to arrange for a more extensive medical evaluation at the hospital.

Any suspect who resists arrest and is struck with hands, feet, or less lethal weapons should be examined closely. Impact from batons, falls, and less lethal beanbags can produce internal injuries such as rupture of the spleen or liver that are not easily detected and can occasionally be fatal. TASER dart removal should follow the local agency protocols, and if the groin, eyeball, neck, or other sensitive area is involved then the suspect should be transported to a hospital for evaluation and removal of the darts. The wrists and ankles should be examined for compression injuries from handcuffs and it should be documented that there is adequate circulation and that the handcuffs are double locked.

Mental status should be carefully evaluated, as some suspects will be under the influence of drugs or alcohol, or have head trauma. A common criminal tactic is for suspects to feign an altered mental status (pretending to be sleepy or comatose) and then attempt to escape when given the opportunity. Always maintain a high degree of suspicion any time you approach a criminal suspect, as it is a high-risk situation. Always take appropriate protective precautions.

Suspects may swallow illegal substances as a way to smuggle them or to hide them from police. This is another common criminal tactic. If the container leaks or ruptures, sudden illness or death may result. Another tactic is to hide illegal drugs by inserting a latex balloon filled with the substance in the rectum or vagina. On occasion these packets have ruptured and released a lethal amount of illegal drugs into the suspect's body. Be aware of the potential signs and symptoms of an illegal substance overdose and provide stabilizing care per your local protocols, if needed.

Be cautious and maintain close observation of these persons, monitor and document the patient's vital signs, and conduct an appropriate examination. Remember that suspects may not give reliable medical histories. If the circumstances warrant it, a full-body cavity search may be indicated. If any doubt exists, err on the side of caution and take the suspect to a hospital for a complete evaluation. Follow your local protocols.

Crime Scene Considerations

Preserving Evidence

Generally, there are two types of evidence: testimonial and real or physical. **Testimonial evidence** is the oral documentation by a witness of the facts. Real or **physical**

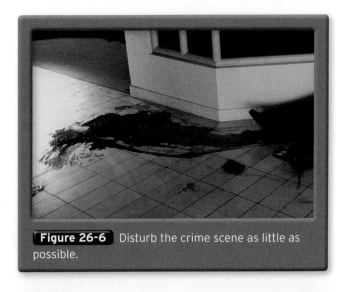

Figure 26-6 Disturb the crime scene as little as possible.

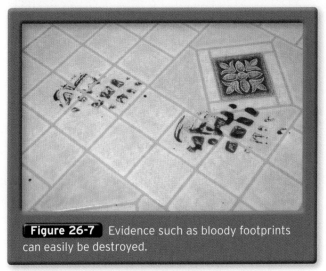

Figure 26-7 Evidence such as bloody footprints can easily be destroyed.

evidence ties a suspect or a victim to a crime and includes blood and other body fluids, objects, and impressions.

Once you are at your patient's side, make an effort to alter the scene as little as possible. Be mindful of bullet casings, weapons, blood spatter, and puddles **Figure 26-6**. Do not step on or move any physical evidence if possible **Figure 26-7**. Whenever possible, walk around such evidence. Do not pick up expended cartridge casings to determine the caliber. When you remove clothes to expose a wound, avoid cutting through bullet holes, knife cuts, or tears if possible. Do not shake clothing you have removed because valuables, including valuable trace evidence, may fall from the pockets to the floor. Each item is placed in an individual paper bag to avoid cross contamination. Consider securing a paper bag over the hands of patients who are victims of violent assaults. They may have gun powder residue on their hands or DNA evidence under their fingernails from their attacker.

You may be called to provide testimonial evidence in court regarding what you saw or heard at the scene of a crime. Because a criminal case might not go to trial for a year or more, it is imperative that the incident be properly documented. Writing a complete and accurate report is the mark of a professional TMP. Ideally, the TEMS unit will have a standard callout documentation form, separate from the patient care report, to be completed after the callout.

Documentation should include a description of the scene. How many patients? Was the victim supine or prone? Where was the weapon? Were any characteristics of the crime scene noteworthy? Do not draw conclusions. Reports should include facts, not speculation.

Any statements made by the patient during transfer to a medical facility should be documented. It is not your duty to interrogate the patient unless knowing what happened pertains to their medical care or that of others. Do not ask, "Who did this to you?" However, if the patient mentions a specific name or detail, then record that information. These statements may be key evidence for a successful prosecution, especially if the patient dies.

Chain of Custody

The chain of custody starts with the original discoverer. In many cases, this may be you, the TMP providing medical care. Any weapons, drugs, or other materials removed from patients should be properly documented on the patient care report. Any evidence should be handed off directly to a nearby SWAT officer or kept nearby within direct control by a SWAT officer. If a SWAT officer or law enforcement officer is not available, then the evidence may be temporarily kept in your physical possession. At an appropriate time, this evidence should be signed over to investigating law enforcement officers to maintain the chain of custody. In your documentation, note the date, time, and the name of the officer taking possession of the evidence.

Eventually the evidence will be gathered by the investigating detectives and properly stored in containers (paper bags for any biologic specimens) with accurate labels and tamper-resistant seals, according to the agency's policies.

If medical care is provided, any gear that is left at the scene such as laryngoscopes or medical packs may be considered crime scene evidence and may possibly be placed in an evidence locker until the trial or whenever the detectives are done with their investigation, which may be several days to potentially years later. Always keep your essential gear close to you during patient care. Before leaving the scene, quickly gather your gear and bring it along with you during evacuation and transport.

Physical Signs of Death

As a TMP, you are responsible for adhering to appropriate medical standards of care and making reasonable, common-sense efforts to preserve life in tactically challenging situations. In the absence of injuries that are incompatible with life, resuscitative measures should be attempted if there is any chance that life exists. However, there are conditions when death is obvious and no resuscitation is indicated:

- Devastating head injury with severe brain trauma
- Rigor mortis
- Dependent lividity **Figure 26-8**
- Decapitation
- Hemicorporectomy (body cut in half)
- Decomposition

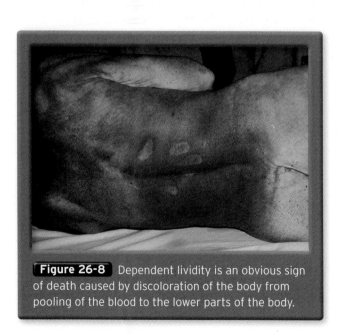

Figure 26-8 Dependent lividity is an obvious sign of death caused by discoloration of the body from pooling of the blood to the lower parts of the body.

At the Scene

Safety and patient care are your primary and secondary concerns; however, you should also do what you can to protect evidence at the scene. Evidentiary items may prove to be critical in the successful prosecution of a criminal case. Consider carrying paper bags, a permanent marker, and other items you might need in order preserve evidence at the scene.

At the Scene

A special consideration in providing resuscitation to patients with signs of very recent death is an obviously pregnant woman. The fetus may be viable after 22 to 24 weeks of gestation. Continue CPR and use towels or other materials under the right side of the backboard in order to tilt the patient to her left side to improve circulation to the fetus. Rapidly transport the patient to an emergency department where a cesarean section may be performed.

Resuscitation should also be limited or stopped if multiple victims are present and triage deems that resources would be more beneficial for use on other patients.

The decision of who, when, and where death may be pronounced differs from state to state. You should be familiar with your local protocols and procedures. If the deceased patient died as a result of a known or possible crime, then the scene is deemed a crime scene and therefore the patient should be left as is with minimal disturbance of the crime scene. Many states only allow a physician to pronounce a patient dead. However, EMS personnel, including many TMPs, have standing orders for termination of resuscitative efforts in the field and/or may contact medical control to obtain direction on when to cease medical care and to contact the medical examiner. Once death has been declared, the medical examiner assumes responsibility of the scene and supersedes all others at the scene.

Special Considerations

If a SWAT officer suffers major trauma on scene, then aggressive resuscitation efforts and transportation will be instituted immediately, regardless of a low or nonexistent likelihood of survival. This is expected and permissible if circumstances allow, as the SWAT unit will want the maximal medical care performed for their fellow officer. Anything less may leave the surviving SWAT officers with emotionally damaging second thoughts. However, this natural tendency should be tempered in other circumstances, as it is unacceptable to risk and possibly lose additional lives while attempting a futile rescue and resuscitation. For example, if a SWAT officer receives a gunshot wound to the head from a large-caliber rifle and is lying motionless and without respiratory effort in full view of a barricaded and armed suspect, then an immediate downed officer rescue that would risk additional lives for a minimal or zero chance of a good outcome likely would not be attempted. As always, follow your local policies and procedures.

Ready for Review

- The suspect must be subdued and restrained to some degree before TMPs can approach and get involved. Legs should also be restrained. If possible, pad and position the patient, taking into consideration the condition of the patient, so that no damage occurs in the joints, the neurovascular structures, and the skin.

- A patient should be carefully restrained onto his or her back with one wrist handcuffed to the upper board near the neck or head, and the other hand secured to the spine board or scoop stretcher at waist level on the opposite side. If the patient's medical condition permits, search the patient for weapons and handcuff keys prior to starting the formal evaluation.

- Patients with ExDS may be impervious to pain and extremely combative. Additional symptoms include a patient making nonsensical statements, constant activity, delirium, profuse sweating, rapid breathing, and failing to respond to a police presence.

- The screening examination follows the standard patient assessment process of checking the ABCs, taking a medical history, and performing a rapid physical examination.

- As you provide patient care at a crime scene, be mindful of evidence and avoid altering and destroying it.

- Any weapons, drugs, or other materials removed from patients should be properly documented on the patient care report.

- Any evidence should be handed off directly to a nearby SWAT officer or kept nearby within direct control of a SWAT officer.

- If a SWAT officer or law enforcement officer is not available, then the evidence may temporarily be kept in your physical possession.

- If a SWAT officer suffers major trauma on scene, then aggressive resuscitation efforts and transportation will be instituted immediately, regardless of a low or nonexistent likelihood of survival. This course of action should be reevaluated if additional lives may be lost or others harmed by attempting a futile rescue and resuscitation.

Vital Vocabulary

excited delirium syndrome (ExDS) A syndrome where the patient displays hyperaggressive, combative behavior; symptoms include rapid breathing, profuse sweating, and delirium.

physical evidence Evidence such as blood, objects, or impressions that ties a suspect or victim to a crime.

screening examination An on-site patient assessment of a suspect to determine if the suspect should be transported to jail or to a hospital for further examination and treatment.

testimonial evidence Oral documentation of the facts by a witness.

K-9 Management

Police Dog Emergency Medical Gear

Many SWAT teams use police dogs and K-9 officers during missions. During SWAT missions K-9 units are used to establish and secure the outer perimeter and to help catch any fleeing suspect(s). Often the police dog is sent in first in highly dangerous urban settings to locate hidden suspects. Police dogs also may be specially trained and used to detect illegal drugs and identify explosives. Overall, police dogs are very useful members of a law enforcement agency. In many states they are considered to be police officers, and shooting a police dog is considered a felony crime equivalent to shooting a human police officer. The cost for a trained police dog is $15,000 to $40,000; therefore, these are valuable and useful creatures **Figure A-1**.

Due to the nature of their work, police dogs are at high risk of injury. Suspects will punch, kick, stab, poison, or shoot police dogs. In addition, extreme heat and cold may cause environmental injuries. It may be difficult to locate a veterinarian to care for police dogs during the weekends and at night. A SWAT callout at

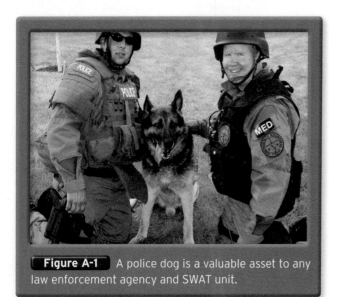

Figure A-1 A police dog is a valuable asset to any law enforcement agency and SWAT unit.

At the Scene

Part of obtaining medical intelligence is collecting the name, number, and location of the closest veterinarian hospital. You should have the contact information and hours of operation for nearby veterinary hospitals, especially those that offer 24-hour care. In addition, you should be aware of the type of police dog(s) that are being utilized, their weight, and their unique medical issues, and acquire the medical supplies needed to stabilize a dog.

a remote location may involve a long transport time for injured police dogs to reach a veterinary hospital. As a tactical medical provider (TMP), you should be trained and equipped to provide first aid to police dogs. Fortunately, many of the assessment skills, medications, medical procedures, and resuscitation principles are very similar to those for humans.

Preparing for Police Dog Emergencies

During training and callouts, it will be extremely difficult to arrange for the police dog's veterinarian to be present. The K-9 officer often has completed training in basic canine medical emergencies and should have a medical kit and basic canine medical management skills. You should work together to assemble and place medical kits for canines in the SWAT vehicles, the K-9 patrol car, and your TEMS backpack.

Canine Tactical Assessment

Call-A

The Call-A-CAB 'N Go tactical assessment applies equally well to police dogs. If an injury occurs, then call out and inform fellow personnel and command. Seek appropriate help while threats are being abolished. The actions of an injured dog are unpredictable. Although police dogs are highly intelligent, they will be confused and in pain if injured. As a result, an injured police dog may not respond to the commands from the K-9 officer. A wounded dog's first instinct is to run and hide, and it may not understand that you are trying to help.

Most injured dogs in pain will attempt to bite any approaching person as a defensive reflex. This hazard must be properly abolished by calmly and carefully leashing and muzzling the police dog. When approaching an injured police dog, speak softly. Approach slowly. Do not make any sudden movements. Stop your approach when you are several feet away. Extend your closed hand, knuckles upward. If there is no aggression, pet the dog and then apply the muzzle. The muzzle should fit over the long nose and mouth (snout) of the police dog with a strap around the back of the head to hold it in place **Figure A-2**. The muzzle is usually made of leather, and if it is not available, you or the K-9 officer can use a makeshift muzzle made from a roll of medical gauze. Arrange for familiar officers to gently and calmly talk to the dog so that it calms down.

If the police dog is too aggressive to safely approach and muzzle, then the use of two loops of rope around the dog's neck held by K-9 or SWAT officers on opposite sides may be required in order to control the dog. In extreme situations, the use of pepper spray or a TASER may be indicated to neutralize the wounded police dog.

Keep in mind that sometimes both police dog and K-9 officer are patients, and you must be mentally and physically prepared to treat an injured police dog alone. If the police dog and the K-9 officer are both injured, then the priority will be to treat and stabilize the human officer first, remembering that the police dog may act defensively and attempt to protect the injured K-9 officer. If this occurs, then use common sense to safely calm the police dog, apply a muzzle, and treat the K-9 officer accordingly. Other K-9 officers or SWAT officers at the scene may know the injured dog and can assist.

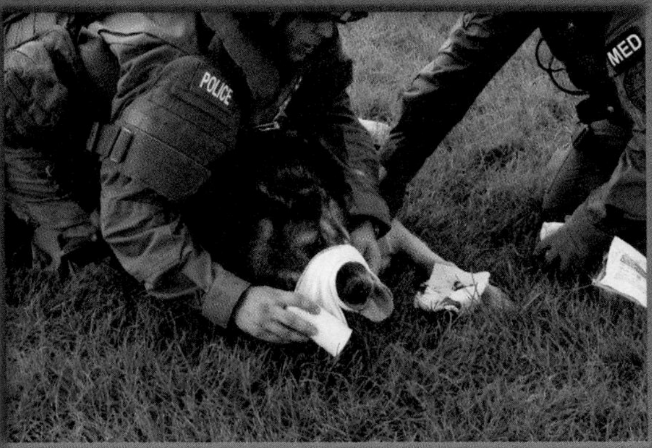

Circulation

It is critical to assess and stabilize the dog's circulation and stop any bleeding. Assess the pulse by pressing in on the inside of the upper front leg or back leg. TMPs should practice this on normal healthy police dogs during routine training in order to learn where the arteries are. If the pulse is thready and weak, the injured dog is likely in shock. The heart can be heard by placing a stethoscope on the mid-lower chest just behind the left shoulder, or by placing your ear directly onto the chest to listen.

Any major bleeding from the extremities should be stopped with a tourniquet. If a standard tourniquet does not work, then use your available materials to make one using at least 1- to 2-inch wide material if possible. Practice this on a healthy and happy police dog during training so you will be able to apply the tourniquet during an emergency **Figure A-3**.

If the police dog has a penetrating injury to the body, neck, or head, then apply direct pressure over the bleeding site and recognize this as a load-and-go situation. Rapidly evacuate your canine patient to transportation. It may take several SWAT or K-9 officers to evacuate the injured dog. The dog will be in pain and confused and may not cooperate by being still.

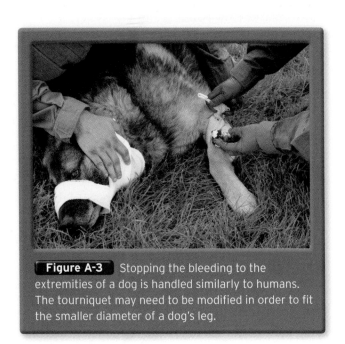

Figure A-3 Stopping the bleeding to the extremities of a dog is handled similarly to humans. The tourniquet may need to be modified in order to fit the smaller diameter of a dog's leg.

Figure A-2 A muzzle is required prior to further assessment and treatment.

Airway and Breathing

A dog can be ventilated by blowing into the nose with your mouth. To provide artificial ventilation to a dog, follow these steps:

1. Position the dog on its side. Gently align the head and neck.
2. Open the dog's mouth and pull the tongue forward so it does not block the throat.
3. Close the dog's mouth and apply the muzzle.
4. Inhale and put your mouth over the dog's nose, forming a good tight seal. Exhale and breathe into the dog's nose and lungs. Remove your mouth and allow your breath to leave the dog.
5. Repeat about once every 6 to 7 seconds (10 to 15 times per minute)
6. If the dog's gum color improves and the dog starts to fight the procedure, then the dog's breathing is improving.

If you need to ventilate the dog for an extended period of time, it is best to intubate the dog with a 9- to 12-mm endotracheal tube and a number 3 or 4 Miller blade. This is a two-person technique and is typically done with the dog in a prone position. One person holds the upper jaw while you place the ET tube with the assistance of a 3 or 4 Miller laryngoscope blade. The anatomy is similar to humans' and placement of the tube through the vocal cords and inflation of the ET cuff should result in good bilateral breath sounds if the lungs are inflated. This should only be performed if you are authorized to intubate human patients. A bag-mask device can then be used to gently ventilate the dog.

Load and Go

Load-and-go indications for dogs are similar to humans and include penetrating trauma to the head, neck, and torso; severe burns; fall from significant height; severe dehydration; altered mental status; and possible or proven poisoning or ingestion of toxic agents. If possible, call a veterinarian or veterinary hospital prior to arrival so the staff can adequately prepare.

It may be more difficult to determine if the police dog has a load-and-go-injury. The presence of thick fur may limit visualization of any penetrating trauma.

Pain Management

Dogs have a high pain tolerance, but pain and sedation medication should be carried and administered per veterinary protocols. One of the most effective medicines for pain control is morphine, and it is dosed at 0.05 to 0.12 mg/lb or 0.25 mg/kg given IM or IV push. Repeat approximately every 15 to 30 minutes as needed acutely, and later every 2 to 4 hours as needed. Some dogs may break out in a reddish rash or experience itching; if so, administer 1 mg/kg of Benadryl. Medications such as fentanyl may be administered at the same dosage per kilogram as humans.

Fractures

Leg fractures are the most common broken bones in canines. The splinting process is similar to humans with a few exceptions. To apply a splint, follow these steps:

1. Before splinting or realigning the leg, administer pain medicine and sedation when indicated. Follow local veterinary protocols.
2. When splinting, use thin soft material to initially gently wrap over the fracture site. If there is bleeding near the fracture, then it is considered to be an open fracture requiring sterile bandages.
3. Use firm, straight splint material such as a SAM splint to lay alongside the extremity, above and below the fracture site. Use tape or a compression bandage to keep the splint in place and try to realign the extremity.
4. Check the distal pulse and ensure that the splint is not applied too tightly.
5. Keep the dog from walking. Evacuate the dog to transport.
6. Arrange for continued sedation and pain medication for the dog. Start IV fluids while en route if conditions allow it. Consult an appropriate veterinarian. Note that complex fractures and other injuries may require transportation to a regional veterinary center for treatment.

Heat Emergencies

Heatstroke and other heat emergencies are a risk in hot weather. Dogs do not have sweat glands and can only pant and breathe through their nose to cool themselves. Move an overheated dog out of the sun and into an air-conditioned location. Cool the dog with water and fans to speed evaporation. Apply ice packs to the neck, groin, and head. Rapidly transport to a veterinarian if the dog shows signs of significant heat injury such as lying down with lethargy or altered mental status, appearance of dry mouth and dehydration, or a heart rate of more than 120 beats/min.

If possible, start an IV of normal saline or Ringer's lactate and infuse a 15 mL/kg IV fluid bolus over 20 to 30 minutes. Follow with additional IV fluids as needed for the first hour and then reassess. Consider additional IV fluids if the urine output is insufficient or other signs of continued dehydration exist.

When starting an IV in a dog, the cephalic vein is the most commonly used vein by veterinarians. It is accessed by applying a mild constriction band midway up a front leg, just below the elbow joint, shaving the fur off the front of the lower leg, identifying the vein under the skin anteriorly to the lower leg bone, and then placing a 20- or 18-gauge IV into the vein. Release the compression band and the IV should flush and infuse easily. If this vein is not accessible in one leg, then use the other or the lateral saphenous vein in the lateral lower rear leg. Clip the fur prior to starting an IV if it interferes with visualizing the veins.

IV access is often difficult in dehydrated dogs (and in dogs in shock). A subcutaneous IV may also be given to a dehydrated dog. Insert a 16-gauge catheter under the skin, just over the top of the shoulder blades. Rapidly infuse 15 mL/kg IV fluid bolus. Consider using intraosseous (IO) lines. The IO line can be placed in a proximal leg tibia, similar to humans. To insert an IO line in a dog, follow these steps:

Medical Gear

Practically all of the first aid gear and medications carried by TMPs may be used in treating canine injuries. However, due to the relatively smaller diameter of a dog's leg, a tourniquet device for a dog's extremities should be made ahead of time. A muzzle and a small disposable razor should be included in your equipment if you work with K-9 units.

1. Provide pain medication.
2. Identify an unfractured leg. Shave and prep the insertion site, located at the medial upper aspect of the tibia a finger-width distance from the knee joint. If time allows, place several milliliters of 1% lidocaine at this site subcutaneously.
3. Using a Jamshidi bone marrow needle (or other intraosseous needle), apply firm pressure to the needle tip with alternating clockwise and counterclockwise pressure and drill into the marrow. Stop rotations when sudden resistance is decreased.
4. Check the placement by brief aspiration of 1 mL of blood followed by immediate flushing of the IO device, and then hook up to the IV.
5. Secure the IO device as best as possible and transport.

Poisoning

Poisoning of dogs may occur, either intentionally or by accident. The most common is ingestion of rodenticide (rat poison). If this occurs, then entice the dog to drink activated charcoal in order to bind and absorb the poison and prevent it from being absorbed into the bloodstream. If poisoning is known or suspected, call the National Animal Poison Control Center at Champaign-Urbana College of Veterinary Medicine, 1-800-548-2423.

TEMS Forms

Personal Medical Data Form

Date: _____

Agency/Employer: _____ Rank/Title: _____

Badge # _____ Agency Mailing Address: _____

Personal Information

Name (Last, First): _____

Age: _____ Sex: M F   Date of Birth: _____

Home Phone: _____

Work Phone: _____

Cell Phone: _____

Medical Information

Height: _____ Weight: _____ Blood Type (if known): _____

Primary Care Physician: _____ Phone: _____

Date of Last Physical Exam: _____ Doctor/Location: _____

Medications (Type and Dose): _____

_____

Immunization Status (Date of last update/test):

　　TB/PPD Tuberculosis Test: _____

　　Tetanus: _____

　　Hepatitis B: Last Immunization: _____

　　Hepatitis B: Last Test: _____

Allergies (If you answer yes to any item, please list all allergies.):

　　Medications　　　　　No　　Yes _____

　　X-ray Contrast or Iodine　No　　Yes _____

　　Food Allergies　　　　No　　Yes _____

　　Please list any additional allergies here: _____

Do you wear: Glasses? No   Yes   Contact Lenses?   No   Yes

List any previous surgeries: _____

Have you or your family members had any serious side effects or reactions to anesthesia or any operations? No   Yes

If yes, then explain further: _____

_____

List any medical issues: _____

Organ Donor Status: No   Yes

If yes, list the location of your Organ Donor Card or your Living Will: _____

_____

Emergency Contact

     Name: _____

     Relationship: _____

     Address: _____

               _____

     Phone: _____

Medical Threat Assessment Form

Medical Contacts		
Hospitals		
Medical Center	Location:	Phone:
Trauma/Burn Centers		
Medical Center	Location:	Phone:
MEDEVAC		
Air Ambulance	Contact Name:	Landing Zone Location: GPS Coordinates:
Support Services		
HAZ MAT Agency	Contact Name:	Phone:
FIRE Agency	Contact Name:	Phone:
EMS Agency	Contact Name:	Phone:
Disaster/Med Comm	Contact Name:	Phone:
Poison Control	Contact Name:	Phone:
Child Protective Services	Contact Name:	Phone:
Social Services	Contact Name:	Phone:
Animal Control	Contact Name:	Phone:
Food Support/Red Cross	Contact Name:	Phone:
Sewage/Port-a-potty	Contact Name:	Phone:
Utilities		
Electric Company	Contact Name:	Phone:
Water Company	Contact Name:	Phone:
Environmental Factors		
Temperature Expected:		
Precipitation Expected:		
Cold Weather Gear?	Warm Weather Gear?	Rain Gear?
Threat of Ticks?	Threat of Snakes?	Threat of Insects/Mosquitoes?
Rehabilitation Station		
Heat Sources		
Hydration/Cooling Sources		
Dogs		
Police Dog:	K-9 Officer:	Vet/Animal Hospital:
Operation Classification		
Other Threats:		
Additional Supplies:		

GLOSSARY

2-chlorobenzalmalononitrile (CS) tear gas A tearing and/or irritant chemical agent; a fine yellow powder that has a pungent, pepper-like odor.

abrasion Loss or damage of the superficial layer of skin as a result of a body part rubbing or scraping across a rough or hard surface.

acute radiation syndrome The clinical course that usually begins within hours of exposure to a radiation source. Symptoms include nausea, vomiting, diarrhea, fatigue, fever, and headache. The long-term symptoms are dose-related and hematopoietic and gastrointestinal.

advanced EMT (AEMT) An individual who has training in specific aspects of advanced life support, such as intravenous therapy and the administration of certain emergency medications.

advanced life support (ALS) Advanced lifesaving procedures, such as cardiac monitoring, administration of IV fluids and medications, and use of advanced airway adjuncts.

air-purifying respirator (APR) A gas mask worn to filter particulates and contaminants from the air.

alpha radiation Type of energy that is emitted from a strong radiologic source; it is the least harmful penetrating type of radiation and cannot travel fast or through most objects.

ambient temperature The temperature of the surrounding environment.

amputation An injury in which part of the body is completely severed.

anaphylaxis An extreme, life-threatening systemic allergic reaction that may include shock and respiratory failure.

anchor sleep A specific period of time at least 4 hours long, during which a responder sleeps every day, both on-duty and off-duty, while on a particular shift rotation.

anthrax A deadly bacterium (*Bacillus anthracis*) that lies dormant in a spore (protective shell); the germ is released from the spore when exposed to the optimal temperature and moisture. The route of entry is inhalation, cutaneous, or gastrointestinal (from consuming food that contains spores).

antivenin A serum that counteracts the effect of venom from an animal or insect.

apneic Not breathing.

aspiration In the context of airway, the introduction of vomitus or other foreign material into the lungs.

auditory exclusion A temporary loss of hearing that occurs as part of the fight-or-flight stress response during confrontation with danger; serves to remove background noise allowing for a sole focus on survival.

AVPU scale A method of assessing level of consciousness by determining whether the patient is alert, responsive to verbal stimuli or pain, or unresponsive; used principally early in the assessment.

avulsion An injury in which soft tissue either is torn completely loose or is hanging as a flap.

bacteria Microorganisms that reproduce by binary fission. These single-cell creatures reproduce rapidly. Some can form spores (encysted variants) when environmental conditions are harsh.

bag-mask device A device with a one-way valve and a face mask attached to a ventilation bag.

balaclava Black or camouflage-colored stocking-hat type of head cover that slips over the head and neck, covering the entire head except for the eyes, nose, and possibly mouth.

ballistic vest Designed to stop many types of bullets, help defeat shrapnel, and resist puncture by other projectiles; worn underneath other protective garments and gear.

barotrauma Injury resulting from pressure disequilibrium across body surfaces; for example, from too much pressure in the lungs.

barricaded subjects People who are not suspected of committing a crime but are the focus of a legitimate police intervention effort, most often involving threats of suicide and/or self-destructive behavior involving the mentally ill.

barricaded suspects Criminal suspects who have taken a position in a physical location, most often a structure or vehicle, fortified or not, that does not allow immediate police access and who are refusing police orders to exit; may be known to be armed, thought to be armed, have access to weapons in the location, or be in an unknown weapons status.

barrier device A protective item, such as a pocket mask with a valve, that limits exposure to a patient's body fluids.

battering ram A tool made of hardened steel with handles on the sides used to force open doors and to breach walls. Larger versions may be used by as many as four people; smaller versions are made for one or two people.

Beck's triad The combination of narrowed pulse pressure, muffled heart tones, and jugular vein distention associated with cardiac tamponade; usually resulting from penetrating chest trauma.

beta radiation Type of energy that is emitted from a strong radiologic source, is slightly more penetrating than alpha, and requires a layer of clothing stop it.

bilateral command structure A command structure for a TEMS unit that has law enforcement assume command in the field, while medical direction is given remotely during a mission.

bloodborne pathogens Pathogenic microorganisms that are present in human blood and can cause disease in humans. These pathogens include, but are not limited to, hepatitis B virus and human immunodeficiency virus (HIV).

bomb squad Specially trained police officers and specialists with unique equipment and protective gear to assist in the recognition and inactivation or neutralization of explosive threats.

botulinum Produced by bacteria, this is a very potent neurotoxin. When introduced into the body, this neurotoxin affects the nervous system's ability to function and causes botulism.

breacher SWAT officer who carries a heavy metal battering ram and other tools to force open doors or walls.

buboes Enlarged lymph nodes (up to the size of tennis balls) that were characteristic of people infected with the bubonic plague.

bubonic plague An epidemic that spread throughout Europe in the Middle Ages, causing over 25 million deaths, also called the Black Death, transmitted by infected fleas and characterized by acute malaise, fever, and the formation of tender, enlarged, inflamed lymph nodes that appear as lesions, called buboes.

bulla An elevated lesion containing fluid.

caliber The measurement of the inside diameter of the barrel of a firearm; may be measured in hundredths of an inch or millimeters.

cardiopulmonary resuscitation (CPR) mask A portable face mask used as a standard precaution to protect emergency care providers administering rescue breaths to a patient.

casualty collection point (CCP) The point outside of the outer perimeter where civilian EMS meet the patient and TMPs to initiate transportation to an appropriate local hospital.

cavitation A temporary cavity that forms from the pressure wake from a bullet that stretches the skin and other tissues outward.

CBRN Acronym that stands for chemical, biologic, radiologic, and nuclear threats.

cerebral edema Swelling of the brain.

cerebrospinal fluid (CSF) Fluid produced in the ventricles of the brain that flows in the subarachnoid space and bathes the meninges.

chlorine (CL) The first chemical agent ever used in warfare. It has a distinct odor of bleach and creates a green haze when released as a gas. Initially it produces upper airway irritation and a choking sensation.

Class 1 dental fracture A fracture to the tooth that involves only the enamel portion of the tooth.

Class 2 dental fracture A fracture to the tooth that includes the enamel and the dentin but not the pulp.

Class 3 dental fracture A fracture to the tooth that includes the enamel, the dentin, and the pulp chamber.

Class 4 dental fracture A fracture to the tooth that involves the root and may destabilize the tooth.

closed abdominal injury An injury in which there is soft-tissue damage inside the body but the skin remains intact.

closed wound Wound in which damage occurs beneath the skin or mucous membrane but the surface remains intact.

Combitube A multilumen airway device that consists of a single tube with two lumens, two balloons, and two ventilation ports; an alternative airway device if endotracheal intubation is not possible or has failed.

communicability Describes how easily a disease spreads from one human to another human.

compartment syndrome Swelling in a confined space that produces dangerous pressure; may cut off blood flow or damage sensitive tissue; frequently seen in fractures below the elbow or knee in children.

compressed-air technology Use of a paintball marker firearm (.68-caliber) to shoot small projectiles of variable contents, but most involve use of oleoresin capsicum (OC), which is a powder or liquid irritant that will cause suspects to stop their actions and retreat.

conduction The loss of heat by direct contact (eg, when a body part comes into contact with a colder object).

contact dermatitis Skin inflammation caused by exposure to irritants or allergens.

contact hazard A hazardous agent that gives off very little or no vapors; the skin is the primary route for this type of chemical to enter the body; also called a skin hazard.

contagious A person infected with a disease that is highly communicable.

contamination The presence of infective organisms or foreign bodies such as dirt, gravel, or metal.

contusion A bruise from an injury that causes bleeding beneath the skin without breaking the skin.

convection The loss of body heat caused by air movement (eg, breeze blowing across the body).

core temperature The temperature of the central part of the body (eg, the heart, lungs, and vital organs).

coup-contrecoup injury Dual impacting of the brain into the skull; coup injury occurs at the point of impact; contrecoup injury occurs on the opposite side of impact, as the brain rebounds.

cricoid pressure Pressure on the cricoid cartilage; applied to occlude the esophagus in order to inhibit gastric distention and regurgitation of vomitus in the unconscious patient.

cricothyroid membrane A thin sheet of fascia that connects the thyroid and the cricoid cartilages that make up the larynx.

critical incident Any situation faced by an emergency services worker that generates an unusually strong emotional response (internal and/or external), which overwhelms the ability to cope with the experience, either at the scene or later.

critical incident stress debriefing (CISD) A confidential peer group discussion in which specially trained teams work with emergency personnel who have been involved in traumatic calls or other painful incidents; CISDs usually occur within 24 to 72 hours of the incident.

critical incident stress management (CISM) A process that confronts the responses to critical incidents and defuses them, directing the emergency services personnel toward physical and emotional equilibrium.

cross-contamination Occurs when a person is contaminated by an agent as a result of coming into contact with another contaminated person.

crush syndrome Significant metabolic derangement that develops when crushed extremities or body parts remain trapped for prolonged periods. This can lead to renal failure and death.

Cushing's reflex The combination of a slowing pulse, rising blood pressure, and erratic respiratory patterns; a grave sign for patients with head trauma.

cyanide Agent that affects the body's ability to use oxygen. It is a colorless gas that has an odor similar to almonds. The effects begin on the cellular level and are very rapidly seen at the organ system level.

decay A natural process in which a material that is unstable attempts to stabilize itself by changing its structure.

decompression sickness A painful condition seen in divers who ascend too quickly, in which gas, especially nitrogen, forms bubbles in blood vessels and other tissues; also called "the bends."

deep partial-thickness burn A burn in which the skin is blistered but not charred and is painful to the touch, usually the result of steam, oil, or flames and involving the deeper layers of the dermis.

derringers Small, concealable pistols with one or two barrels, usually loaded by a hinge-style, break-open breech; named after a famous nineteenth century pocket pistol maker, Henry Deringer.

dignitary protection Providing personal protective services to very important persons (VIPs).

disease vector An animal that spreads a disease, once infected, to another animal.

dissemination The means with which a terrorist will spread an agent, for example, by poisoning the water supply or aerosolizing the agent into the air or ventilation system of a building.

dynamic entries Rapid entries by an entry team into an incident scene; designed to overwhelm those inside.

emergency medical responder (EMR) The first trained individual, such as a police officer, fire fighter, lifeguard, or other rescuer, to arrive at the scene of an emergency to provide initial medical assistance.

emergency medical services (EMS) A multidisciplinary system that represents the combined efforts of several professionals and agencies to provide prehospital emergency care to the sick and injured.

emergency medical technician (EMT) An individual who has training in basic life support, including automated external defibrillation, use of a definitive airway adjunct, and assisting patients with certain medications.

emotionally disturbed persons (EDPs) People who are functionally impaired due to a mental, behavioral, physical, or emotional disorder.

endotracheal (ET) tube Tube that is inserted into the trachea; equipped with a distal cuff, proximal inflation port, a 15/22-millimeter adapter, and centimeter markings on the side.

endotracheal intubation Insertion of an endotracheal tube directly through the larynx between the vocal cords and into the trachea to maintain and protect an airway.

entry team Four to eight SWAT officers who are primarily responsible for finding and arresting suspects and clearing the building.

evacuation Timely, efficient movement of patients from hard cover to transportation.

evaporation Conversion of water or another fluid from a liquid to a gas.

excited delirium syndrome (ExDS) A syndrome where the patient displays hyperaggressive, combative behavior; symptoms include rapid breathing, profuse sweating, and delirium.

executive protection Techniques and tactics used to mitigate the threat of violence or kidnapping of a very important person or family member with a large amount of money, power, or fame.

executive protection detail team Group of professionals tasked with the job of protecting a very important person or family member from harm or kidnapping.

expandable baton Commonly known as the ASP; a less-lethal, handheld device.

Explosive Ordnance Disposal (EOD) search Methods and techniques used by specially trained experts to search for, neutralize, and prevent bombs from detonating.

external ballistics The study of projectiles in the phase between the weapon and the intended target. This includes velocity, trajectory, and many other factors.

extraction The process of moving the patient from the point of injury to a point of relative safety.

extrication The process of safely disentangling a patient who is trapped in a motor vehicle crash, building collapse, or explosion debris.

extubation Removal of a tube after it has been placed.

fight-or-flight response The sympathetic nervous system's automatic response to fear: stress hormones are released, which temporarily increase the blood flow to the skeletal muscles, thereby increasing the body's ability to run or fight, and focusing the mind purely on survival.

flail chest A condition in which two or more ribs are fractured in two or more places or in association with a fracture of the sternum so that a segment of the chest wall is effectively detached from the rest of the thoracic cage.

flares Bright bursts of light used to communicate or illuminate; used in shotguns and survival pistols to mark a position.

flechettes Pointed steel projectiles with an appearance of a small nail and with small tails for stable flight; used in shotguns and other weapons in the military.

frostbite Damage to tissues as the result of exposure to cold; frozen body parts.

full-thickness burn A burn that affects all skin layers and may affect the subcutaneous layers, muscle, bone, and internal organs, leaving the area dry, leathery, and white, dark brown, or charred; traditionally called a third-degree burn.

fuse A mechanical or electrical device used for setting off (detonating) an explosive charge or mechanism.

G agents Early nerve agents that were developed by German scientists in the period after WWI and into WWII. There are three such agents: sarin, soman, and tabun.

gag reflex A normal reflex mechanism that causes retching; activated by touching the soft palate or the back of the throat.

gamma (X-rays) Type of energy that is emitted from a strong radiologic source that is far faster and stronger than alpha and beta rays. These rays easily penetrate through the human body and require either several inches of lead or concrete to prevent penetration.

gasman SWAT officer who may shoot or throw chemical agents into a building to force suspects to leave the building.

gastric distention A condition in which air fills the stomach, often as a result of high volume and pressure during artificial ventilation.

gauge The diameter of a shotgun barrel.

Glasgow Coma Scale (GCS) score An evaluation tool used to determine level of consciousness, which evaluates and assigns point values (scores) for eye opening, verbal response, and motor response, which are then totaled; effective in helping predict patient outcomes.

grains Weight unit used for measuring bullets; the heavier the bullet, the larger the grains.

handguns Firearms designed to be held and operated with one hand.

hard body armor inserts Rigid inserts made of steel, ceramics, aluminum, or titanium that are used for added frontal-torso protection in addition to soft body armor; available in threat protection Levels III and IV.

hazardous materials Any substances that are toxic, poisonous, radioactive, flammable, cause infections, or explode resulting in illness, injury, or death due to exposure.

hazardous materials (hazmat) incident An incident in which a hazardous material is no longer properly contained and isolated.

head tilt-chin lift maneuver A combination of two movements to open the airway by tilting the forehead back and lifting the chin; not used for trauma patients.

Health Insurance Portability and Accountability Act (HIPAA) Federal legislation passed in 1996. Its main effect in EMS is in limiting availability of patients' health care information and penalizing violations of patient privacy.

heat cramps Painful muscle spasms usually associated with vigorous activity in a hot environment.

heat exhaustion A form of heat injury in which the body loses significant amounts of fluid and electrolytes because of heavy sweating; also called heat prostration or heat collapse.

heatstroke A life-threatening condition of severe hyperthermia caused by exposure to excessive natural or artificial heat, marked by warm, dry skin; severely altered mental status; and often irreversible coma.

hematemesis Vomited blood.

hemopneumothorax The accumulation of blood and air in the pleural space of the chest.

hemorrhage The escape of blood cells and plasma from capillaries, veins, and arteries; bleeding.

hemostatic agent Powder, packet, gauze, or other dressing that is specially mixed with or coated with an agent or material that increases the speed and efficiency of the body to form clots and stop bleeding.

hemothorax A collection of blood in the pleural cavity.

hepatitis Inflammation of the liver, usually caused by a viral infection, that causes fever, loss of appetite, jaundice, fatigue, and altered liver function.

high-risk prisoner transport medicine When a TMP is tasked with accompanying a protective detail transporting a high-risk prisoner.

human immunodeficiency virus (HIV) Acquired immunodeficiency syndrome (AIDS) is caused by HIV, which damages the cells in the body's immune system so that the body is unable to fight infection or certain cancers.

hymenoptera A family of insects that includes bees, wasps, ants, and yellow jackets.

hyperkalemia An abnormally high level of potassium in the blood.

hyperthermia A condition in which the body's core temperature rises to 101°F (38.3°C) or more.

hypothermia A condition in which the body's core temperature falls below 95°F (35°C) after exposure to a cold environment.

hypovolemia An abnormal decrease in blood volume.

hypovolemic shock A condition in which low blood volume, due to massive internal or external bleeding or extensive loss of body water, results in inadequate tissue perfusion.

immediate action drill (IAD) A tactic or approach to a situation that is planned and practiced in drills by the SWAT unit so it may be performed smoothly and efficiently if needed during a callout.

immediate reaction team A group of five to seven SWAT officers and at least two TMPs who stand ready to immediately respond to the incident while detailed tactical plans involving the entire SWAT unit are being created.

incident command center The location at the scene of an emergency where incident command is located and where command, coordination, control, and communications are centralized.

incident commander An upper-level law enforcement officer who supervises the entire tactical operation from the incident command center.

incision A sharp, smooth cut.

incubation The period of time from a person being exposed to a disease to the time when symptoms begin.

individual first aid kit (IFAK) A medical kit that contains the essential first aid supplies for a tactical officer or TMP, and is usually located on the vest or in a cargo pocket that is supposed to be carried in the same location.

infrared flashlight Device that emits infrared light, which is invisible to the human eye; may be used to illuminate an area, allowing SWAT and TEMS officers to discern the presence of objects and humans more than 400 yards away.

inner perimeter The most dangerous area at a tactical callout, where the suspect can potentially attack and use weapons to cause casualties.

internal ballistics The study of projectiles and their effect on human tissue.

intraosseous (IO) infusion Administration of fluids and medication into the bone.

intravenous (IV) therapy The delivery of medication directly into a vein.

ionizing radiation Energy that is emitted in the form of rays or particles.

jaw-thrust maneuver Technique to open the airway by placing the fingers behind the angle of the jaw and bringing the jaw forward; used for patients who may have a cervical spine injury.

JumpSTART triage A sorting system for pediatric patients younger than 8 years or weighing less than 100 lb. There is a minor adaptation for infants since they cannot walk on their own.

K-9 officer Law enforcement officer who trains and deploys police dogs.

kinetic energy The energy of motion; this energy is transferred to anything that the projectile comes in contact with.

King LT A supraglottic airway used as an alternative to tracheal or mask ventilation.

laceration A jagged open wound.

laryngeal mask airway (LMA) An advanced airway device that is blindly inserted into the mouth to isolate the larynx for direct ventilation; consists of a tube and a mask or cuff that inflates to seal around the laryngeal opening.

law enforcement officers Personnel who are armed and authorized to use negotiation and physical force under certain conditions when carrying out their duties to prevent, protect against, detect, investigate, and prosecute criminal behavior.

less-lethal weapons Weapons designed to incapacitate a person while limiting the exposure of officers to undesirable situations. During normal use, these types of weapons do not penetrate the body, with the exception of small, TASER fish-hook-like probes.

Lewisite (L) A blistering agent that has a rapid onset of symptoms and produces immediate intense pain and discomfort on contact.

Lund and Browder chart A detailed version of the rule of nines chart that takes into consideration the changes in body surface area brought on by growth.

luxation injury An injury where the tooth is displaced within the socket, usually as a result of a direct blow to the front of the mouth.

marksmanship Acquired ability to shoot a firearm and accurately place a bullet or other projectile into the target.

marksmen (snipers) SWAT officers trained in precision long-range threat neutralization.

mass gathering event A gathering of more than 1,000 people at a single site for an event that is planned in advance.

mechanism of injury (MOI) The way in which traumatic injuries occur; the forces that act on the body to cause damage.

medical control Physician instructions that are given directly by radio or cell phone (online/direct) or indirectly by protocol/guidelines (off-line/indirect), as authorized by the medical director of the service program.

medical director The physician who authorizes or delegates to the TMP the authority to provide medical care in the tactical environment.

medical intelligence Gathering of data and medical information about prospective patients and mission conditions that may impact tactical medical care and decision making.

medical plan A medical predeployment plan that coordinates the interaction of all medical assets to include both those internal to the SWAT unit and those accessible within the surrounding medical community.

medical threat assessment (MTA) An assessment that identifies the threats that can have an impact on the physiological and psychological health and performance of the SWAT and TEMS units.

Molotov cocktails Improvised weapons made of glass bottles filled with gasoline with a cloth rag acting as a wick.

multilumen airway Advanced airway devices, such as the esophageal tracheal Combitube and the pharyngeotracheal lumen airway, that have multiple tubes to aid in ventilation and will work whether placed in the trachea or esophagus.

mutagen A substance that mutates, damages, and changes the structure of the DNA in the body's cells.

mutual aid agreement A contract entered into by a group of medical providers (eg, a TEMS unit) to provide medical support for another public safety entity or government organization.

myocardial contusion A bruise of the heart muscle.

myoglobin An oxygen-carrying protein present in high concentrations of the cardiac and skeletal muscles.

nasopharyngeal airway (NPA) Airway adjunct inserted into the nostril of a conscious patient who is unable to maintain airway patency independently.

National Incident Management System (NIMS) A Department of Homeland Security system designed to enable federal, state, and local governments and private-sector and nongovernmental organizations to effectively and efficiently prepare for, prevent, respond to, and recover from domestic incidents, regardless of cause, size, or complexity.

needle cricothyrotomy Insertion of a 14- to 16-gauge over-the-needle IV catheter through the cricothyroid membrane and into the trachea.

negotiations team Law enforcement officers with special training in crisis negotiations and psychology.

nerve agents A class of chemical called organophosphates; they function by blocking an essential enzyme in the nervous system, which causes the body's organs to become overstimulated and burn out.

neurotoxins Biologic agents that are the most deadly substances known to humans; they include botulinum toxin and ricin.

neutron radiation Type of energy that is emitted from a strong radiologic source; neutron energy is the fastest moving and most powerful form of radiation. Neutrons easily penetrate through lead, and require several feet of concrete to stop them.

night vision equipment Devices that enable humans to see in the dark, using infrared or ambient light to identify objects and people up to several hundred yards away.

nightstick A plastic or wood baton or stick that is used by law enforcement to force the compliance of a suspect.

nitrile gloves Inner gloves, made of synthetic latex. They are more durable and chemical-repellant than rubber gloves, and do not cause problems for officers or citizens with latex allergies.

noise-flash distraction devices (NFDDs) Devices that use a flash powder charge to produce a bright flash and extremely loud explosion to stun, distract, and disorient suspects, allowing entry team members to safely enter the room to contain and deal with any threats; sometimes called "flash-bangs" or flash-sound diversionary devices (FSDDs).

observer SWAT officer who assists marksmen and provides area security.

off-gassing The emitting of an agent after exposure, for example from a person's clothing that has been exposed to the agent.

oleoresin capsicum (OC) spray A derivative of cayenne pepper; classified as an inflammatory agent. It is used to force compliance with instructions.

open abdominal injury An injury in which there is a break in the surface of the skin or mucous membrane, exposing deeper tissue to potential contamination.

open cricothyrotomy Also referred to as a surgical cricothyrotomy; an emergent procedure that involves incising the cricothyroid membrane with a scalpel and inserting an endotracheal or tracheostomy tube directly into the subglottic area of the trachea.

open pneumothorax An injury that extends from the surface of the skin into the peritoneal cavity. It may be associated with internal organ damage and creates the potential for contamination of the deeper tissues.

open wound Wound in which there is a break in the surface of the skin, exposing deeper tissue to potential contamination.

oropharyngeal airway (OPA) Airway adjunct inserted into the mouth to keep the tongue from blocking the upper airway and to facilitate suctioning the airway.

orotracheal intubation Endotracheal intubation through the mouth.

outer perimeter The area at a tactical callout felt to be safe from weapons and violence; boundary generally enforced by perimeter patrol officers to keep bystanders out and to watch for and apprehend any potential suspects trying to escape.

over-the-counter (OTC) medications Medications that do not require the authorization of a physician.

paramedic An individual who has extensive training in advanced life support, including endotracheal intubation, emergency pharmacology, cardiac monitoring, and other advanced assessment and treatment skills.

Parkland formula A formula that recommends giving 4 mL of lactated Ringer's solution or normal saline for each kilogram of body weight, multiplied by the percentage of body surface area burned; sometimes used to calculate fluid needs during lengthy transport times.

partial-thickness burn A burn affecting the epidermis and some portion of the dermis but not the subcutaneous tissue characterized by blisters and skin that is white to red, moist, and mottled; traditionally called a second-degree burn.

patent Open, clear of obstruction.

pelargonyl vanillyamide (PAVA) capsaicin II A powder irritant used by law enforcement to force compliance with instructions.

perceptual narrowing A temporary reduction of higher brain center processing of sensory information that occurs as part of the fight-or-flight stress response during confrontation with danger; serves to simplify decision-making and help a person focus on survival.

pericardial tamponade Impairment of diastolic filling of the right ventricle as a result of significant amounts of fluid in the pericardial sac surrounding the heart, leading to a decrease in the cardiac output.

pericardiocentesis A procedure in which a needle is introduced into the pericardial sac to remove fluid and relieve a pericardial tamponade.

perimeter security team Uniformed patrol officers and undercover officers who provide outer-perimeter security to ensure no suspects leave and no bystanders enter the callout site.

permissive hypotension The limited use of IV fluids to maintain a radial pulse or normal level of consciousness without excessively raising the patient's blood pressure past 90 mm Hg systolic in order to prevent further hemorrhaging.

persistency Term used to describe how long a chemical agent will stay on a surface before it evaporates.

personal protective equipment Protective equipment that OSHA requires to be made available to emergency medical providers. In the case of infection risk, PPE blocks entry of an organism into the body.

personal protective equipment (PPE) levels Measures of the amount and type of protective equipment that an individual needs to avoid injury during contact with a hazardous material.

pharynx Chamber that connects the oral cavity with the esophagus.

phenacyl chloride (CN) tear gas A type of tear gas that is used in grenades and projectiles for aerosol delivery. It is reliable and offers many advantages when faced with a noncompliant suspect(s).

phosgene oxime (CX) A blistering agent that has a rapid onset of symptoms and produces immediate intense pain and discomfort on contact.

phosgene A pulmonary agent that is a product of combustion, such as might be produced in a fire at a textile factory or house, or from metalworking or burning Freon.

physical evidence Evidence such as blood, objects, or impressions that ties a suspect or victim to a crime.

pistols Handguns that do not hold ammunition in a revolving cylinder.

pneumonic plague A lung infection, also known as plague pneumonia that is the result of inhalation of plague bacteria.

pneumothorax Partial or complete accumulation of air in the pleural space.

point man SWAT officer who guides the entry team to the deployment area and enters the building or other structure first.

point of relative safety An area located at either the outer perimeter or just inside it in the tactical warm zone, where TMPs can more safely provide stabilizing medical care.

post-incident analysis A routine critique following an incident when information surrounding the response is reviewed and discussed in an effort to learn lessons to improve future responses.

post-traumatic stress disorder (PTSD) A delayed stress reaction to a prior incident. This delayed reaction is often the result of one or more unresolved issues concerning the incident, which if untreated, can lead to short-term and long-term difficulties with job performance and family life.

powered air-purifying respirator (PAPR) A battery-operated air filter device that supplies filtered air to the wearer and removes contaminants.

prescription medications Medications requiring the authorization of a physician.

primary high explosive materials Explosives that are extremely sensitive to stimuli such as impact, friction, heat, static electricity, or electromagnetic radiation; often used to help trigger an explosion.

pulmonary blast injuries Pulmonary trauma resulting from short-range exposure to the detonation of high explosives.

pulmonary contusion Severe blunt injury to a lung resulting in swelling and bleeding within the lung tissue itself.

quick peeks A method for observing a specific setting while minimizing exposure.

radiation The transfer of heat to colder objects in the environment by radiant energy—for example, being warmed by a fire.

radioactive material Any material that emits radiation.

radiologic dispersal device (RDD) Any container that is designed to disperse radioactive material.

rapid decontamination The process of removing clothing and flushing victims with water in the field when a formal decontamination line is unavailable.

rapid sequence intubation (RSI) A specific set of procedures, combined in rapid succession, to induce sedation and paralysis and intubate a patient quickly.

rear guard SWAT officer who provides rear security for the entry team.

rehabilitation station A protected location in the outer perimeter where SWAT officers and TMPs can rest, recover, and be medically evaluated for a short period of time during a prolonged callout or significantly challenging training session.

rem A unit of measure that quantifies the amount of radiation exposure to the human body.

remote assessment medicine (RAM) Visually assessing injured patients from a safe distance with a goal of determining if the patient is dead or alive.

rescue team Team of tactical officers who stand by, ready to come to the aid of or supplement the primary entry team.

respiration The loss of body heat as warm air in the lungs is exhaled into the atmosphere and cooler air is inhaled.

reverse triage A triage process in which efforts are focused on those who are in respiratory and cardiac arrest, and different from conventional triage where such patients would be classified as deceased. Used in triaging multiple victims of a lightning strike.

revised trauma score A trauma scoring system that rates injury severity by comparing the Glasgow Coma Scale score, the systolic blood pressure, and the respiratory rate and assigning a score between 1 and 13 based on those factors.

revolvers Handguns with a revolving cylinder that rotates and holds rounds of ammunition.

rhabdomyolysis The destruction of muscle tissue leading to a release of potassium and myoglobin, which then accumulate in the blood and urine and impair filtration; occurs often with crush injuries.

ricin Neurotoxin derived from mash that is left from the castor bean; causes pulmonary edema and respiratory and circulatory failure, leading to death.

rifles Firearms designed to be fired from the shoulder, with a barrel that has a helical groove or pattern of grooves and lands cut into the barrel that increase the accuracy of the bullet.

riot A public act of violence by an unruly mob, or state of disorder involving group violence.

round The entire unit that consists of a case that holds the propellant, primer, and the bullet.

route of exposure Manner by which a toxic substance enters the body.

rule of nines A system that assigns percentages to sections of the body, allowing calculation of the amount of skin surface involved in the burn area.

SAMPLE history A brief history of a patient's condition to determine signs and symptoms, allergies, medications, pertinent past history, last oral intake, and events leading to the injury or illness.

sarin (GB) A nerve agent that is one of the G agents; a highly volatile, colorless and odorless liquid that turns from liquid to gas within seconds to minutes at room temperature.

screening examination An on-site patient assessment of a suspect to determine if the suspect should be transported to jail or to a hospital for further examination and treatment.

secondary device An additional explosive used by terrorists, set to explode after the initial bomb.

secondary explosive materials Explosive compounds that are less sensitive to handling and require more energy for an explosion to occur.

self-contained breathing apparatus (SCBA) Respirator with independent air supply used by fire fighters to enter toxic and otherwise dangerous atmospheres.

Sellick maneuver A technique that is used to prevent gastric distention in which pressure is applied to the cricoid cartilage; also referred to as cricoid pressure.

septum The central divider in the nose.

shank A makeshift knife made out of various materials including wood, metal, plastic, glass shard, and others.

shock waves Waves of pressure from muzzle velocities above 2,000 feet per second that precede the bullet and compress the tissue ahead of and around the bullet. Shock waves can reach pressures above 200 atmospheres.

shotgun beanbag rounds Small sacks of lead pellets designed to be shot at noncompliant suspects, causing pain and bruising, enabling the law enforcement officers to arrest and manage a difficult situation.

shotshell A self-contained cartridge loaded with shot or a slug designed to be fired from a shotgun.

sleep deficit The result of several days going by with a responder only getting 4 to 6 hours of sleep per night. Sleep deficit leads to decreased performance and increased risks of multiple hazards such as falling asleep at the wheel while driving, memory deficits, increased risks of infections and poor health, and sleep disturbances.

slugs Large bullets typically fired from a shotgun; primarily used for hunting deer or other large animals.

smallpox A highly contagious disease; it is most contagious when blisters begin to form.

smoke grenade A device that emits hexachloroethane (HC), which is a solid that may be chemically colored in a variety of ways. It smells like smoke and is used to provide cover during tactical movement.

soft body armor A ballistic-resistant fabric worn concealed under the uniform or over the uniform, made from polyethylene fiber.

soman (GD) A nerve agent that is one of the G agents; twice as persistent as sarin and five times as lethal; it has a fruity odor, as a result of the type of alcohol used in the agent, and is both a contact and inhalation hazard that can enter the body through skin absorption and through the respiratory tract.

Special Weapons and Tactics (SWAT) unit Specialized law enforcement units who deal with a variety of critical incidents including barricaded felony suspects, hostage rescue scenarios, perpetrators armed with military-style weapons, organized crime, methamphetamine laboratories with chemical and explosive threats, terrorist acts, bomb threats, dignitary protection, riots, and other hazards.

sprain A joint injury involving damage to supporting ligaments and sometimes partial or temporary dislocation of bone ends.

stab-resistant ballistic vest A vest designed to be resistant against puncture from knives, shanks, and other pointed or edged weapons.

stack formation Single-file formation of SWAT officers designed to allow rapid entry and overwhelming response; used during the entry phase.

standard precautions An infection control concept and practice that assumes that all body fluids are potentially infectious.

START triage A patient sorting process that stands for Simple Triage and Rapid Treatment and uses a limited assessment of the patient's ability to walk, breathing status, circulation status, and mental status.

state-sponsored terrorism Terrorism that is funded and/or supported by nations that hold close ties with terrorist groups.

stealth entries Slow and silent entries by an entry team into an incident scene; often used if there is no time urgency.

strain Stretching or tearing of a muscle; also called a muscle pull.

subdermal burn A severe, life-threatening burn involving the deep structures of muscle, bone, larger blood vessels, and nerves; also called a fourth-degree burn.

subglottic area The area of the trachea below the vocal cords.

subungual hematoma An accumulation of blood underneath the fingernail or toenail, usually due to a compression force that causes bleeding under the nail; usually treated using the trephination technique.

sucking chest wound An open or penetrating chest wall wound through which air passes during inspiration and expiration, creating a sucking sound. See also open pneumothorax.

sulfur mustard (agent H) A blister agent; it is a brownish-yellowish oily substance that is generally considered very persistent; has the distinct smell of garlic or mustard and, when released, it is quickly absorbed into the skin and/or mucous membranes and begins an irreversible process of damaging the cells.

SWAT officer data cards Cards carried by TMPs and SWAT unit leaders; contain essential medical and personal data for each SWAT officer in case of injury.

tabun (GA) A nerve agent that is one of the G agents; is 36 times more persistent than sarin and approximately half as lethal; has a fruity smell and is unique because the components used to manufacture the agent are easy to acquire and the agent is easy to manufacture.

tactical compression dressings Gauze that is already attached to elastic wrapping with prerigged cinching and fastening devices; should be vacuum-packed, sterile, lightweight, and easily deployed.

tactical emergency medical support (TEMS) Prehospital emergency care during special weapons and tactics training and tactical missions.

tactical medical providers (TMPs) Medically trained persons whose mission it is to support the wellness of the SWAT officers and perform emergency medical care in the tactical environment for anyone in need.

tactical medicine The services and emergency medical support needed to preserve the safety, health, and overall well-being of SWAT officers.

tactical operations center (TOC) Location at the scene of a critical incident involving the SWAT unit, which is where the SWAT officers and SWAT unit leaders meet and make plans and preparations.

tactical operations leader Directs the details of the callout from either the incident command center or from a tactical operations center.

tactical personal protective equipment (TPPE) Personal protective equipment designed to protect TMPs from medical and violent threats in the tactical environment, including clear goggles, protective mask, nitrile gloves, and head and boot protection.

tactical tourniquet A medical device used to stop arterial and venous bleeding from the arms and legs (extremities) and compresses the blood vessels so that no blood flows distal to (past) the device, thus significantly slowing or stopping hemorrhage.

tactical warm zone Located between the inner and outer perimeters, this is an area of increased threat and risk, but does not have direct risk due to the contained suspects within the hot zone.

tactics, techniques, and procedures (TTP) Unique methods, tools, and description of medical and other types of procedures that are utilized by TMPs and SWAT officers to complete a mission.

team leader Directs the SWAT officers personally as a member of the entry team when entering buildings, often located in the middle of the entry team line.

tension pneumothorax A life-threatening collection of air within the pleural space; the volume and pressure have both collapsed the involved lung and caused a shift of the mediastinal structures to the opposite side.

testimonial evidence Oral documentation of the facts by a witness.

thermal imaging devices Electronic devices that detect differences in temperature based on infrared energy and then generate images based on those data; commonly used in obscured environments to locate victims and/or suspects.

toxicity level Measure of the risk that a hazardous material poses to the health of an individual who comes into contact with it.

trachea The windpipe; the main trunk for air passing to and from the lungs.

translaryngeal catheter ventilation A procedure that provides oxygenation and temporary ventilation to patients with a needle cricothyrotomy by injecting air using a high-pressure jet ventilator to the hub of the catheter.

trench foot Cold injury similar to frostbite caused by prolonged exposure to cool, wet conditions (up to 60°F [16°C]).

triage The process of establishing treatment and transportation priorities according to severity of injury and medical need.

tularemia An infection caused by a bacterium called *Francisella tularensis*; common in wild rodents.

tunnel vision A temporary reduction in the field of vision that occurs as part of the fight-or-flight stress response during confrontation with danger.

tympanic membrane The eardrum; a thin, semitransparent membrane in the middle ear that transmits sound vibrations to the internal ear by means of the auditory ossicles.

V agent (VX) One of the G agents; it is a clear, oily agent that has no odor and looks like baby oil; over 100 times more lethal than sarin and is extremely persistent.

vapor hazard An agent that enters the body through the respiratory tract.

velocity The rate of change of position or speed. Commonly measured in meters per second (m/s) or feet per second (fps).

viral hemorrhagic fevers (VHFs) A group of diseases that include the Ebola, Rift Valley, and Yellow Fever viruses among others. This group of viruses causes the blood in the body to seep out from the tissues and blood vessels.

viruses Germs that require a living host to multiply and survive.

volatility Term used to describe how long a chemical agent will stay on a surface before it evaporates.

weaponization The creation of a weapon from a biologic agent generally found in nature and that causes disease; the agent is cultivated, synthesized, and/or mutated to maximize the target population's exposure to the germ.

weapons of mass destruction (WMDs) Any agent designed to bring about mass death, casualties, and/or massive damage to property and infrastructure (bridges, tunnels, airports, and seaports).

INDEX

Figures and tables are indicated by f and t following page numbers.

CREDITS

Chapter 1
1-2 © National Library of Medicine

Chapter 2
2-2 Courtesy of USDA; **2-3** © Photos.com; **2-4** © Lucian Coman/ShutterStock, Inc; **2-5** © 4774344sean/Dreamstime.com; **2-6** © BananaStock/age fotostock; **2-7** © Monkey Business Images/Dreamstime.com

Chapter 3
3-2 © Sam Mircovich/Reuters/Landov; **3-9** TASER® X26™ photo courtesy of TASER International, Scottsdale, AZ–USA; **3-11** Used with permission of Randy Montoya, Sandia National Laboratories

Chapter 4
4-10 Courtesy of CamelBak; **4-15** Courtesy of Z-Medica Corporation. Used with permission; **4-21** Courtesy of RAE Systems

Chapter 5
5-2A © Fibobjects/Dreamstime.com; **5-2B** © Akulova/ShutterStock, Inc; **5-3** Photo © Grazvydas/Dreamstime.com; **5-4** Photo © Dimitar Marinov/Dreamstime.com; **5-5** © Neo Edmund/ShutterStock, Inc; **5-6** © michael ledray/ShutterStock, Inc; **5-7** Photo © Mcoddington/Dreamstime.com; **5-8A** Used with permission of Rossi USA; **5-8B** Courtesy of Sig Sauer, Inc; **5-8C** © Raynald Bélanger/Dreamstime.com; **5-8D** Courtesy of Rock River Arms, Inc; **5-8E** Used with permission of Remington Arms Company; **5-14** Courtesy of Liberty Safe & Security Products, Inc. [http://www.libertysafe.com]

Chapter 6
6-1 Reproduced from *When Violence Erupts: A Survival Guide for Emergency Responders*, courtesy of Dennis R. Krebs; **6-3** Courtesy of Kai USA, Ltd; **6-4, 6-5, 6-6** Reproduced from *When Violence Erupts: A Survival Guide for Emergency Responders*, courtesy of Dennis R. Krebs; **6-7** © Radar Bali/AP Photos

Chapter 7
7-3A © Joao Estevao A Freitas (jefras)/Shutterstock, Inc; **7-3B** Courtesy of James Gathany/CDC; **7-4A** Courtesy of Kenneth Cramer, Monmouth College; **7-4B, 7-4C** Courtesy of Department of Entomology, University of Nebraska; **7-5** Courtesy of Mass Communication Specialist 2nd Class Kristopher Wilson/US Navy

Chapter 10
10-2 © Alan Kim, *The Roanoke Times*/AP Photos; **10-5** © Angela E. Kershner, *The Morning News*/AP Photos; **10-6** Courtesy of Officer Navin Sharma (ret), Vancouver Police Department; **10-7** © Stephen Chernin/AP Photos; **10-9** Courtesy of Christopher A. Ebdon, av8pix.com

Chapter 12
12-7 Courtesy of Tactical Medical Solutions, Inc; **12-8** Used with permission of PerSys Medical; **12-13** Courtesy of Z-Medica Corporation. Used with permission

Chapter 14
14-7 Courtesy of James P. Thomas, MD; **14-14** Courtesy of King Systems

Chapter 15
15-10 Used with permission of PerSys Medical

Chapter 16
16-5 Courtesy of North American Rescue, LLC; **16-6** Photo of the Sling-Link® system used with permission of Groves Incorporated [www.sling-link.com]; **16-10** Courtesy of Ferno, Inc; **16-20** Courtesy of Sean McKay

Chapter 17
17-6A © Chuck Stewart, MD; **17-6B** © D. Willoughby/Custom Medical Stock Photo; **17-11** Courtesy of Lt. David Roger, Peoria Police Department

Chapter 18
18-25 Courtesy of Pyng Medical Corp.

Chapter 19
19-16 © Stan Kujawa/Alamy Images; **19-17** © Cordelia Molloy/Photo Researchers, Inc; **19-18** © commercial collection/Alamy Images

Chapter 20
20-4 Courtesy of Ferno, Inc; **20-8** © Chuck Stewart, MD; **20-9A** © Chuck Stewart, MD; **20-13** © Sean Gladwell/Dreamstime.com

Chapter 21
21-1A © Amy Walters/ShutterStock, Inc; **21-1B** © E.M. Singletary, MD. Used with permission; **21-1C** © John Radcliffe Hospital/Photo Researchers, Inc; **21-1D** © Chuck Stewart, MD; **21-6A, 21-6B**

© Chuck Stewart, MD; **21-15** © Marcin Pwainski/ Dreamstime.com; **21-16, 21-17** Courtesy of Dr. Lucille K. Georg/CDC; **21-18** © Custom Medical Stock Photo/Alamy Images; **21-19** Courtesy of Adam Buchbinder

Chapter 22

22-4A Courtesy of Neil Malcom Winkelmann; **22-4C** © Chuck Stewart, MD; **22-7** Courtesy of Dr. Jack Poland/CDC; **22-10** © Crystal Kirk/ShutterStock, Inc; **22-11** Courtesy of Kenneth Cramer, Monmouth College; **22-12** Courtesy of Department of Entomology, University of Nebraska; **22-13A** © manfredxy/ShutterStock, Inc; **22-13B** © Heintje Joseph T. Lee/ShutterStock, Inc; **22-14A** Courtesy of Dey, LP; **22-14B** Courtesy of Shionogi Pharma, Inc; **22-15A** © Photos.com; **22-15B** Courtesy of Ray Rauch/US Fish and Wildlife Service; **22-15C** Courtesy of Luther C. Goldman/US Fish and Wildlife Service; **22-15D** © SuperStock/Alamy Images; **22-18** © EcoPrint/ShutterStock, Inc; **22-19** © Joao Estevao A. Freitas (jefras)/ShutterStock, Inc; **22-20** Courtesy of James Gathany/CDC; **22-22A** © Thomas Photography LLC/Alamy Images; **22-22B** © Thomas J. Peterson/ Alamy Images; **22-22C** Courtesy of US Fish & Wildlife Service

Chapter 23

23-3 Photo provided by a private source; **23-4** Courtesy of Cephalon, Inc.

Chapter 24

24-1 Courtesy of Dr Saeed Keshavarz/RCCI, Research Center of Chemical Injuries/IRAN; **24-3** Courtesy of CDC; **24-4** Courtesy of Professor Robert Swanepoel/ National Institute for Communicable Disease, South Africa; **24-5** Courtesy of James H. Steele/CDC; **24-6A, 24-6B** Courtesy of CDC; **24-7** Courtesy of Sperian Protection; **24-8** Courtesy of Brian Pretchel/USDA; **24-10** Courtesy of S.E. International, Inc. [www.sientl.com]

Chapter 25

25-2C Courtesy of the DuPont Company; **25-4** Courtesy of DEA

Chapter 26

26-2 Courtesy of ASP, Inc; **26-7** Reproduced from *When Violence Erupts: A Survival Guide for Emergency Responders,* courtesy of Dennis R. Krebs.

Unless otherwise indicated, all photographs and illustrations are under copyright of Jones & Bartlett Learning, courtesy of Maryland Institute for Emergency Medical Services Systems, courtesy of the American Academy of Orthopaedic Surgeons, or have been provided by the authors.